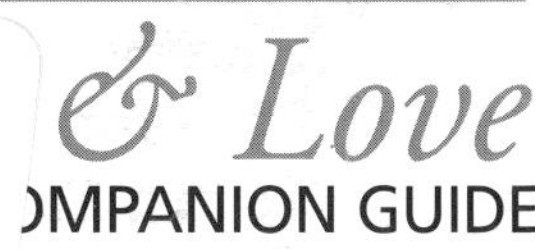

& Love
MPANION GUIDE

MCQs and
EM
Su

AN HACHETTE UK COMPANY

First published in Great Britain in 2010 by
Hodder Arnold, an imprint of Hodder Education,
part of Hachette UK, 338 Euston Road, London NW1 3BH

http://www.hodderarnold.com

British Library Cataloguing in Publication Data
A catalogue record for this book is available from the British Library

Library of Congress Cataloging-in-Publication Data
A catalog record for this book is available from the Library of Congress

ISBN 978-0-340-99067-4

1 2 3 4 5 6 7 8 9 10

Commissioning Editor: Gavin Jamieson
Project Editor: Francesca Naish
Production Controller: Joanna Walker
Cover Design: Helen Townson
Indexer: Laurence Errington

Typeset in 9.5/11.5 Formata Light Condensed by MPS Limited, A Macmillan Company.
Printed and bound in India by Replika Press

Contents

Foreword ix

Contributors x

Preface xi

Acknowledgements xii

List of Abbreviations Used xiii

Introduction xvi

PART 1: PRINCIPLES **1**

1 The metabolic response to injury 3
Pradip Datta

2 Shock and blood transfusion 8
Bandipalyam Praveen

3 Wounds, tissue repair and scars 16
Bandipalyam Praveen

4 Surgical infection 22
Bandipalyam Praveen

5 Tropical surgery 31
Pawanindra Lal, Sanjay De Bakshi

6 Paediatric surgery 75
Pradip Datta

7 Oncology 84
Bandipalyam Praveen

8 Surgical audit and research 90
Bandipalyam Praveen

9 Surgical ethics 94
Pradip Datta

10 Diagnostic imaging 96
Pradip Datta

PART 2: INVESTIGATION AND DIAGNOSIS **101**

11 Gastrointestinal endoscopy 103
Bandipalyam Praveen

12 Tissue diagnosis 107
■ Pradip Datta

PART 3: PERIOPERATIVE CARE **111**

13 Preoperative preparation 113
■ Bandipalyam Praveen

14 Anaesthesia and pain relief 118
■ Nigel Webster

15 Care in the operating room 122
■ Pradip Datta

16 The high-risk surgical patient 124
■ Bandipalyam Praveen

17 Nutrition and fluid therapy 127
■ Nandini Rao

18 Basic surgical skills and anastomosis 135
■ Pradip Datta

19 Laparoscopic and robotic surgery 137
■ Bandipalyam Praveen

20 Postoperative care 144
■ Pradip Datta

PART 4: TRAUMA **151**

21 Introduction to trauma 153
■ Pradip Datta

22 Trauma epidemiology 156
■ Christopher Bulstrode

23 Head injury 160
■ Lynn Myles

24 Neck and spine 166
■ Christopher Bulstrode

25 Trauma to the face and mouth 171
■ Charles Perkins

26 Trauma to the chest and abdomen 176
■ Pradip Datta

27 Extremity trauma 185
Christopher Bulstrode

28 Burns 195
John McGregor

29 Plastic and reconstructive surgery 205
John McGregor

30 Disaster surgery 212
Christopher Bulstrode

PART 5: ELECTIVE ORTHOPAEDICS **217**

31 Elective orthopaedics: musculoskeletal examination 219
Christopher Bulstrode

32 Sports medicine 224
Christopher Bulstrode

33 The spine 233
Christopher Bulstrode

34 The upper limb 238
Christopher Bulstrode

35 The hip and knee 246
Christopher Bulstrode

36 The foot and ankle 252
Christopher Bulstrode

37 Infection and tumours 257
Christopher Bulstrode

38 Paediatric orthopaedics 264
Christopher Bulstrode

PART 6: SKIN AND SUBCUTANEOUS TISSUE **271**

39 Skin and subcutaneous tissue 273
Pradip Datta

PART 7: HEAD AND NECK **281**

40 Elective neurosurgery 283
Lynn Myles

41 The eye and orbit 292
■ Brian Fleck

42 Cleft lip and palate: developmental abnormalities of face, mouth and jaws 302
■ John McGregor

43 The nose and sinuses 309
■ Iain J Nixon

44 The ear 319
■ Iain J Nixon

45 Pharynx, larynx and neck 330
■ Iain J Nixon

46 Oropharyngeal cancer 341
■ Iain J Nixon

47 Disorders of the salivary glands 351
■ Iain J Nixon

PART 8: BREAST AND ENDOCRINE **361**

48 Thyroid and the parathyroid gland 363
■ Nandini Rao

49 Adrenal glands and other endocrine disorders 375
■ Nandini Rao

50 The breast 385
■ Pradip Datta

PART 9: CARDIOTHORACIC **389**

51 Cardiac surgery 391
■ Dumbor Ngaage

52 The thorax 397
■ Dumbor Ngaage

PART 10: VASCULAR **403**

53 Arterial disorders 405
■ Peter McCollum

54 Venous disorders 411
■ Peter McCollum

55 Lymphatic disorders 416
■ Peter McCollum

PART 11: ABDOMINAL **421**

56 History and examination of the abdomen 423
■ Pradip Datta

57 Hernia, umbilicus and abdominal wall 425
■ Bandipalyam Praveen

58 The peritoneum, omentum, mesentery and retroperitoneal space 432
■ Pradip Datta

59 The oesophagus 437
■ Pradip Datta

60 Stomach and duodenum 441
■ Bandipalyam Praveen

61 The liver 451
■ Pradip Datta

62 The spleen 458
■ Pradip Datta

63 The gall bladder and bile ducts 461
■ Bandipalyam Praveen

64 The pancreas 468
■ Pradip Datta

65 The small and large intestines 474
■ Pradip Datta

66 Intestinal obstruction 488
■ Bandipalyam Praveen

67 The vermiform appendix 495
■ Pradip Datta

68 The rectum 499
■ Pradip Datta

69 The anus and anal canal 504
■ Bandipalyam Praveen

PART 12: GENITOURINARY **513**

70 Urinary symptoms and investigations 515
- Pradip Datta

71 The kidneys and ureters 521
- Pradip Datta

72 The urinary bladder 533
- Pradip Datta

73 The prostate and seminal vesicles 541
- Pradip Datta

74 The urethra and penis 546
- Pradip Datta

75 The testis and scrotum 549
- Pradip Datta

76 Gynaecology 554
- Pradip Datta

PART 13: TRANSPLANTATION **559**

77 Transplantation 561
- Bandipalyam Praveen

Index 569

Foreword

This innovative companion volume will certainly be considered as an essential complement to *Bailey & Love's Short Practice of Surgery*. The authors and contributors have recognised the fundamental changes that have occurred in surgical training and assessment where greater knowledge must be acquired in a shorter period of time, not only to ensure success in examinations but also to provide the comprehensive foundations on which to build clinical expertise. The Silver Jubilee edition of *Bailey & Love* in 2008 emphasised its enduring importance for generations of surgeons internationally. *MCQs and EMQs in Surgery* will define the indispensable elements for today's surgical practitioners.

John D Orr, FRCS (Ed)

Contributors

Sanjay De Bakshi MS FRCS (Eng & Ed)
Consultant Surgeon, Calcutta Medical Research Institute (CMRI), Kolkata, India

Brian W Fleck FRCS (Ed), MD Consultant Ophthalmic Surgeon, Princess Alexandra Eye Pavilion and Royal Hospital for Sick Children, Edinburgh

Professor Pawanindra Lal MS DNB MNAMS FRCS (Ed & Eng)
Professor of Surgery, Maulana Azad Medical College, New Delhi, India

Professor Peter McCollum MCh, FRCS (Ed), FRCSI
Professor of Vascular Surgery, Hull/York Medical School

John C McGregor BSc (Hons) MBChB (with commendation) FRCS, FRCS (Edin)
Former Consultant in Plastic, Reconstructive and Cosmetic Surgery, St John's Hospital, West Lothian

Lynn Myles BSc (Hons), MB ChB, MD, FRCS (SN)
Consultant Neurosurgeon, Department of Clinical Neurosciences, Western General Hospital, Edinburgh

Dumbor L Ngaage MB BS FRCS (Ed), FWACS, FRCS (C-Th), FETCS (Cardiovascular), FETCS (Thoracic), MS
Specialist Registrar in Cardiothoracic Surgery, Castle Hill Hospital, Hull. Honorary Clinical Tutor, Hull York Medical School, Universities of Hull & York

Iain J. Nixon MBChB FRCS (Edin.) Specialist Registrar in Otolaryngology Head and Neck Surgery, West of Scotland Rotation. Clinical Research Fellow, Memorial Sloan Kettering Cancer Center, New York, USA

Charles S Perkins FDSRCS, FFDRCSI, FRCS
Consultant Oral and Maxillofacial Surgeon, Gloucestershire Royal and Cheltenham General Hospitals, Gloucestershire

Nandini P Rao, MRCP, Msc
Specialist Registrar in Chemical Pathology/Metabolic Medicine, Royal Free Hospital, London

Professor N R Webster MB ChB PhD FRCA FRCP FRCS
Institute of Medical Sciences, Foresterhill, Aberdeen

Preface

First published in 1932, *Bailey & Love's Short Practice of Surgery* has stood the test of time. Perhaps this is an understatement, considering that all three of us have used the book as medical students! This book has been the result of good foresight on the part of Hodder Arnold to keep up with the changing trends in the pattern of surgical examinations, both at undergraduate and postgraduate levels. The publishers should be congratulated in bringing out this book – converting the original Silver Jubilee (25th) edition – all 77 chapters of it – as Multiple Choice Questions (MCQs) and Extended Matching Questions (EMQs).

The book is aptly titled as a companion to *Bailey & Love*. We would therefore hope that the reader, specifically preparing for a written examination, would use this book as the major reading material, referring to the original for detailed elucidation of a particular point or operative detail.

Most of the contributors are different from *Bailey & Love's Short Practice of Surgery* except for chapters 5, 25 the section on orthopaedics and part of trauma. Thus while retaining the essence of the original material, this book has been seasoned by different authors, thus giving it a fresh flavour without losing any of its original ingredients. We are grateful to all the contributors for their prompt response in spite of the pressures of work in the National Health Service.

The images and pictures are mostly different to those in the original book, giving this tome an added attraction. While the MCQs test knowledge, the EMQs with the illustrations give a good format for a self-assessment exercise. The chapters are specifically geared towards helping the reader with preparation for the written papers of the MRCS and FRCS(Gen) examinations. The undergraduate will also find this book equally stimulating for the same reasons. In surgical examinations in the English-speaking world, where essays have been replaced by short-answer questions (short notes of yesteryear), the reader will find the EMQs ideal preparation.

Any book must be dynamic, much more so a new venture such as this. It was said in the preface of the parent book, "Whereas the past informs the present, it must never enslave the future." As authors of this very exciting project we can stay true to the spirit of this statement only with help from you – our readers. Therefore we look forward to your suggestions and constructive criticisms for the next edition.

Pradip K Datta
Christopher J K Bulstrode
B V Praveen

November 2009

Acknowledgements

An email from Gavin Jamieson to one of us (PKD) was the inspiration behind this publication, he being the catalyst who set alight our enthusiasm to write this book. Thus to him we owe a huge debt of gratitude for getting this project off the ground. Indeed it is a tribute to all concerned that this book was published in just over a year since the idea was born as his brainchild.

All the contributors have done a tremendous job not only in producing comprehensive chapters but also delivering them on time – and this, in spite of the pressures of the present-day National Health Service; to them we are grateful. Francesca Naish, as editorial manager, has kept the team on track by liaising with us all on a regular basis, thus bringing our efforts to fruition. We give our thanks to her. To Jane Utting we are grateful for her meticulous proofreading. Thanks are also due to Adam Campbell for his efficient and prompt copy-editing.

We are very grateful to Mr John D Orr, immediate Past President of the Royal College of Surgeons of Edinburgh for writing the foreword. Finally, our great appreciation goes to our families (Swati, Sandip, Victoria, Harry, John-James, Jenny, Nandini and Prakruti) for their encouragement and support. We dedicate this book to them.

PKD
CJKB
BVP

List of Abbreviations Used

5-FU 5-fluorouracil
5-HIAA 5-hydroxyindoleacetic acid
AAAs abdominal aortic aneurysms
ABCD airways, breathing, circulation and disability
ABGs arterial blood gases
ACS abdominal compartment syndrome
ACTH adrenocorticotrophic hormone
ADH antidiuretic hormone
ADP adenosine diphosphate
AF atrial fibrillation
AFP alpha-fetoprotein
AIN anal intraepithelial neoplasia
ALG antilymphocytic globulin
ALP alkaline phosphatase
ALS antilymphocytic serum
ALT alanine transaminase
ANCA antineutrophil cytoplasmic antibodies
ANDI aberrations of normal development and involution
ANF atrial natriuretic factor
ANP atrial natriuretic peptide
AP anteroposterior
APC adenomatous polyposis coli
ARDS acute respiratory distress syndrome
AST aspartate transaminase
ATLS Advanced Trauma Life Support
AVC adrenal vein catheterisation
AVMs arteriovenous malformations
BCC basal cell carcinoma
BCG Bacillus Calmette Guérin
BMI body mass index
BOO bladder outflow obstruction
BP blood pressure
BPH Benign prostatic hypertrophy
BPPV benign paroxysmal positional vertigo
CABG coronary artery bypass graft
CAH congenital adrenal hyperplasia
CBD common bile duct
CCD charge-coupled device
CCK cholecystokinin
CD Crohn's disease
CEA carcinoembryonic antigen
CECT contrast-enhanced computed tomography
CHD common hepatic duct
CJD Creutzfeldt–Jakob Disease
CMV cytomegalovirus
CNS central nervous system
COAD Chronic obstructive airways disease
COPD chronic obstructive pulmonary disease
CRF corticotrophin-releasing factor
CRF chronic renal failure
CRH Cortisol-releasing hormone
CRP C-reactive protein
C/S cervical spine
CSF cerebrospinal fluid
CRH Cortisol-releasing hormone
CT Computed tomography
CVA cardiovascular accident
CVP central venous pressure
DHEA dehydroepiandrosterone
DHT dihydrotestosterone
DIC disseminated intravascular coagulation
DISH diffuse idiopathic spinal hyperostosis
DKA diabetic ketoacidosis
DL diagnostic laparoscopy
DLC differential leucocyte count
D-PAS diastase periodic acid-Schiff/diastase PAS
DPL diagnostic peritoneal lavage
DRE digital rectal examination
DTPA diethyltriaminepentacetic acid
DVT deep vein thrombosis
EBV Epstein–Barr virus
ECF enterochromaffin
ECG electrocardiogram
EDTA ethylenediaminetetra-acetic acid
ECL enterochromaffin-like
ELISA enzyme-linked immunosorbent assay
ERCP endoscopic retrograde cholangiopancreatography
ERP Enhanced Recovery Programme
ESR erythrocyte sedimentation rate
ESWL extracorporeal shock wave lithotripsy
EUA examination under anaesthesia

EuroSCORE	European System for Cardiac Operative Risk Evaluation
EUS	endoluminal ultrasound
EUS	Endosonography
EVLT	endovascular laser treatment
FAP	familial adenomatous polyposis
FAST	focused assessment with sonography for trauma
FB	foreign body
FBC	full blood count
FDG	flurodeoxyglucose
FEV_1	forced expiratory volume in 1 sec
FFP	fresh frozen plasma
FHH	familial hypocalciuric hypocalcaemia
FISH	fluorescence in-situ hybridisation
FNAC	fine-needle aspiration cytology
FSH	follicle-stimulating hormone
fT3	free T3
fT4	free T4
GALT	gut-associated lymphoid tissue
GCS	Glasgow Coma Scale
GDT	goal-directed therapy
GGT	gamma-glutamyl transpeptidase
GH	growth hormone
GI	gastrointestinal
GIST	gastrointestinal stromal tumours
GIT	gastrointestinal tract
GOO	gastric outlet obstruction
GORD	gastro-oesophageal reflux disease
GRH	gonadotrophin-releasing hormone
GSI	genuine stress incontinence
GTN	glyceryl trinitrate
GVHD	graft-versus-host disease
HAART	Highly Active Anti-Retroviral Therapy
HAI	health care-associated infection
Hb	haemoglobin
HCC	hepatocellular carcinoma
HCG	human chorionic gonadotrophin
HH	hiatus hernia
HHT	hereditary haemorrhagic telangiectasia
HLA	human leucocyte antigen
HNPCC	hereditary non-polyposis colorectal cancer
HPV	human papillomavirus
ICP	intracranial pressure
ICU	intensive care unit
IHD	ischaemic heart disease
IM	intramuscular
INR	international normalised ratio
IPSS	International Prostate Symptom Score
ITP	idiopathic thrombocytopenic purpura
ITU	intensive treatment unit
IUCD	intrauterine contraceptive device
IV	intravenous
IVC	inferior vena cava
IVU	intravenous urogram
JVP	jugular venous pressure
KUB	kidney, ureter and bladder
LDH	lactate dehydrogenase
LFTs	liver function tests
LH	luteinising hormone
LHRH	luteinising hormone-releasing hormone
LIF	left iliac fossa
LMA	laryngeal mask airway
LMP	last menstrual period
LOCM	low-osmolality contrast media
LOS	lower oesophageal sphincter
LP	lumbar puncture
LUTS	lower urinary tract symptoms
LV	left ventricular
MALT	mucosa-associated lymphoid tissue
MAMA	microsomal antibody
MAS	minimal access surgery
MEN-1	multiple endocrine neoplasia type 1
MI	myocardial infarction
MIBI	technetium-99m-labelled sestamibi isotope
MM	malignant melanoma
MODS	multiple organ dysfunction syndrome
MOF	multiple organ failure
MRA	magnetic resonance angiography
MRCP	magnetic resonance cholangiopancreatography
MRI	magnetic resonance imaging
MRSA	methicillin-resistasnt *Staphylococcus aureus*
MSH	melanocyte-stimulating hormone
MSOF	multiple system organ failure

MUST Malnutrition Universal Screening Tool
NAI non-accidental injury
NETs neuroendocrine tumours
NOTES natural orifice transluminal surgery
NRES National Research Ethics Service
NSAIDs non-steroidal anti-inflammatory drugs
OCP oral contraceptive pill
OGD oesophagogastroduodenoscopy
OPSI opportunist post-splenectomy infection
OPT orthopantomogram
ORIF open reduction and internal fixation
PAS periodic acid-Schiff
PCA patient-controlled analgesia
PCNL percutaneous nephrolithotomy
PCR polymerase chain reaction
PDGF platelet-derived growth factor
PE pulmonary embolism
PET positron emission tomography
PETs pancreaticoduodenal endocrine tumours
PHA primary hyperaldosteronism
PID pelvic inflammatory disease
POC Per-Operative Cholangiogram
PPIs proton pump inhibitors
PSA prostate-specific antigen
PSARP posterior sagittal anorectoplasty
PSC primary sclerosing cholangitis
PT prothrombin time
PTC percutaneous transhepatic cholangiography
PTH parathyroid hormone
PTLD post-transplant lymphoproliferative disorder
PTT partial thromboplastin time
PUJ pelviureteric junction
PVP polyvinylpropylene
RT radiotherapy
RTA road traffic accident
RUQ right upper quadrant
RV right ventricular
SAH subarachnoid haemorrhage
SCC squamous cell carcinoma
SIADH syndrome of inappropriate antidiuretic hormone hypersecretion
SIRS systemic inflammatory response syndrome
SLE systemic lupus erythematosus
SLNB sentinel lymph node biopsy
SOD sphincter of Oddi dysfunction
SPECT single photon emission computed tomography
SPKT simultaneous pancreas and kidney transplant
SRUS solitary rectal ulcer syndrome
SSIs surgical site infections
SUFE slipped upper femoral epiphysis
SVC superior vena cava
TAPP transabdominal preperitoneal repair
TBSA total body surface area
TBW total body water
TED thromboembolic deterrent (stockings)
TEP total extraperitoneal repair
TFTs thyroid function tests
TGF transforming growth factor
TIA transient ischaemic attack
TIPSS transjugular intrahepatic portosystemic stent shunt
TIVA total intravenous anaesthetic
TLC total leucocyte count
TNF tumour necrosis factor
TNM classification of malignant tumours (tumour, nodes, metastasis)
TPN total parenteral nutrition
TPO thyroid peroxidase antibodies
TRUS transrectal ultrasound-guided biopsy
TSH thyroid-stimulating hormone
TURP transurethral resection of the prostate
U&E urea and electrolytes
UC ulcerative colitis
UICC Union Internationale Contre le Cancer
US ultrasound
UTI urinary tract infection
VAC vacuum-assisted closure
VATS video-assisted thoracoscopy
VP ventriculoperitoneal
VPC vapour pulse coagulation
WCC white cell count
WHO World Health Organization

Introduction

Bailey & Love's Short Practice of Surgery celebrated the publication of its Silver Jubilee edition in 2008. It has certainly come a long way since the first edition was published in 1932. As authors of this book (CJKB being one of the editors of *Bailey & Love*), dare we say that the title of the book is a misnomer. It is anything but a 'Short Text Book'. Editions of yesteryear consisted of some 1300 pages of single column text. The current edition consists of over 1500 pages, each containing a double column.

Arguably *Bailey & Love* is not just a text book. Many students and teachers of surgery the world over use it as a reference book too. Today both postgraduate and undergraduate examinations lay emphasis on knowledge rather than presentation and the nuances of essay writing. Thus for many years, the candidate's test of theory knowledge in examinations has been based on Multiple Choice Questions (MCQs) and Extended Matching Questions (EMQs), sometimes supplemented by Single Best Answers (SBAs).

Therefore for the first time in this book, all 77 chapters of *Bailey & Love* have been converted into MCQs and EMQs. We, as authors, along with the other contributors, have reproduced the original text in this form of MCQs and EMQs. We hope that we have accurately mirrored the subject matter. Most of the images in this book are not from *Bailey & Love*, but are from the personal collection of one of the authors (PKD).

We hope that this book will be useful for medical students studying surgery in the English-speaking world and for those doing MRCS and FRCS (Gen) examinations in the UK. As authors of the very first such undertaking, we would welcome suggestions for future editions from our readers.

PKD
CJKB
BVP

PART 1 Principles

1 The metabolic response to injury 3

2 Shock and blood transfusion 8

3 Wounds, tissue repair and scars 16

4 Surgical infection 22

5 Tropical surgery 31

6 Paediatric surgery 75

7 Oncology 84

8 Surgical audit and research 90

9 Surgical ethics 94

10 Diagnostic imaging 96

1 The metabolic response to injury

Multiple choice questions

→ Homeostasis

1. Which of the following statements about homeostasis are false?

A It is defined as a stable state of the normal body.

B The central nervous system, heart, lungs, kidneys and spleen are the essential organs that maintain homeostasis at a normal level.

C Elective surgery should cause little disturbance to homeostasis.

D Emergency surgery should cause little disturbance to homeostasis.

E Return to normal homeostasis after an operation would depend upon the presence of co-morbid conditions.

→ Stress response

2. In stress response, which of the following statements are false?

A It is graded.

B Metabolism and nitrogen excretion are related to the degree of stress.

C In such a situation there are physiological, metabolic and immunological changes.

D The changes cannot be modified.

E The mediators to the integrated response are initiated by the pituitary.

→ Mediators

3. Which of the following statements about mediators are true?

A They are neural, endocrine and inflammatory.

B Every endocrine gland plays an equal part.

C They produce a model of several phases.

D The phases occur over several days.

E They help in the process of repair.

→ The recovery process

4. With regard to the recovery process, identify the statements that are true.

A All tissues are catabolic, resulting in repair at an equal pace.

B Catabolism results in muscle wasting.

C There is alteration in muscle protein breakdown.

D Hyperalimentation helps in recovery.

E There is insulin resistance.

→ Optimal perioperative care

5. Which of the following statements are true for optimal perioperative care?

A Volume loss should be promptly treated by large intravenous (IV) infusions of fluid.

B Hypothermia and pain are to be avoided.

C Starvation needs to be combated.

D Avoid immobility.

E Helpful measures can be taken.

Answers: Multiple choice questions

Homeostasis

1. D

The normal physiological state of the human body is referred to as homeostasis – a normal internal environment (the *milieu intérieur* of Claude Bernard). All the vital organs – the brain, heart, lungs, kidneys and, to a lesser extent, the spleen – play an important role in its maintenance. These organs are interdependent and thus help to maintain a normal fluid and acid–base balance.

In the elective situation, the patient is always optimised prior to any operation, thereby minimising the homeostatic disturbance. The extent of surgery also plays a part. Disturbance in the homeostasis to some degree occurs in emergency surgery; this depends upon the extent of injury, presence of sepsis and any ongoing insults. If the patient has co-morbid conditions, postoperatively the return to normal homeostasis would take longer than in those with no co-morbidity. In such cases, care in a high-dependency or intensive care unit (ICU) is essential.

Stress response

2. D

The stress response is graded according to the injury inflicted. An elective operation in a fit patient, such as a laparoscopic cholecystectomy in a 30-year-old female, will elicit a minor transient stress response from which the patient recovers quite quickly. On the other hand, a severely injured patient of 70 will elicit a major response, requiring care in the ICU (see Fig. 1.1). There is an increase in metabolism and nitrogen excretion in direct proportion to the injury. There are immunological and metabolic changes which are reflected in the physiology – pyrexia, tachycardia and tachypnoea. The body's innate defence mechanisms can combat mild stress, and return to normal physiology occurs very soon.

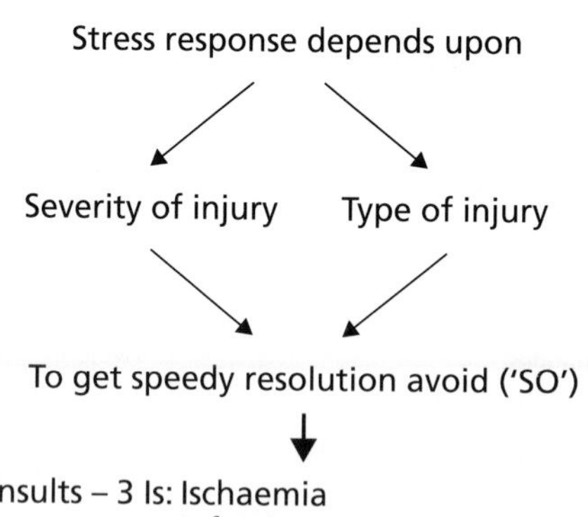

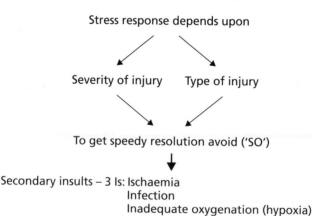

Figure 1.1 Metabolic response to severe trauma.

In severe injury, the stress response can be modified by anticipating complications and preventing them by judicious management in an ICU, i.e. attention to nutrition and anticipation and prevention of secondary insults such as ischaemia, infection, hypoxia and compartment syndrome.

The pituitary gland, rightly referred to as 'the leader in the endocrine orchestra' (Sir Walter Langdon-Brown, 1931), sets in motion the entire synchronous response. The body will bring into play neural, endocrine and inflammatory responses. The neural response that initiates and acts in concert with the endocrines is referred to as the neuroendocrine response to trauma.

Mediators

3. A, B, E

Stress from injury travels along afferent pathways of the spinal cord to the hypothalamus which secretes the corticotrophin-releasing factor (CRF) that acts on the pituitary to secrete adrenocorticotrophic hormone (ACTH) and growth hormone (GH). This creates the 'flight or fight' response. The pancreas increases glucagon secretion. Other endocrines, thyroid and gonads play a minor role. This concerted neuroendocrine response results in lipolysis, hepatic gluconeogenesis, protein breakdown, pyrexia and hypermetabolism. Cytokines, interleukins (IL-1, IL-6) and tumour necrosis factor-alpha (TNFα) are simultaneously released (see Fig. 1.2).

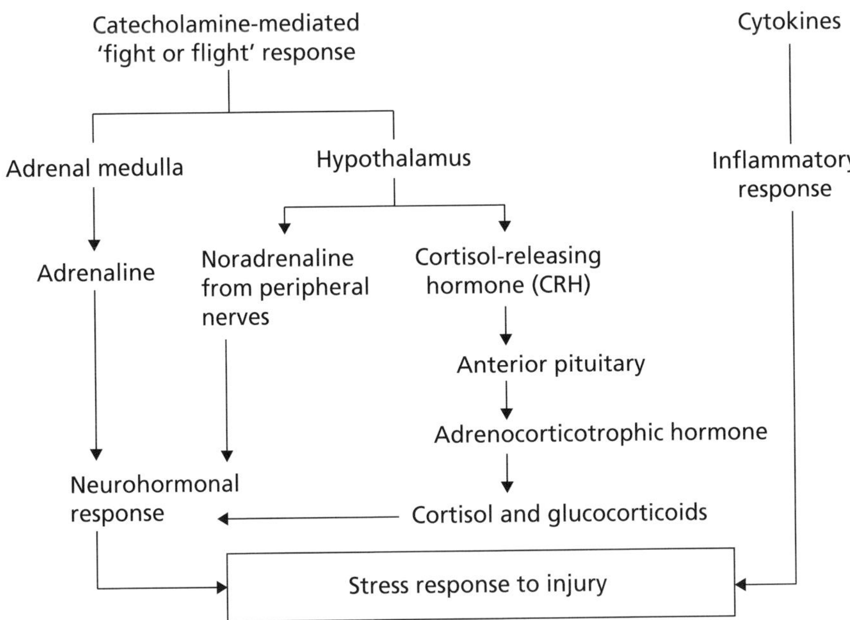

Figure 1.2 Neuroendocrine response to trauma.

A model of two phases, 'ebb and flow', is created. The term was coined by Sir David Cuthbertson in 1930. The ebb, or early, phase helps initiate a 'holding pattern' within the first 12 hours (clinically manifesting as shock). The flow phase lasts much longer depending upon the extent of damage. It can be divided into a catabolic phase lasting several days, followed by a recovery and repair phase lasting several weeks. The time factor depends upon the extent of initial injury and any ongoing insults. The mediators do help in the repair process by endogenous cytokine antagonists, which controls the proinflammatory response, commonly called the systemic inflammatory response syndrome (SIRS). If the response to SIRS is inadequate, multiple organ dysfunction syndrome occurs (MODS), which is just a step away from death.

The recovery process

4. B, C, E

Catabolism is an important aspect of recovery. However, the body's stress response has a capacity to triage the catabolic effect. The catabolic effect concentrates away from the peripheries, such as muscle fat and skin, to the more important parts – the liver, the immune system and the wound. During catabolism, muscle wasting occurs from muscle protein breakdown and a decrease in muscle protein synthesis. The major site for such a change is peripheral skeletal muscle; sometimes respiratory muscles are affected, resulting in hypoventilation with resultant pulmonary problems; gut muscle may be affected to produce paralytic ileus. Therefore, clinically, patients are weak with malaise and function suboptimally with increased risk of hospital-acquired infections.

Hyperalimentation is not advisable as it enhances the metabolic stress. Nutritional support should therefore be at a modest level. Hyperglycaemia is a normal response to stress. This is due to increased glucose production and decreased uptake in peripheral tissues as a result of insulin resistance, a temporary effect of stress. The severity of the stress determines the duration of the hyperglycaemic state – stress-induced diabetes. The patient is therefore at increased risk of diabetic complications: sepsis, renal impairment and polyneuropathy. Intravenous insulin infusion in the ICU setting using a sliding scale has been shown to reduce morbidity and mortality.

Optimal perioperative care

5. B, C, D, E

As a result of hypovolaemia, receptors in the carotid artery, aortic arch and left atrium act to release aldosterone and antidiuretic hormone (ADH). Aldosterone is also released by the renin–angiotensin system activated by the juxtaglomerular apparatus (see Fig. 1.3). Aldosterone and ADH help in sodium and water retention. Therefore large volumes of fluid infusion should not be used, as it will result in oedema, peripheral and visceral, the latter causing delayed gastric emptying.

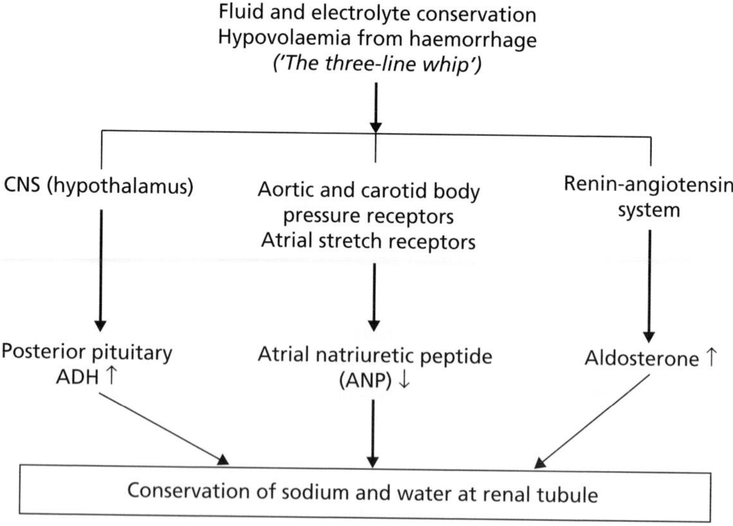

Figure 1.3 Hypovolaemia in trauma.

Hypothermia, due to increased production of adrenal steroids and catecholamines, causes greater risk of cardiac arrythmias. Therefore all efforts must be made to conserve heat in the stressed patient.

As a result of starvation, the body needs to produce glucose to sustain cerebral function. This is done by mobilising glycogen stores by hepatic gluconeogenesis. Fat is mobilised from adipose tissue followed by loss of lean tissue. At least 2 L of 5 per cent dextrose intravenously provides 100 g of glucose a day; this has a protein-sparing effect. Early institution of nutrition by the most appropriate route will avoid loss of body mass.

Immobility should be avoided as it induces muscle wasting. Inactivity of skeletal muscle impairs protein synthesis. Early mobilisation therefore helps in preventing muscle wasting besides minimising the dreaded complications of deep vein thrombosis and pulmonary embolism.

Perioperative care can be optimised by attention to feeding and preventing fluid overload. Epidural analgesia not only reduces stress from pain but also reduces the insulin resistance, by blocking the cortisol stress response. Beta-blockers and statins have a role in improving long-term survival after recovery from a major stress response.

2 Shock and blood transfusion

Multiple choice questions

➜ Cell metabolism

1. Which of the following statements are true?

A Cells change from aerobic to anaerobic metabolism when perfusion to tissues is reduced.
B The product of aerobic respiration is lactic acid.
C The product of anaerobic respiration is carbon dioxide.
D The accumulation of lactic acid in the blood produces systemic respiratory acidosis.
E Lack of oxygen and glucose in the cell will eventually lead to failure of sodium/potassium pumps in the cell membrane and intracellular organelles.

➜ Hypovolaemic shock

2. Which of the following statements regarding hypovolaemic shock are true?

A It is associated with high cardiac output.
B The vascular resistance is high.
C The venous pressure is low.
D The mixed venous saturation is high.
E The base deficit is low.

➜ Ischaemia-reperfusion syndrome

3. Which of the following statements about ischaemia-reperfusion syndrome is correct?

A This refers to the cellular injury because of the direct effects of tissue hypoxia.
B It is seen after the normal circulation is restored to the tissues following an episode of hypoperfusion.
C The increased sodium load can lead to myocardial depression.
D This is influenced by the duration and extent of tissue hypoperfusion.
E It usually does not cause death.

➜ Responses in shock

4. In which of the following cases might tachycardia accompany shock?

A Hypovolaemia due to gastrointestinal (GI) bleeds
B Patients on alpha-blockers
C Patients with implanted pacemakers
D Fit young adults with normal pulse rate of 50/min
E Cardiogenic shock.

5. Which of the following regarding blood pressure in shock are false?

A Elderly patients who are normally hypertensive may present with a 'normal' blood pressure.
B Children and fit young adults are able to maintain blood pressure until the final stages of shock.
C Hypotension is one of the first signs of shock.
D Beta-blockers may prevent a tachycardic response.
E Blood pressure is increased by reduction in stroke volume and peripheral vasoconstriction.

➜ Compensated shock

6. Which of the following statements about compensated shock are false?

A The preload is preserved by the cardiovascular and endocrinal compensatory responses.
B Tachycardia and cool peripheries may be the only clinical signs.
C The perfusion to the skin, muscle and GI tract is increased.

D Systemic respiratory acidosis is seen.
E Patients with occult hypoperfusion for more than 12 hours have a significantly higher mortality rate.

Resuscitation in shock

7. Which of the following statements are false?

A Administration of inotropic agents to an empty heart will help to increase diastolic filling and coronary perfusion.
B In all cases, regardless of classification, hypovolaemia and preload must be addressed first.
C Long, wide-bore catheters allow rapid infusion of fluids.
D The oxygen-carrying capacity of both colloids and crystalloids is zero.
E Hypotonic solutions are poor volume expanders and should not be used in shock except in conditions of free water loss or sodium overload.

Inotropic support in shock

8. Which of the following are true regarding inotropic support in shock?

A This is the first-line therapy in hypovolaemic shock.
B Phenylephrine and noradrenaline are indicated in distributive shock states.
C Dobutamine is the agent of choice in cardiogenic shock or septic shock complicated by low cardiac output.
D Vasopressin may be used when the vasodilatation is resistant to catecholamines.
E Use in the absence of adequate preload may be harmful.

Mixed venous saturation

9. Which of these statements about mixed venous saturation are false?

A The percentage saturation of oxygen returning to the heart from the body is a measure of the oxygen delivery and extraction by the tissues.
B The normal mixed oxygen saturation levels are 30–40 per cent.
C Accurate measurements are via analysis of blood drawn from a line placed in the superior vena cava (SVC).
D Levels below 50 per cent indicate inadequate oxygen delivery consistent with hypovolaemic shock.
E High mixed venous saturation levels are seen in sepsis.

Reactionary haemorrhage

10. Which of the following about reactionary haemorrhage are false?

A This is delayed haemorrhage occurring within 24 h after operation.
B It is usually caused by dislodgement of clot, normalisation of blood pressure or slippage of ligature.
C It is associated with infection.
D It can be significant, requiring re-exploration.
E It is usually venous.

Blood transfusion

11. Which of the following about blood transfusion are false?

A A haemoglobin level of 10 g/dL or less is now considered a typical indication.
B Fresh frozen plasma (FFP) is considered as the first-line therapy in coagulopathic haemorrhage.
C Cryoprecipitate is useful in low-fibrinogen states and in factor VIII deficiency.
D Platelets have a shelf life of 3 weeks.
E Patients can pre-donate blood up to 3 weeks before surgery for autologous transfusion.

12. Which of the following is a complication of massive blood transfusions?

A Coagulopathy
B Hypercalcaemia
C Hyperkalaemia
D Hypokalaemia
E Hypothermia.

Extended matching questions

1. Types of shock

A Septic shock
B Cardiogenic shock
C Hypovolaemic shock – haemorrhagic
D Neurogenic shock
E Anaphylactic shock
F Endocrinal shock
G Hypovolaemic shock – non-haemorrhagic

Choose and match the correct diagnosis with each of the scenarios given below:

1 A 7-year-old boy with nut allergy develops stridor and collapses after eating a snack. He requires airway and breathing support. His BP is 60/38 mmHg.

2 A 78-year-old man with known ischaemic heart disease (IHD) complains of chest pain and collapses. His pulse is irregular and BP is 74/48 mmHg. ECG shows features of an anterolateral myocardial infarction (MI).

3 A 76-year-old male is brought to the hospital with persistent diarrhoea and vomiting for the past 4 days. He has been unable to keep his food down and feels very tired. On examination he is very dehydrated. His pulse is 128/min and his BP is 88/52 mmHg.

4 A 55-year-old woman with poorly controlled hypothyroidism is found comatose. She is hypothermic. Her pulse is irregular and her BP is 96/70 mmHg.

5 An 86-year-old male has been complaining of increasing lower abdominal pain for the past week. On examination he looks very unwell with warm peripheries. He has signs of generalised peritonitis. His pulse is 130/min and his BP 84/50 mmHg.

6 A 28-year-old motorist is brought to the A&E after a road traffic accident (RTA). He has sustained an isolated injury to his back and has motor and sensory deficits in both lower limbs. His pulse is 122/min and his BP 100/62 mmHg.

7 A 19-year-old male is brought to the hospital after sustaining an abdominal injury while playing rugby. He is complaining of left upper abdominal pain and has some bruising over the same area. His pulse is 140/min and his BP is 100/82 mmHg.

2. Vasopressor and inotropic support in shock

A Noradrenaline
B No role for vasopressor or inotropic agent
C Phenylephrine
D Dobutamine
E Vasopressin

Choose and match the correct intervention with each of the scenarios given below:

1 Cardiogenic shock when myocardial depression complicates shock state.

2 Distributive shock due to sepsis.

3 Vasodilatation resistant to catecholamines due to relative or absolute steroid deficiency.

4 Hypovolaemic shock due to splenic injury.

5 Distributive shock due to spinal cord injury.

3. Complications of blood transfusion

A Haemolytic transfusion reaction due to incompatibility
B Fluid overload
C Disseminated intravascular coagulation (DIC)
D Hypocalcaemia
E Infection

Choose and match the correct diagnosis with each of the scenarios given below:

1 A 86-year-old woman is admitted with a haemoglobin (Hb) of 5.6 g/dL. The HO prescribes 4 units of blood. These 4 units are transfused over a period of 6 h. Four hours later the patient is found to be having difficulty in breathing. Chest examination reveals fine creps bilaterally. Chest X-ray confirms pulmonary oedema.

2 A 28-year-old male is taken to a nearby hospital after sustaining injuries while on a safari in Africa. He has lost a lot of blood and is hence given 2 units of blood transfusion. He develops fever and chills with rigors the next day. Peripheral blood smear demonstrates malarial parasite.

3 A 38-year-old man requires several units of blood transfusion due to multiple injuries sustained as a result of a fall. He develops tetany and complains of cicumoral tingling.

4 A 34-year-old motorcyclist sustains multiple injuries after an RTA. He is brought to the hospital in severe shock and requires multiple blood transfusions. It is observed that the bleeding is still uncontrolled and the blood fails to clot.

5 The ward is very busy and quite a few staff have phoned in sick. There are two patients (with the same surnames) needing blood transfusions. The staff nurse points to the blood units on the table and asks the HCA to start them as she is just going off for her break. The blood transfusion is started. Within a few minutes the patient is unwell and his urine is haemorrhagic. He collapses and becomes anuric. He is also found to be jaundiced.

Answers: Multiple choice questions

Cell metabolism

1. A, E

Cells switch from aerobic to anaerobic metabolism when deprived of oxygen. The product of aerobic respiration is carbon dioxide. This is eliminated efficiently through the lungs. The product of anaerobic respiration is lactic acid. When enough tissue is underperfused, the accumulation of lactic acid in the blood produces systemic metabolic acidosis. As tissue ischaemia progresses, the immune and complement systems are activated. This also results in the complement and neutrophil priming with the generation of oxygen-free radicals and cytokines. This leads to injury of the epithelial and endothelial cells, which leads to loss of integrity and 'leaky' walls. The resultant oedema further increases tissue hypoxia. As glucose within the cells is exhausted, anaerobic respiration ceases and there is a failure of the sodium/potassium pump. Intracellular lysosomes release autodigestive enzymes and cell lysis ensues. Intracellular contents, including the potassium, are released into the bloodstream.

Hypovolaemic shock

2. B, C (see Table 2.1)

Table 2.1 Response in different types of shock

Parameter	Type of shock			
	Hypovolaemia	Cardiogenic	Obstructive	Distributive
Cardiac output	Low	Low	Low	High
Vascular resistance	High	High	High	Low
Venous pressure	Low	High	High	Low
Mixed venous saturation	Low	Low	Low	High
Base deficit	High	High	High	High

Ischaemia-reperfusion syndrome

3. B, D

During the period of reperfusion, cellular and organ damage progresses as a result of direct effects of tissue hypoxia and local activation of inflammation. Further injury occurs once the normal circulation is restored. This is termed ischaemia-reperfusion syndrome. The acid and potassium load that has built up can lead to direct myocardial depression, vascular dilatation and further hypotension. The cellular and humoral components flushed back into circulation cause further endothelial injury and organ damage. This can lead to multiple organ failure (MOF) and death. Ischaemia-reperfusion injury can be reduced by limiting the extent and duration of tissue hypoperfusion.

Responses in shock

4. A, B

Tachycardia is an early warning sign in hypovolaemic shock. The tachycardic response is not seen in patients on beta-blockers.

5. C, E

Hypotension may not be seen until the shock is well established. The heart compensates initially to maintain cardiac output by increasing both the rate and the stroke volume.

Compensated shock

6. C, D

Systemic metabolic acidosis is seen in shock (also see Table 2.2)

Table 2.2 Responses in different degrees of shock

Parameter	Degree of shock			
	Compensated	Mild	Moderate	Severe
Lactic acidosis	+	++	++	+++
Urine output	Normal	Normal	Reduced	Anuric
Level of consciousness	Normal	Mild anxiety	Drowsy	Comatose
Respiratory rate	Normal	Increased	Increased	Laboured
Pulse rate	Mild increase	Increased	Increased	Increased
Blood pressure	Normal	Normal	Mild hypotension	Severe hypotension

Resuscitation in shock

7. A, C

Resuscitation should not be delayed in order to definitively diagnose the cause of the shocked state. The first-line therapy is intravenous (IV) access administration of IV fluids using short, wide-bore catheters that allow rapid infusion of fluids. Hypotonic fluids are poor volume expanders and should not be used in the treatment of shock (an exception is free water loss, as in diabetes insipidus and sodium overload, e.g. cirrhosis). If there is an initial doubt about the cause of shock, it is safer to assume that it is hypovolaemia and begin with fluid resuscitation, followed by an assessment of the response. In patients who are actively bleeding (major trauma, ruptured abdominal aortic aneurysm, GI bleed), it is counterproductive to institute high-volume fluid therapy without controlling the site of bleeding. Resuscitation should proceed in parallel with surgery. Conversely, a patient with bowel obstruction and hypovolaemic shock should be adequately resuscitated before undergoing surgery. Administration of inotropic agents to an empty heart will rapidly and permanently deplete the myocardium of oxygen stores and dramatically reduce diastolic filling and therefore coronary perfusion.

➜ Inotropic support in shock

8. B, C, D, E

The first-line therapy in hypovolaemic shock is IV access and administration of fluids. Phenylephrine and noradrenaline are helpful in distributive shock states, such as those due to sepsis and neurogenic causes. These states are characterised by peripheral vasodilatation, a low systemic vascular resistance and a high cardiac output. If the vasodilatation is resistant to these agents (e.g. absolute or relative steroid deficiency), vasopressin may be used.

➜ Mixed venous saturation

9. B, C

The percentage saturation of oxygen returning to the heart from the body is a measure of the oxygen delivery and extraction by the tissues. Accurate measurement is by a long line placed in the right atrium. Samples from the SVC give slightly higher values. Normal mixed venous oxygen saturation levels are 50–70 per cent. Levels below 50 per cent indicate inadequate oxygen delivery and increased oxygen extraction by the cells. This is consistent with hypovolaemic or cardiogenic shock. High mixed venous saturation levels (>70 per cent) are seen in sepsis and some forms of distributive shock.

➜ Reactionary haemorrhage

10. C, E

The bleeding is usually arterial. It is not associated with infection, unlike secondary haemorrhage.

➜ Blood transfusion

11. A, D

The transfusion trigger was historically 10 g/dL. It is now believed, however, that a level of 6 g/dL is acceptable in patients who are not bleeding, not symptomatic and not about to undergo major surgery. Levels between 6 and 8 g/dL are selectively transfused. Also see Table 2.3.

12. A, C, D, E

Hypocalcaemia is another complication of massive transfusion. People who receive repeated transfusions over long periods of time develop iron overload.

Complications from a single transfusion include incompatibility haemolytic transfusion reaction, febrile transfusion reaction, allergic reaction, infection, air embolism, thrombophlebitis and transfusion-related acute lung injury (usually from FFP).

Table 2.3 Components used in blood transfusions

Component	Parameter: Constituents	Indications	Storage	Shelf life
Packed red cells	Red blood cells spun down and concentrated	Chronic anaemia	SAG-M solution 2–6°C	5 weeks
Fresh frozen plasma (FFP)	Coagulation factors	Coagulopathic haemorrhage	−40 to −50°C	2 years
Cryoprecipitate	Supernatant precipitate of FFP – rich in factor VIII and fibrinogen	Low fibrinogen states, factor VIII deficiency	−30°C	2 years
Platelets	Platelet concentrates	Thrombocytopenia, platelet dysfunction	20–24°C (special agitator)	5 days
Prothrombin complex concentrates	Purified concentrates of factors II, IX, X; factor VII is also included/separate	Emergency reversal of anticoagulant (Warfarin) in uncontrolled haemorrhage	–	–

Answers: Extended matching questions

1. Types of shock

1E, 2B, 3G, 4F, 5A, 6D, 7C

2. Vasopressor and inotropic support in shock

1D, 2A (or 5), 3E, 4B, 5C (or 2)

3. Complications of blood transfusion

1B

Extreme caution should be exercised in prescribing transfusions/fluids to elderly patients. Packed cells are preferable to whole blood and the patient must be closely monitored for signs of fluid overload. Administration of frusemide following transfusion of units may be needed.

2E

The other infections that can be transmitted through blood transfusion are hepatitis B and C, bacterial infections, HIV and new-variant Creutzfeldt–Jakob Disease (CJD).

3D

Hypocalcaemia is a known complication after massive transfusions.

4C

Coagulopathy is a known complication after massive multiple transfusions. This should be aggressively treated and, better still, avoided. The standard guidelines are:

- FFP, if prothrombin time (PT) and partial thromboplastin time (PTT) > 1.5 times normal values
- cryoprecipitate, if fibrinogen < 0.8 g/L
- platelets, if platelet count < 50×10^9/L.

5A

This is completely avoidable and hence should never happen. While prescribing and administering blood, it is essential that the correct patient receives the correct transfusion. Care should be taken to ensure correct labelling of samples. Two individuals should check the patient's details against the prescription and the label of the donor blood. Additionally the donor blood serial number should be checked against the issue slip for that patient.

3 Wounds, tissue repair and scars

Multiple choice questions

➜ Wound healing

1. **Which of these factors influences healing of a wound?**

A Vascular insufficiency
B Diabetes mellitus
C Malnutrition
D Site of wound
E Smoking.

2. **Which of the following statements about the process of wound healing are true?**

A The inflammatory phase begins 2–3 days after the injury.
B The proliferative phase lasts from 3 days to 3 weeks following the injury.
C The remodelling phase involves fibroblast activity and production of collagen and ground substance.
D Fibroblasts require vitamin C to produce collagen.
E The white cells stick to the damaged endothelium and release adenosine diphosphate (ADP) and cytokines.

3. **Which of the following statements are true?**

A Healing by primary intention results in minimum inflammation and the best scar.
B Granulation, contraction and epithelialisation are seen in healing by secondary intention.
C Tertiary intention involves immediate closure of the wound.
D A crushed and contaminated wound is best suited for healing by primary intention.
E Primary repair of all structures should be attempted in an untidy wound.

➜ Management of wounds

4. **Which of the following statements regarding management of the acute wound are correct?**

A A bleeding wound should be elevated and a pressure pad applied.
B Clamps may sometimes need to be put on bleeding vessels blindly.
C Anaesthesia is usually not required in the assessment of wounds.
D A thorough debridement is essential.
E Repair of all damaged structures may be attempted in a tidy wound.

5. **Which of the following statements regarding the management of specific wounds are true?**

A A haematomata should never require release.
B Anaerobic and aerobic organism prophylaxis is needed in bite wounds.
C Puncture wounds should always be explored.
D Degloving injuries will require serial excision until viable tissue is confirmed.
E Compartment syndrome typically occurs in a closed lower limb injury.

➜ Chronic wounds

6. **Which of the following statements are true?**

A The most common chronic wound in developed countries is the leg ulcer.
B Pressure sores occur in approximately 5 per cent of all hospitalised patients.
C Surgical treatment is usually required in the treatment of leg ulcers.
D Bed-bound patients should be turned every 4 h to prevent pressure sores.

E Risk of tissue necrosis increases if the external pressure exceeds the capillary occlusive pressure (30 mmHg).

Pressure sores

7. Pressure sores can occur over which of the following areas?

A Sacrum
B Heel
C Occiput
D Greater trochanter
E Ischium.

Necrotising soft-tissue infections

8. Which of the following statements about necrotising soft-tissue infections are true?

A They are usually polymicrobial infections.
B The onset is usually gradual and they run a chronic course.
C 'Dishwater pus' is a characteristic feature.
D Clostridial species cause toxic shock syndrome.
E Treatment is essentially medical using antibiotics.

Scars

9. Which of the following statements are true?

A Scars continue maturing for 3 months.
B Keloids contain an excess of type B collagen.
C Suture marks can be reduced by using polyfilament sutures.
D The tensile strength of the scar never reaches that of the normal skin.
E A hypertrophied scar extends beyond the boundaries of the previous incision.

Keloids

10. Which of the following are useful in the treatment of keloids?

A Elasticated garments
B Silicone gel sheeting
C Excision and steroid injection
D Excision and radiotherapy
E Vitamin D preparations.

Extended matching questions

1. Types of wound

A Tidy
B Puncture
C Degloving
D Untidy
E Compartment syndrome
F Pressure sore

Choose and match the correct diagnosis with each of the scenarios given below:

1 This occurs when the skin and subcutaneous fat are stripped from the underlying fascia by avulsion, leaving the neurovascular structures, tendon or bone exposed.

2 This is caused by crush or avulsion forces and usually has variable amount of tissue loss. It is invariably contaminated and has devitalised tissues.

3 These are wounds caused by sharp objects such as needles. X-ray may be needed to rule out a retained foreign body.

4 These wounds are defined as tissue necrosis with ulceration due to prolonged pressure. They should be regarded as preventable.

5 These typically occur in closed lower limb injuries and are characterised by severe pain, pain on passive movement, distal sensory disturbance and, finally, absent pulses.

6 These are clean wounds and usually incised. The tissues are healthy with seldom tissue loss.

2. Management of wounds and related conditions

A Tidy wounds
B Degloving wounds
C Compartment syndrome
D Untidy wounds
E Pressure sore
F Keloids
G Necrotising infections
H Contractures

Choose and match the correct diagnosis with each of the scenarios below:

1 Multiple debridements followed by definitive closure/repair.

2 Multiple Z-plasties or use of skin grafts/flaps.

3 Primary repair of all structures – bone, tendon, vessel and nerve.

4 Intralesional steroid injection and intralesional excision.

5 Fasciotomy.

6 Debridement and vacuum-assisted closure (VAC).

7 Surgical excision with tissue biopsies sent for culture. Skin graft may be needed later on.

8 Examination under anaesthesia (EUA) with radical excision of all non-bleeding skin. Serial excision is usually done until punctuate dermal bleeding is seen. This is followed by split skin graft.

3. Phases of wound healing

A Early inflammatory phase
B Late inflammatory phase
C Proliferative phase
D Remodelling phase
E Mature scar

Choose and match the correct diagnosis with each of the scenarios below:

1 This phase is characterised by replacement of type 3 collagen by type 1 until a ratio of 4:1 is achieved. Realignment of collagen fibres along the lines of tension, decreased vascularity and wound contraction are also seen in this phase.

2 Platelet-enriched blood clot and dilated vessels are a feature of this phase.

3 The contraction of the scar is now complete. The vascularity has reduced and growth ceases.

4 This phase has increased vascularity with plenty of neutrophils and lymphocytes.

5 This phase consists mainly of fibroblast activity and collagen production. The collagen produced during this phase is type 3.

4. Wound dressings

A Debriding agent
B Hydrogel
C Hydrocolloid
D Foam
E Polymeric film

F Fibrous polymer
G Biological membranes

Choose and match the correct description with each of the wound dressings below:

1 Kaltostat, Sorbsan

2 Intrasite, Lyofoam

3 Porcine skin, amnion

4 Benoxyl-benzoic acid

5 Granuflex

6 Opsite, Tegaderm

7 Silastic (Elastomer).

Answers: Multiple choice questions

Wound healing

1. A, B, C, D, E

Wound healing is also influenced by other factors, including structures involved, mechanism of wounding (incision, crush or crush avulsion), contamination, loss of tissue, previous radiation, pressure, vitamin and mineral deficiencies, medications (steroids, chemotherapy), HIV and any other cause of immunodeficiency.

2. B, D

The inflammatory phase begins immediately after the wounding and lasts 2–3 days. Platelets stick to the damaged endothelial lining of the vessels and release ADP and cytokines such as platelet-derived growth factor (PDGF), platelet factor 4 and transforming growth factor (TGF)-beta. These attract inflammatory cells such as polymorphonuclear lymphocytes and macrophages.

The proliferative phase lasts from the third day to the third week, consisting mainly of fibroblast activity with the production of collagen and ground substance, the growth of new blood vessels as capillary loops and re-epithelialisation of the wound surface. The remodelling phase is characterised by maturation of collagen, with type 1 *replacing* type 3 until a ratio of 4:1 is achieved. There is realignment of collagen fibres along the line of tension, decreased wound vascularity and wound contraction due to fibroblast and myofibroblast activity.

3. A, B

Tertiary intention is also called delayed primary intention and in this the wound is initially left open and the edges later opposed when healing conditions are favourable. A crushed and contaminated wound is best managed by debridement on one or several occasions before definitive repair can be carried out. Primary repair of all structures should be attempted in a tidy wound.

Management of wounds

4. A, D, E

The surgeon should remember to examine the whole patient according to the Advanced Trauma Life Support (ATLS) guidelines. The wound itself should be examined, taking into consideration the site and possible structures damaged. Clamps should not be applied blindly as nerve damage is likely and vascular anastomosis is rendered impossible. In order to facilitate examination, adequate analgesia and/or anaesthesia (local, regional or general) are required. General anaesthesia is preferred in children. In limb injuries, particularly those of the hand, a tourniquet should be used.

5. B, C, D, E

If large, painful or causing neural deficit, a haematoma may require release by incision or aspiration.

Chronic wounds

6. A, B, E

An ulcer is defined as a break in the epithelial continuity. A prolonged inflammatory phase leads to an overgrowth of granulation tissue, and attempts to heal by scarring leaves a fibrotic margin. Necrotic tissue, often at the ulcer centre, is called slough. Most ulcers are managed by dressings and simple treatments. An ulcer not responsive to this treatment should be biopsied to rule out malignant change (Marjolin's ulcer). Effective treatment of any ulcer depends on treating the cause, and diagnosis is hence vital. Surgical treatment is only indicated if non-operative methods have failed and the patient has intractable pain. Meshed skin grafts are more successful than sheet grafts.

Pressure sores

7. A, B, C, D, E

A pressure sore is defined as tissue necrosis with ulceration due to prolonged pressure. They occur in about 5 per cent of all hospitalised patients and the incidence is higher in paraplegic patents, in the elderly and the severely ill patients. The stages of pressure sore are as follows:

- stage 1: non-blanchable erythema without a breach in the epidermis
- stage 2: partial-thickness skin loss involving the epidermis and dermis
- stage 3: full-thickness skin loss extending into the subcutaneous tissue but not through underlying fascia
- stage 4: full-thickness skin loss through fascia with extensive tissue destruction, possibly involving muscle, tendon, bone or joint.

If external pressure exceeds the capillary occlusion pressure (over 30 mmHg), blood flow to the skin ceases, causing tissue anoxia, necrosis and ulceration. Prevention is the best treatment with good skin care, special pressure, dispersion cushions or foams, the use of low air-loss and air-fluidised beds and urinary/faecal diversion in appropriate cases. The bed-bound patient should be turned every 2 h, with the wheelchair-bound patient being taught to lift themselves off their seat for 10 s every 10 min.

Care of pressure sores follows the principles of acute wound management. Debridement, use of VAC and skin flaps may be helpful in achieving healing.

Necrotising soft-tissue infections

8. A, C

These are rare but often fatal infections that are usually seen after trauma or surgery with wound contamination. They are polymicrobial infections involving Gram-positive aerobes (*S. aureus*, *S. pyogenes*), Gram-negative aerobes (*E. coli*, *P. aeruginosa*), *Clostridia*, *Bacteroides* and beta-haemolytic *Streptococcus*. The infections are characterised by sudden presentation and rapid progression. There are two main types of necrotising infections – clostridial and non-clostridial (streptococcal gangrene and necrotising fasciitis). *Streptococcus pyogenes* causes toxic shock syndrome and is often called 'flesh-eating bug'. Treatment is surgical excision with tissue being sent for culture. Wide raw areas are often left behind which may require skin graft.

Scars

9. B, D

The maturation phase of healing results in scarring. The mature scar becomes mature over a period of a year or more. At first, it is pink, hard, raised and itchy. As the scar matures, it becomes almost acellular as the fibroblasts and blood vessels reduce. The scar then becomes paler, flat and soft. Most of the changes take place over the first 3 months but a scar will continue to mature for 1–2 years. The strength gradually increases but will never reach that of normal skin. Suture marks can be reduced by using monofilament sutures. A hypertrophic scar is defined as excessive scar tissue that does not extend beyond the boundary of the original incision or wound. It results from a prolonged inflammatory phase of wound healing and from unfavourable siting of the scar.

➜ Keloids

10. A, B, C, D

A keloid is defined as excessive scar tissue that extends beyond the boundaries of the original incision or wound. Its aetiology is unknown but it is associated with elevated levels of growth factor, deeply pigmented skin, an inherited tendency and certain areas of the body (a triangle whose points are the xiphisternum and each shoulder tip). Histology shows excess collagen with hypervascularity and increased B type of collagen.

Answers: Extended matching questions

➜ 1. Types of wound

1C, 2D, 3B, 4F, 5E, 6A

➜ 2. Management of wounds and related conditions

1D, 2H, 3A, 4F, 5C, 6E, 7G, 8B

➜ 3. Phases of wound healing

1D, 2A, 3E, 4B, 5C

➜ 4. Wound dressings

1F, 2B, 3G, 4A, 5C, 6E, 7D

4 Surgical infection

Multiple choice questions

➜ Koch's postulates

1. Which of the following are part of Koch's postulates?

A It must be found in considerable numbers in the septic focus.
B A reduction in the organisms should be achieved by using appropriate antibiotics.
C It should be possible to culture it in a pure form from the septic focus.
D Healing of a wound is possible without pus formation.
E It should be able to produce similar lesions when injected into another host.

➜ Natural barriers to infection

2. Which of the following is a natural barrier to infection?

A Intact epithelial surface
B High gastric pH
C Antibodies
D Antibiotics
E Macrophages.

➜ Host resistance to infection

3. Which of the following is a cause of reduced host resistance to infection?

A Malnutrition
B Heart failure
C Cancer
D AIDS
E Systemic sclerosis.

➜ Risk factors for wound infection

4. Which of the following is a risk factor for wound infection?

A Poor perfusion
B Use of skin clips for wound closure.
C Poor surgical technique
D Not using prophylactic antibiotics
E Uraemia.

➜ Secondary infections

5. Which of the following is a cause of secondary (or exogenous) infection?

A Poor hand-washing technique
B Community
C Perforated diverticular disease
D Anastomotic leak
E Inadequate air filtration in the theatre.

➜ Surgical site infections

6. Which of the following statements about surgical site infections (SSIs) are true?

A Infection in the musculofascial tissues is known as deep SSI.
B The patient may have systemic signs in a minor SSI.
C Infection causing delay in hospital discharge is a major SSI.
D The differentiation between major and minor SSIs is not important.
E Surveillance for surgical site infection should be done for a year after implanted joint surgery.

➜ Abscesses

7. Which of the following statements regarding abscesses are true?

A *Staphylococcus aureus* is one of the most common causative organisms.
B The abscess wall is composed of epithelium.
C Most wound-site abscesses occur before the patient is discharged from the hospital.
D Antibiotics are indicated if there is evidence of cellulitis.
E *Actinomyces* can cause a chronic abscess.

Cellulitis

8. Which of the following statements regarding cellulitis are true?

A This is non-suppurative invasive infection of tissues.
B It is poorly localised.
C It is commonly caused by *Clostridium perfringens*.
D Systemic signs are not present.
E Blood culture is usually positive.

Systemic inflammatory response syndrome (SIRS)

9. Which if the following can be seen in SIRS?

A Hypothermia (<36° C)
B White cell count (WCC) $< 4 \times 1000$/dL
C No documented infection
D Tachycardia (>90/min)
E Tachypnoea (>20/min).

Severe sepsis (sepsis syndrome)

10. Which of the following statements about severe sepsis (sepsis syndrome) are true?

A Acute respiratory distress syndrome (ARDS) is common.
B There is absence of documented infection.
C Multiple organ dysfunction syndrome (MODS) is the systemic effect of infection.
D Multiple system organ failure (MSOF) is the end stage of uncontrolled MODS.
E MSOF is mediated by released cytokines such as interleukins (IL-6) and tumour necrosis factor (TNF)-alpha.

Clostridial wound infections

11. Which of the following statements regarding clostridial wound infections are true?

A Clostridia are Gram-positive aerobic spore-bearing cocci.
B Thin, brown and sweet-smelling exudate is seen in gas gangrene.
C Necrotic and foreign material in wounds increase risk.
D The spores are widely spread in soil and manure.
E The signs and symptoms are due to the endotoxins.

Treatment of surgical infections

12. Which of the following statements are true?

A Identification of the causative organism should be done before starting antibiotics.
B Wounds are best managed by delayed primary or secondary closure.
C Subcuticular continuous skin closure decreases the incidence of wound infection.
D Polymeric films can be useful in infected wounds.
E Administration of antibiotic preparations locally is more effective than the oral route.

Prophylactic antibiotics

13. Which of the following affects the choice of prophylactic antibiotic?

A The expected spectrum of organisms likely to be encountered
B Cost
C Personal preference
D Hospital policies
E Local resistance strains.

14. Which of the following may require more than one dose of prophylactic antibiotic?

A Prolonged operations
B Excessive blood loss
C Gastrointestinal surgery
D Insertion of prosthesis
E Unexpected contamination.

Surgical wound infection

15. Which of the following measures is useful in reducing surgical wound infection?

A Antiseptic skin preparation
B Shaving of area

C Avoid hypothermia perioperatively
D Increasing hospital stay to detect more infections
E Supplemental oxygen in recovery room.

Different types of wounds

16. Which of the following statements about types of wounds are true?

A The infection rate in a 'clean wound' is between 1 and 2 per cent.
B The wound after a biliary surgery is classified as 'contaminated'.
C A 'clean-contaminated wound' has an infection rate of less than 10 per cent.
D Antibiotic prophylaxis would be mandatory in 'dirty wounds'.
E The role of prophylactic antibiotics in non-prosthetic clean surgery is controversial.

Infection causing bacteria

17. Which of the following statements regarding bacteria in surgical infection are true?

A Beta-haemolytic *Streptococcus* is always associated with infection.
B All streptococci are sensitive to penicillin and erythromycin.
C Staphylococci are normally resident in the nasopharynx of up to 15 per cent of the population.
D Staphylococcal epidermidis is a commensal and does not cause clinical infection.
E Gram-negative bacilli are a major cause of infection related to urethral catheterisation.

Principles of antimicrobial treatment

18. Which of the following statements regarding antimicrobial treatment of surgical infections are true?

A Antibiotics are mandatory in all SSIs.
B Antibiotics should not be started before knowing the causative organism and sensitivity.
C A 'broad-spectrum' approach is used while treating methicillin-resistant *Staphylococcus aureus* (MRSA) infections.
D Antibiotics can be used as a replacement for surgical drainage.
E Rotating antibiotics may be required in the treatment of 'resident opportunists'.

Antibiotics in surgical infections

19. Which of the following statements regarding antibiotics in surgical infections are true?

A Tetracycline is a bactericidal antibiotic.
B Flucloxacillin is useful in treating community-acquired staphylococcal infections.
C Cephalosporins are not effective against *Streptococcus faecalis*.
D Serum levels should be monitored if aminoglycoside therapy is continued for more than 1 week.
E Vancomycin is effective against both MRSA and *Clostridium difficile*.

AIDS

20. Which of the following statements regarding AIDS are true?

A After exposure, the virus binds to CD4 receptors.
B The gut-associated lymphoid tissue (GALT) is not affected.
C The HIV transmission risk is low during the stage of seroconversion.
D Most antiviral drugs (HAART) act by inhibiting reverse transcriptase and protease synthesis.
E Within 2 years, progression of HIV infection to AIDS is seen in 25–35 per cent of patients.

Extended matching questions

→ 1. Prophylactic antibiotics regimen

A Vascular
B Orthopaedic
C Biliary
D Colorectal.

Choose and match the correct systems with each of the antibiotics below:

1 Second-generation cephalosporin (or gentamicin) and metronidazole

2 Broad-spectrum cephalosporin (with anti-staphylococcal action) or gentamicin beads

3 Flucloxacillin with or without gentamicin, vancomycin or rifampicin, if MRSA is a risk

4 Second-generation cephalosporin.

→ 2. Bacteria involved in surgical infection

A *Streptococcus*
B *Staphylococcus*
C *Clostridium*
D *E. coli*
E *Proteus*
F *Pseudomonas*
G *Bacteroides.*

Choose and match the correct organism with each of the descriptions below:

1 Lactose-fermenting Gram-negative bacillus, which is the most common cause of UTI.

2 Gram-negative bacillus, which tends to colonise burns and tracheostomy wounds. These can also case UTI. Hospital strains can acquire resistance transferred through plasmids.

3 Non-spore-bearing anaerobes that colonise the colon, vagina and oropharynx.

4 Gram-positive cocci which form chains; causes cellulitis and spreading tissue destruction by release of enzymes.

5 Non-lactose-fermenting Gram-negative bacillus which is a normal resident of the colon and is a cause of intra-abdominal infection after bowel surgery.

6 Gram-positive, obligate anaerobes which produce spores; causes serious infections such as gas gangrene, tetanus and pseudomembranous colitis.

7 Gram-positive aerobic coccus, which forms grape-like clumps; causes wound and prosthesis infection. Resistant strains (MRSA) can cause epidemics.

→ 3. Specific infections

A Gas gangrene
B Necrotising fasciitis
C Pseudomembranous colitis
D Tetanus

E Surgical wound infection
F Pelvic abscess
G Diverticular abscess.

Choose and match the correct diagnosis with each of the scenarios below:

1 A 78-year-old nursing home resident who has finished a course of antibiotics recently presents with severe diarrhoea for the past 3 days. On examination, he is very unwell and in shock. Abdominal examination reveals generalised distension and tenderness.

2 A 16-year-old boy who had an appendicectomy for a gangrenous appendix 1 week ago presents with diarrhoea, fever and lower abdominal pain.

3 An 80-year-old male presents with a week-long history of left iliac fossa (LIF) pain. This has increased significantly over the last couple of days and is associated with fever and urinary irritation. On examination he is very unwell and has signs of peritonitis over the LIF with a vaguely palpable tender mass.

4 A young soldier injured in combat develops severe pain over his leg wound. Examination reveals thin, brown, sweet-smelling exudate with oedema and crepitus.

5 An immunocompromised patient develops rapidly spreading infection of the abdominal wall after a laparotomy for peritonitis. He complains of severe pain. Examination reveals extensive cellulitis with crepitus. Culture swab reveals mixed aerobic and anaerobic growth.

6 A 45-year-old male who sustained minor injury 3 weeks ago while gardening presents with difficulty in swallowing and jaw movements followed by generalised motor spasms. He is finding it difficult to breathe. On examination you find opisthotonus and respiratory failure.

7 A 30-year-old female underwent an appendicectomy for an inflamed appendix 4 days ago. The wound appears red with some seropurulent discharge at one end. She has been febrile over the past couple of days.

→ 4. Different types of operations and infection rates

A Clean
B Clean-contaminated
C Contaminated
D Dirty.

Choose the correct operation type for each of the scenarios below:

1 Drainage of an abscess

2 No viscus opened

3 Gastric and biliary surgery

4 Wound infection rate 1–2 per cent

5 Open viscus surgery or gross spillage or inflammatory bowel disease

6 Wound infection rate 15–20 per cent

7 Wound infection rate < 40 per cent

8 Wound infection rate < 10 per cent.

Answers: Multiple choice questions

Koch's postulates

1. A, C, E

Surgical infection has always been a major complication of surgery and trauma and has been documented for 4000–5000 years. The Hippocratic teachings described the use of antimicrobials, such as wine and vinegar, to irrigate wounds. Galen recognised that localisation of infection heralded recovery. Microbes had been seen under the microscope but it was Koch who laid down the first definition of infectious disease.

Natural barriers to infection

2. A, C, E

The breakdown of the intact epithelial surface by surgery and trauma increases the risk of infection. The other natural barriers are low gastric pH, complements, opsonins, phagocytic cells, polymorphonuclear cells and killer lymphocytes.

Host resistance to infection

3. A, C, D

The other causes of reduced host resistance include diabetes, uraemia, jaundice, obesity, radiotherapy, chemotherapy and steroids.

Risk factors for wound infection

4. A, C, E

The factors that increase the risk of wound infection include malnutrition (obesity and weight loss), metabolic conditions such as diabetes and jaundice, immunosuppression due to cancer, AIDS, steroids, chemotherapy and radiotherapy, colonisation and translocation in the gut, poor perfusion due to systemic shock or local ischaemia, foreign body material and poor surgical technique, such as dead space and haematoma.

Secondary infections

5. A, D, E

The sources of infection are classified as primary and secondary (exogenous). The primary sources include infection acquired from a community or endogenous source (e.g. perforated peptic ulcer). Secondary or exogenous sources include infections acquired from the operation theatre (such as inadequate air filtration) or the ward (e.g. poor hand-washing compliance) or from contamination at or after surgery (e.g. anastomotic leak). Infection that follows surgery or admission to hospital is termed health care-associated infection (HAI). There are four main groups of HAI: respiratory infections, including ventilator-associated pneumonia, urinary tract infection (UTI), bacteraemia (mostly associated with indwelling vascular catheters) and SSIs.

Surgical site infections

6. A, C, E

A major SSI is defined as a wound that either discharges significant quantities of pus spontaneously or needs a secondary procedure to drain it. The patient may have systemic signs such as tachycardia, pyrexia and a raised white count (SIRS). It results in delayed return home.

A minor wound infection may discharge pus or infected serous fluid but should not be associated with excessive discomfort, systemic signs or delay in return home. The differentiation between major and minor infections and the definition of SSI is important in audit or trials of antibiotic prophylaxis. There are scoring systems (Southampton and ASEPSIS) for the severity of wound infection which are particularly useful in surveillance and research (see Table 4.1)

Table 4.1 ASEPSIS wound score

Criterion	Points
Additional treatment – antibiotics/drainage/debridement	10/5/10
Serous discharge	Daily 0–5
Erythema	Daily 0–5
Purulent exudate	Daily 0–10
Separation of deep tissues	Daily 0–10
Isolation of bacteria from wound	10
Stay as in-patient prolonged over 14 days as a result of wound infection.	5

Accurate surveillance can only be achieved using trained, unbiased and blinded assessors. Most include surveillance for a 30-day postoperative period for non-prosthetic surgery and 1 year after implanted hip and knee surgery.

Abscesses

7. A, D, E

An abscess presents all features of acute inflammation – calor (heat), rubor (redness), dolour (pain) and tumour (swelling). To this is added functio laesa (loss of function). Pyogenic organisms cause suppuration and necrosis. Pus is composed of dead and dying white blood cells that release damaging cytokines, oxygen free radicals and other molecules. An abscess is surrounded by an acute inflammatory response and a pyogenic membrane composed of fibrinous exudate and oedema and the cells of acute inflammation. Abscesses contain hyperosmolar material that draws in fluid. This increases pressure and causes pain. Most abscesses relating to surgical wounds take 7–10 days to form after surgery. As many as 75 per cent of SSIs present after the patient has left the hospital.

Abscess cavities need cleaning out/curettage after incision and drainage. Modern imaging techniques may allow guided aspiration. Antibiotics are indicated if the abscess is not localised, i.e. there is evidence of cellulitis. Healing by secondary intention is encouraged.

Cellulitis

8. A, B, C, E

Spreading infection presenting in surgical practice is typically caused by organisms such as beta-haemolytic *Streptococcus*, *Staphylococcus* and *C. perfringens*. Tissue destruction, gangrene and ulceration may follow, which are caused by release of proteases. Systemic signs – SIRS, chills, fever and rigors, are common. Blood cultures are often negative.

Systemic inflammatory response syndrome (SIRS)

9. A, B, C, D, E

Sepsis is defined as the systemic manifestation of SIRS with a documented infection. The other components of SIRS are hyperthermia (>38°C), WCC > 12 × 1000/dL.

Severe sepsis (sepsis syndrome)

10. A, C, D, E

Severe sepsis or sepsis syndrome is sepsis with evidence of one or more organ failures.

Clostridial wound infections

11. B, C, D

Clostridia are anaerobic, terminal, spore bearing, Gram-positive bacteria. The spores are widespread in soil and manure. The signs and symptoms are mediated by the release of the exotoxin tetanospasmin, which affects the myoneural junctions and the motor neurons of the anterior horn cells. Prophylaxis with tetanus toxoid is the best preventive treatment, but, in an established infection, minor debridement of the wound may be needed along with antibiotic treatment with benzylpenicillin. The use of antitoxin using human immunoglobulin ought to be considered for both at-risk wounds and established infection.

➜ Treatment of surgical infections

12. B

The choice of antibiotics may need to be empirical initially as it is illogical to withhold antibiotics until the organisms and their sensitivities are known. If an infected wound is under tension, or there is clear evidence of suppuration, sutures or clips need to be removed, with curettage if necessary, to allow pus to drain adequately. In severely contaminated wounds, it is logical to leave the wound open. Polymeric films are used as incision drapes and also to cover sutured wounds but are not indicated for use in wound infections. The use of topical antibiotics should be avoided because of the risks of allergy and resistance.

➜ Prophylactic antibiotics

13. A, B, D, E

When using antibiotics for prophylaxis, ideally, maximum blood and tissue levels should be present at the time at which the first incision is made and before contamination occurs. Intravenous administration at induction of anaesthesia is optimal.

14. A, B, D, E

➜ Surgical wound infection

15. A, C, E

A short preoperative hospital stay lowers the risk of acquiring MRSA and acquisitions of HAI. Medical staff should always wash hands between patients. Preoperative shaving should be avoided except for aesthetic reasons or to prevent adherence of dressings. If it is to be undertaken, shaving should be done immediately before surgery as the SSI rate after clean wound surgery may be doubled if it is performed the night before, because minor skin injury enhances superficial wound colonisation.

➜ Different types of wounds

16. A, C, E

Wounds are classified into clean (no viscus opened), clean-contaminated (viscus opened, minimal spillage), contaminated (open viscus with spillage or inflammatory disease) and dirty (pus or perforation or incision through an abscess). There is undisputed evidence that prophylactic antibiotics are effective in clean-contaminated and contaminated operations. The infection rates in a contaminated and dirty wound are 15–20 and <40 per cent, respectively. A dirty wound is already associated with infection and hence prophylaxis is not the issue.

➜ Infection causing bacteria

17. B, C, E

Beta-haemolytic *Streptococcus* resides in the pharynx of 5–10 per cent of the population. Staphylococcal epidermidis was regarded as a commensal but is now recognised as a major threat in prosthetic (vascular and orthopaedic) surgery and in indwelling vascular catheters.

Principles of antimicrobial treatment

18. E

Antibiotics are needed to treat SSIs if there is evidence of spreading infection, bacteraemia or systemic complications (SIRS or MODS). Antibiotics should not be held back if indicated, the choice being empirical, and later modified depending on the microbiological findings. Antibiotics do not replace surgical drainage of infection. The appropriate treatment of localised SSIs is interventional radiological drainage or open drainage and debridement.

A narrow-spectrum antibiotic may be used to treat a known infection, e.g. MRSA. A broad-spectrum antibiotic can be used when the organism is not known or when it is suspected that several bacteria, acting in synergy, may be responsible for the infection.

Antibiotics in surgical infections

19. B, C, E

Penicillins and aminoglycosides are bactericidal, whilst tetracycline and erythromycin are bacteriostatic. Serum levels immediately before and 1 h after intramuscular administration must be taken 48 h after the start of aminoglycoside therapy.

AIDS

20. A, D, E

The HIV virus is a retrovirus that has become increasingly prevalent through sexual transmission, IV drug addiction and infected blood. After exposure, the virus binds to CD4 receptors. There is a subsequent loss of CD4+ cells, T-helper cells and other cells involved in cell-mediated immunity, antibody production and delayed hypersensitivity. Macrophages and GALT are also affected. In the early weeks of infection there may be a flu-like illness and the patients present the greatest risk of transmission during the phase of seroconversion.

Answers: Extended matching questions

1. Prophylactic antibiotics regimen

1D, 2B, 3A, 4C

2. Bacteria involved in surgical infection

1D, 2F, 3G, 4A, 5E, 6C, 7B

3. Specific infections

1C, 2F, 3G, 4A, 5B, 6D, 7E

4. Different types of operations and infection rates

1D, 2A, 3B, 4A, 5C, 6C, 7D, 8B

5 Tropical surgery

Multiple choice questions

➜ Ascariasis

1. **Which of the following are caused by *Ascaris lumbricoides*?**
A Intestinal symptoms as a larva
B Pulmonary symptoms as a larva
C Intestinal symptoms as an adult worm
D Pulmonary symptoms primarily as an adult worm
E Biliary disease as a larva.

2. **What percentage of the world's population is affected by roundworms (*Ascaris lumbricoides*)?**
A 2 per cent
B 10 per cent
C 25 per cent
D 50 per cent
E 75 per cent.

3. **How is roundworm disease transmitted?**
A Inadvertent ingestion of the larva in soil
B Inadvertent ingestion of the fertilised egg in soil
C The larva penetrates unbroken skin
D Inadvertent ingestion of fertilised eggs in contaminated meat
E The larva is transmitted to the lung as a droplet infection.

4. **Which of the following are true of the life cycle of the *Ascaris lumbricoides*?**
A Eggs release larva in the lumen of the intestine which then develop into adult worms.
B Eggs release larva into the portal blood and thereafter into the liver and then the lungs.
C Eggs penetrate the intestinal wall and travel to the liver where they develop into adult worms and are released into the intestinal lumen via the biliary tract.
D The larvae are released in the lungs. The developing larvae are swallowed in sputum and complete their maturation in the intestine.
E Eggs are released into the environment in stool as cysts which survive.

5. **How is Loeffler's syndrome characterised?**
A Chest pain with productive cough the presence of friction rub and a chest X-ray showing pleural effusion
B Retrosternal burning, discomfort on ingestion of food, fever and mediastinal widening on chest X-ray
C Epigastric pain radiating to the right, a tender palpable liver and an elevated right dome of the diaphragm
D Chest pain, dry cough, dyspnoea and fever with fluffy exudates on chest X-ray.

6. **Which of the following are caused by roundworm infestation?**
A Malnutrition and failure to thrive
B Mechanical obstruction of the intestine
C Perforation of the intestine
D Ascending cholangitis, obstructive jaundice and acute pancreatitis
E Chest symptoms
F All of the above.

7. **Which of the following may be found in roundworm infestations?**
A A high eosinophil count
B Charcot–Leyden crystals in stool
C Larvae in sputum or bronchoscopic lavage
D Fluffy exudates on chest X-rays
E Barium meal may show the worm lying freely in the lumen.

8. Which of the following are valid for the treatment of a diagnosed uncomplicated roundworm intestinal obstruction?

A Urgent laparotomy

B Nasogastric suction, intravenous (IV) saline and hypertonic saline enemas

C Kneading a worm bolus into the large intestine at laparotomy, to be subsequently treated with hypertonic saline enemas

D Gastrojejunostomy

E A long-standing small intestinal perforation may require exteriorisation in the presence of a heavy worm load.

9. A patient presents with sudden severe upper abdominal pain with chills and rigors. He has icterus and is diffusedly tender over the right upper abdomen. His blood tests shows that he has an elevated white cell count (WCC) with high polymorphs and an obstructive jaundice. The ultrasound scan (Fig. 5.1) shows stones in the gall bladder and a linear shadow in a dilated common bile duct (CBD). The magnetic resonance cholangiopancreatography (MRCP) shows a linear shadow in the CBD which in real time is found to change its position. Which of the following statements are true?

A The most likely diagnosis is a line of stones in the CBD.

B The condition is likely to be due to a live worm in the CBD.

C The condition should be treated with pyrantel palmoate, an anthelmintic which kills worms by causing tetanic convulsion.

D The condition should be treated with albendazole.

E Following an anthelmintic, the condition may be treated by endoscopic removal of the roundworm followed by cholecystectomy.

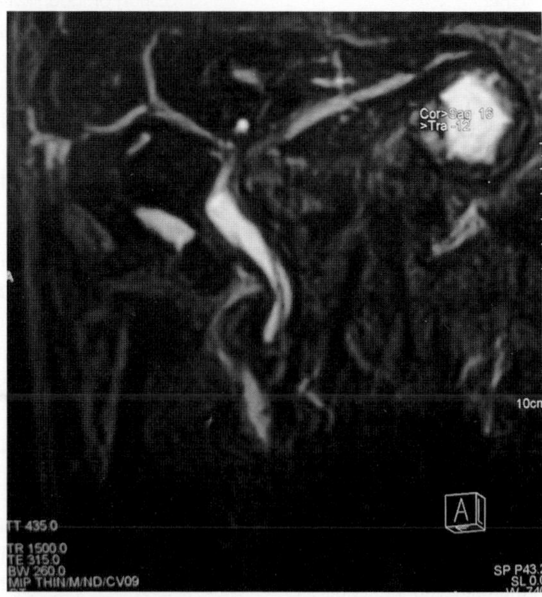

Figure 5.1 Stones in the gall bladder and a linear shadow in a dilated common bile duct.

Hydatid disease

10. Which of the following are true with regard to hydatid disease caused by *Echinococcus granulosus*?

A Man is the definitive host.

B Dogs are the definitive host.

C Sheep and cattle are intermediate hosts.

D The disease causes cystic lesions mainly in the liver but may affect any organ.

E The disease causes an infiltration of the liver without any definite margin.

11. How is hydatid disease transmitted?

A By eating infected meat and it therefore affects only non-vegetarians
B By the faeco-oral route through ingestion of eggs
C Through penetration of the skin of unshod feet by larvae
D It may be vector-borne
E It spreads by droplet infection.

12. Which of the following statements regarding cystic hydatid disease are true?

A It contains an outer pericyst made up of spreading living parasites.
B It contains an intermediate ectocyst which is non-infective.
C It contains an inner endocyst which has a germinal membrane containing viable parasites.
D The germinal envelope may give rise to daughter cysts.
E It spreads to the liver by travelling along the intestinal lymphatics.

13. Which of the following features may hydatid disease present with?

A Chest symptoms of a dry cough with fluffy exudates called Loeffler's syndrome
B A dull aching pain in the upper right abdomen
C Abdominal pain, anaphylactic shock and collapse after trivial trauma
D Patients often complain of passing live worms in stool
E Features of obstructive jaundice.

14. Which ultrasound scan features characterise a hepatic hydatid cyst?

A A cyst with multiple septations
B A cyst wall with shaggy and irregular outlines
C A cyst wall with calcifications
D A solid lesion with a surrounding rim of oedema
E A cyst with split walls.

15. A young girl was dancing in school and felt a dull pain in the abdomen. In the evening the mother noticed a diffuse skin rash and started her on a course of antihistamines to which she responded and the pain reduced in intensity. A week later she underwent an ultrasound scan, which showed a cystic lesion with a split wall. Blood tests showed a high eosinophil count and a CT scan is shown (Fig. 5.2). Which of the following are true of this clinical scenario?

A The feature is compatible with a ruptured simple cyst of the liver.
B The feature suggests a ruptured hydatid cyst.
C Treatment is with masterly inactivity.
D Treatment is with exploratory laparotomy under cover of albendazole.
E Anaphylaxis can occur during laparotomy.

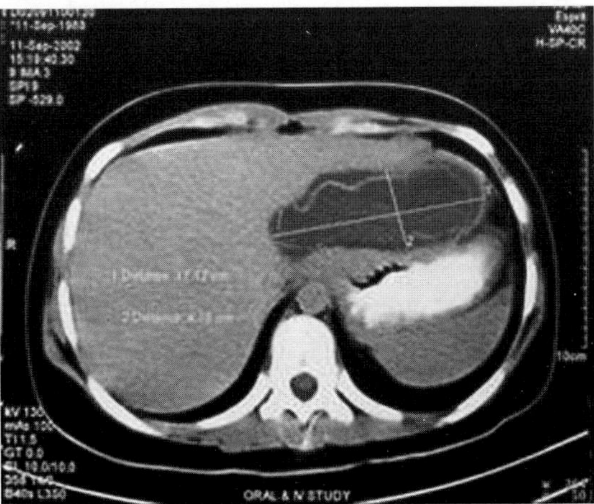

Figure 5.2 CT scan of schoolgirl with a dull pain in her abdomen.

16. A young woman presents with pain in her upper abdomen with chills and rigors followed by high-coloured urine. She is jaundiced and tender over the upper abdomen. An ultrasound scan (Fig. 5.3) shows gall bladder calculi, a dilated CBD with echogenic material and a septated cyst in the left lobe of the liver. A CT scan shows a septated cyst of the left lobe of the liver (Fig. 5.4). At endoscopic retrograde cholangiopancreatography (ERCP), multiple membranous structures were delivered after sphincterotomy. Which of the following are true of this condition?

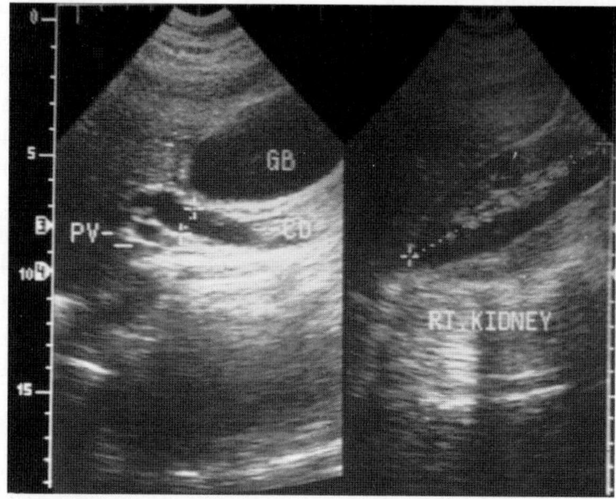

Figure 5.3 Ultrasound showing gall bladder calculi, a dilated common bile duct with echogenic material and a septated cyst in the left lobe of the liver.

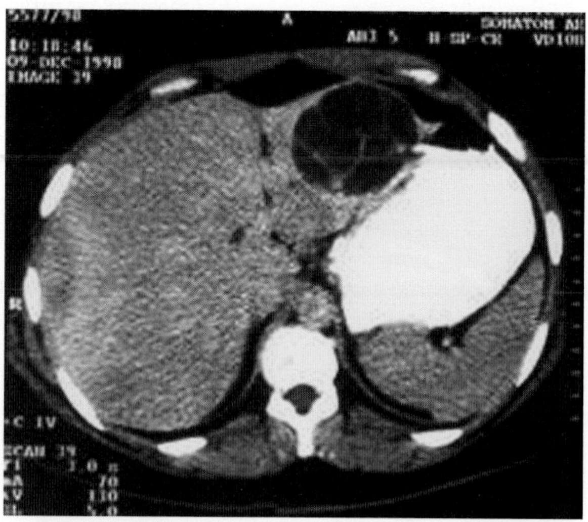

Figure 5.4 CT scan showing a septated cyst of the left lobe of the liver.

A The likely diagnosis is cholecystitis and choledocholithiasis with an incidental liver cyst.
B The likely diagnosis is a multiseptated hydatid cyst with biliary communication, causing daughter cysts in the CBD and gall bladder calculi, due to hydatid sand.
C Treatment following endoscopic clearance of the CBD should only require a cholecystectomy.
D Treatment following endoscopic clearance of the CBD should be with a cholecystectomy followed by injection of sclerosants into the cyst.
E Treatment of the cyst by injection of scolicidal solutions has a risk of causing sclerosing cholangitis because of the presence of biliary communications.

17. Which of the following statements are true of hydatid cysts?
A Anaphylactic shock is commoner in the treatment of unilocular hydatid cyst than in the treatment of multiloculated cysts.
B Sclerosing cholangitis is more common following injection of scolicidal solutions into multiloculated hydatid cysts.
C Small deep cysts which show calcification in their walls may be watched and treated with albendazole.
D Surgical curettage of the cyst wall is mandatory.
E Rupture of a cyst may cause dissemination of the disease.

→ Poliomyelitis

18. Which of the following are true of poliomyelitis?
A It is an enteroviral infection that spreads by inhalation or ingestion.
B It is a rotavirus that spreads by the faeco-oral route.
C It targets the anterior horn cells of the spinal cord.
D It causes sensory loss which spreads cranially.
E It causes a lower motor neuron type of flaccid paralysis.

→ Tuberculosis of the small intestine

19. Which of the following types of infection may be caused by intestinal infection with *Mycobacterium tuberculosis*?
A Transverse ulcers with undermined edges in the ileum
B Tubercles on the serosal aspect of the intestine
C Apple-core lesions of the colon
D Hyperplasia and thickening of the terminal ileum
E Transmural inflammation with a propensity for fistula formation.

20. What presenting features do patients with tuberculosis of the small intestine show?
A Weight loss, vague abdominal pain and evening rise of temperature
B A doughy feel of the abdomen from area of localised ascites
C A mass in the right iliac fossa
D A watering-can perineum with undermined edges and a watery discharge
E Characteristically, a non-caseating granuloma on histology.

21. A 24-year-old female from a poor socioeconomic background in a developing country presents with repeated attacks of abdominal pain with abdominal distension. A barium meal X-ray is carried out (Fig. 5.5). Which of the following should make you consider a diagnosis of tuberculosis?
A Residence in a developing country from a poor socioeconomic background
B Presence of active tuberculosis of the lungs
C Skip lesions of the intestine
D The barium meal X-ray shows a narrowing of the terminal ileum with a normally placed caecum
E The barium meal X-ray shows a narrowing of the terminal ileum with a pulled up subhepatic caecum.

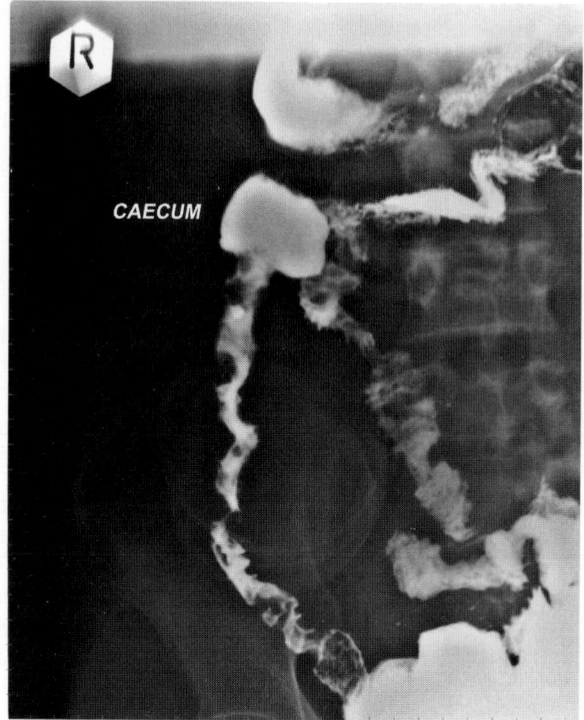

Figure 5.5 Barium meal X-ray in a 24-year-old female who presents with repeated attacks of abdominal pain with abdominal distension.

22. Surgery for ileal and ileocaecal tuberculosis may involve:

A Stricturoplasty
B Limited ileocolic resection
C Right hemicolectomy
D Ileo-transverse anastomosis
E All of the above.

23. Which of the following are true in tuberculous perforation?

A Free gas under the diaphragm is always present.
B It is treated by resuscitation followed by resection of the affected segment.
C It may be treated by resuscitation, followed by stricturoplasty through the perforation.
D It may be treated by resection and exteriorisation as a first step, followed by restoration of bowel continuity after completion of antituberculous chemotherapy.
E It should always be treated conservatively.

→ Amoebiasis

24. Which of the following are true of amoebiasis?

A The disease is common in the Indian subcontinent, Africa and parts of Central and South America.
B The majority produce symptoms of some kind.
C Amoebic liver abscess, the commonest extraintestinal manifestation, occurs in more than 50 per cent of people affected.
D The mode of infection is via the faeco-oral route, the disease occurring where there is a breakdown of standards of hygiene or sanitation
E The organism enters the gut via contaminated food and water.

25. *Entamoeba histolytica*, the causative organism behind amoebiasis, enters the body as cysts contaminating water or food. Which of the following occurs?

A The cysts hatch in the large bowel and colonise the colon.
B The cysts cause flask-shaped ulcers in the colon.
C The trophozoites may invade the wall of the colon and pass to the liver via the portal circulation, causing focal infarction and liquefactive necrosis in the liver.
D Cysts may form which are passed in the faeces as an infective form.
E The right lobe of the liver is affected in 10 per cent of cases, the left in 80 per cent and the rest are multiple.

26. An alcoholic, middle-aged man presents with pain in the upper right abdomen. He has had fever, night sweats, anorexia, malaise, cough and weight loss. He is found to be toxic, anaemic and mildly jaundiced. He has a tender hepatomegaly with tenderness over the right lower intercostal spaces. An ultrasound scan had shown a hypoechoic lesion in the right lobe of the liver and his CT scan is shown (Fig. 5.6). Which of the following statements are true?

A While the clinical features are all suggestive of amoebiasis, travel to an endemic area and a history of bloody diarrhoea may also have been given.
B The CT scan is compatible with an amoebic liver abscess.
C The abscess cavity contains blackcurrant jelly-like fluid.
D The collection is normally odourless and sterile but becomes smelly if secondarily infected.
E Trophozoites may be found in the wall of the abscess cavity in a minority of cases.

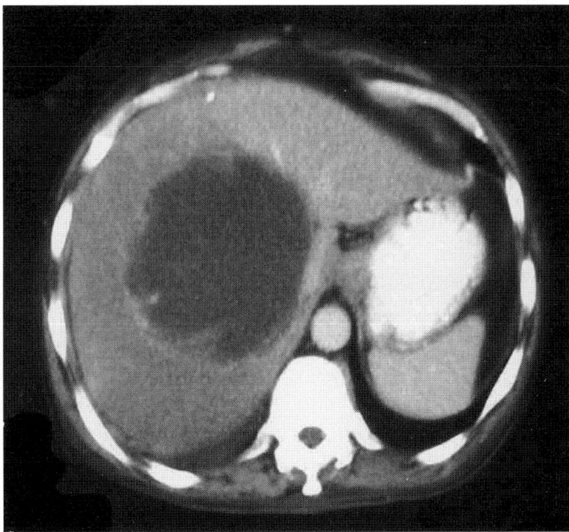

Figure 5.6 CT scan of an alcoholic, middle-aged man with pain in the upper right abdomen.

27. Which of the following are presenting features of amoebiasis?

A Chronic diarrhoea, often bloodstained, with colicky abdominal pain
B Pain in the upper right abdomen with right shoulder-tip pain, hiccoughs and a painful dry cough
C An apple-core lesion on barium enema due to the formation of a chronic granuloma. This is most commonly seen in the caecum
D Features of peritonitis with shock
E All of the above.

28. What is the treatment for an amoebic abscess?

A Urgent laparotomy upon diagnosis
B Medical treatment with metronidazole or tinidazole
C Medical treatment with diloxanide furoate is sufficient

D Aspiration may be carried out for abscesses which present with features of imminent rupture

E Surgical treatment for amoebiasis is indicated for a ruptured liver abscess, for patients with severe haemorrhage and toxic megacolon and for a suspected amoeboma, which is not responding to treatment or where carcinoma cannot be excluded.

➜ Asiatic cholangiohepatitis

29. Asiatic cholangiohepatitis, also called 'Oriental cholangiohepatitis', results from infestation of the hepatobiliary system by *Clonorchis sinensis*, a liver fluke. Which of the following pertain to the disease?

A The disease occurs in humans, who act as the intermediate host, by the ingestion of infected fish and snails, who are the definitive host.

B The parasite matures into an adult worm in the intrahepatic biliary channel, causing epithelial hyperplasia and periductal fibrosis.

C The eggs or dead worms may form the nidus for stone formation in the biliary system.

D Changes around the intrahepatic biliary channels often cause dysplasia, which may lead to cholangiocarcinoma.

E Ultrasound scan characteristically shows uniform dilatation of small peripheral intrahepatic ducts with only minimal dilatation of the common duct system.

30. What is the treatment of Asiatic cholangitis?

A Praziquantel and albendazole are the drugs of choice.

B Cholecystectomy, exploration of the bile duct and choledochoduodenostomy may be done.

C A Roux-en-Y choledochojejunostomy with or without an access loop may be performed.

D The disease should ideally be diagnosed and treated in its subclinical form.

E All of the above.

➜ Filariasis

31. Which of the following statements about filariasis are true?

A It is mainly caused by the parasite *Brugia malayi* and *Brugia timori*. In some 10 per cent of sufferers, the parasite *Wuchereria bancrofti* also causes the disease.

B Once inoculated by a mosquito bite, the matured eggs enter the circulation to hatch and grow into adult worms.

C The adult worms cause lymphatic blockage, resulting in massive limb oedema. This is often compounded by streptococcal secondary infection, leading to additional fibrosis of the lymphatic channels and further leading to elephantiasis.

D Chyluria and chylous ascites seen in cancers blocking lymphatics are never seen in filariasis.

E A mild form of the disease which affects the respiratory tract and presents with dry cough is called tropical pulmonary eosinophilia.

32. Which of the following statements about filariasis are true?

A Blood tests often reveal an elevated lymphocyte count.

B Immature worms can be seen in nocturnal peripheral blood smear.

C Medical treatment with diethylcarbamazepine is effective even when huge elephantiasis occurs.

D Hydroceles are treated in the usual way but excess skin may need trimming.

E Elephantiasis can be easily treated with operations to reduce the size of the limb.

➜ Leprosy

33. A 33-year-old female comes to the outpatients department of a hospital with the following facial features: loss of eyebrows, collapse of the nasal bridge and lifting of the tip of the nose, paralysis of the left orbicularis oculi causing exposure keratitis and

blindness (Fig. 5.7). A diagnosis of leprosy is made. Which of the following features are relevant to the disease?**

A The disease is caused by the acid-fast bacillus, *Mycobacterium tuberculosis*.

B The disease is transmitted by sexual contact.

C The disease is broadly classified into two groups, lepromatous and tuberculoid, depending on the immune response of the patient to the disease.

D The disease is slowly progressive and affects the skin, upper respiratory tract and peripheral nerves.

E The deformities produced are divided into primary, which are caused by leprosy or its reactions, and secondary, resulting from effects such as anaesthesia of the hands and feet.

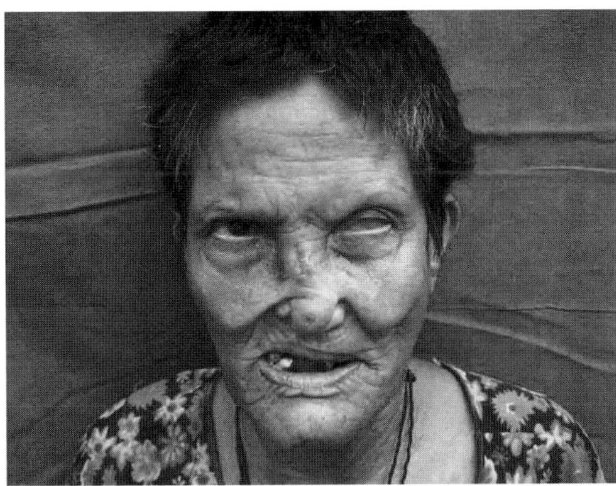

Figure 5.7 A 33-year-old woman presenting with leprosy.

34. Which of the following statements about leprosy (also called Hansen's disease) are true?

A Patients have neural involvement characterised by thickening of the nerves, which are tender.

B Patients may present with 'leprids', which are asymmetrical, well-defined, anaesthetic, hypopigmented or erythematous macules with elevated edges and a dry rough surface.

C There are often nodular lesions on the patient's face in the acute phase of the lepromatous variety. The characteristic facies thus produced is known as 'leonine facies' (looking like a lion).

D The condition is diagnosed by demonstrating the bacilli in urine.

E The patient is treated by a multidisciplinary team of infection disease specialist, plastic surgeon, ophthalmologist, hand and orthopaedic surgeon.

→ Tropical chronic pancreatitis

35. Tropical chronic pancreatitis is a disease which affects the younger generation from poor socioeconomic strata in developing countries. Which of the following statements about the condition are true?

A It is caused by ingestion of cassava (tapioca), a root vegetable, which contains derivatives of cyanide. The concurrent absence of sulphur-containing amino acid in the diet prevents the cyanide from being detoxified in the liver, leading to cyanogen toxicity and the disease.

B It is caused by alcoholism.

C Patients present with extensive pancreatic periductal fibrosis, intraductal calcium carbonate stones and type I diabetes mellitus.

D Patients show pancreatic calcification in the form of discrete stones on straight abdominal X-ray. Ultrasound and CT scanning of the pancreas confirm the disease.

E Patients need medical support for exocrine and endocrine pancreatic insufficiency and treatment for pain. Some require surgery.

Typhoid

36. Typhoid fever is caused by *Salmonella typhi*, which is a Gram-negative bacillus. Which of the following are true of the disease?

A The bacteria enter the body through infected blood or contaminated needles.

B The organism colonises the Peter's patches in the terminal ileum, initially causing hyperplasia and later necrosis and ulceration.

C If left untreated or inadequately treated, the ulcers may bleed or perforate.

D A typical patient may present with high fever for 2–3 weeks after a visit to an endemic area, with abdominal distension due to paralytic ileus.

E Patients may present as an emergency due to melaena and hypovolaemia or with features of peritonitis and shock.

37. How is typhoid diagnosed?

A It is diagnosed by positive blood and stool cultures.

B The Widal test is often carried out in the Indian subcontinent, although it has become obsolete in the UK. The test looks for the presence of bacteria in red blood cells.

C In the scenario of inadequately carried out treatment, where blood cultures are often negative, special kits may be used, such as Multi-Test Dip-S-Ticks to detect immunoglobulin G, Tubex to detect immunoglobulin M and TyphiDot to detect both IgG and IgM.

D In the second or third week, any patient who shows signs of deterioration accompanied by abdominal pain should be considered to have a perforation unless proved otherwise.

E Abdominal distension in typhoid disease in the second or third week of the fever should be treated by high-bowel washout to get rid of the toxins.

38. What is the treatment for typhoid perforation?

A Treatment involves vigorous resuscitation with IV fluids and antibiotics in an intensive care unit.

B Chloramphenicol is the drug of choice.

C Several surgical options can be carried out, depending on the condition of the patient, the site and number of perforations and the amount of peritoneal soiling.

D The skin and subcutaneous tissue are often kept open for delayed closure, as wound infection inevitably happens, leading to wound dehiscence.

E Perforation occurring in the first week of typhoid fever has a better prognosis as the patient's nutritional and immunological status is better.

Extended matching questions

1. Upper abdominal pain

A Amoebiasis

B Typhoid fever

C Lobar pneumonia

D Tropical chronic pancreatitis

E Myocardial infarction

Choose and match the correct diagnosis with each of the scenarios below:

1 A 35-year-old male patient resident of southern India presents with complaints of episodic severe upper abdominal pain radiating to the back for the last 5 months. He has also noticed

increased thirst with polyuria and passage of bulky pale stools. He consumes tapioca as a staple diet. On examination, the abdomen is unremarkable with no palpable abnormality. His fasting blood sugar level is 180 mg/dL and plain X-ray of the abdomen shows linear calcification in the upper abdomen extending across the spine.

2 A 45-year-old male patient presents with anorexia, gradually increasing pain in the upper abdomen associated with high-grade fever with night sweats and general malaise for the last 5 days. The pain has been constant and mainly in the right upper abdomen since the previous day and is aggravated with movement and coughing. He gives a history of having suffered from bloody diarrhoea about 3–4 weeks previously. On examination there is tender hepatomegaly 5 cm below the costal margin in the right midclavicular line, and there is intercostal tenderness in the right 5th, 6th and 7th spaces. The liver span is increased to 20 cm on percussion.

3 A 50-year-old male with a history of heavy smoking complains of feeling unwell for a week. He reports cough productive of yellow-coloured sputum, shortness of breath, pain over the left upper abdomen and high-grade fever. The examination reveals a respiratory rate of 18/min, with the presence of bronchial breathing over the left lower zone and a crunching sound with each respiration. The abdomen is normal on examination.

4 A 25-year-old female gives a history of high-grade fever with chills for the last 2 weeks, and diarrhoea for the last 10 days. She is a resident of a working women's hostel and complains that several of her colleagues have also been unwell. She also complains of a dragging pain in the upper left abdomen that gets relieved on taking rest. On examination, she is dehydrated and febrile. Abdominal examination reveals the presence of a firm splenomegaly almost reaching the umbilicus.

5 A 55-year-old male presents with complaints of pain in the upper central abdomen for the last 3 hours, associated with heaviness in the left side of the chest and shortness of breath. There is also associated sweating and a feeling of weakness. The patient has been a smoker for 20 years and has a history of occasional heaviness along the inner side of the left arm. On examination, the pulse rate is 80/min and regular, and blood pressure (BP) is 110/60 mmHg. Abdomen is soft on palpation and there is no tenderness. Respiratory examination reveals the presence of normal breath sounds.

→ 2. Lump in the abdomen

A Amoebic liver abscess
B Acute typhoid fever
C Hyperplastic ileocaecal tuberculosis
D Hydatidosis
E Acute cholecystitis

Choose and match the correct diagnosis with each of the scenarios below:

1 A 45-year-old sheep farmer complains of a gradually enlarging painful mass in the right upper abdomen over the last 3 months. He is otherwise healthy. Physical examination reveals firm enlargement of the liver which is somewhat tender on palpation. There is no other significant finding in the abdominal examination. A blood count reveals a total leucocyte count (TLC) of 8600 with a differential leucocyte count (DLC) showing eosinophils constituting 12 per cent.

2 A 51-year-old male patient, residing in Bangladesh, presents with anorexia, gradually increasing pain in the right upper abdomen associated with high-grade fever, with night sweats and general malaise for the last 5 days. He has also noticed the presence of a swelling in the upper abdomen, which is tender to touch. The pain is aggravated with movement and coughing.

On examination there is tender hepatomegaly 5 cm below the costal margin in the right midclavicular line, and there is intercostal tenderness in the right 5th, 6th and 7th spaces. The liver span is increased to 20 cm on percussion.

3 A 45-year-old female complains of pain in the right upper abdomen since the previous night, which is severe in intensity and only partially relieved on taking analgesics. The pain is also radiating to the back on the right side and is associated with nausea and vomiting. She gives a history of intolerance to fatty foods in the past, associated with slight discomfort in the right upper abdomen. On examination there is tenderness on palpation at the tip of the ninth costal cartilage in the midclavicular line on the right side, and a lump is palpable in the same region. The rest of the abdomen is normal.

4 A 25-year-old female gives a history of a high-grade fever with chills for the past 2 weeks, and diarrhoea over the past 10 days. She is a resident of a working women's hostel and complains that several of her colleagues have also been unwell. She also complains of a dragging sensation in the upper left abdomen that is relieved by rest. On examination, she is dehydrated and febrile. Abdominal examination reveals the presence of a firm splenomegaly, almost reaching the umbilicus.

5 A 19-year-old female patient presents with a history of off-and-on colicky central abdominal pain for the past 6 months. There is a history of diarrhoea alternating with constipation over this period. She has also had irregular menstruation over the past 4–5 months. Her father died 2 years previously of a prolonged respiratory ailment. On examination, the patient is pale, and the abdomen has a slight fullness in the right iliac fossa, and on palpation, a firm lump is palpable in the same region that is tender. A barium meal follow-through reveals string sign of terminal ileum.

→ 3. Vomiting

A Subacute intestinal obstruction – Koch's
B Ascariasis
C Typhoid enteritis
D Gastric outlet obstruction – chronic duodenal ulcer

Choose and match the correct diagnosis with each of the scenarios below:

1 A 40-year-old male smoker presents with history of projectile non-bilious vomiting for the past week. The vomitus contains residue of food items eaten previously and is foul-smelling. The vomiting is associated with bouts of severe upper abdominal colicky pain that are relieved after vomiting. He gives history of episodes of upper abdominal gnawing pain in the past. On examination, the patient is dehydrated and has a pulse rate of 100/min and a BP of 100/60 mmHg. There is distension in the epigastrium and umbilical regions with presence of a succussion splash on auscultation.

2 A 25-year-old male patient, residing in Sri Lanka, presents with history of off-and-on colicky central abdominal pain over the past 12 months, associated with weight loss that is not documented. There is a history of diarrhoea alternating with constipation during this period. Over the last 2 weeks there has been a history of projectile bilious vomiting associated with a bout of colic. On examination, the patient is pale and dehydrated, and the abdomen has central fullness with visible bowel loops. The bowel sounds are markedly diminished and there is no clinically evident free fluid in the abdomen. An erect X-ray of the abdomen reveals the presence of central abdominal air fluid levels.

3 A 17-year-old boy gives a history of high-grade fever with chills for the past 2 weeks, and diarrhoea for the past 10 days. In the last 2 days the colour of the stools has become darker,

and on two occasions there was frank blood in the stools. He studies in a boarding school and complains that several of his friends have been suffering from fever and diarrhoea in the last few weeks. On examination, he is dehydrated and febrile. Abdominal examination reveals the presence of a palpable spleen just below the costal margin. There is associated central abdominal tenderness.

4 A 13-year-old boy is brought to the hospital by his mother with complaints of failure to thrive. The boy's height is much less than that of his classmates. There is also a history of episodes of colicky abdominal pain that are relieved on their own. On examination, the boy is found to be pale and underweight for his age. The abdominal examination is normal. His haemoglobin (Hb) is 10.2 g/dL and there are 10 per cent eosinophils in differential count.

→ 4. Abdominal distension

A Acute intestinal obstruction
B Multiple hydatidosis
C Ascariasis
D Paralytic ileus
E Adhesive intestinal obstruction

Choose and match the correct diagnosis with each of the scenarios below:

1 A 30-year-old man had an extensive retroperitoneal lymph node dissection for testicular malignancy 2 days previously. The house surgeon, after having seen the patient in the ward, is worried as the abdomen seems to be full, with no bowel sounds. Abdominal X-rays show the presence of multiple air-fluid levels all over the length of the small bowel and the serum electrolyte levels are within normal limits.

2 A 45-year-old owner of a dog-breeding farm complains of a gradual abdominal distension over the last 6 months that has become painful of late. He is otherwise healthy and has no bowel complaints. Physical examination reveals firm distension of the abdomen which is somewhat tender on palpation and dull on percussion. There is no other significant finding in the abdominal examination. A blood count reveals a TLC of 8600 with a DLC showing eosinophils constituting 12 per cent. An abdominal ultrasound (US) shows the presence of multiple fluid-filled structures spread all over the abdominal viscera.

3 A 35-year-old man presents with severe central abdominal colicky pain for the past 8 hours. It is associated with vomiting and abdominal distension. He has also not moved his bowels since the onset of pain. He underwent an appendicectomy as a child. On examination the abdomen has central distension that is resonant on percussion. The abdomen is tense but non-tender. The bowel sounds are exaggerated and high-pitched. Abdominal X-rays show the presence of multiple air-fluid levels distributed mainly in the central abdomen.

4 A 10-year-old boy is brought to the hospital by his mother with complaints of a sudden onset of severe colicky abdominal pain associated with several episodes of vomiting. There is a history of failure to thrive and also of the passage of worms per rectum in the past. On examination, the boy is found to be pale and underweight for his age. The abdomen is distended with palpable bowel loops. The bowel sounds are exaggerated. His Hb is 10.2 g/dL and there are 12 per cent eosinophils in differential count.

→ 5. Acute abdomen

A Appendicular perforation
B Ruptured liver abscess
C Typhoid perforation

D Duodenal ulcer perforation
E Tubercular peritonitis

Choose and match the correct diagnosis with each of the scenarios below:

1 A 25-year-old female patient gives a history of high-grade fever with chills over the past 3 weeks, and diarrhoea 10 days previously, which lasted for about 1 week. She also gives a history of abdominal pain for the past 4–5 days that started in the lower abdomen and later became severe as well as generalized. On examination, she is severely dehydrated and febrile. Abdominal examination reveals a board-like rigidity with absent bowel sounds. There is free gas under the diaphragm on erect abdominal radiograph.

2 A 30-year-old male presents with history of sudden-onset severe abdominal pain that started in the upper abdomen and later became generalized. He has been a chronic smoker for 15 years and gives a history of episodes of upper abdominal gnawing pain in the past. On examination, the patient is dehydrated, has a pulse rate of 100/min and a BP of 100/60 mmHg. There is rigidity in the abdomen and rebound tenderness. An erect film of the abdomen reveals free gas under the diaphragm.

3 A 30-year-old female patient presents with a history of off-and-on colicky central abdominal pain for the past 10 months, associated with weight loss and amenorrhoea over the last 3 months. There is a history of diarrhoea alternating with constipation during this period. In the last week the pain has been continuous and is increasing in severity progressively. There is also a history of absolute constipation over the last 2 days. Her husband suffered from pulmonary tuberculosis in the recent past. On examination, the patient is pale and dehydrated, and the abdomen is distended with the absence of bowel sounds. There is rigidity all over the abdomen with the presence of free fluid. An erect X-ray of the abdomen reveals free gas under the diaphragm.

4 A 45-year-old male patient presents with anorexia, gradually increasing pain in the upper abdomen associated with high-grade fever, with night sweats and general malaise for the past 5 days. The pain suddenly worsened and became generalized over the last day. He gives a history of having suffered from diarrhoea about 3–4 weeks previously. On examination there is tender hepatomegaly 5 cm below the costal margin. The liver span is increased to 20 cm on percussion. There is evidence of free fluid in the peritoneal cavity. The abdominal X-rays are essentially normal.

5 A 20-year-old married female presents with pain in the right lower abdomen during the past 4–5 days that has, of late, become severe and generalized in the last 24 h. She says that the pain was better for a couple of days after she was started on some drugs by a private practitioner. There is associated vomiting, loose stools and high-grade fever in the last 2 days. The menstrual history is unremarkable. On examination, the patient is febrile, dehydrated and has tachycardia and tachypnoea. There is rigidity and tenderness all over the abdomen, more so in the lower abdomen. The bowel sounds are absent. Total counts are raised and abdominal X-rays are normal. Abdominal US reveals presence of free fluid in the abdomen.

➜ 6. Swollen leg

A Filariasis
B Deep vein thrombosis (DVT)
C Pelvic tumour – vein congestion
D Primary lymphoedema
E Cellulitis

Choose and match the correct diagnosis with each of the scenarios below:

1 A 60-year-old postmenopausal woman complains of vague discomfort in the lower abdomen over the last 3 months, associated with occasional instances of spotting per vaginum. She has also noticed heaviness and swelling of the left lower limb over the last 2 months. There is no history of fever or any trauma to the limb. On examination, there is a firm to hard mass in the left lower abdomen, the lower limit of which cannot be reached. The rest of the abdomen is unremarkable. The left lower limb is swollen and shows the presence of pitting oedema extending from the thigh down to the foot.

2 A 40-year-old male resident of Bihar, India, complains of progressive swelling of his right leg over the last 6 months. He has also been having episodes of high-grade fever over the last 4 months, during which the leg becomes red and painful, and the swelling also increases. On examination, the girth of the affected limb is found to be increased and the skin is very thick and rough. The swelling of the limb does not pit with pressure. Blood examination reveals the presence of marked eosinophilia.

3 A 70-year-old female with a history of recent surgery for fractured neck of femur complains of pain associated with swelling in the opposite leg for 2 days. She has been on bed rest for the past 2 weeks. On examination, the local temperature of the limb is raised and the swelling is involving mainly the calf region. The pain is aggravated by passive dorsiflexion of the foot as well as compression of the thigh.

4 A 13-year-old girl is brought by her mother with complaints of insidious onset of painless unilateral lower limb swelling of 1 year's duration that is progressive in its course. The girl attained menarche 1 year ago. There is no history of any fever or trauma. On examination, the swelling is non-pitting and is limited to the leg below the knee. The local temperature is not raised and the draining nodes are not enlarged.

5 A 45-year-old diabetic presents with history of a small prick on his right foot 1 week ago, following which he developed progressive swelling over the foot and leg associated with pain and fever. On examination, the limb is warm, erythematous, swollen and tender. All the peripheral pulses are palpable and are normal.

→ 7. Scrotal swelling

A Filariasis
B Congestive heart failure
C Hydrocele
D Hernia
E Varicocele

Choose and match the correct diagnosis with each of the scenarios below:

1 A 30-year-old male patient complains of swelling in the right side of his scrotum over the last 2 years, which has been progressively increasing in size. It is painless and there is no history of scrotal trauma. On examination, the swelling is limited to the scrotum, is transilluminant and the testis is not felt separately from it.

2 A 70-year-old male patient complains of progressively increasing swelling in his right scrotum over the past 10 years. The size of the swelling increases on straining and decreases on lying down. On examination, an inguinoscrotal swelling is seen to be present which is separate from the testis and reduces with a gurgle when manipulated by the patient.

3 A 55-year-old male resident of Bangladesh complains of progressive swelling of his lower limbs over the past 6 months. It is associated with painless enlargement of his scrotum over the past

3 months. He has also been having episodes of high-grade fever for 3–4 months. There is no history of trauma to the legs or scrotum. On examination, the girth of the affected limb is found to be increased and the skin is very thick and rough. The scrotal swelling is transilluminant, fluctuant and the testis cannot be palpated separate from it.

4 A 50-year-old male who is a known chronic obstructive pulmonary disease (COPD) patient complains of sudden onset of increased breathlessness and easy fatiguability over the past 2 weeks. It is associated with progressive distension of the abdomen over the past 2 weeks and swelling of bilateral scrotum in the last week. On examination, he has bilateral fine crepitations at the lung bases, the jugular venous pressure (JVP) is raised and he is dyspnoeic at rest. There is tender enlargement of the liver with free fluid in the peritoneal cavity. The scrotum is transilluminant and the swelling decreases on elevation of the scrotum.

5 A 23-year-old military recruit complains of a dragging sensation in left hemiscrotum over the past year. There is no history of trauma. He has been married for 2 years but has no children. On examination, the left scrotum is found to be lower than the right one. There is bag of worms feel to the cord and the testis is also smaller and flabby on the same side.

➜ 8. Claw hands

A Leprosy
B Ulnar nerve palsy
C Median nerve palsy
D Poliomyelitis
E Dupuytren's contracture

Choose and match the correct diagnosis with each of the scenarios below:

1 A 47-year-old woman is admitted to hospital for a major abdominal surgery. On discharge 2 weeks after the operation she complains to the operating surgeon that she has developed tingling and weakness affecting the ring and little fingers of her left hand. On examination there is some numbness and weakness of flexion in the medial two fingers. There is also mild flexion deformity affecting these two digits.

2 A 20-year-old male patient presents with a history of weakness and deformity of the lateral three digits of the right hand over the past month. A month previously he sustained a cut injury from window glass just above the wrist joint. There are no other complaints. On examination, there is hyperextension of metacarpophalangeal joints and flexion of the interphalangeal joints of the lateral three digits of the right hand. The thenar eminence seems to be flat and the power of the lateral three digits is decreased in flexion movements. There is also hypoasthaesia over the palmar aspect of lateral three digits.

3 A 40-year-old female resident of Myanmar (Burma) complains of progressive deformity affecting both her hands over the past 3–4 years. She also complains of numbness of the tips of her fingers and non-healing ulcers involving several of them. There is no history of any trauma. On examination, there is bilaterally symmetrical clawing of all the digits of both the hands with non-healing ulcers over the tips of several of the digits. There are multiple hypoaesthetic and anaesthetic areas involving both the forearms and hands. Incidentally, she is also found to have lost her eyebrows.

4 A 50-year-old male complains of progressive flexion deformity of the ring finger of his left hand over the past 3 months. He also had a painless enlargement of both the parotid glands 2 months previously. On examination there is fixed flexion deformity involving the metacarpophalangeal, proximal and distal interphalangeal joints of the ring finger of the

affected hand. The skin of the palm also appears to be thicker with subcutaneous nodules. The sensory and motor examinations are normal.

5 A 6-year-old boy is brought by the parents with the complaints of sudden-onset fever, with severe headache and weakness and deformities of both the upper limbs. He is a resident of a small village in Sri Lanka. On examination, the boy is malnourished, with no neck rigidity. There is weakness of the muscles of shoulders, elbows and wrist, more on the left side. There is also accompanying flattening of the thenar eminence with weakness of flexion of the fingers and apposition of the thumb. The sensory examination is normal.

→ 9. Limb deformity

A Filariasis
B Poliomyelitis
C Leprosy
D Psoas abscess

Choose and match the correct diagnosis with each of the scenarios below:

1 A 6-year-old boy is brought by his parents with the complaints of sudden-onset fever, with severe headache and weakness and deformity of the left lower limb. He lives in a remote village and has not been immunised. On examination, the boy is malnourished, with no neck rigidity. There is flaccid paralysis of the muscles of the left lower limb with flail knee, foot drop and talipes equines. The deep tendon reflexes are unelicitable. The sensory examination is normal.

2 A 40-year-old female resident of Myanmar (Burma) complains of progressive deformity affecting both her hands over the past 3–4 years. She also complains of numbness of the tips of her fingers and non-healing ulcers involving several of them. There is no history of any trauma. On examination, there is bilaterally symmetrical clawing of all the digits of both the hands with non-healing ulcers over the tips of several of the digits. There are multiple hypoaesthetic and anaesthetic areas involving both the forearms and hands. Incidentally she is also found to have lost her eyebrows.

3 A 40-year-old male resident of Bihar, India, complains of progressive swelling and deformity of his right leg over the past 6 months. He also has been having episodes of high-grade fever over the past 4 months, during which the leg swelling increases. On examination, the girth of the affected limb is found to be increased and the skin is very thick and rough. The swelling of the limb does not pit with pressure. The affected limb appears to be greatly deformed, but the bony structure on the X-ray is normal. Blood examination reveals the presence of marked eosinophilia.

4 A 30-year-old female presents complaining of an inability to straighten her left lower limb at the hip joint for the last 2 weeks. The deformity was preceded by a history of backache for 6–7 months for which she did not take any treatment. She also has history of low-grade evening fever over the past 4–5 months. On examination there is flexion deformity of the left hip joint with evidence of fullness in the abdomen over the left iliac fossa. There is also a gibbus deformity of the upper lumbar spine which is tender with fullness along the left paravertebral region.

→ 10. Paralysis

A Poliomyelitis
B Pott's spine
C Traumatic paraplegia
D Cerebrovascular accident
E Acute embolic limb ischaemia

Choose and match the correct diagnosis with each of the scenarios below:

1 A 30-year-old female presents with complaints of slowly progressive weakness of both her lower limbs over the past 2 months. This was preceded by a history of severe backache for 6–7 months for which she did not take any treatment. She also has a history of low-grade evening fever over the past 4–5 months. On examination there is a gibbus deformity of the lumbar spine which is tender with fullness along both paravertebral regions. There is bilateral sensorimotor loss below the level of L2–L3. An X-ray of the lumbar spine shows complete destruction of the L2 vertebra with loss of lumbar lordosis.

2 A 55-year-old male smoker is admitted with complaints of sudden-onset pain, numbness and inability to move his left leg and foot for half an hour. He is a known cardiac patient with history of myocardial infarction 6 months previously. On examination, the pulse is 60/min and BP is 130/90. The affected limb is cold, mottled and there is a loss of sensation below the knee. The motor power is also 1/5 in the affected part. In this limb only the femoral pulse is palpable and is bounding.

3 A 65-year-old smoker, who is a known hypertensive, is brought to the hospital with a history of sudden-onset slurring of speech and an inability to move his left upper and lower limbs over the past hour. There is no history of previous similar episodes and there is no history of trauma. On examination, the patient is conscious, BP is 210/160 and Glasgow Coma Score is 14/15. There is no neck rigidity. All the cranial nerves are normal and the motor power of the left-sided limbs is 3/5 compared with 5/5 on the right side. The sensory faculties are normal.

4 A 5-year-old girl is brought in by her father with complaints of sudden-onset fever, with severe headache and inability to move both the lower limbs over the past 2 weeks. She has not received any vaccines. On examination, the girl is malnourished, with no neck rigidity. There is flaccid paralysis of the muscles of bilateral hips, thighs and legs with bilateral foot drop. The deep tendon reflexes are unelicitable. The sensory examination is normal.

5 A 25-year-old male patient is brought with a history of sudden-onset loss of sensation and inability to move the lower half of his body and the lower limbs after falling on his back from a height the previous day. There is no history of loss of consciousness. He is able to move the upper half of his body normally. On examination, there is a step deformity at the junction of thoracolumbar spine. There is flaccid paralysis of all the muscles below the level of T12, and there is complete loss of all sensations below T10 level.

Answers: Multiple choice questions

→ Ascariasis

1. B, C

The life cycle of ascariasis is as follows. The ingested eggs release larva, which penetrate the intestinal wall and get carried via the bloodstream to the lungs. In the lung, the larvae penetrate to the bronchioles. This causes inflammation with a dry cough, chest pain and fluffy exudates on chest X-ray called Loeffler's syndrome. The larvae are swallowed in sputum and complete their maturation in the intestine. In the intestine they mature and cause intestinal symptoms.

2. C

Some 25 per cent of the world's population, principally in the developing world, harbour ascariasis in their intestines. The vast majority are asymptomatic or have transient ill-defined symptoms.

3. B

The egg of the *Ascariasis lumbricoides* survives in the external environment even under hostile conditions. Hot and humid conditions are ideally suited for the eggs to turn into embryos. The fertilised eggs are present in the soil contaminated with infected faeces. Faeco-oral contamination causes human infection.

4. B, D

The life cycle of ascariasis is as follows. The ingested eggs release larva, which penetrate the intestinal wall and get carried via the portal circulation to the liver and then to the lungs. In the lung the larva penetrate to the bronchioles. This causes inflammation with a dry cough, chest pain and fluffy exudates on chest X-ray called Loeffler's syndrome. The larva are swallowed in sputum and complete their maturation in the intestine. In the intestine, they mature and cause intestinal symptoms.

5. D

The release of larva of ascaris causes an inflammation of the lung characterised by dry cough, chest pain, dyspnoea and fever with fluffy exudates on chest X-ray. This combination of symptoms combined with characteristic features on chest X-ray is called Loeffler's syndrome.

6. F

Roundworms cause problem in the lungs when larvae are released into the bronchioles from circulating blood. Additionally, they colonise the intestine and if the infestation is very heavy, compete for nutrients. This may lead to malnutrition and failure to thrive. A worm bolus may cause intestinal obstruction and even perforation. The worms may travel up the papilla of Vater, causing ascending cholangitis, obstructive jaundice and even acute pancreatitis.

7. A, C, D, E

Worm infestation is often associated with a high eosinophil count as in most parasitic infestations. Bronchoscopic lavage may show larvae or Charcot–Leyden crystals. In Loeffler's syndrome, chest X-ray shows fluffy exudates. A barium meal often demonstrates roundworms in the intestine either by a negative shadow or a linear streak lying parallel to the intestine. This represents barium ingested by the worm.

8. B, C, E

An uncomplicated roundworm obstruction of the intestine should always be treated conservatively with nasogastric suction, IV fluids and hypertonic saline enemas. When laparotomy is indicated, there is never a situation of an actual pyloric narrowing and therefore a gastrojejunostomy is not indicated. Kneading the bolus of worms into the large bowel and subsequent treatment with hypertonic saline enemas is sometimes a way of treating the condition. A long-standing perforation in a malnourished patient may sometimes ideally require exteriorisation of the bowel.

9. B, D, E

The imaging in real time is found to change its position. It is more likely to be due to a roundworm in the common bile duct. Pyrantel palmoate, an anthelmintic, kills worms by causing tetanic convulsion and makes subsequent removal extremely difficult. Therefore this should not be used in this condition. Following the use of albendazole, an anthelmintic, the worm may be extricated by an endoscope.

Hydatid disease

10. B, C, D

Echinococcus granulosus, the parasite which causes cystic echinococcal disease, infects dogs and grow in their intestine. They are the definitive host. The eggs infect sheep, cattle and humans. The worms spread into the blood stream via the portal system. Therefore, the liver is the commonest site of infection, but may infect any organ. The lesions are cystic and spread by expanding rather than by direct invasion.

11. B

In the dog, the adult worm reaches the small intestine and the eggs are passed in the faeces. The ovum gains access to humans by being ingested. On excystation, the parasite penetrates the intestine to reach and spread through the portal system.

12. B, C, D

The cyst is characterised by three layers, an outer pericyst derived from compressed host organ tissues, an intermediate hyaline ectocyst which is non-infective and an inner endocyst that is the germinal membrane and contains viable parasites which can separate forming daughter cysts.

13. B, C, E

Hydatid disease commonly affects the liver. Hence, patients commonly present with a dull aching pain in the upper right abdomen due to the enlargement of the liver. Exposure to the hydatid antigen means that patients often present with anaphylactic shock and collapse in addition to pain as trivial trauma sometimes causes a rupture of the cyst. A large cyst may exert pressure on the CBD, and additionally daughter cysts may communicate with the biliary tract, causing obstructive jaundice.

14. A, C, E

Hydatid cysts are characterised by the presence of multiple septations, calcification in the wall and, when the lamellar membrane separates from the exocyst, split walls. In addition, the presence of multiple daughter cysts sometimes gives rise to the characteristic 'cartwheel' appearance.

15. B, D, E

The clinical scenario of abdominal pain after a trivial trauma, followed by skin rash which responded to antihistamines, is suggestive of a ruptured hydatid cyst. The blood tests reveal an elevated eosinophil count and imaging shows a cyst with a split wall. The cyst, having already ruptured, needs immediate treatment with albendazole followed by laparotomy. As the patient is already exposed to the hydatid antigen, a repeat exposure during exploration of the cyst could initiate a violent anaphylactic attack. This needs to be anticipated and appropriate prophylactic measures initiated.

16. B, E

ERCP revealed multiple membranous structures in the CBD. The imaging revealed a septated hydatid cyst. A septated cyst, often caused by trivial trauma, is more likely to communicate with the biliary channel. Therefore, the likely diagnosis is that the entire biliary system has become colonised by hydatid disease. Injecting scolicidal solutions into this patient runs a real risk of the solution escaping into the biliary channel and causing sclerosing cholangitis.

17. B, C, E

Multiloculated cysts often occur after insignificant trauma. They are more likely to communicate with the biliary channels and thus injection of scolicidal solutions is more likely to cause sclerosing cholangitis. Moreover, the host is more likely to have been exposed to hydatid antigen, and anaphylactic reactions are more common in multiloculated hydatid cysts. Some of these cysts are large and the ectocyst often has a thin layer of compressed tissue spread over vital structures such as the intrahepatic inferior vena cava. Surgical curettage of the cyst wall is often fraught with danger. Deep cysts which show calcification signify that the parasite may be dying or dead and need only be treated with albendazole.

→ Poliomyelitis

18. A, C, E

Poliomyelitis is an enteroviral disease which enters the body by ingestion or inhalation. The disease targets the anterior horn cells, causing lower motor neuron paralysis. It does not cause sensory loss, a fact that distinguishes it from the Guillain–Barré syndrome, which also presents with fever and muscle weakness.

Tuberculosis of the small intestine

19. A, B, D

Typically when a patient with pulmonary tuberculosis swallows infected sputum, the organism colonises the lymphatics of the terminal ileum, causing transverse ulcers with undermined edges. The other variety, called the hyperplastic type, occurs when the host resistance is stronger than the virulence of the organism. It is often caused by drinking infected unpasteurised milk. There is a marked inflammatory reaction, causing hyperplasia and thickening of the terminal ileum because of the abundance of lymphoid follicles. Transmural inflammation with a propensity for fistula formation is a feature of Crohn's disease.

20. A, B, C, D

A patient with tuberculosis of the intestine may present with weight loss, vague abdominal pain and evening rise of temperature. They may also present with a doughy feel of the abdomen from the area of localised ascites or a mass in the right iliac fossa. The patient may also present as an emergency with distal small-bowel obstruction or peritonitis from perforation. The disease may also present as multiple perianal fistulae, sometimes causing a typical watering-can perineum. Caseation on histology is the *sine qua non* of tubercular infection.

21. A, B, E

Tuberculosis is often endemic in people from developing countries with poor socio-economic background. There is often a co-existent pulmonary tuberculosis. While tuberculosis may affect multiple sites of the intestine, 'skip lesions' are characteristic of Crohn's disease. Narrowing of the terminal ileum on a barium study is present in Crohn's disease as in tuberculosis. However, because of intense fibrosis of the intestine and around draining lymph nodes, the caecum in tuberculosis often gets pulled up into the subhepatic position.

22. E

Tuberculosis affects various sites and amounts of the intestine, and therefore all the noted surgical procedures may be carried out for a patient with intestinal tuberculosis.

23. B, D

For patients from developing countries and with poor socioeconomic background, a high index of suspicion for tubercular perforation needs to be maintained. Rarely, patients present with features of peritonitis and, because of a localised perforation due to adhesions, gas under the diaphragm is often absent. These patients often present very late. While laparotomy is almost always indicated, resection and anastomosis may not be feasible in a septic, undernourished patient with severe adhesions. In these individuals, resection and exteriorisation as a first step is followed by restoration of bowel continuity after completion of antituberculous chemotherapy.

Amoebiasis

24. A, D, E

The disease is common in the Indian subcontinent, Africa and parts of Central and South America. The majority produce no symptoms and amoebic liver abscess occurs in less than 10 per cent of patients affected with amoebiasis. The mode of infection is via the faeco-oral route through contaminated food or water.

25. B, C, D

The cysts hatch in the small intestine and large numbers of trophozoites are released and carried to the colon. Here they attach themselves to the mucosa and may penetrate to cause flask-shaped ulcers, or invade the portal vein to be carried to the liver. Here they affect the right lobe in 80 per cent of cases, the left lobe in 10 per cent and the rest are multiple. A large number in the intestine form cysts which are passed in stool that can infect other humans as well.

26. A, B, D, E

The clinical features are all those of an amoebic liver abscess. The CT scan features of a hypodense lesion with irregular walls showing peripheral enhancement are characteristic of an abscess. The fluid is chocolate-coloured, odourless and 'anchovy sauce'-like fluid, a mixture of blood and necrotic liver tissue. This fluid becomes smelly when secondarily infected. The abscess is usually high in the diaphragmatic surface of the right lobe. This may cause pulmonary symptoms. Untreated abscesses are likely to rupture.

27. E

A large majority of patients will present with bloody diarrhoea due to colonic infestation. A liver abscess often presents with upper abdominal and chest symptoms. Rupture of the abscess causes peritonitis and shock. A chronic granuloma, called an amoeboma may form, commonly on the right side of the colon, where the patient has had a long history of repeated indiscriminate and inadequate self-medication. This condition may mimic a carcinoma. While being from an endemic background, a history of blood-stained mucoid diarrhoea and a history of altered bowel habit in a right sided lesion is suggestive of an amoeboma, carcinoma must be excluded. The condition often co-exists with a carcinoma of the colon which is why it is mandatory to take repeated biopsies and repeat the colonoscopy after adequate treatment.

28. B, D, E

The primary and very effective treatment for an amoebic liver abscess is medical. Metronidazole and tinidazole are the effective drugs. After treatment with metronidazole or tinidazole, diloxanide furoate, which is not effective against hepatic infestation, is used for 10 days to destroy any intestinal amoeba. Aspiration not only prevents rupture, but also promotes the penetration of amoebicidal drugs. Surgery is carried out for complications of amoebiasis. However, the general principles of vigorous resuscitation must be applied to these very sick patients.

➜ Asiatic cholangiohepatitis

29. B, C, D, E

Clonorchis sinensis infects snails and fish, which act as the intermediate host. Ingestion of infected fish and snails when eaten raw or partly cooked causes infection in humans and other fish-eating mammals. The disease may remain dormant for years. It often presents with non-specific symptoms but can also present with features of ascending cholangitis, obstructive jaundice and even acute pancreatitis.

30. E

Patients from endemic areas should be offered screening by ultrasonography of the biliary system. Stool examination for eggs or worms is diagnostic. The disease can be cured when treated in its subclinical form. Therefore, the risk of developing the disease of cholangiocarcinoma is eliminated.

➜ Filariasis

31. B, C, E

The disease is mainly caused by *Wuchereria bancrofti* and in 10 per cent is caused by the parasite *Brugia malayi* and *Brugia timori*. Chyluria and chylous ascites may be seen in filariasis.

32. B, D

Blood tests reveal an eosinophilia. Treatment with diethylcarbamazepine is very effective but only in the early stages before the gross deformity of elephantiasis sets in. Once elephantiasis sets in, the condition is rarely treated with surgery as none of the operations described are universally successful.

Leprosy

33. C, D, E

The disease is caused by a *Mycobacterium leprae*, which is weakly acid-fast compared with *Mycobacterium tuberculosis*. It is transmitted by the nasal secretions of a patient, the infection being contracted in childhood or early adolescence. After an incubation of several years, the disease presents with skin and upper respiratory or neurological manifestations. The deformities are therefore a direct cause of the disease or its reactions, and secondary, resulting from effects such as anaesthesia of hands and feet causing repeated unrecognised trauma and damage to the hands and feet. The tissue damage is proportional to the host's immune response, with a plethora of grades between tuberculoid, where there is a strong immune response with scanty bacteria and epithelioid granuloma formation, to lepromatous, where there is a poor immune response, with widespread dissemination of abundant bacilli in the tissues with macrophages and few lymphocytes.

34. A, B, C, E

The disease is diagnosed by obtaining a skin smear, which often demonstrates the acid-fast bacillus, and by a skin biopsy, which shows the characteristic histology. Treatment is carried out according to WHO guidelines with rifampicin, dapsone and clofazimine. Deformities formed need a multidisciplinary approach to their solution.

Tropical chronic pancreatitis

35. A, C, D, E

The disease is not caused by alcohol ingestion but is caused by derivatives of cyanide in cassava (tapioca), which is eaten by the poor as a staple diet. The disease is thus present in families. Patients present with abdominal pain, thirst, polyuria, weight loss due to malnutrition and features of gross pancreatic insufficiency. ERCP is used as a therapeutic procedure. Surgery is necessary for intractable pain, particularly for stones in a dilated pancreatic duct. The choice of procedure is usually a lateral pancreaticojejunostomy. Resectional surgery is used as a last resort for intractable pain.

Typhoid

36. B, C, D, E

The bacillus is ingested in contaminated food and drink and is a result of poor hygiene and inadequate sanitation. The clinical features and a history of a visit to an endemic area should raise suspicions about the disease.

37. A, C, D

The Widal test, which is obsolete in the UK, tests for the presence of agglutinins to O and H antigens of the *Salmonella typhi* and *paratyphi* in the patients' serum. The risk of a perforation is high in cases of untreated typhoid fever. Therefore, a patient who has abdominal symptoms and shows signs of deterioration in the second or third week should be investigated appropriately, using an erect chest X-ray or an abdominal X-ray in lateral decubitus, if the patient is very sick, to exclude free gas in the abdomen.

38. A, C, D, E

Metronidazole, cephalosporins and gentamycin are used in combination in the treatment of typhoid perforation. Chloramphenicol, though very specific for typhoid infection, is used very sparingly, as it can cause aplastic anaemia. Surgical options for treatment of typhoid perforation can vary, including, closure of the perforation after freshening the edges, wedge resection of the perforated segment, resection of bowel with anastomosis or exteriorisation of ileum or colon and closure of the perforation with side-to-side ileo-transverse anastomosis. Delayed wound closure to prevent wound infection is an accepted procedure, as is creating a laparotomy in the presence of rampant infection.

Answers: Extended matching questions

→ 1. Upper abdominal pain

1D

Tropical chronic pancreatitis is a disease affecting the younger generation from poor socioeconomic strata in developing countries, seen mostly in southern India. The aetiology remains obscure, with malnutrition, dietary, familial and genetic factors being possible causes.

Cassava (tapioca) is a root vegetable that is readily available and inexpensive and is therefore consumed as a staple diet by people from a poor background. Several members of the same family have been known to suffer from this condition; this strengthens the theory that cassava toxicity is an important cause, because family members eat the same food.

The patient, usually male, is almost always younger than 40 years and from a poor background. The clinical presentation is abdominal pain, thirst, polyuria and features of gross pancreatic insufficiency, causing steatorrhoea and malnutrition. He looks ill and emaciated.

Initial routine blood and urine tests confirm that the patient has type 1 diabetes mellitus. Plain abdominal X-ray shows typical pancreatic calcification in the form of discrete stones in the duct. Ultrasound and CT scan of the pancreas confirm the diagnosis.

2A

Amoebiasis is caused by *Entamoeba histolytica*. The disease is common in the Indian subcontinent, Africa and parts of Central and South America where almost half the population is infected. The majority remain asymptomatic carriers. Amoebic liver abscess, the commonest extraintestinal manifestation, occurs in less than 10 per cent of the infected population and, in endemic areas, is much more common than pyogenic abscess.

The typical patient with amoebic liver abscess is a young adult male with a history of pain and fever and insidious onset of non-specific symptoms such as anorexia, fever, night sweats, malaise, cough and weight loss, which gradually progress to more specific symptoms of pain in the right upper abdomen, shoulder tip pain, hiccoughs and a non-productive cough. A past history of bloody diarrhoea or travel to an endemic area raises the index of suspicion.

Examination reveals a patient who is toxic and anaemic. The patient will have upper abdominal rigidity, tender hepatomegaly, tender and bulging intercostal spaces, overlying skin oedema, a pleural effusion and basal pneumonitis – the last symptom is usually a late manifestation. Occasionally, a tinge of jaundice or ascites may be present. Rarely, the patient may present as an emergency due to the effects of rupture into the peritoneal, pleural or pericardial cavity.

3C

Most patients with pneumonia experience an acute or subacute onset of fever, cough with or without sputum production, and dyspnoea. Other common symptoms include rigors, sweats, chills, chest discomfort, pleurisy, haemoptysis, fatigue, myalgias, anorexia, headache and abdominal pain.

- Symptoms and signs of an acute lung infection are fever or hypothermia, cough with or without sputum, dyspnoea, chest discomfort, sweats or rigors.
- Bronchial breath sounds or rales are frequent auscultatory findings.
- Parenchymal infiltrate on chest radiograph.

Common physical findings include fever or hypothermia, tachypnoea, tachycardia and mild arterial oxygen desaturation. Many patients will appear acutely ill. Chest examination is often remarkable for altered breath sounds and rales. Dullness to percussion may be present if a parapneumonic pleural effusion is present.

Occasionally, a patient with involvement of lower zones of the lungs may present with symptoms attributable to the upper abdomen only and can be misdiagnosed by the callous examiner as having an abdominal pathology.

4B

Typhoid fever is caused by *Salmonella typhi*, also called the typhoid bacillus. This is a Gram-negative organism. The organism gains entry into the human gastrointestinal tract as a result of poor hygiene and inadequate sanitation. It is a disease normally managed by physicians, but the surgeon is called upon to treat the patient with typhoid fever because of perforation of a typhoid ulcer.

A typical patient is from an endemic area or someone who has recently visited such a country and suffers from a high temperature for 2–3 weeks. The patient may be toxic with abdominal distension from paralytic ileus. The patient may have melaena due to haemorrhage from a typhoid ulcer; this can lead to hypovolaemia.

In the second or third week of the illness, if there is severe generalised abdominal pain, this heralds a perforated typhoid ulcer. The patient, who is already very ill, deteriorates further with classical features of peritonitis. An erect chest X-ray or a lateral decubitus film (in the very ill, as they usually are) will show free gas in the peritoneal cavity. In fact, any patient being treated for typhoid fever who shows a sudden deterioration accompanied by abdominal signs should be considered to have a typhoid perforation until proven otherwise.

5E

Primary thoracic conditions like acute myocardial infarction and lobar pneumonia, especially of the lower zone, may present with signs and symptoms referred to the upper abdomen. An unwary physician may incorrectly attribute the findings to an intra-abdominal condition, whereas there may be none. The key to diagnosis lies in a meticulous history and careful examination, including the cardiovascular and respiratory systems.

Thus acute myocardial infarction and lobar pneumonia must be kept in differential diagnosis of upper abdominal symptoms, especially in a patient who can have any of these conditions as well in order not to miss these potentially lethal but treatable conditions.

→ 2. Lump in the abdomen

1D

Commonly called dog tapeworm, hydatid disease is caused by *Echinococcus granulosus*. While it is common in the tropics, in the UK the occasional patient may come from a rural sheep farming community. The dog is the definitive host and, as a pet, is the commonest source of infection transmitted to the intermediate hosts: humans, sheep and cattle.

As the parasite can colonise virtually every organ in the body, the condition can be protean in its presentation. When a sheep farmer, who is otherwise healthy, complains of a gradually enlarging painful mass in the right upper quadrant with the physical findings of a liver swelling, a hydatid liver cyst should be considered. The liver is the organ most often affected. The pulmonary hydatid is the next most common. The parasite can affect any organ or several organs in the same patient.

The disease may be asymptomatic and discovered coincidentally at postmortem or when an ultrasound or CT scan is done for some other condition. Symptomatic disease presents with a swelling causing pressure effects. Thus, a hepatic lesion causes dull pain from stretching of the liver capsule, and a pulmonary lesion, if large enough, causes dyspnoea.

The patient may present as an emergency with severe abdominal pain following minor trauma when the CT scan may be diagnostic. Rarely, a patient may present as an emergency with features of anaphylactic shock without any obvious cause.

2A

Amoebiasis is caused by *Entamoeba histolytica*. The disease is common in the Indian subcontinent, Africa and parts of Central and South America where almost half the population is infected. The majority remain asymptomatic carriers. Amoebic liver abscess, the most common extraintestinal manifestation, occurs in less than 10 per cent of the infected population and, in endemic areas, is much more common than pyogenic abscess.

The typical patient with amoebic liver abscess is a young adult male with a history of pain and fever and insidious onset of non-specific symptoms such as anorexia, fever, night sweats, malaise, cough and weight loss, which gradually progress to more specific symptoms of pain in the right upper abdomen, shoulder tip pain, hiccoughs and a non-productive cough. A past history of bloody diarrhoea or travel to an endemic area raises the index of suspicion.

Examination reveals a patient who is toxic and anaemic. The patient will have upper abdominal rigidity, tender hepatomegaly, tender and bulging intercostal spaces, overlying skin oedema, a pleural effusion and basal pneumonitis – the last symptom is usually a late manifestation. Occasionally, a tinge of jaundice or ascites may be present. Rarely, the patient may present as an emergency due to the effects of rupture into the peritoneal, pleural or pericardial cavity.

3E

Classically a fat, fertile, flatulent female of 40 has been described as a patient of gallstone disease. Of the various presentations of this condition, acute biliary colic and acute cholecystitis are the most common. Whereas acute biliary colic refers to a self-limiting pain in right upper abdomen associated with nausea, and is seen as short recurring episodes, acute cholecystitis is a more elaborate manifestation. Here the patient has a more pronounced pain which may last for more than a day and is associated with severe systemic symptoms. The pain may be referred to the tip of the right shoulder and may also radiate to the inferior angle of right scapula.

The classical findings on abdominal examination are tenderness in the right hypochondrium, specifically at the tip of the ninth costal cartilage on the right side (Murphy's sign), and not infrequently a palpable tender lump in the same region which is constituted by the inflamed gall bladder along with adherent omentum.

4B

Typhoid fever is caused by *Salmonella typhi*, also called the typhoid bacillus. This is a Gram-negative organism. The organism gains entry into the human gastrointestinal tract as a result of poor hygiene and inadequate sanitation. It is a disease normally managed by physicians, but the surgeon is called upon to treat the patient with typhoid fever because of perforation of a typhoid ulcer.

A typical patient is from an endemic area or someone who has recently visited such a country and suffers from a high temperature for 2–3 weeks. The patient may be toxic with abdominal distension from paralytic ileus. The patient may have melaena due to haemorrhage from a typhoid ulcer; this can lead to hypovolaemia.

In the second or third week of the illness, if there is severe generalised abdominal pain, this heralds a perforated typhoid ulcer. The patient, who is already very ill, deteriorates further with classical features of peritonitis. An erect chest X-ray or a lateral decubitus film (in the very ill, as they usually are) will show free gas in the peritoneal cavity. In fact, any patient being treated for typhoid fever who shows a sudden deterioration accompanied by abdominal signs should be considered to have a typhoid perforation until proven otherwise.

5C

Infection by *Mycobacterium tuberculosis* is common in the tropics. Any patient, particularly one who has recently arrived from an endemic area and who has features of generalised ill health and altered bowel habit, should arouse the suspicion of intestinal tuberculosis.

Patients present electively with weight loss, chronic cough, malaise, evening rise in temperature with sweating, vague abdominal pain with distension and alternating constipation and diarrhoea. As an emergency, they present with features of distal small-bowel obstruction from strictures of the small bowel, particularly the terminal ileum. Rarely, a patient may present with features of peritonitis from perforation of a tuberculous ulcer in the small bowel. Examination shows a chronically ill patient with a 'doughy' feel to the abdomen from areas of localised ascites.
In the hyperplastic type, a mass may be felt in the right iliac fossa.

As this is a disease mainly seen in developing countries, patients may present late as an emergency from intestinal obstruction. Abdominal pain and distension, constipation, and bilious and faeculent vomiting are typical of such a patient who is in extremis.

Raised erythrocyte sedimentation rate (erythrocyte sedimentation rate) and C-reactive protein (C-reactive protein), low haemoglobin and a positive Mantoux test are usual, although the last is not significant in a patient from an endemic area. Sputum for culture and sensitivity (the result may take several weeks) and staining by the Ziehl–Neelsen method for acid-fast bacilli (the result is obtained much earlier) should be done. A barium meal and follow-through (or small bowel enema) will show strictures of the small bowel, particularly the ileum, typically with a high subhepatic caecum with the narrow ileum entering the caecum directly from below upwards in a straight line rather than at an angle.

In the patient presenting as an emergency, urea and electrolytes show evidence of gross dehydration. Plain abdominal X-ray shows typical small bowel obstruction – valvulae conniventes of dilated jejunum and featureless ileum with evidence of fluid between the loops.

➜ 3. Vomiting

1D

The two common causes of gastric outlet obstruction are gastric cancer and pyloric stenosis secondary to peptic ulceration. Previously the latter was more common. Now, with the decrease in the incidence of peptic ulceration and the advent of potent medical treatments, gastric outlet obstruction should be considered malignant until proven otherwise, at least in the West.

The term pyloric stenosis is normally a misnomer. The stenosis is seldom at the pylorus. Commonly, when the condition is due to underlying peptic ulcer disease, the stenosis is found in the first part of the duodenum, the most common site for a peptic ulcer.

Clinical features. In benign gastric outlet obstruction there is usually a long history of peptic ulcer disease. In some patients the pain may become unremitting and in other cases may largely disappear. The vomitus is characteristically unpleasant in nature and is totally lacking in bile. Very often it is possible to recognise foodstuff taken several days previously. The patient commonly complains of losing weight, and appears unwell and dehydrated. Examining the patient it may be possible to see the distended stomach, and a succussion splash may be audible on shaking the patient's abdomen.

2A

Infection by *Mycobacterium tuberculosis* is common in the tropics. Any patient, particularly one who has recently arrived from an endemic area and who has features of generalised ill health and altered bowel habit, should arouse the suspicion of intestinal tuberculosis.

Patients present electively with weight loss, chronic cough, malaise, evening rise in temperature with sweating, vague abdominal pain with distension and alternating constipation and diarrhoea. As an emergency, they present with features of distal small-bowel obstruction from strictures of the small bowel, particularly the terminal ileum. Rarely, a patient may present with features of peritonitis from perforation of a tuberculous ulcer in the small bowel. Examination shows a chronically ill patient with a 'doughy' feel to the abdomen from areas of localised ascites. In the hyperplastic type, a mass may be felt in the right iliac fossa.

As this is a disease mainly seen in developing countries, patients may present late as an emergency from intestinal obstruction. Abdominal pain and distension, constipation, bilious and faeculent vomiting are typical of such a patient who is in extremis.

Raised ESR and CRP, low Hb and a positive Mantoux test are usual, although the last is not significant in a patient from an endemic area. Sputum for culture and sensitivity (the result may take several weeks) and staining by the Ziehl–Neelsen method for acid-fast bacilli (the result is obtained much earlier) should be done. A barium meal and follow-through (or small bowel enema) will show strictures of the small bowel, particularly the ileum, typically with a high subhepatic caecum with the narrow ileum entering the caecum directly from below upwards in a straight line rather than at an angle.

In the patient presenting as an emergency, urea and electrolytes show evidence of gross dehydration. Plain abdominal X-ray shows typical small-bowel obstruction – valvulae conniventes of dilated jejunum and featureless ileum with evidence of fluid between the loops.

3C

Typhoid fever is caused by *Salmonella typhi*, also called the typhoid bacillus. This is a Gram-negative organism. The organism gains entry into the human gastrointestinal tract as a result of poor hygiene and inadequate sanitation. It is a disease normally managed by physicians, but the surgeon is called upon to treat the patient with typhoid fever because of perforation of a typhoid ulcer.

A typical patient is from an endemic area or someone who has recently visited such a country and suffers from a high temperature for 2–3 weeks. The patient may be toxic with abdominal distension from paralytic ileus. The patient may have melaena due to haemorrhage from a typhoid ulcer; this can lead to hypovolaemia.

In the second or third week of the illness, if there is severe generalised abdominal pain, this heralds a perforated typhoid ulcer. The patient, who is already very ill, deteriorates further with classical features of peritonitis. An erect chest X-ray or a lateral decubitus film (in the very ill, as they usually are) will show free gas in the peritoneal cavity. In fact, any patient being treated for typhoid fever who shows a sudden deterioration accompanied by abdominal signs should be considered to have a typhoid perforation until proven otherwise.

4B

Ascaris lumbricoides, commonly called the roundworm, is the commonest intestinal nematode to infect the human and affects a quarter of the world's population. The parasite causes pulmonary symptoms as a larva and intestinal symptoms as an adult worm.

The adult worm can grow up to 45 cm long. Its presence in the small intestine causes malnutrition, failure to thrive and abdominal pain. Small intestinal obstruction can occur, particularly in children, due to a bolus of adult worms incarcerated in the terminal ileum. This is a surgical emergency. Rarely, perforation of the small bowel may occur from ischaemic pressure necrosis from the bolus of worms.

A high index of suspicion is necessary if one is not to miss the diagnosis. If a person from a tropical developing country, or one who has recently returned from an endemic area, presents with pulmonary, gastrointestinal, hepatobiliary and pancreatic symptoms, ascariasis infestation should be high on the list of possible diagnoses.

Increase in the eosinophil count is common, in keeping with most other parasitic infestations. Stool examination may show ova. Sputum or bronchoscopic washings may show Charcot–Leyden crystals or the larvae.

→ 4. Abdominal distension

1D

Paralytic ileus is a state in which there is failure of transmission of peristaltic waves secondary to neuromuscular failure. The resultant stasis leads to accumulation of fluid and gas within the bowel, with associated distension, vomiting, absence of bowel sounds and absolute constipation.

Varieties of paralytic ileus are:

- postoperative
- infection
- reflex ileus
- metabolic.

Clinical features. It takes clinical significance if 72 h after laparotomy there has been no return of bowel sounds and no passage of flatus. Abdominal distension becomes more marked and tympanitic. Pain is not a feature. Radiologically, the abdomen shows gas-filled loops of intestine with multiple air-fluid levels.

2B

Commonly called dog tapeworm, hydatid disease is caused by *Echinococcus granulosus*. While it is common in the tropics, in the UK the occasional patient may come from a rural sheep farming community. The dog is the definitive host and, as a pet, is the commonest source of infection transmitted to the intermediate hosts, humans, sheep and cattle.

As the parasite can colonise virtually every organ in the body, the condition can be protean in its presentation. When a sheep farmer who is otherwise healthy complains of a gradually enlarging painful mass in the right upper quadrant with the physical findings of a liver swelling, a hydatid liver cyst should be considered. The liver is the organ most often affected. The pulmonary hydatid is the next most common. The parasite can affect any organ or several organs in the same patient.

The disease may be asymptomatic and discovered coincidentally at post mortem or when an ultrasound or CT scan is done for some other condition. Symptomatic disease presents with a swelling causing pressure effects. Thus, a hepatic lesion causes dull pain from stretching of the liver capsule, and a pulmonary lesion, if large enough, causes dyspnoea.

The patient may present as an emergency with severe abdominal pain following minor trauma when the CT scan may be diagnostic. Rarely, a patient may present as an emergency with features of anaphylactic shock without any obvious cause.

3A

There are four cardinal features of acute intestinal obstruction:

- pain
- vomiting
- distension
- constipation.

These features vary according to:

- location of the obstruction
- age of the obstruction
- underlying pathology
- presence or absence of intestinal ischaemia.

Late manifestations that may be encountered include dehydration, oliguria, hypovolaemic shock, pyrexia, septicaemia, respiratory embarrassment and peritonism. (Note that peritonism refers to the signs of rebound tenderness in the abdomen on clinical examination, due to bowel ischaemia, when intestinal obstruction can lead to strangulation and gangrene. In the very late stages, there can be bowel perforation leading to overt clinical peritonitis.) In all cases of suspected intestinal obstruction, all hernial orifices must be examined.

Radiological diagnosis. This is based on a supine abdominal film. When distended with gas, the jejunum, ileum, caecum and remaining colon have a characteristic appearance that allows them to be distinguished radiologically, as follows:

- The obstructed small bowel is characterized by straight segments that are generally central and lie transversely. No gas is seen in the colon.
- The jejunum is characterized by its valvulae conniventes that completely pass across the width of the bowel and are regularly spaced giving a 'concertina' or ladder effect.
- Ileum – the distal ileum has been piquantly described by Wangensteen as featureless.

- Caecum – a distended caecum is shown by a rounded gas shadow in the right iliac fossa.
- Large bowel – except for the caecum, it shows haustral folds which, unlike valvulae conniventes, are spaced irregularly and the indentations are not placed opposite one another.

3E

In Western countries where abdominal operations are common, adhesions and bands are the commonest cause of intestinal obstruction. Any source of peritoneal irritation results in local fibrin production, which produces adhesions between opposed surfaces. Early fibrinous adhesions may disappear when the cause is removed or they may become vascularised and replaced by mature fibrous tissue.

Adhesions may he classified into various types by virtue of whether they are early (fibrinous) or late (fibrous) or by the underlying aetiology. From a practical perspective, there are only two types: 'easy' flimsy ones and 'difficult' dense ones.

Postoperative adhesions giving rise to intestinal obstruction usually involve the lower small bowel. Operations for appendicitis and gynaecological procedures are the most common precursors and are an indication for early intervention.

Usually only one band is culpable. This may be:

- congenital, e.g. obliterated vitellointestinal duct
- a string band following previous bacterial peritonitis
- a portion of greater omentum usually adherent to the parietes.

4C

Ascaris lumbricoides, commonly called the roundworm, is the commonest intestinal nematode to infect the human and affects a quarter of the world's population. The parasite causes pulmonary symptoms as a larva and intestinal symptoms as an adult worm.

The adult worm can grow up to 45 cm long. Its presence in the small intestine causes malnutrition, failure to thrive and abdominal pain. Small intestinal obstruction can occur, particularly in children, due to a bolus of adult worms incarcerated in the terminal ileum. This is a surgical emergency. Rarely, perforation of the small bowel may occur as a result of ischaemic pressure necrosis from the bolus of worms.

A high index of suspicion is necessary if one is not to miss the diagnosis. If a person from a tropical developing country, or one who has recently returned from an endemic area, presents with pulmonary, gastrointestinal, hepatobiliary and pancreatic symptoms, ascariasis infestation should be high on the list of possible diagnoses. Increase in the eosinophil count is common, in keeping with most other parasitic infestations. Stool examination may show ova. Sputum or bronchoscopic washings may show Charcot–Leyden crystals or the larvae.

→ 5. Acute abdomen

1C

Typhoid fever is caused by *Salmonella typhi*, also called the typhoid bacillus. This is a Gram-negative organism. The organism gains entry into the human gastrointestinal tract as a result of poor hygiene and inadequate sanitation. It is a disease normally managed by physicians, but the surgeon is called upon to treat the patient with typhoid fever because of perforation of a typhoid ulcer.

A typical patient is from an endemic area or someone who has recently visited such a country and suffers from a high temperature for 2–3 weeks. The patient may be toxic with abdominal distension from paralytic ileus. The patient may have melaena due to haemorrhage from a typhoid ulcer; this can lead to hypovolaemia.

In the second or third week of the illness, if there is severe generalised abdominal pain, this heralds a perforated typhoid ulcer. The patient, who is already very ill, deteriorates further with classical features of peritonitis. An erect chest X-ray or a lateral decubitus film (in the very ill, as they usually are) will show free gas in the peritoneal cavity. In fact, any patient being treated for typhoid fever who shows a sudden deterioration accompanied by abdominal signs should be considered to have a typhoid perforation until proven otherwise.

2D

Despite the widespread use of gastric antisecretory agents and eradication therapy, the incidence of perforated peptic ulcer has changed little. Anteriorly placed ulcers tend to perforate and, by contrast, posterior duodenal ulcers tend to bleed, sometimes by eroding a large vessel such as a gastroduodenal artery.

Clinical features. The classical presentation of perforated duodenal ulcer is instantly recognisable. The patient, who may have a history of peptic ulceration, develops sudden-onset severe generalised abdominal pain due to the irritant effect of gastric acid on the peritoneum. Although the contents of an acid-producing stomach are relatively low in bacterial load, bacterial peritonitis supervenes over a few hours usually accompanied by a deterioration in the patient's condition. The abdomen exhibits a board-like rigidity and the patient is disinclined to move because of the pain. The abdomen does not move with respiration. Patients with this form of presentation need an operation without which the patient will deteriorate with a septic peritonitis.

An erect plain chest radiograph will reveal free gas under the diaphragm in excess of 50 per cent of cases with perforated peptic ulcer.

3E

Infection by *Mycobacterium tuberculosis* is common in the tropics. Any patient, particularly one who has recently arrived from an endemic area, who has features of generalised ill health and altered bowel habit should arouse the suspicion of intestinal tuberculosis.

Patients present electively with weight loss, chronic cough, malaise, evening rise in temperature with sweating, vague abdominal pain with distension and alternating constipation and diarrhoea. As an emergency, they present with features of distal small-bowel obstruction from strictures of the small bowel, particularly the terminal ileum. Rarely, a patient may present with features of peritonitis from perforation of a tuberculous ulcer in the small bowel. Examination shows a chronically ill patient with a 'doughy' feel to the abdomen from areas of localised ascites. In the hyperplastic type, a mass may be felt in the right iliac fossa.

As this is a disease mainly seen in developing countries, patients may present late as an emergency from intestinal obstruction. Abdominal pain and distension, constipation, bilious and faeculent vomiting are typical of such a patient who is in extremis.

Raised ESR and CRP, low haemoglobin and a positive Mantoux test are usual, although the last is not significant in a patient from an endemic area. Sputum for culture and sensitivity (the result may take several weeks) and staining by the Ziehl–Neelsen method for acid-fast bacilli (the result is obtained much earlier) should be done. A barium meal and follow-through (or small bowel enema) will show strictures of the small bowel, particularly the ileum, typically with a high subhepatic caecum with the narrow ileum entering the caecum directly from below upwards in a straight line rather than at an angle.

In the patient presenting as an emergency, urea and electrolytes show evidence of gross dehydration. Plain abdominal X-ray shows typical small-bowel obstruction – valvulae conniventes of dilated jejunum and featureless ileum with evidence of fluid between the loops.

4B

Amoebiasis is caused by *Entamoeba histolytica*. The disease is common in the Indian subcontinent, Africa and parts of Central and South America where almost half the population is infected. The majority remain asymptomatic carriers. Amoebic liver abscess, the commonest extraintestinal manifestation, occurs in less than 10 per cent of the infected population and, in endemic areas, is much more common than pyogenic abscess.

The typical patient with amoebic liver abscess is a young adult male with a history of pain and fever and insidious onset of non-specific symptoms such as anorexia, fever, night sweats, malaise, cough and weight loss, which gradually progress to more specific symptoms of pain in the right upper abdomen, shoulder tip pain, hiccoughs and a non-productive cough. A past history of bloody diarrhoea or travel to an endemic area raises the index of suspicion.

Examination reveals a patient who is toxic and anaemic. The patient will have upper abdominalrigidity, tender hepatomegaly, tender and bulging intercostal spaces, overlying skin oedema, a pleural effusion and basal pneumonitis – the last symptom is usually a late manifestation. Occasionally, a tinge of jaundice or ascites may be present. Rarely, the patient may present as an emergency due to the effects of rupture into the peritoneal, pleural or pericardial cavity.

5A

The pain of classical appendicitis is initially periumbilical (visceral: derivative of midgut) and later shifts to right iliac fossa at McBurney's point (parietal). The treatment of an established case of appendicitis is appendicectomy and not antibiotics.

The natural course of appendicitis, if allowed to progress as a result of incorrect diagnosis, can be resolution or it may progress to a fulminant inflammation. The inflammation spreads transmurally, and the pressure inside the lumen of appendix rises. Ultimately, the wall of the appendix gives way, and the contents, loaded with bacteria and inflammatory cells which are under pressure, are disseminated in the general peritoneal cavity.

If by now the omentum has walled off the appendix, it results in a localized abscess. On the other hand, generalised dissemination causes a fulminant bacterial peritonitis. This is evident clinically as a patient who initially presents with typical right iliac fossa pain, receives some medical treatment on which the pain seems to be improving, and then suddenly experiences a worsening of the pain which now becomes generalized along with deterioration in the clinical status of the patient.

On examination, there will be classical signs of peritonitis, which in the initial stages are limited to the lower abdomen, before becoming generalized.

6. Swollen leg

1C

Venous congestion is an important cause of limb swelling. It can arise due to an interference with the normal venous return out of the limb. This in turn could be because of an intrinsic block in the veins (due to thrombosis) or extrinsic compression (veins being thin-walled are prone to extrinsic compression; compartment syndrome, tumours).

The findings in a limb with venous congestion are:

- pitting oedema
- dusky in colour
- warmth
- engorged superficial veins
- normal pulsations and neurological examination.

2A

Filariasis is mainly caused by the parasite *Wuchereria bancrofti* carried by the mosquito. A variant of the parasite called *Brugia malayi* and *Brugia timori* is responsible for causing the disease in about 10 per cent of sufferers. The condition affects more than 90 million people worldwide, two-thirds of whom live in India, China and Indonesia.

It is mainly males who are affected because females in general cover a greater part of their bodies, thus making them less prone to mosquito bites. In the acute presentation, there are episodic attacks of fever with lymphadenitis and lymphangitis. Occasionally, adult worms may be felt subcutaneously.

Chronic manifestations appear after repeated acute attacks over several years. The adult worms cause lymphatic obstruction, resulting in massive lower limb oedema. Obstruction to the cutaneous lymphatics causes skin thickening, not unlike the 'peau d'orange' appearance in breast cancer, thus exacerbating the limb swelling. Secondary streptococcal infection is common. Recurrent attacks of lymphangitis cause fibrosis of the lymph channels, resulting in a grossly swollen limb with thickened skin, producing the condition of elephantiasis.

Bilateral lower limb filariasis is often associated with scrotal and penile elephantiasis. Early on, there may be a hydrocele underlying scrotal filariasis.

Eosinophilia is common, and a nocturnal peripheral blood smear may show the immature forms or microfilariae. The parasite may also be seen in chylous urine, ascites and hydrocele fluid.

3B

Venous thrombosis of the deep veins is a serious life-threatening condition which may lead to sudden death in the short term or to long-term morbidity due to the development of a post-thrombotic limb and venous ulceration. The deep veins of the lower extremities and pelvis are most frequently involved. The process begins approximately 80 per cent of the time in the deep veins of the calf, although it can arise in the femoral or iliac veins.

Clinical manifestations of DVT, which may develop up to 2 weeks postoperatively, occur in about 3 per cent of patients undergoing major general surgical procedures (in the absence of effective prophylaxis). Certain operations, such as total hip replacement, are associated with appreciably higher incidences of thromboembolic complications. Illnesses that involve periods of bed rest, such as cardiac failure or stroke, are also associated with a high incidence of DVT. Use of oral contraceptive drugs, especially by women over 30 and by those who smoke, may be associated with hypercoagulability, resulting in DVT in some women. These drugs should not be prescribed for women with a history of DVT. Hypercoagulability is also observed in cancer, particularly adenocarcinoma, and especially in tumours of the pancreas, prostate, breast and ovary. Finally, hereditary factors such as factor V Leiden, protein C and S deficiencies, and antithrombin III deficiency should be considered in young patients with positive family histories and recurrent venous thrombosis. Homocystinuria and paroxysmal nocturnal haemoglobinuria are also associated with venous hypercoagulability.

Approximately half of patients with DVT have no symptoms or signs in the extremity in the early stages. The patient may suffer a pulmonary embolism, presumably from the leg veins, without symptoms or demonstrable abnormalities in the extremities.

Symptoms and signs. The patient may complain of a dull ache, a tight feeling or frank pain in the calf or, in more extensive cases, the whole leg, especially when walking. Typical findings include a slight swelling in the involved calf, distension of the superficial venous collaterals, slight fever and tachycardia. These symptoms are often absent or may occur in the absence of DVT. The skin may be cyanotic if venous obstruction is severe or pale and cool with massive swelling and restriction of blood flow or a reflex arterial spasm is superimposed.

4D

The underlying mechanism in lymphoedema is impairment of the lymph flow from an extremity. When lymphoedema is the result of congenital developmental abnormalities consisting of hypoplastic or hyperplastic involvement of the proximal or distal lymphatics, it is referred to as the primary form. The secondary form of lymphoedema involves inflammatory or mechanical lymphatic obstruction from trauma, regional lymph node resection or irradiation, or extensive involvement of regional nodes by malignant disease or filariasis.

The essentials of diagnosis are: painless persistent oedema of one or both lower extremities, primarily in young women; and pitting oedema, which rarely becomes brawny and non-pitting.

History. The age of onset of painless swelling, together with the presence or absence of a family history or coexistent pathology, will allow differentiation of primary from secondary lymphoedema to be made in most cases.

Lymphoedema praecox (onset from 1 to 35 years of age) is three times more common in females than in males, has a peak incidence shortly after menarche, is three times more likely to be unilateral than bilateral, usually only extends to the knee and accounts for about 20 per cent of primary lymphoedema. The familial form is referred to as Meige's disease and represents about one-third of all cases.

Signs. Unlike other types of oedema, lymphoedema characteristically involves the foot. Lymphoedema usually spreads proximally to knee level and less commonly affects the whole leg. Lymphoedema will pit easily at first but, with time, fibrosis and dermal thickening prevent pitting except following prolonged pressure.

5E

Cellulitis is a diffuse inflammation of connective tissue with severe inflammation of dermal and subcutaneous layers of the skin. Cellulitis can be caused by normal skin flora or by exogenous bacteria, and often occurs where the skin has previously been broken: cracks in the skin, cuts, blisters, burns, insect bites, surgical wounds or sites of intravenous catheter insertion. Skin on the face or lower legs is most commonly affected by this infection, although cellulitis can occur on any part of the body.

Cellulitis is caused by bacteria entering the skin, usually by way of a cut, abrasion or break in the skin. This break does not need to be visible. Group A *Streptococcus* and *Staphylococcus* are the most common of these bacteria, which are part of the normal flora of the skin but cause no actual infection while on the skin's outer surface. Predisposing conditions for cellulitis include insect bite, blistering, animal bite, tattoos, pruritic skin rash, recent surgery, athlete's foot, dry skin, eczema, injecting drugs (especially subcutaneous or intramuscular injection), pregnancy, diabetes and obesity, which can affect circulation, as well as burns and boils, although there is debate as to whether minor foot lesions contribute.

Cellulitis usually begins as a small area of tenderness, swelling and redness. As this red area begins to enlarge, the person may develop a fever – sometimes with chills and sweats – and swollen lymph nodes near the area of infected skin. The signs of cellulitis include redness, warmth, swelling and pain in the involved tissues. Any skin wound or ulcer that exhibits these signs may be developing cellulitis.

→ 7. Scrotal swelling

1C

A hydrocele is an abnormal collection of serous fluid in some part of the processus vaginalis, usually the tunica.

Aetiology. A hydrocele can be produced in four ways:

- by excessive production of fluid within the sac, e.g. secondary hydrocele
- by defective absorption of fluid. This appears to be the explanation for most primary hydroceles although the reason why the fluid is not absorbed is obscure
- by interference with lymphatic drainage of scrotal structures
- by connection with a hernia of the peritoneal cavity in the congenital variety.

Hydrocele fluid is amber-coloured and sterile, and contains albumin and fibrinogen. If the contents of a hydrocele are allowed to drain into a collecting vessel, the liquid does not clot, but the fluid coagulates if it is mixed with even a small quantity of blood that has been in contact with damaged tissue. In long-standing cases, hydrocele fluid is sometimes opalescent with cholesterol and may occasionally contain crystals of tyrosine

Clinical features. Hydroceles are almost invariably translucent and it is possible to 'get above the swelling' on examination of the scrotum.

2D

Males are 20 times more commonly affected by inguinal hernias than females. The patient complains of pain in the groin or pain referred to the testicle when performing heavy work or taking strenuous exercise. When asked to cough, a small transient bulging may be seen and felt together with an expansile impulse. When the sac is still limited to the inguinal canal, the bulge may be better seen by observing the inguinal region from the side or even looking down the abdominal wall while standing behind the respective shoulder of the patient.

As an indirect inguinal hernia increases in size, it becomes apparent when the patient coughs and persists until reduced. As time goes on, the hernia comes down as soon as the patient stands up. In large hernias there is a sensation of weight, and dragging on the mesentery may produce epigastric pain. If the contents of the sac are reducible, the inguinal canal will be found to be commodious.

Differential diagnosis in the male is as follows:

- vaginal hydrocele
- encysted hydrocele of the cord
- spermatocele
- femoral hernia
- incompletely descended testis in the inguinal canal – an inguinal hernia is often associated with this condition
- lipoma of the cord – this is often a difficult, but unimportant, diagnosis. It is usually not settled until the parts are displayed by operation.

Examination using finger and thumb across the neck of the scrotum will help to distinguish between a swelling of inguinal origin and one which is entirely intrascrotal.

Differential diagnosis in the female is as follows:

- hydrocele of the canal of Nuck is the most common differential diagnostic problem
- femoral hernia.

3A

Filariasis is mainly caused by the parasite *Wuchereria bancrofti* carried by the mosquito. A variant of the parasite called *Brugia malayi* and *Brugia timori* is responsible for causing the disease in about 10 per cent of sufferers. The condition affects more than 90 million people worldwide, two-thirds of whom live in India, China and Indonesia.

It is mainly males who are affected because females in general cover a greater part of their bodies, thus making them less prone to mosquito bites. In the acute presentation, there are episodic attacks of fever with lymphadenitis and lymphangitis. Occasionally, adult worms may be felt subcutaneously.

Chronic manifestations appear after repeated acute attacks over several years. The adult worms cause lymphatic obstruction, resulting in massive lower limb oedema. Obstruction to the cutaneous lymphatics causes skin thickening, not unlike the 'peau d'orange' appearance in breast cancer, thus exacerbating the limb swelling. Secondary streptococcal infection is common. Recurrent attacks of lymphangitis cause fibrosis of the lymph channels, resulting in a grossly swollen limb with thickened skin, producing the condition of elephantiasis.

Bilateral lower limb filariasis is often associated with scrotal and penile elephantiasis. Early on, there may be a hydrocele underlying scrotal filariasis.

Eosinophilia is common, and a nocturnal peripheral blood smear may show the immature forms or microfilariae. The parasite may also be seen in chylous urine, ascites and hydrocele fluid.

4B
Heart failure may be right-sided or left-sided (or both). Patients with left heart failure have symptoms of low cardiac output and elevated pulmonary venous pressure; dyspnoea is the predominant feature. Signs of fluid retention predominate in right heart failure, with the patient exhibiting oedema, hepatic congestion and, on occasion, ascites. Most patients exhibit symptoms or signs of both right- and left-sided failure, and left ventricular (LV) dysfunction is the primary cause of right ventricular (RV) failure.

Essentials of diagnosis. These are as follows:

- LV failure – exertional dyspnoea, cough, fatigue, orthopnoea, paroxysmal nocturnal dyspnoea, cardiac enlargement, rales, gallop rhythm and pulmonary venous congestion
- RV failure – elevated venous pressure, hepatomegaly, dependent oedema, usually due to LV failure.

Many patients with heart failure, including some with severe symptoms, appear comfortable at rest. Others will be dyspnoeic during conversation or minor activity, and those with long-standing severe heart failure may appear cachectic or cyanotic. The vital signs may be normal, but tachycardia, hypotension and reduced pulse pressure may be present.

Important peripheral signs of heart failure can be detected by examination of the neck, lungs, abdomen and the extremities. Right atrial pressure may be estimated through the height of the pulsations in the jugular venous system. In the lungs, crackles at the lung bases reflect transudation of fluid into the alveoli. Patients with severe right heart failure may have hepatic enlargement – tender or non-tender – due to passive congestion. Systolic pulsations may be felt in tricuspid regurgitation. Ascites may also be present. Peripheral pitting oedema is a common sign in patients with right heart failure and may extend into the scrotum, thighs and abdominal wall.

5E
Varicocele is a relatively common condition (affecting approximately 10 per cent of men) that tends to occur in young men, usually during the second or third decade of life. Typical varicocele symptoms are mild and many do not require treatment. Treatment may be necessary if the varicocele is causing discomfort or any of the other problems listed below.

Symptoms of a varicocele may include:

- dragging-like or aching pain within the scrotum
- feeling of heaviness in the testicle(s)
- atrophy (shrinking) of the testicle(s)
- visible or palpable (able to be felt) enlarged vein, likened to feeling a bag of worms
- infertility.

Fertility problems. There is an association between varicoceles and infertility or subfertility, but it is difficult to be certain if a varicocele is the cause of fertility problems in any one case. In one study, as many as 40 per cent of men who were subfertile were found to have a varicocele. Other signs of varicoceles can be a decreased sperm count; decreased motility, or movement, of sperm; and an increase in the number of deformed sperm. It is not known for certain how varicoceles contribute to these problems, but a common theory is that the condition raises the temperature of the testicles and affects sperm production. Studies have shown that 50–70 per cent of men with fertility problems will have a significant improvement in the quality and/or quantity of sperm production after they have undergone varicocele repair.

Testicular atrophy. Atrophy, or shrinking, of the testicles is another of the signs of varicocele. The condition is often diagnosed in adolescent boys during a sports physical examination. When the affected testicle is smaller than the other one, repair of the varicocele is often recommended. The repaired testicle will return to its normal size in many cases.

Upon palpation of the scrotum, a non-tender, twisted mass along the spermatic cord is felt. Palpating a varicocele can be likened to feeling a bag of worms. When lying down, gravity may allow the drainage of the pampiniform plexus such that the mass is not obvious. This is especially true in primary varicocele, and absence may be a sign for clinical concern. The testicle on the side of the varicocele may or may not be smaller than that on the other side.

Varicocele can be reliably diagnosed with ultrasound, which will show dilatation of the vessels of the pampiniform plexus to greater than 2 mm. The patient being studied should undergo a provocative manoeuvre, such as Valsalva's manoeuvre (straining, like he is trying to have a bowel movement) or standing up during the examination, both of which are designed to increase intra-abdominal venous pressure and increase the dilatation of the veins. Doppler ultrasound is a technique of measuring the speed at which blood is flowing in a vessel. An ultrasound machine that has a Doppler mode can see blood reverse direction in a varicocele with a Valsalva, increasing the sensitivity of the examination.

8. Claw hands

1B

The ulnar nerve is most commonly damaged by lacerations in the forearm or entrapment as it passes behind the medial epicondyle of the humerus, in which case decompression or anterior transposition may be indicated.

Clinical features include:

- Motor – paralysis of the small muscles of the hand, with the exception of the thenar muscles and lateral two lumbricals. The patient is unable to abduct and adduct the fingers, or indeed grip a piece of paper between them. Weakness of flexion of the metacarpophalangeal joints and extension of the interphalangeal joints result in a claw-type deformity. If the patient pinches a piece of paper between the thumb and the index finger, the distal phalanx of the thumb assumes a flexed position, as weakness of the adductor pollicis permits over-action of flexor pollicis longus (Froment's sign). In longer-standing cases, muscle wasting will be evident in the interosseous spaces and along the medial border of the hand. Lesions proximal to the elbow also cause paralysis of the flexor carpi ulnaris and medial half of the flexor digitorum profundus
- Sensory – sensation is lost on the medial one and a half fingers.

2C

The median nerve is classically injured at the elbow or wrist. Injuries at the elbow are due to fractures of the distal humerus or dislocation of the elbow joint.

Clinical features include:

- Motor – paralysis of the pronators of the forearm and flexors of the wrist and fingers, with the exception of the flexor carpi ulnaris and the medial part of the flexor digitorum profundus. The index finger and thumb cannot be flexed at the interphalangeal joints, but flexion of the other fingers is performed by the portion of the flexor digitorum profundus which is supplied by the ulnar nerve. The thenar muscles are paralysed with resulting loss of abduction and opposition of the thumb
- Sensory – sensation is lost over the palmar aspect of the thumb, index, middle and the radial half of the ring fingers, as well as part of the palm.

Damage to the median nerve at the wrist is comparatively common as a result of lacerations, fractures of the distal radius or compression in the carpal canal. Clinical features include paralysis of the thenar muscles and loss of sensation on the palmar aspect of the radial three and a half fingers.

3A

Leprosy, also called Hansen's disease, is a chronic infectious disease caused by the acid-fast bacillus, *Mycobacterium leprae*, that is widely prevalent in the tropics. Globally, India, Brazil, Nepal,

Mozambique, Angola and Myanmar (Burma) account for 91 per cent of all the cases; India alone accounts for 78 per cent of the world's disease.

The disease is broadly classified into two groups, lepromatous and tuberculoid. In lepromatous leprosy, there is widespread dissemination of abundant bacilli in the tissues with macrophages and a few lymphocytes. This is a reflection of the poor immune response, resulting in depleted host resistance from the patient. In tuberculoid leprosy, on the other hand, the patient shows a strong immune response with scant bacilli in the tissues, epithelioid granulomas, numerous lymphocytes and giant cells. The tissue damage is proportional to the host's immune response.

The disease is slowly progressive and affects the skin, upper respiratory tract and peripheral nerves. In tuberculoid leprosy, the damage to tissues occurs early and is localised to one part of the body with limited deformity of that organ. Neural involvement is characterised by thickening of the nerves, which are tender. There may be asymmetric well-defined anaesthetic hypopigmented or erythematous macules with elevated edges and a dry and rough surface – lesions called leprids. In lepromatous leprosy, the disease is symmetrical and extensive. Cutaneous involvement occurs in the form of several pale macules that form plaques and nodules called lepromas. The deformities produced are divided into primary, which are caused by leprosy or its reactions, and secondary, resulting from effects such as anaesthesia of the hands and feet.

There is loss of eyebrows and destruction of the lateral cartilages and septum of the nose with collapse of the nasal bridge and lifting of the tip of the nose. There may be paralysis of the branches of the facial nerve in the bony canal or of the zygomatic branch.

The hands are typically clawed because of involvement of the ulnar nerve at the elbow and the median nerve at the wrist. Anaesthesia of the hands makes these patients vulnerable to frequent burns and injuries. Similarly, clawing of the toes occurs as a result of involvement of the posterior tibial nerve. When the lateral popliteal nerve is affected, it leads to foot drop, and the nerve can be felt to be thickened behind the upper end of the fibula. Anaesthesia of the feet predisposes to trophic ulceration, chronic infection, contraction and auto-amputation. Involvement of the testes causes atrophy, which in turn results in gynaecomastia.

4E

Dupuytren's contracture (also known as Morbus Dupuytren, Dupuytren's disease or palmar fibromatosis) is a fixed flexion contracture of the hand where the fingers cannot be fully extended. It is named after Baron Guillaume Dupuytren, the surgeon who described an operation to correct the affliction.

Dupuytren's contracture is caused by underlying contractures of the palmar fascia. The ring and little fingers are those most commonly affected. The middle finger may be affected in advanced cases, but the index finger and the thumb are nearly always spared. Dupuytren's contracture progresses slowly and is usually painless. In patients with this condition, the tissues under the skin on the palm of the hand thicken and shorten so that the tendons connected to the fingers cannot move freely. The palmar aponeurosis becomes hyperplastic and undergoes contracture.

It usually has a gradual onset, often beginning as a tender lump in the palm. Over time, pain associated with the condition tends to go away, but tough bands of tissue may develop. These bands, which are the source of the reduced mobility commonly associated with the condition, are visible on the surface of the palm and may appear similar to a small callus. It commonly develops in both hands and has no connection to dominant or non-dominant hands, nor any correlation with right- or left-handedness. Incidence increases after the age of 40; at this age men are affected more often than women. After the age of 80 the distribution is about even.

Dupuytren's disease is a very specific affliction, and primarily affects:

- people of Scandinavian or northern European ancestry; it has been called the 'Viking disease', although it is also widespread in some Mediterranean countries (e.g. Spain and Bosnia) and in Japan

- men rather than women (men are 10 times as likely to develop the condition)
- people over the age of 40
- people with a family history (60–70 per cent of those afflicted have a genetic predisposition to Dupuytren's contracture)
- people with liver cirrhosis.

Some suspected, but unproven, causes of Dupuytren's contracture include trauma, diabetes, alcoholism, epilepsy therapy with phenytoin and liver disease. There is no proven evidence that hand injuries or specific occupational exposures lead to a higher risk of developing Dupuytren's disease, although there is some speculation that Dupuytren's may be caused, or at least the onset may be triggered, by physical trauma, such as manual labour or other over-exertion of the hands. However, the fact that Dupuytren's is not connected with handedness casts some doubt on this claim.

5D

Poliomyelitis is an enteroviral infection that affects children in developing countries. The virus enters the body by inhalation or ingestion. Clinically, the disease manifests itself in a wide spectrum of symptoms, from a few days of mild fever and headache to the extreme variety consisting of extensive paralysis of the bulbar form that may not be compatible with life because of involvement of the respiratory and pharyngeal muscles.

The disease targets the anterior horn cells, causing lower motor neuron paralysis. Muscles of the lower limb are affected twice as frequently as those of the upper limb. Only 1–2 per cent of sufferers develop paralytic symptoms but, when they do occur, the disability causes much misery. When a patient develops fever with muscle weakness, the Guillain–Barré syndrome needs to be excluded. The latter has sensory symptoms and signs, and cerebrospinal fluid (CSF) analysis should help to differentiate the two conditions.

Foot and ankle. The most common deformities are claw toes, cavovarus foot, dorsal bunion, talipes equines, talipes equinovarus, talipes cavovarus, talipes equinovalgus and talipes calcaneus.

Knee. The common knee deformities are flexion contracture, quadriceps paralysis, genu recurvatum and flail knee.

Hip. Common problems are flexion and abduction contractures, hip instability due to paralysis of the gluteal muscles and paralytic hip dislocation.

Trunk. Unbalanced paralysis causes scoliosis along with pelvic obliquity.

Shoulder, elbow, wrist and hand. Common problems are shoulder weakness, wrist drop and claw hands.

→ 9. Limb deformity

1B

Poliomyelitis is an enteroviral infection that affects children in developing countries. The virus enters the body by inhalation or ingestion. Clinically, the disease manifests itself in a wide spectrum of symptoms – from a few days of mild fever and headache to the extreme variety consisting of extensive paralysis of the bulbar form that may not be compatible with life because of involvement of the respiratory and pharyngeal muscles.

The disease targets the anterior horn cells causing lower motor neuron paralysis. Muscles of the lower limb are affected twice as frequently as those of the upper limb. Only 1–2 per cent of sufferers develop paralytic symptoms but, when they do occur, the disability causes much misery. When a patient develops fever with muscle weakness, the Guillain–Barré syndrome needs to be excluded. The latter has sensory symptoms and signs, and CSF analysis should help to differentiate the two conditions.

Foot and ankle. The most common deformities are claw toes, cavovarus foot, dorsal bunion, talipes equines, talipes equinovarus, talipes cavovarus, talipes equinovalgus and talipes calcaneus.

Knee. The common knee deformities are flexion contracture, quadriceps paralysis, genu recurvatum and flail knee.

Hip. Common problems are flexion and abduction contractures, hip instability due to paralysis of the gluteal muscles and paralytic hip dislocation.

Trunk. Unbalanced paralysis causes scoliosis along with pelvic obliquity.

Shoulder, elbow, wrist and hand. Common problems are shoulder weakness, wrist drop and claw hands.

2C

Leprosy, also called Hansen's disease, is a chronic infectious disease caused by the acid-fast bacillus, *Mycobacterium leprae*, that is widely prevalent in the tropics. Globally, India, Brazil, Nepal, Mozambique, Angola and Myanmar (Burma) account for 91 per cent of all the cases; India alone accounts for 78 per cent of the world's disease.

The disease is broadly classified into two groups – lepromatous and tuberculoid. In lepromatous leprosy, there is widespread dissemination of abundant bacilli in the tissues with macrophages and a few lymphocytes. This is a reflection of the poor immune response, resulting in depleted host resistance from the patient. In tuberculoid leprosy, on the other hand, the patient shows a strong immune response with scant bacilli in the tissues, epithelioid granulomas, numerous lymphocytes and giant cells. The tissue damage is proportional to the host's immune response.

The disease is slowly progressive and affects the skin, upper respiratory tract and peripheral nerves. In tuberculoid leprosy, the damage to tissues occurs early and is localised to one part of the body with limited deformity of that organ. Neural involvement is characterised by thickening of the nerves, which are tender. There may be asymmetric well-defined anaesthetic hypopigmented or erythematous macules with elevated edges and a dry and rough surface – lesions called leprids. In lepromatous leprosy, the disease is symmetrical and extensive. Cutaneous involvement occurs in the form of several pale macules that form plaques and nodules called lepromas. The deformities produced are divided into primary – which are caused by leprosy or its reactions – and secondary, resulting from effects such as anaesthesia of the hands and feet.

There is loss of eyebrows and destruction of the lateral cartilages and septum of the nose, with collapse of the nasal bridge and lifting of the tip of the nose. There may be paralysis of the branches of the facial nerve in the bony canal or of the zygomatic branch.

The hands are typically clawed because of involvement of the ulnar nerve at the elbow and the median nerve at the wrist. Anaesthesia of the hands makes these patients vulnerable to frequent burns and injuries. Similarly, clawing of the toes occurs as a result of involvement of the posterior tibial nerve. When the lateral popliteal nerve is affected, it leads to foot drop, and the nerve can be felt to be thickened behind the upper end of the fibula. Anaesthesia of the feet predisposes to trophic ulceration, chronic infection, contraction and auto-amputation. Involvement of the testes causes atrophy, which in turn results in gynaecomastia.

3A

Filariasis is mainly caused by the parasite *Wuchereria bancrofti* carried by the mosquito. A variant of the parasite called *Brugia malayi* and *Brugia timori* is responsible for causing the disease in about 10 per cent of sufferers. The condition affects more than 90 million people worldwide, two-thirds of whom live in India, China and Indonesia.

It is mainly males who are affected because females in general cover a greater part of their bodies, thus making them less prone to mosquito bites. In the acute presentation, there are episodic attacks of fever with lymphadenitis and lymphangitis. Occasionally, adult worms may be felt subcutaneously.

Chronic manifestations appear after repeated acute attacks over several years. The adult worms cause lymphatic obstruction, resulting in massive lower limb oedema. Obstruction to the cutaneous lymphatics causes skin thickening, not unlike the 'peau d'orange' appearance in breast cancer, thus exacerbating the limb swelling. Secondary streptococcal infection is common. Recurrent attacks of lymphangitis cause fibrosis of the lymph channels, resulting in a grossly swollen limb with thickened skin, producing the condition of elephantiasis.

Bilateral lower limb filariasis is often associated with scrotal and penile elephantiasis. Early on, there may be a hydrocele underlying scrotal filariasis.

Eosinophilia is common, and a nocturnal peripheral blood smear may show the immature forms or microfilariae. The parasite may also be seen in chylous urine, ascites and hydrocele fluid.

4D

Psoas abscess is a condition in which an abscess develops in the fascial sheath of the psoas major. The source of infection may be from the adjacent vertebral bodies (tubercular spine is the most common), haematogenous, or from the overlying peritoneal cavity.

The abscess remains silent for a long time due to the deep-seated location of the muscle. At this time the patient may have systemic features of the infection such as fever or malaise, or may have symptoms attributable to the spine such as backache or neurological complaints. The infection tracks along the muscle sheath and may involve the iliacus muscle, which joins the psoas for a common insertion, to form an iliopsoas abscess. This may be palpable as a lump in the iliac fossa. Rarely, the abscess may point on the medial side of the thigh at the point of insertion of the muscle on the femur. The affected muscle may go into spasm, causing flexion deformity of the hip joint.

The clinical signs may include tenderness of the affected vertebrae, fullness of the paravertebral space and scoliosis with concavity towards the affected side, mass in the iliac fossa, flexion deformity of the hip, and lump on the upper medial thigh. An X-ray of the dorsolumbar spine, and an US or CT scan may help in arriving at a diagnosis.

→ 10. Paralysis

1B

Pott's spine, a manifestation of bony tuberculosis, is one of the causes of non-neoplastic compressive myelopathy. It results in the formation of an epidural abscess and presents as a clinical triad of midline dorsal pain, fever and progressive limb weakness. Prompt recognition of this distinctive process will in most cases prevent permanent sequelae. Aching pain is almost always present, either over the spine or in a radicular pattern. The duration of pain prior to presentation is generally 2 weeks but may on occasion be several months or longer. Fever is usual, accompanied by elevated white blood cell count and sedimentation rate. As the abscess expands, further spinal cord damage results from venous congestion and thrombosis. Once weakness and other signs of myelopathy appear, progression may be rapid.

Two-thirds of epidural infections are a result of haematogenous spread of bacteria from the skin (furunculosis), soft tissue (pharyngeal or dental abscesses) or deep viscera (bacterial endocarditis). The remainder arise from direct extension of a local infection to the subdural space; examples of local predisposing conditions are vertebral osteomyelitis, decubitus ulcers, lumbar puncture, epidural anaesthesia and spinal surgery. Most cases are due to *Staphylococcus aureus*; Gram-negative bacilli, *Streptococcus*, anaerobes and fungi can also cause epidural abscesses. Tuberculosis from an adjacent vertebral source, Pott's disease, remains an important cause in the underdeveloped world.

2E

Acute limb ischaemia is most often due to either an acute thrombotic occlusion of a previously partially occluded, thrombosed arterial segment, or an embolus. Without surgical revascularisation, complete acute ischaemia leads to extensive tissue necrosis within 6 h. The effects of sudden arterial occlusion depend on the state of collateral supply. The collateral supply in the leg is usually inadequate unless there has been pre-existing occlusive disease. On the other hand, the subclavian artery has many collateral vessels so that occlusion of a major artery does not necessarily make a limb non-viable.

Causes of acute limb ischaemia are:

- embolism – e.g. left atrium in patients in atrial fibrillation, mural thrombus after myocardial infarction, prosthetic and abnormal heart valves, aneurysm (aorta, femoral or popliteal), proximal atheromatous stenosis, malignant tumour or foreign body
- thrombosis – most cases of leg ischaemia result from the presence of thrombus at sites of atherosclerotic narrowing
- trauma
- Raynaud's syndrome
- compartment syndrome – occurs when perfusion pressure falls below tissue pressure in a closed anatomical space
- congenital causes of early-onset leg ischaemia, e.g. aortic hypoplasia.

Presentation of acute limb ischaemia

- History and examination should identify the severity of ischaemia and whether it is likely to be embolic or thrombotic.
- Important features to differentiate include rapidity of onset of symptoms, features of pre-existing chronic arterial disease, potential source of embolus and the state of pulses in the contralateral limb.
- The affected part becomes pale, pulseless, painful, paralysed, paraesthetic and poikilothermic ('the 6 Ps').
- The onset of fixed mottling of the skin implies irreversible changes.
- The limb may be red when dependent, leading to a misdiagnosis of inflammation, e.g. gout or cellulitis.

Investigations

- Hand-held Doppler ultrasound – may help to demonstrate any residual arterial flow
- Blood tests – for full blood count (ischaemia is aggravated by anaemia), ESR (inflammatory disease, e.g. giant cell arteritis, other connective tissue disorders), glucose (diabetes), lipids and thrombophilia screen.
- If diagnosis is in doubt, perform urgent arteriography
- Identify source of embolus – ECG, echocardiogram; ultrasound of aorta, popliteal and femoral arteries.

3D

Cerebrovascular diseases include some of the most common and devastating disorders: ischaemic stroke, haemorrhagic stroke and cerebrovascular anomalies such as intracranial aneurysms and arteriovenous malformations (AVMs). They are a major cause of disability. The incidence of cerebrovascular diseases increases with age and the number of strokes is projected to increase as the elderly population grows.

The various risk factors associated with cerebrovascular diseases are hypertension, smoking, diabetes, hyperlipidaemia, carotid artery stenosis and atrial fibrillation.

Most cerebrovascular diseases are manifest by the abrupt onset of a focal neurological deficit. A stroke, or cerebrovascular accident, is defined by this abrupt onset of a neurological deficit that is attributable to a focal vascular cause. Thus the definition of stroke is clinical, and laboratory studies including brain imaging are used to support the diagnosis.

The clinical manifestations of stroke are highly variable because of the complex anatomy of the brain and its vasculature. Cerebral ischaemia is caused by a reduction in blood flow that lasts longer than several seconds. Neurological symptoms are manifest within seconds because neurons lack glycogen, so energy failure is rapid. If the cessation of flow lasts for more than a few minutes, infarction or death of brain tissue results. When blood flow is quickly restored, brain tissue can recover fully and the patient's symptoms are only transient: this is called a transient ischaemic attack (TIA). The standard definition of TIA requires that all neurological signs and symptoms resolve within 24 h regardless of whether there is imaging evidence of new permanent brain injury; stroke has occurred if the neurological signs and symptoms last for >24 h. Focal ischaemia or infarction is usually caused by thrombosis of the cerebral vessels themselves or by emboli from a proximal arterial source or the heart. Intracranial haemorrhage is caused by bleeding directly into or around the brain; it produces neurological symptoms by producing a mass effect on neural structures, from the toxic effects of blood itself or by increasing intracranial pressure.

Most of the patients experience the sudden onset of the following: loss of sensory and/or motor function on one side of the body (nearly 85 per cent of ischaemic stroke patients have hemiparesis); change in vision, gait, or ability to speak or understand; or a sudden, severe headache.

4A

Poliomyelitis is an enteroviral infection that affects children in developing countries. The virus enters the body by inhalation or ingestion. Clinically, the disease manifests itself in a wide spectrum of symptoms – from a few days of mild fever and headache to the extreme variety consisting of extensive paralysis of the bulbar form that may not be compatible with life because of involvement of the respiratory and pharyngeal muscles.

The disease targets the anterior horn cells, causing lower motor neuron paralysis. Muscles of the lower limb are affected twice as frequently as those of the upper limb. Only 1–2 per cent of sufferers develop paralytic symptoms but, when they do occur, the disability causes much misery. When a patient develops fever with muscle weakness, the Guillain–Barré syndrome needs to be excluded. The latter has sensory symptoms and signs, and CSF analysis should help to differentiate the two conditions.

Foot and ankle. The most common deformities are claw toes, cavovarus foot, dorsal bunion, talipes equines, talipes equinovarus, talipes cavovarus, talipes equinovalgus and talipes calcaneus.

Knee. The common knee deformities are flexion contracture, quadriceps paralysis, genu recurvatum and flail knee.

Hip. Common problems are flexion and abduction contractures, hip instability due to paralysis of the gluteal muscles and paralytic hip dislocation.

Trunk. Unbalanced paralysis causes scoliosis along with pelvic obliquity.

Shoulder, elbow, wrist and hand. Common problems are shoulder weakness, wrist drop and claw hands.

5C

Diseases of the spinal cord are frequently devastating. They produce quadriplegia, paraplegia and sensory deficits far beyond the damage they would inflict elsewhere in the nervous system because the spinal cord contains, in a small cross-sectional area, almost the entire motor output and sensory input of the trunk and limbs. Many spinal cord diseases are reversible if recognized and treated at an early stage.

The presence of a horizontally defined level below which sensory, motor and autonomic function is impaired is a hallmark of spinal cord disease. This sensory level is sought by asking the patient to identify a pinprick or cold stimulus (e.g. a dry tuning fork after immersion in cold water) applied to the proximal legs and lower trunk and sequentially moved up toward the neck on each side. Lesions that transect the descending corticospinal and other motor tracts cause paraplegia or quadriplegia, with the evolution over time of increased muscle tone, heightened deep tendon reflexes and Babinski signs (the upper motor neuron syndrome). Such lesions also typically produce autonomic disturbances consisting of absent sweating below the implicated cord level, and bladder, bowel and sexual dysfunction.

The uppermost level of a spinal cord lesion can also be localized by attention to the segmental signs corresponding to disturbed motor or sensory innervation by an individual cord segment. A band of altered sensation (hyperalgesia or hyperpathia) at the upper end of the sensory disturbance, fasciculations or atrophy in muscles innervated by one or several segments, or a muted or absent deep tendon reflex may be noted at this level. These signs also occur with focal root or peripheral nerve disorders; thus, segmental signs are most useful when they occur together with signs of long tract damage. With severe and acute transverse lesions, the limbs may initially be flaccid rather than spastic. This state of 'spinal shock' lasts for several days, rarely for weeks, and should not be mistaken for extensive damage to many segments of the cord or for an acute polyneuropathy.

The main features of transverse damage at each level of the spinal cord are outlined below.

Cervical cord. Upper cervical cord lesions produce quadriplegia and weakness of the diaphragm. Lesions at C4–C5 produce quadriplegia; at C5–C6, there is loss of power and reflexes in the biceps; at C7 weakness is found only in finger and wrist extensors and triceps; and at C8, finger and wrist flexion is impaired. Horner's syndrome (miosis, ptosis and facial hypohidrosis) may accompany a cervical cord lesion at any level.

Thoracic cord. Lesions here are localized by the sensory level on the trunk and by the site of midline back pain if it accompanies the syndrome. Useful markers for localization are the nipples (T4) and umbilicus (T10). Leg weakness and disturbances of bladder and bowel function accompany the paralysis. Lesions at T9–T10 paralyse the lower – but not the upper – abdominal muscles, resulting in upward movement of the umbilicus when the abdominal wall contracts (Beevor's sign).

Lumbar cord. Lesions at the L2–L4 spinal cord levels paralyse flexion and adduction of the thigh, weaken leg extension at the knee and abolish the patellar reflex. Lesions at L5–S1 paralyse only movements of the foot and ankle, flexion at the knee and extension of the thigh, and abolish the ankle jerks (S1).

Sacral cord/conus medullaris. The conus medullaris is the tapered caudal termination of the spinal cord, comprising the lower sacral and single coccygeal segments. The conus syndrome is distinctive, consisting of bilateral saddle anaesthesia (S3–S5), prominent bladder and bowel dysfunction (urinary retention and incontinence with lax anal tone) and impotence. The bulbocavernosus (S2–S4) and anal (S4–S5) reflexes are absent. Muscle strength is largely preserved.

By contrast, lesions of the cauda equina, the cluster of nerve roots derived from the lower cord, are characterized by low back and radicular pain, asymmetric leg weakness and sensory loss, variable areflexia in the lower extremities, and relative sparing of bowel and bladder function. Mass lesions in the lower spinal canal often produce a mixed clinical picture in which elements of both cauda equina and conus medullaris syndromes coexist.

6 Paediatric surgery

Multiple choice questions

General surgical management

1. Which of the following statements are false?

A A neonate is a baby up to 4 weeks old.
B The urinary bladder is an intra-abdominal organ in infants and children.
C An infant's head accounts for 20 per cent of the body surface area.
D Gluconeogenesis in infants is as good as in adults.
E The infant's immune system is immature.

2. Which of the following statements are true?

A Children are regarded as small adults and therefore their surgical management is adjusted according to their size.
B Attention to thermoregulation is very important.
C Postoperative management requires extreme care because of inadequate stress response.
D Postoperatively children do not recover as quickly as adults.
E Minimal access surgery (MAS) can be used at all ages.

Paediatric trauma

3. Which of the following statements regarding paediatric trauma are true?

A Follow usual Advanced Trauma Life Support (ATLS) rules as in an adult.
B Usual rules of resuscitation apply.
C Blunt trauma is more common than penetrating trauma.
D Splenic injury in the majority should be treated by splenectomy.
E Consideration must be given to non-accidental injury (NAI).

Inguinoscrotal swellings

4. Which of the following statements about inguinoscrotal swellings are false?

A A hydrocele is a patent processus vaginalis as is a hernia.
B Hernia is always indirect.
C Hernia can be direct or indirect.
D In incarcerated hernia, reduction should be attempted by taxis followed by operation 24 h later.
E A hydrocele always needs an operation.

Undescended testis

5. Which of the following are true for undescended testis?

A Orchidopexy in a subdartos pouch is the treatment of choice.
B The operation is recommended at the age of 2 years.
C When a testis is impalpable and therefore intra-abdominal, laparotomy should be done.
D Laparoscopy is the gold standard procedure for an intra-abdominal testis.
E Orchidopexy reduces the chance of malignancy.

Acute scrotal pain

6. Which of the following statements are true with regard to acute scrotal pain?

A Acute testicular pain can be from torsion of the testis, torsion of the hydatid of Morgagni or acute epididymitis.

B Pain of testicular torsion may originate in the groin or suprapubic area.
C Doppler ultrasound should be done in suspected testicular torsion.
D Incarcerated hernia may cause similar symptoms.
E In case of any doubt, exploration of the scrotum must be carried out.

7. What is the operation for congenital hypertrophic pyloric stenosis called?
A Hartmann
B Whipple
C Heller
D Ramstedt
E Ivor-Lewis.

Extended matching questions

→ 1. Vomiting

A Congenital hypertrophic pyloric stenosis
B Intussusception
C Incarcerated inguinal hernia
D Duodenal atresia
E Intestinal malrotation +/– volvulus

Choose and match the correct diagnosis with each of the scenarios given below:

1 A 2-year-old boy has been sent in as an emergency with vomiting for 24 h. According to the parents the vomitus was greenish to start with but over the last few hours has consisted of dirty brownish fluid. There has been no bowel action. On examination the child looks toxic and is dehydrated – sunken eyes, depressed fontanelles, loss of skin turgor. There is a tympanitic abdomen with a red, irreducible swelling in the left groin not noticed by the parents.

2 Jonathan, a 5-week-old boy, has been vomiting intermittently for 2 weeks. This has become incessant for the last 24 h. The vomitus is clear fluid. The infant seems hungry and takes its feed only to bring it up within a short while. The mother noticed some twitching of muscles. The baby is dehydrated. The paediatrician felt a lump in the upper abdomen when Jonathan was being fed by his mother.

3 Mary-Ann, a 10-month-old girl, has been brought in with occasional vomiting for a couple of days. The parents noticed that the vomitus is sometimes green and at other times brownish. They feel that Mary-Ann is in pain intermittently because she screams, flexing her knees and elbows, denoting spasms. They noticed that the nappy has bloodstained mucus. On examination she looks ill and dehydrated and the right side of the abdomen feels empty.

→ 2. Acute abdomen

A Non-specific abdominal pain
B Acute appendicitis
C Constipation
D Urinary tract infection
E Right lower-lobe pneumonia

Choose and match the correct diagnosis with each of the scenarios given below:

1 A 10-year-old boy has been brought in with abdominal pain, vomiting, pyrexia and diarrhoea for the last 24 h or so. He has been off his food for a couple of days. He has pyrexia of 39°C, tachycardia, looks toxic and has marked lower abdominal tenderness, rigidity and rebound tenderness, and the abdominal wall does not move with respiration.

2 Millie, a 10-year-old girl, has been admitted with generalised abdominal pain, vomiting and anorexia for 2 days. She has missed school a few times because of similar attacks of abdominal pain in the past, which subsided on its own within 24 h. On this occasion it has persisted. Examination revealed a well-looking, introspective child with generalised abdominal tenderness without any rigidity or rebound tenderness, with the abdominal wall moving freely with respiration.

3 Kerry, a 5-year-old girl, has been brought by her parents with generalised abdominal pain which has been recurrent over 6 months or so. On this occasion she looks ill, out of sorts, anorexic and has been vomiting. She has marked urinary frequency. On examination she has a temperature of 100°C, looks toxic, listless and dehydrated and has generalised abdominal and bilateral loin tenderness.

→ 3. Congenital malformations

A Tracheo-oesophageal fistula
B Congenital diaphragmatic hernia
C Intestinal atresia
D Intestinal malrotation
E Biliary atresia
F Hirschsprung's disease
G Necrotising enterocolitis

Choose and match the correct diagnosis with each of the scenarios given below:

1 A 2-month-old Down's syndrome baby has been brought in with gradual abdominal distension, intermittent bilious vomiting with a history of delayed passage of meconium. The parents feel that the baby is unduly constipated. Examination shows a baby that has not been thriving normally, with a hugely distended abdomen and gross dehydration.

2 A prenatal ultrasound scan alerted the paediatricians to a congenital abnormality affecting the abdomen and chest. The premature neonate has been born with severe respiratory compromise and is on ventilatory support in the neonatal ICU.

3 A neonate is born with frothy saliva and episodes of cyanosis. Any attempt to feed makes the symptoms worse. A fine orogastric tube is arrested. A plain X-ray shows that the tube is curled up in the chest and there is gas in the abdomen. The condition was suspected on prenatal ultrasound.

4 A mother who suffered from polyhydramnios has given birth to a baby who has Down's syndrome. The baby has bilious vomiting. The plain abdominal X-ray shows a 'double-bubble' appearance and the condition was suspected on prenatal ultrasound.

5 A neonate has bile-stained vomiting with passage of bloodstained stools. The baby is very sick and a contrast meal shows the bowel mostly on the right side with a subhepatic caecum.

6 A 2-week-old neonate who was born with jaundice has exhibited increasing yellowish discoloration of skin and conjunctiva ever since birth. There are some superficial skin bruises.

7 A few days after birth, a neonate has developed abdominal distension, bloodstained stools and bilious vomiting. The baby is toxic with septic shock.

Answers: Multiple choice questions

➜ General surgical management

1. D

In paediatric surgery, it is important to have a clear idea about the various age groups. A baby born before 37 weeks is called a preterm; one born between 37 and 42 weeks is full term. A baby is called a neonate up to 4 weeks in age; an infant up to 1 year; a pre-school child below 5 years; and a child and adolescent up to 16 years.

As infants and small children have a shallow pelvis, the urinary bladder is intra-abdominal. The head in infants accounts for 20 per cent of body surface and this does not equal an adult proportion of 9 per cent until the age of 14 years.

The ability for gluconeogenesis is much impaired in infants, which renders them hypoglycaemic very easily in the postoperative period. An immature immune system renders them more susceptible to infection, which may manifest with non-specific features.

2. B, C, E

Children should never be regarded as small adults. Conditions that afflict children by and large are different from those in adults. In children the thermoregulatory system is immature. They have little subcutaneous fat (hence no natural insulation) and an undeveloped vasomotor centre. Therefore the theatre must be well heated, their head and neck well covered (the head is almost a fifth of the body's surface area), infusions need to be warmed, a warm air blanket used and the core temperature closely monitored.

The metabolic response to stress is inadequate because of the immature neurohormonal and immune systems. The effects of clotting deficiencies need to be prevented with intramuscular vitamin K. Ability to concentrate urine and conserve sodium is impaired; therefore fluid and sodium needs are high. Gastro-oesophageal reflux may result in aspiration, causing pulmonary problems.

With meticulous attention to detail along with good pain relief, children recover more quickly than adults under similar circumstances. Intravenous fluids – 0.45 per cent saline with 2.5 per cent dextrose or isotonic saline – help to maintain optimum fluid and electrolyte balance. Minimal access surgical techniques have all the advantages as seen in the adults; obviously the instruments and insufflation pressures have to be tailored.

➜ Paediatric trauma

3. B, C, E

In the West, injury is the most common cause of death and disability in childhood; most of the deaths are avoidable. Adult ATLS guidelines cannot be followed because of the smaller body mass of children. Therefore trauma results in a larger force applied per unit of body area. The effects are far more serious because the body has less fat, less elastic connective tissue, there is proximity of vital organs to the skin and a poor thermoregulatory system. Because of the elasticity of the child's skeleton, underlying solid organs can be damaged without overlying skeletal damage: cardiac, pulmonary, hepatic, pancreatic and splenic injury can occur without any fractured ribs or sternum.

Blunt rather than penetrating trauma is more common. If the child is stable, contrast-enhanced computed tomography (CECT) is the investigation of choice. Liver, pancreatic, splenic and renal injuries are usually managed conservatively with close clinical monitoring supplemented by serial CECT or ultrasound. The team must be prepared to anticipate the need for immediate operation as the child who is being observed can suddenly deteriorate.

A child's blood volume is 80 mL/kg. In shock (systolic blood pressure falls after loss of 25 per cent of blood volume) 20 mL/kg Ringer's lactate solution is used as a bolus to be repeated judiciously. Interosseous access into the upper tibia may be necessary in infants.

When the severity of trauma is at variance with the degree of injury, when there has been undue delay in seeking medical advice following trauma, when there is repeated trauma and inconsistent history between family members, NAI should be strongly suspected and paediatricians should be involved forthwith.

Inguinoscrotal swellings

4. C, E

An inguinal hernia in a child is indirect as it occurs in a patent processus vaginalis. Sometimes it may be incarcerated, resulting in vomiting and irreducibility. In the early stages of obstruction, manual reduction under analgesia (taxis) can be attempted so that the operation can be done as an elective procedure 24 h later to allow the oedema to settle down. However, if the infant is ill, dehydrated and toxic with a distended abdomen, strangulation is imminent or present. This requires IV fluid resuscitation followed by emergency operation.

A congenital hydrocele is a patent processus vaginalis where the patency at the internal ring is too narrow to allow any bowel through; only normal peritoneal fluid comes into the scrotum, causing the hydrocele. This does not require any surgical treatment. If it is persistent after the age of 2 years, the persistent processus is ligated through a groin incision.

Undescended testis

5. A, B, D

When a testis is arrested in the normal path of descent, it is called an undescended testis. On the other hand, when the testis is found at a site away from its normal path of descent, such as in the superficial inguinal pouch, root of the scrotum or femoral triangle, it is then regarded as an ectopic testis.

When the scrotum is empty but well developed, and the testis can be coaxed down into the scrotum, the infant has a retractile testis. This does not require any treatment except reassurance to the parents. When a testis is palpable in the line of descent and is not a retractile testis, the child requires an orchidopexy operation. This is ideally carried out before the age of 2 years and the testis is fixed in a subdartos pouch.

When the testis is not palpable, it means that the testis is intra-abdominal. Laparoscopy is the procedure of choice. The testis can then be localised and mobilised as a staged procedure for orchidopexy. A maldescended testis should be brought down to prevent torsion, trauma, infertility and to enable earlier diagnosis of a tumour when any abnormality of a scrotal testis is much more easily identifiable. Orchidopexy does not reduce the chance of malignancy but increases the chances of early detection.

Acute scrotal pain

6. A, B, D, E

Torsion of the testis can occur at any age. There may be a history of intermittent pain in the past. On clinical suspicion, the scrotum should be explored as an emergency forthwith. Colour Doppler ultrasound, an investigation not usually carried out, to show reduced blood flow may be used, provided it does not compromise promptness of treatment. Torsion of the testicular appendage occurs in prepubertal boys. Sometimes the bluish appendage can be seen on top of the testis. It can be left alone if the diagnosis is certain. Excision is preferable as it results in early cure of the problem while at the same time excluding the serious condition of testicular torsion. Incarcerated hernia will present with vomiting and abdominal distension from intestinal obstruction.

7. D

Answers: Extended matching questions

1. Vomiting

1C

Bilious vomiting in an infant is a sign of intestinal obstruction. An irreducible lump in the groin indicates an incarcerated inguinal hernia as the cause. Incarceration indicates intraluminal obstruction, whereas strangulation means compromise of the blood supply to the bowel. As the child is toxic, incarceration may be proceeding to strangulation. Brownish or faeculent vomitus is a sinister sign. The infant should be resuscitated with intravenous fluids, nasogastric suction and prophylactic antibiotics. Once optimised, an emergency operation should be carried out.

2A

Jonathan suffers from congenital (idiopathic) hypertrophic pyloric stenosis. This occurs during the first 6 weeks of life usually in a first-born male infant. Typically the baby has non-bilious vomiting, is hungry and, in late cases, may have muscle spasms from alkalotic tetany.

Examination shows a dehydrated baby with a hard mass ('pyloric tumour') felt in the epigastrium on test feed. Confirmation, if necessary, may be obtained on ultrasound or a gastrograffin swallow (Fig. 6.1).

The biochemical abnormality of hypochloraemic, hypokalaemic, metabolic alkalosis is corrected. After optimum resuscitation, a Ramstedt's pyloromyotomy (an operation first performed by German surgeon Wilhelm Conrad Ramstedt, 1867–1963, in 1911) is done through a transverse right upper quadrant incision.

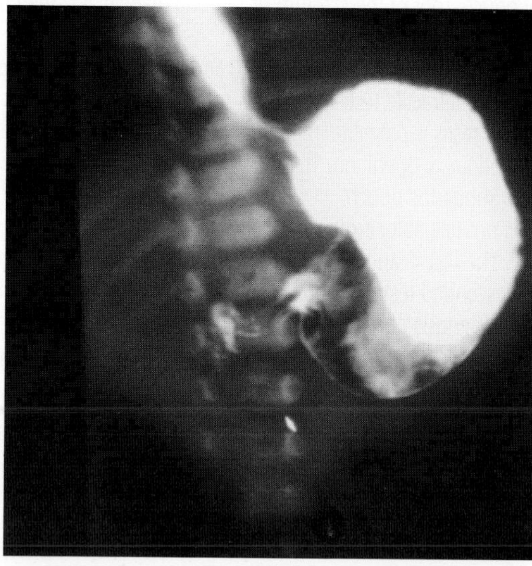

Figure 6.1 A gastrograffin swallow showing no flow of contrast past the pylorduodenal junction: Congenital hypertrophic pyloric stenosis.

3B

Mary-Ann suffers from intussusception. This is the invagination of a proximal part of the bowel into the adjacent distal part, resulting in strangulating intestinal obstruction. Usually the ileum invaginates into the caecum and ascending colon. There is bloodstained mucus from the anus ('redcurrant jelly stools'), an empty right iliac fossa and sometimes a sausage-shaped mass may be felt which might migrate with concavity towards the umbilicus. Confirmation is by ultrasound or a gastrograffin enema which shows a typical crab claw deformity (Fig. 6.2).

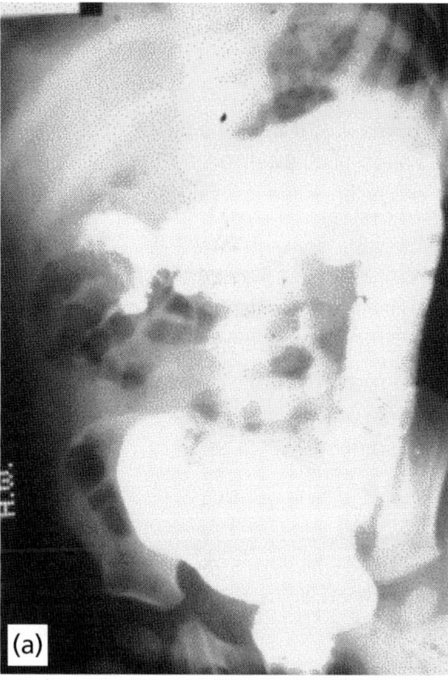

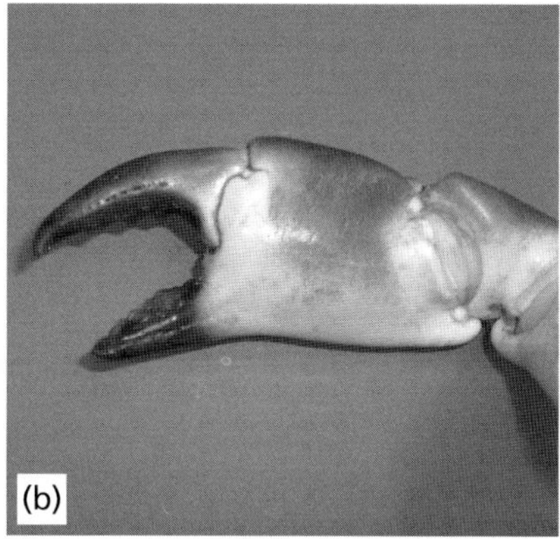

Figure 6.2 Barium enema showing typical crab-claw deformity of acute ileo-caeco-colic intussusception.

After full resuscitation, radiological reduction with air or contrast enema is attempted; if unsuccessful, laparotomy is undertaken and manual reduction or bowel resection is done according to the findings.

2. Acute abdomen

1B

He has acute appendicitis. In children the history may be atypical. Diarrhoea denotes a pelvic position of the appendix. The abdominal signs are typical of peritonitis. Perforation in children is common because of their inability to localise intra-abdominal infection as a result of poorly developed omentum. Complete examination of the chest should be done in all cases of acute abdominal pain in children to exclude right lower-lobe pneumonia.

2A

Millie has features suggestive of non-specific abdominal pain – recurrent attacks, generalised abdominal symptoms, no signs of peritonism and missing school on more than one occasion, the latter denoting psychosocial problems. This is a diagnosis made in 30–50 per cent of children admitted to hospital with acute abdomen. Sometimes constipation may be a cause.

3D

Kerry has urinary tract infection. Children usually have an underlying urinary tract abnormality such as pelviureteric junction obstruction or vesicoureteric reflux. Such conditions should be promptly diagnosed and treated so as to prevent long-term deleterious effects of renal scarring from ascending pyelonephritis. Clinical examination usually does not reveal any abnormality. Urine examination and renal ultrasound are the initial investigations. This is followed by micturating cystogram and/or isotope renogram.

→ 3. Congenital malformations

1F

Congenital megacolon, first described by Harald Hirschsprung in 1911, occurs due to congenital absence of intramural ganglion cells causing large bowel obstruction: in 3 out of 4 patients the abnormality is restricted to the rectum and colon. Enterocolitis is a dreaded complication. The diagnosis is established by a contrast enema which shows the exact site and extent of the diseased segment; it is confirmed by biopsy.

2B

This is a congenital diaphragmatic hernia (Fig. 6.3). Respiratory embarrassment is the key presentation with an empty feeling of the abdomen. The diagnosis is usually made prenatally; therefore the team is ready to intervene soon after birth. Respiratory support is the keynote in the initial management. Repair is carried out if adequate oxygenation is obtained. Almost a third of cases succumb to respiratory failure due to severe pulmonary hypoplasia.

3A

Soon after birth when a neonate presents with frothy saliva and cyanosis, oesophageal atresia is the diagnosis, the commonest variety being a blind proximal pouch with a distal tracheo-oesophageal fistula. Associated anomalies affecting the heart, kidneys and skeletal system may be present. After confirmation of diagnosis, referral to a paediatric surgeon is made. Operation is carried out within a day or two of birth.

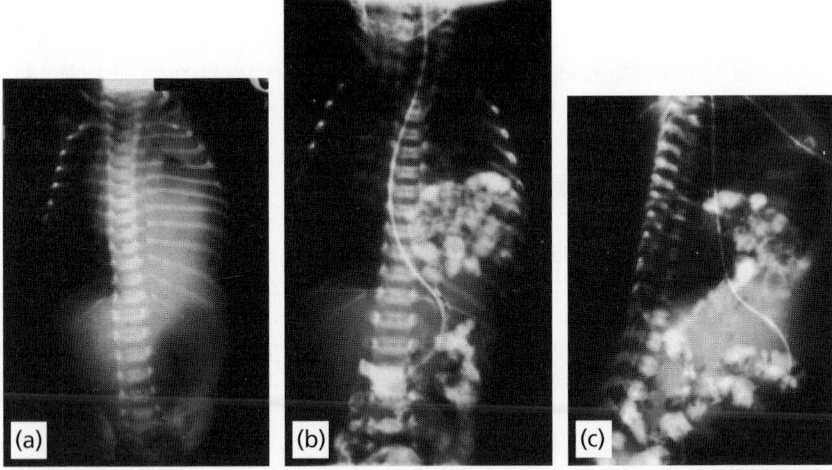

Figure 6.3(a) Plain X-ray of neonate showing absence of left dome of diaphragm and collapsed left lung with gas shadows in the left hemi-thorax. **(b)** Anterior posterior view of a gastrograffin swallow showing loops of bowel in the left hemi-thorax: Congenital diaphragmatic hernia. **(c)** Lateral view of a gastrograffin swallow showing loops of bowel in the left hemi-thorax: Congenital diaphragmatic hernia.

4C

This is duodenal atresia which may be a part of intestinal atresia. The 'double-bubble' appearance on plain X-ray is diagnostic (Fig. 6.4). Bile-stained vomiting differentiates it from congenital hypertrophic pyloric stenosis. It is caused by a complete membrane. The operation is duodenoduodenostomy.

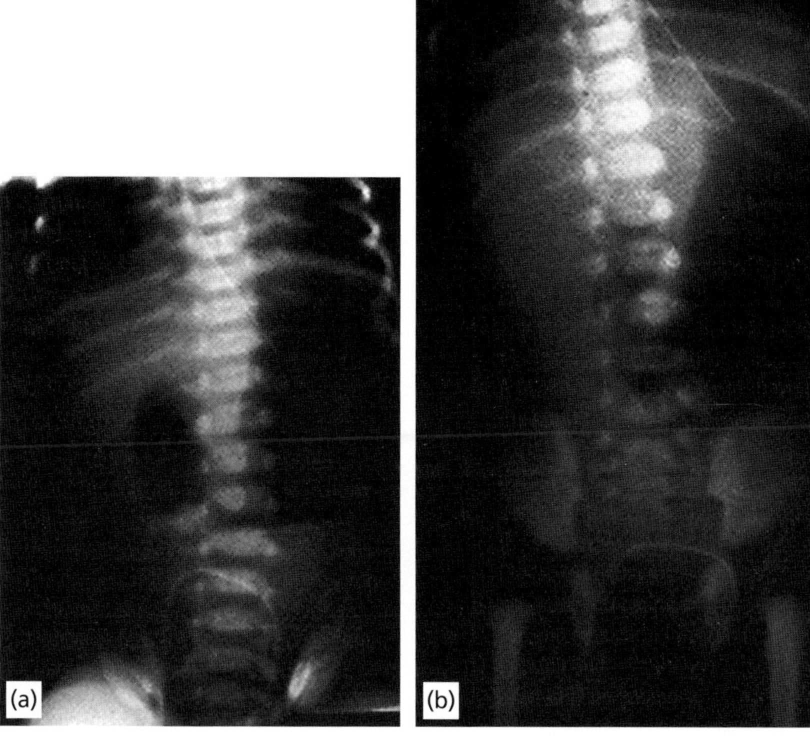

Figure 6.4(a) and (b) Double-bubble appearance of duodenal atresia on plain X-ray.

5D

The neonate has bile-stained vomiting, which is a sign of intestinal obstruction. A contrast meal shows a high caecum with the duodenojejunal flexure on the right side. The small bowel mesentery has a narrow base predisposing to a midgut volvulus.

6E

Congenital biliary atresia should be suspected if the jaundice in the newborn does not subside within 2 weeks. The incidence is 1 in 17 000. In the presence of conjugated hyperbilirubinaemia, coagulopathy is a problem which needs to be combated with vitamin K. An ultrasound scan, radioisotope scan and liver biopsy are the investigations of choice.

7G

Necrotising enterocolitis is an inflammatory bowel disease occurring in the premature neonate. The baby presents with features of toxic shock, abdominal distension, bloodstained stools and bilious vomiting and aspirate. A variable length of the intestine is affected.

7 Oncology

Multiple choice questions

Malignant transformation

1. **Which of the following statements about malignant transformation in cells are true?**

A Cells become immortal.
B Cells acquire angiogenic competence.
C Cells increase apoptosis.
D Cells resist signals that inhibit growth.
E Cells evade detection/elimination.

Gompertzian growth

2. **Which of the following statements are true with regard to Gompertzian growth?**

A The majority of the growth of the tumour occurs before it is clinically detectable.
B 'Early tumours' are genetically old.
C The rate of regression of a tumour depends upon its age.
D By the time of clinical detection, the window during which tumours are most sensitive to antiproliferative drugs would have passed.
E The growth of the tumour has an exponential relationship.

Causation of cancer

3. **Which of the following statements about the causation of cancer are true?**

A Environmental factors have been implicated in more than 80 per cent of cancers.
B HPV infection is associated with cancer of the penis.
C Familial breast cancer involving BRCA1 and BRCA2 has an autosomal recessive inheritance.
D Wood dust is associated with paranasal sinus cancers.
E Pituitary tumours are a part of MEN type 2A syndrome.

Cancers associated with obesity

4. **Which of the following cancers is associated with obesity?**

A Breast
B Kidney
C Colon
D Oesophagus
E Endometrium.

Cancer screening

5. **Which of the following are criteria for cancer screening?**

A Sensitive and specific test
B Acceptable to the screened population
C Rare disorders
D Recognisable early stage
E Treatment at an early stage to be as effective as that at a later stage.

Staging of colorectal cancer

6. **Which of the following concerning the staging of colorectal cancer are true?**

A T3b refers to invasion of between 5 and 15 mm beyond the muscularis propia.
B N2 means involvement of four or more regional lymph nodes.
C V1 means intramural vascular invasion.
D T0 means tumour limited to mucosa.
E R0 means complete surgical resection with adequate margins.

Treatment of cancer

7. **Which of the following statements regarding surgery for cancer are true?**

A The diagnosis of cancer should always be confirmed before surgery.
B Ultraradical surgery has a significant role in reducing the incidence of distant metastases.

C Up to one-third of patients can expect long-term survival after successful resection of colorectal liver metastases.
D Surgery has no role in palliation.
E Laparoscopic approach has been shown to be equally effective as open surgery in colorectal cancer.

8. Which of the following statements regarding radiotherapy (RT) for cancer are true?
A Delivering RT in fractions facilitates cell repair.
B Hypoxic cells are more radiosensitive than others.
C Repopulation phenomenon suggests that longer overall treatment time is more beneficial than shorter.
D The fractions should be timed to coincide with the late G2 and M phases of the cell cycle.
E Early laryngeal cancers can be cured by RT alone.

9. Which of the following can be cured without surgery?
A Leukaemia
B Lymphoma
C Breast cancer
D Anal cancer
E Medulloblastoma.

10. Which of the following statements regarding chemotherapy in cancer treatment are true?
A Cytotoxic drugs are usually used as single agents.
B Cis-platinum acts by inhibition of thymidylate synthase.
C Imatinib is useful in gastrointestinal stromal tumours (GIST).
D Spatial cooperation refers to the combined use of chemotherapy and radiotherapy.
E Synergy refers to use of agents with different modes of actions.

➜ Palliative therapy in cancer

11. Which of the following statements regarding palliative therapy in cancer are true?
A It may involve surgery.
B An early referral may be distressing and hence should be delayed as much as possible.
C Quality-of-life assessment is an important aspect.
D Spiritual support is outside its remit.
E Palliative care is essentially pain control.

➜ End-of-life issues

12. Which of the following are end-of-life issues?
A Active intervention with curative intent
B Euthanasia
C Living wills
D Spirituality
E Bereavement.

Extended matching questions

➜ 1. Treatment options in cancer

A Curative surgery
B Neoadjuvant chemoradiotherapy followed by surgery
C Chemoradiotherapy
D Palliative surgery
E Adjuvant chemotherapy
F Surgery for secondaries
G Palliative care

Choose and match the correct treatment option with each of the scenarios below:

1 A 60-year-old man has had a right hemicolectomy for a caecal carcinoma. The pathologist has graded it to be a Duke's C tumour T3 N1 (2/20) M0 R0. He is fit and keen on any further treatment if indicated.

2 A 92-year-old man who underwent a previous operation for rectal cancer presents with symptoms of intestinal obstruction. CT scan reveals disseminated intra-abdominal cancer with multiple liver and lung metastases.

3 A 50-year-old female presents with anaemia. Colonoscopy reveals a small caecal tumour confirmed on biopsy to be malignant. CT scan does not show any evidence of local or distant spread.

4 A 56-year-old fit male who underwent surgery for colonic carcinoma 3 years ago is observed to have raised carcinoembryonic antigen (CEA) levels. CT scan shows a small solitary left-lobe metastasis. Positron emission tomography (PET) scan does not show any evidence of extrahepatic spread.

5 A 68-year-old male presents with rectal bleeding and alteration in his bowels. Investigations reveal a low rectal cancer and MRI scan stages this as T3b N1. There is no evidence of distant spread.

6 A 78-year-old male presents with a lump at the anal margin. Biopsies from these confirm a squamous cell carcinoma (SCC). He is very keen to avoid a stoma.

7 A 46-year-old female with known ovarian carcinoma presents with features of intestinal obstruction. CT suggests a localised mass which is causing the obstruction. She is otherwise fit and keen on any treatment for her bowel problem.

→ 2. Mechanisms of action of drugs used in cancer

A Cis-platinum
B Vincristine
C 5-Fluorouracil (5-FU)
D Methotrexate
E Cyclophosphamide
F Irinotecan
G Imatinib
H Tamoxifen

Choose and match the correct drug with each of the mechanisms of action below:

1 Inhibition of mutant c-KIT

2 Interferes with the formation of microtubules – spindle poisons

3 Blocks oestrogen receptor

4 This is a prodrug which, on conversion, causes DNA cross-linkages

5 Forms adducts between DNA strands and interferes with replication

6 Inhibits topoisomerase 1 and hence prevents DNA from unwinding and repairing during replication

7 Inhibition of dihydrofolate reductase

8 Inhibition of thymidylate synthase.

→ 3. Appropriate chemotherapeutic agent selection

A Goserelin
B Tamoxifen
C Imatinib

D Vincristine
E Cis-platinum
F Oxaliplatin

Choose and match the correct drug with each of the conditions below:

1 Breast cancer

2 Colorectal cancer

3 GIST

4 Prostate cancer

5 Lymphomas

6 Ovarian cancer.

Answers: Multiple choice questions

➜ Malignant transformation

1. A, B, D, E

The other aspects of malignant transformation include the following: cells establish an autonomous lineage, acquire independence from signals stimulating growth, evade apoptosis, acquire the ability to invade, acquire the ability to disseminate and implant, genomic instability, jettison excess baggage and subvert communication to and from the environment/milieu.

➜ Gompertzian growth

2. A, B, C, D, E

The growth of a typical human tumour can be described by an exponential relationship, the doubling time of which increases exponentially – so-called Gompertzian growth. In its early stages growth is exponential, but as the tumour grows, the growth rate slows. The decrease in growth rate is probably because of difficulties in nutrition and oxygenation. The tumour cells are in competition not only with the host cells but also with one another. Ninety-nine per cent of the cells produced may be lost, mainly by exfoliation, during its growth. A tumour 10 mm in diameter will contain about 10^9 cells, which implies it would take 30 generations to reach the threshold of clinical viability. This has several important implications for the diagnosis and treatment of cancer. By the time they are detected, tumours will have had plenty of time for individual cells to detach, invade, implant and form distant metastases.

➜ Causation of cancer

3. A, B, D

Both environment and inheritance (nature and nurture) are important determinants of whether or not an individual develops cancer. Environmental factors have been implicated in more than 80 per cent of cancers. Genetic factors act along these environmental factors to cause cancer. Familial breast cancer involving BRCA1 and BRCA2 has an autosomal dominant inheritance. Pituitary tumours are a part of MEN type 1 syndrome which also consists of parathyroid and islet cell tumours.

➜ Cancers associated with obesity

4. A, B, C, D, E

Maintaining ideal weight and regular exercise may be helpful in the prevention of many cancers.

→ Cancer screening

5. A, B, D

The other criteria include: treatment at an early stage is more effective than at a later stage; it is sufficiently common to warrant screening; there are safe, inexpensive, adequate diagnostic facilities for those with a positive test; there exists high-quality treatment for screen-detected disease to minimise morbidity and mortality; screening will be repeated at intervals if the disease is of insidious onset; and the benefit must outweigh physical and psychological harm.

→ Staging of colorectal cancer

6. B, E

T3b refers to slight invasion of between 1–5 mm beyond the muscularis propia; T3c is between 5 and 15 mm. V1 refers to extramural vascular invasion. T0 means no evidence of primary tumour.

→ Treatment of cancer

7. C, E

In most cases, the diagnosis of cancer has been made before definitive surgery is carried out, but occasionally a surgical procedure is required to make the diagnosis. It is now recognised that ultraradical surgery probably has little effect on the development of metastases. It is important, however, to appreciate that high-quality meticulous surgery, taking care not to disrupt the primary tumour at the time of excision, is of the utmost importance in obtaining a cure and preventing local recurrence. Surgery can be extremely valuable for palliation in some cases.

8. A, D, E

Repair half-times are typically 3–6 h. Fractionation offers a means whereby any differentials in repair capacity between the tumour and normal cells can be exploited. Hypoxic cells are relatively radio-resistant compared with well oxygenated cells. Normal cells are well oxygenated and tumour cells are hypoxic – this is an obvious therapeutic disadvantage. Repopulation is a phenomenon whereby when RT kills cancer cells, rapid proliferation of cancer cells is stimulated. It is thus better if the overall treatment time is as short as possible. The sensitivities of the cells to RT varies within the cell cycle. It is hence beneficial to synchronise the RT with the most vulnerable phases of the cell cycle.

9. A, B, D, E

The other malignancies with potentially curative non-surgical treatment include small-cell lung cancer, tumours of childhood, such as rhabdomyosarcoma and Wilm's tumour, early laryngeal cancer, cancer of the cervix, medulloblastoma and skin cancers.

10. C, D, E

Cytotoxic agents are rarely used as single agents and they are usually used in combinations which are proven to be effective. Agents are selected which have different modes of action and non-overlapping toxicities. Cis-platinum acts by forming adducts between DNA strands and interferes with replication.

→ Palliative therapy in cancer

11. A, C

The aim of palliative therapy will be growth control and improving quality of life rather than extirpation of every last cancer cell. Transition from curative care to palliative care should be seamless. The most important factor in the successful palliative management of a patient is that a referral is made early enough in the course of the disease. Palliative care is much more than pain control and includes several other issues such as symptom relief, quality-of-life assessment, psychosocial interventions, physical and practical support, information and knowledge, nutritional support, social support, financial support and spiritual support.

End-of-life issues

12. B, C, D, E

End-of-life care is distinct from palliative care – end-of-life care concerns the last few months of a patient's life. Many issues such as symptom control are common to both areas. Problems more relevant to the feelings of approaching death include spiritual need, profound fear and the specific needs of those who are facing bereavement. The other issues at the end of life are appropriateness of active intervention, physician-assisted suicide, support to allow death at home and the problem of medicalisation of death.

Answers: Extended matching questions

1. Treatment options in cancer

1E, 2G, 3A, 4F, 5B, 6C, 7D

2. Mechanisms of action of drugs used in cancer

1G, 2B, 3H, 4E, 5A, 6F, 7D, 8C

3. Appropriate chemotherapeutic agent selection

1B, 2F, 3C, 4A, 5D, 6E

8 Surgical audit and research

Multiple choice questions

Audit

1. **Which of the following statements regarding audit are true?**

A It addresses clearly defined questions, aims and objectives.
B It measures against a standard.
C It may involve randomisation.
D Re-audit is not necessary.
E There is no allocation to intervention group.

Research studies

2. **Which of the following statements regarding research are true?**

A A cross-sectional study is one where a series of patients with a particular disease or condition are compared with matched control patients.
B Type 1 error is when benefit is perceived when really there is none (false positive).
C Randomised trials are essential for testing new drugs.
D It is a common practice to set the level of power for the study at 80 per cent with a 5 per cent significance level.
E A single-blind study is when the clinician is unaware of the treatment allocation.

Statistical analysis in research

3. **Which of the following statements regarding statistical analysis in research are true?**

A Range is the value with the highest frequency observed.
B Unpaired *t*-test is used to compare two groups which are numerical and normally distributed.
C A confidence interval which includes zero usually implies a lack of statistical significance.
D A *P*-value of <0.5 is commonly taken to imply a true difference.
E Chi-squared tests are useful in comparing two groups that are categorical.

Research

4. **Which of the following questions should be answered before undertaking research?**

A Why do the study?
B Will it answer a useful question?
C Will there be any financial incentives?
D Is it practical?
E What impact will it have?

Electronic information sites

5. **Which of the following are electronic information sites?**

A Medline
B EMBASE
C ERIC
D NRES
E Omni.

Extended matching questions

1. Types of research study

A Observational
B Case–control

C Cross-sectional
D Longitudinal
E Randomised
F Randomised controlled

Choose and match the correct study with each of the descriptions below:

1 Two randomly allocated treatments are compared.

2 Series of patients with a particular disease or condition are compared with matched control patients.

3 A condition or treatment is evaluated in a defined population. This study can either be prospective or retrospective.

4 This study involves a control group who receives standard treatment.

5 Measurements made on a single occasion, not looking at the whole population but selecting a small similar group and expanding results.

6 Measurements are taken over a period of time, not looking at the whole population but selecting a small similar group and expanding results.

2. Statistical tests

A Paired *t*-test
B Unpaired *t*-test
C Mann-Whitney *U*-test
D Wilcoxon's signed-rank test
E Chi-squared test

Choose and match the correct test with each of the scenarios below:

1 To compare two groups which are numerical but not normally distributed

2 To compare two groups which are categorical

3 To assess whether a variable has changed between two time points in numerical and normally distributed data

4 To assess whether a variable has changed between two time points in numerical but not normally distributed data

5 To compare two groups which are numerical and normally distributed.

Answers: Multiple choice questions

Audit

1. B, E

Clinical audit is a process used by clinicians who seek to improve patient care. The process involves comparing aspects of care (structure, process and outcome) against explicit criteria. An audit study is designed and conducted to produce information to inform the delivery of best care. This is designed to answer the question: Does the service reach a pre-determined standard? This does not involve randomisation or allocation to intervention group, which is seen in a research study. It usually involves analysis of existing data but may include administration of simple interviews or questionnaires. Re-audit is an important part to close the loop.

→ Research studies

2. B, C, D

Research is designed to generate new knowledge and might involve testing a new treatment or regimen. A research study addresses clearly defined questions, aims and objectives. It is of two broad types: quantitative and qualitative. Quantitative research is designed to test a hypothesis, which may involve evaluating or comparing interventions, particularly new ones. The study design may involve allocating patients to intervention groups. Qualitative research identifies/explores themes following established methodology and usually involves the way in which interventions and relationships are experienced. This uses a clearly defined sampling framework underpinned by conceptual or theoretical justifications.

A single-blind study is when the patient is unaware of the treatment allocation. A case–control study is one where a series of patients with a particular disease or condition are compared with matched control patients. A cross-sectional study is one where measurements are made on a single occasion, not looking at the whole population but selecting a small similar group and expanding results.

→ Statistical analysis in research

3. B, C, E

Mean (average) is the result of dividing the total by the number of observations. Median is the middle value with an equal number of observations above and below – used for numerical or ranked data. Mode is the value with the highest frequency observed – used for nominal data collection. Range is the largest to the smallest value.

The most important decision for analysis is whether the distribution of results is normal, i.e. parametric or non-parametric. Normally distributed results have a symmetrical, bell-shaped curve. The mean, median and the mode all lie at the same value.

When analysing numerical and normally distributed data (e.g. blood pressure), *t*-test is used to compare two groups, and a paired *t*-test to assess if a variable has changed between two time points. When analysing numerical but not normally distributed data (e.g. tumour size), a Mann–Whitney *U*-test is used to compare two groups and Wilcoxon's signed-rank test to assess if a variable has changed between two time points.

When dealing with categorical data (e.g. admission to ITU), a chi-squared test is used to compare two groups.

A *P*-value <0.05 is commonly taken to imply a true difference. This simply means that there is only a 1 in 20 chance that the difference between the variables would have happened by chance when there was no real difference.

→ Research

4. A, B, D, E

The other questions to be asked are: 'Can it be accomplished in the available time and with the available resources?' and 'What findings are expected?'

→ Electronic information sites

5. A, B, C, E

National Research Ethics Service (NRES) provides guidance regarding independent ethical review of all health and social care research.

Answers: Extended matching questions

→ 1. Types of research study

1E, 2B, 3A, 4F, 5C, 6D

→ 2. Statistical tests

1C, 2E, 3A, 4D, 5B

9 Surgical ethics

Multiple choice questions

informed consent

1. Which of the following statements are true with regard to Informed consent?

A Consent should be obtained by the person doing the operation.
B The written communication material must always be in English.
C Consent is necessary before physical examination of a patient.
D Every possible hazard, however remote the possibility, should be explained in detail.
E Legally, a signed consent from a patient is proof that valid consent has been properly obtained

Consent in difficult situations

2. In difficult situations, which of the following statements are true?

A There is no need to explain to children the procedures for which consent has already been given by their parent/guardian.
B Children can unconditionally refuse treatment.
C In patients who cannot give consent because of their illness, e.g. they are unconscious or there is psychiatric illness, their legal guardian can give consent.
D Therapy can proceed after consent from a carer in an unconscious patient irrespective of any previous wishes of the patient.

Matters of life and death

3. In matters of life and death, which of the following are true statements?

A The surgeon is always obliged to provide life-sustaining treatment.
B Decision to withhold treatment should be taken along with another senior clinician and recorded in detail.
C In palliation for pain in advanced malignancy, a potential lethal dose of analgesia is appropriate.
D Confidentiality is absolute.

Answers: Multiple choice questions

Informed consent

1. A, C

The surgeon who will carry out the operation should take the consent. The obtaining of consent should not be delegated to a junior member of the team who has not performed the procedure. Informed consent must be obtained before starting treatment. Informed consent denotes that patients understand what they are consenting to. Patients must be given information and choices so that they can make subsequent plans and decisions in future. They must be given appropriate and accurate information to agree to undergo surgical treatment and in a language that they can understand. Information should consist of: the condition and the reason for the operation; the type of operation; the prognosis with anticipated side-effects; unexpected complications; any alternative but successful treatment; and the outcome of not having the procedure carried out. Patients should be given the chance to ask questions and voice any misgivings.

The communication need not always be in English as the patient may not speak or understand English. Written and verbal communication in the patient's preferred language, by the use of an interpreter, should be given with adequate time for patients to mull over the advice given, so as to be able to make up their own mind.

Prior to touching a patient for physical examination, consent must be obtained; otherwise it constitutes battery. However, this is unnecessary every time a patient is to be touched while under the care of the surgeon. Implied consent will have been given by the patient once an initial consent has been taken.

It is not necessary to inform of every possible hazard, however remote the possibility. Surgeons should inform patients of hazards that any reasonable person in their position would like to know. A signed consent form is no proof that a valid consent has been properly obtained. Patients can and do sometimes deny that they were given appropriate information. Surgeons should therefore record in the notes details of information given, particularly about complications.

➜ Consent in difficult situations

2. C

The surgeon must take care to explain to children in layperson's terms the proposed treatment, and where possible their views should be sought. This is in keeping with patient autonomy, for both adults and children. 'Under English law, children can provide their own consent to surgical care, although they cannot unconditionally refuse it until they are 18 years old.' Notwithstanding this statement, the surgeon must respect the child's autonomy with regard to the surgical management.

In the presence of psychiatric illness or mental handicap, the legal guardian can give consent. In patients who are detained for compulsory psychiatric care, their competence to consent to surgical treatment should be assumed and hence consent sought. If they are incompetent to provide consent, then life-saving surgical treatment can proceed. If adult patients are permanently incompetent to give consent for surgery, treatment can proceed to save life or prevent disability. The exception to this rule is when the patient has already drawn up a legally valid document refusing specific intervention – 'a living will'.

➜ Matters of life and death

3. B, C

The surgeon is not obliged to provide or continue life-sustaining treatment in the following cases: if doing so is futile; death is imminent and irreversible; there is permanent brain damage. A decision to withhold treatment should be taken in consultation with a senior colleague. All details of decisions and conversations should be recorded.

There are circumstances when palliation for disseminated and inoperable cancer is becoming increasingly difficult. The management of pain under such circumstances may require analgesia in doses that may cause respiratory depression, thus hastening death. This is legally justifiable on the premise of 'double effect' – pain relief and death might follow.

A surgeon must not discuss a patient's clinical condition with anyone else without the patient's explicit consent; to do so would incur the wrath of the General Medical Council. Nevertheless, this is not absolute. Surgeons may communicate with other members of the multidisciplinary team should this information help in the patient's management. When patients consent to a treatment plan, they have given implied consent. Confidentiality cannot be strictly adhered to if doing so poses a serious threat to the health and safety of others, if there is a court order, or in an attempt to prevent serious crime or protect individuals who may be at risk.

10 Diagnostic imaging

Multiple choice questions

Hazards of imaging and radiation

1. Which of the following statements are true?

A Low-osmolality contrast media (LOCM) are safer than their higher-osmolality counterparts.
B Routine steroid prophylaxis is recommended before use of contrast in the high-risk patient.
C In the diabetic, metformin should be stopped before using contrast.
D The majority of ionising radiation comes from medical exposure from investigations.
E Portable X-ray machines use much more radiation to achieve the same result.

Diagnostic imaging

2. Which of the following statements is false?

A Conventional X-rays will delineate different soft tissues reliably.
B Conventional X-rays can be manipulated.
C Dedicated transducers can help in endocavitary ultrasound (US).
D Change in the frequency of an US wave can be caused by red blood cells.
E The higher the frequency of the US wave, the greater the resolution of the image.

3. Which of the following statements are true about diagnostic imaging?

A US has no disadvantages.
B Computed tomography (CT) scan has a higher resolution than plain radiographs.
C Magnetic resonance imaging (MRI) scans give excellent contrast resolution.
D MRI scan has no disadvantages.
E Radionuclide imaging allows function to be studied.

Orthopaedic imaging

4. In orthopaedic imaging, which of the following statements are false?

A Synovitis can be detected by plain X-ray.
B MR arthrography is the ideal imaging for articular cartilage damage.
C MRI is the ideal method of staging a malignant bone tumour.
D X-ray is the first investigation in destructive bone lesions.
E US is used to examine mass lesions of soft tissues.
F Plain film of a joint is best for suspected acute joint infection.

Imaging in trauma

5. In trauma imaging, which of the following statements are false?

A In a multiply injured patient, CT of head and spine should be the first line of imaging.
B Focused assessment with sonography for trauma (FAST) helps in detecting intraperitoneal fluid and cardiac tamponade.
C CT should not be used when a patient is unstable.
D US is useful for diagnosing occult pneumothorax.
E CT is the main imaging method for intracranial, intra-abdominal and vertebral injuries.
F Use of MRI in trauma is limited.

Imaging in the acute abdomen

6. Which of the following statements are false with regard to imaging of the acute abdomen?

A US is a good first-line investigation.
B CT is the best investigation for acute diverticulitis.
C Plain X-ray of KUB (kidney, ureter, bladder) is the best imaging for suspected ureteric colic.
D US and CT can diagnose the cause and site of bowel obstruction.
E Plain X-ray is the first-line investigation for suspected perforation or obstruction.

Imaging in oncology

7. Which of the following statements about oncological imaging are true?

A Early disease is best staged by endoscopic US.
B Accurate preoperative nodal involvement is not possible.
C Liver and lung metastases are best detected by US and CT.
D Intraoperative US is used in liver resection.

Answers: Multiple choice questions

Hazards of imaging and radiation

1. A, E

For contrast-enhanced computed tomography (CECT) scan, LOCM are much safer than the higher-osmolality agents. The Royal College of Radiologists (RCR) in the UK does not recommend routine steroid prophylaxis for high-risk patients. The use of LOCM and close observation of the patient for 30 min after injection is recommended with the cannula still in situ. Most reactions occur shortly after injection.

The RCR recommend that metformin can be continued and no more than 100 mL of LOCM can be given in the presence of normal renal function. A recent serum creatinine should be done as all contrast media are nephrotoxic. In patients with a history of iodine allergy, gadolinium diethyltriaminepentacetic acid (DTPA) can be used. Mild reactions can occur in 1:200 and severe reactions in 1:10 000 patients.

The majority of ionising radiation in the human comes from natural sources, medical exposure accounting for only 12 per cent. Portable X-ray machines should be avoided as much as possible. Along with fluoroscopy, these imaging equipments use much more radiation to obtain the same result.

Diagnostic imaging

2. A

Different soft tissues cannot be reliably distinguished as all soft tissues contain the same quantity of water. In certain circumstances, however, such as mammography, by manipulating the X-ray systems and X-ray energies, differentiation between the different types of soft tissues can be obtained.

Ultrasound is the second most common method of imaging. Special transducers have been developed for intracavitary imaging, such as transvaginal, transrectal and endoscopic (of oesophagus and stomach). The latter not only allows imaging of the wall of the viscus but also of the adjacent structures such as mediastinal lymph nodes in oesophageal US and the pancreas in gastric US. The higher the frequency of the US wave, the greater is the resolution of the image.

A change in the frequency of the US wave can be caused by moving objects such as red blood cells. This change in frequency helps to measure the speed and direction of movement – the principle of Doppler US (Christian Johann Doppler, a Viennese Professor of experimental physics, articulated his principle in 1842), which can record the speed of blood flow through a vessel or a solid organ – thus diagnosing stenosis within a vessel wall.

3. B, C, E

Ultrasound has its drawbacks: it is very operator-dependent; the information is mostly useful during the actual scanning process so that images cannot be reliably reviewed by looking at static pictures; it does not go through air and bone; resolution depends upon the machine used; and the process has a long learning curve.

Computed tomography scan has a high contrast resolution, allowing the assessment of tissues with similar attenuation characteristics. The injection of contrast allows images at various phases of the blood supply, the early arterial phase, for example, in vascular liver lesions and the delayed pictures for solid renal lesions.

Magnetic resonance imaging gives excellent contrast resolution without any radiation hazard. It lends itself to imaging particularly of tissues with relatively little natural contrast. MRI does have some downsides: there is limited availability because of expense; it is time-consuming; and the patient needs to be motionless, making it difficult in those with pain. Those patients with metallic implants cannot be examined because the investigation entails the use of high-strength magnetic fields.

The use of a radionuclide allows the study of function. The chosen radionuclide – technetium, gallium, thallium, iodine – is coupled with other compounds and administered intravenously for it to be tracked by a gamma camera, thus forming a functional image. Positron emission tomography (PET) is a similar imaging method which is useful in the detection of recurrent cancer, particularly when combined with CT (PET/CT).

→ Orthopaedic imaging

4. A, F

Although radiographs are the first-line imaging used for examination of joints, early synovitis is best detected by gadolinium DTPA-enhanced MRI, which will show up synovial thickening. MRI is the best way to detect articular damage. MR arthrography, where a scan is performed after gadolinium DTPA is injected into the joint, is 'the gold standard'. MRI is the best investigation for staging of bone or soft-tissue malignant tumours. Image-guided (US, CT or MRI) needle biopsy in consultation with the surgeon is then carried out. Bone scan or whole-body MRI is particularly necessary when multiple lesions are suspected.

A plain X-ray is the first imaging technique when a destructive bone lesion is suspected. It also shows up soft-tissue calcification in muscle, tendon and fat. Careful interpretation is essential to distinguish malignant from benign lesions. When malignancy is suspected, further investigations are mandatory to establish a firm diagnosis.

Ultrasound is diagnostic in the majority of mass lesions of soft tissues. When the lesion is cystic, it obviates the need for further imaging. However, if the lesion has a solid element to it, then MRI is performed. In soft-tissue lesions, the routine should be US on all palpable lesions; when there is an unidentifiable mass or the mass is partly solid, then MRI is used.

Ultrasound is the most accurate method of assessing acute inflammation of a joint, as a plain film may be normal unless there is bone erosion. US will detect an effusion which can then be aspirated under US guidance.

→ Imaging in trauma

5. A

Initially plain X-rays and not CT will give a rapid assessment of major injuries. Although the areas to be X-rayed will depend upon the mechanism of injury and the condition of the patient (intubated or not), the initial radiographs are X-rays of the chest, an anteroposterior view of the pelvis and the cervical spine (C/S).

Focused assessment with sonography for trauma (FAST), although operator-dependent, is an extremely efficient method to detect intraperitoneal fluid and cardiac tamponade. FAST may not be helpful in the presence of bowel gas or extensive surgical emphysema. A repeat FAST may be used when the initial test has been negative.

The unstable patient needs to be treated forthwith according to the clinical needs and no time should be lost in arranging a CT, which should only be considered in a patient who is holding his own with adequate resuscitation.

Pneumothorax in a supine chest X-ray can be difficult to see. An US using a high-resolution probe will detect the pleura as an echogenic stripe and its movement can be assessed; the sliding motion of the pleura is lost in a pneumothorax; haemothorax can also be diagnosed.

Computed tomography is the ideal method of imaging intracranial and intra-abdominal injuries and vertebral fractures. Using a multidetector scanner a comprehensive examination of the entire body can be completed in 5 min – in far less time than it takes to organise the investigation. Hence this imaging modality should be reserved only for the stable patient.

The value of emergency MRI is limited because of practical problems of accessibility of the ventilated patient with monitoring equipment and MRI compatibility. It is mainly confined to detailed imaging of spinal injuries.

→ Imaging in the acute abdomen

6. C

Ultrasound is a good initial imaging for most acute abdominal conditions – biliary colic, acute cholecystitis, acute appendicitis, acute pancreatitis and pelvic diseases.

When patients present with left iliac fossa pain and a diagnosis of acute diverticulitis is made, CT is the investigation of choice – showing thickening of the bowel wall, paracolic collection and/or abscess. CT-guided drainage of an abscess can also be done.

In suspected ureteric colic (wrongly called renal colic because one cannot get colic in a solid organ), plain X-ray of the KUB area is of limited value. Faecoliths cannot be distinguished from ureteric stones. Unenhanced helical CT is the most sensitive imaging procedure for ureteric colic.

In intestinal obstruction US and CT are useful in showing up dilated fluid-filled loops and can often identify the site and cause of obstruction. CT colonography is increasingly being used in the confirmation of acute large-bowel closed-loop obstruction from carcinoma.

Clinical suspicion of perforation of a hollow viscus is best confirmed by an erect chest X-ray or an abdominal X-ray to include the diaphragmatic domes or lateral decubitus film (if the patient is too ill).

→ Imaging in oncology

7. A, B, C, D

In the staging of early carcinoma (T1 and T2) of distal large bowel, endoluminal ultrasound (EUS) is the imaging of choice. The same is true of early oesophageal cancer. Biopsy is carried out at the same time; however, this should be done only after the US so as not to distort the US images.

Accurate preoperative nodal staging cannot be obtained by EUS. While the size of nodes (pararectal in rectal cancer or mediastinal in oesophageal cancer) gives an idea of nodal involvement, one cannot be absolutely certain as the enlargement can be due to metastasis or reactive hyperplasia.

Ultrasound and CT are the ideal imaging methods to detect haematogenous spread to the lungs and liver. CT is the most sensitive technique for pulmonary deposits. However, occult lesions may be overlooked in 10–30 per cent of patients.

Intraoperative US is routine during liver resection for metastasis. Deep-seated impalpable secondaries may be missed by the conventional preoperative US and CT, particularly if they are smaller than 1 cm. Good high-resolution imaging will detect secondaries as small as 0.5 cm – a finding that will influence the definitive management.

PART 2

Investigation and diagnosis

11 Gastrointestinal endoscopy 103

12 Tissue diagnosis 107

11 Gastrointestinal endoscopy

Multiple choice questions

➜ Sedation in endoscopy

1. Regarding sedation during endoscopy, which of the following statements are false?

A Sedation has no significant dangers and can be used without restrictions.
B All sedated patients require secure intravenous access.
C Co-administration of opiates and benzodiazepines has a synergistic effect.
D The use of supplementary oxygen is essential in all sedated patients.
E All sedated patients require pulse oximetry to monitor oxygen saturations.

➜ Antibiotic prophylaxis in endoscopy

2. In which of the following should antibiotic prophylaxis not be considered?

A Prosthetic heart valves
B Previous history of endocarditis
C Severe neutropenia
D Chronic liver disease undergoing variceal sclerotherapy
E Previous cholecystectomy.

➜ General issues in endoscopy

3. Which of the following statements regarding endoscopy are true?

A It is easy to get views beyond the ligament of Treitz during an oesophagogastroduodenoscopy (OGD) with a standard endoscope.
B The current state-of-the-art endoscope is the fibreoptic endoscope.
C It is not necessary to stop clopidogrel before a colonoscopic polypectomy.
D Verbal consent for an endoscopy is acceptable practice.
E Perforation and haemorrhage are uncommon but significant complications of the procedure.

➜ Post-ERCP pancreatitis

4. Which of the following are not risk factors for post-ERCP (endoscopic retrograde cholangiopancreatography) pancreatitis?

A Young age
B Difficult cannulation
C Increased bilirubin
D Pancreatic sphincterotomy
E Balloon dilatation of biliary sphincter.

➜ Recent trends in endoscopy

5. Which of the following about recent developments in endoscopy are false?

A Chromoendoscopy involves the use of stains or pigments to improve tissue localisation.
B Narrow-band imaging relies on an optical filter technology that radically improves the visibility of veins and capillaries.
C High-resolution magnifying endoscopy achieves near cellular definition of the mucosa.
D Capsule endoscopy acquires video images during natural propulsion through the gut.
E Balloon enteroscopy permits visualisation of the small bowel but is unable to perform therapeutic procedures.

Extended matching questions

1. Endoscopic diagnosis

A Barrett's oesophagus
B Cancer of the oesophagus
C Mallory–Weiss tear
D Peptic stricture
E Hiatus hernia
F Reflux gastritis
G Oesophageal varices
H Linitis plastica
I Gastrointestinal stromal tumour

Choose and match the correct diagnosis with each of the scenarios below:

1 Abnormal veins are seen at the lower end of the oesophagus which are dilated and 'grape-like'.

2 A smooth, tapering stricture is seen at the lower end of the oesophagus along with inflammation and ulceration.

3 A mucosal tear is seen at the cardia with some fresh blood.

4 The pylorus is seen to be wide open with plenty of bile in the stomach. The antrum shows streaks of erythema.

5 The stomach is difficult to distend and appears to have low capacity. The mucosa appears stretched but no mucosal lesion is seen.

6 A submucosal lump is seen. The mucosa is stretched over this lump but is otherwise normal. The superficial endoscopic biopsies confirm the mucosa to be normal.

7 There is an ulcerated and polypoidal mass at the lower end of the oesophagus, causing obstruction.

8 There is evidence of gastro-oesophageal reflux disease (GORD) and a linear tongue of erythematous mucosa extending for 3 cm into the oesophagus above.

9 The gastro-oesophageal junction is at 34 cm with prolapsing fundal mucosa and increased oesophageal fluid.

2. Endoscopic complications

A Bleeding
B Perforation
C Aspiration
D Sedation overdose
E Dental injury

Choose and match the correct diagnosis with each of the scenarios below:

1 An 80-year-old patient who has just had an OGD after local anaesthetic spray has severe coughing and breathing problems after eating a sandwich in the recovery room.

2 Patient collapses and is found to be hypotensive after an endoscopic polypectomy.

3 An 70-year-old male is rushed to the emergency 8 hours after an endoscopic dilatation of an oesophageal stricture complaining of severe chest pain and change in voice.

4 An 86-year-old female patient has pain and bleeding from mouth following an uneventful OGD.

5 An 86-year-old female patient has severe bradycardia and low Po_2 and is difficult to arouse.

Answers: Multiple choice questions

Sedation in endoscopy

1. A

Medication-induced respiratory depression in elderly patients or those with co-morbidities is the greatest cause of endoscopy-related mortality and hence safe sedation practices are essential. Pharyngeal anaesthesia may increase the risk of aspiration in sedated patients. The use of supplemental oxygen and pulse oximetry is essential in all sedated patients. The current guidelines suggest that the dose of sedation is halved in patients over 70 years of age. A trained assistant should be available for patient monitoring throughout the procedure. Resuscitation equipment and sedation reversal agents must be readily available.

Antibiotic prophylaxis in endoscopy

2. E

The majority of endoscopy can be performed safely without the need for routine antibiotic prophylaxis. However, certain endoscopic procedures are associated with a significant bacteraemia. The incidence rates of bacteraemia after a colonoscopy, diagnostic OGD and ERCP for an occluded common bile duct (CBD) are 2–4, 4 and 11 per cent, respectively. In fact, the incidence of bacteraemia can be between 34 and 54 per cent after an oesophageal dilatation. Patients with high-risk conditions such as severe neutropenia, prosthetic heart valves or a previous history of infective endocarditis should have prophylaxis for all endoscopic procedures. Patients with moderate-risk conditions such as mitral valve prolapse with leaflet pathology or regurgitation only require antibiotics for procedures which cause significant bacteraemia. The antibiotic regimen will depend on local policies but a standard protocol is 1 g of amoxicillin and 120 mg of gentamicin IV 5–10 min prior to the procedure (teicoplanin 400mg IV if allergic to penicillin).

General issues in endoscopy

3. E

A diagnostic OGD usually examines up to the second part of the duodenum. The fibreoptic endoscope was the original workhorse but became obsolete after the introduction of the charge-coupled device (CCD) in the 1960s. The CCD allows the creation of a digital electronic image which is processed by a computer and transmitted to a TV monitor. The patient will need to stop clopidogrel prior to a colonoscopic polypectomy to minimise the risks of bleeding. Although endoscopy is safe, it is still associated with rare but potentially life-threatening complications such as bleeding, perforation and sedation-related problems. It is hence mandatory to explain the procedure and complications clearly to the patient and take a fully informed signed consent prior to the procedure. Approximately 1 per cent of medical negligence claims in the USA are related to endoscopic procedures.

Post-ERCP pancreatitis

4. C

The incidence of post-ERCP pancreatitis is around 4.3 per cent. The additional risk factors for this complication include suspected sphincter of Oddi dysfunction (SOD), normal bilirubin, prior ERCP-related pancreatitis and pancreatic duct contrast injection. Possible factors also include female sex, absent CBD stone and low volume of ERCPs performed.

Recent trends in endoscopy

5. E

Balloon enteroscopy allows the direct visualisation of, and therapeutic intervention for, the entire small bowel and may be attempted via the oral or the rectal route.

Answers: Extended matching questions

→ 1. Endoscopic diagnosis

1G
This may be seen in patients with portal hypertension presenting with haematemesis. The varices are usually injected or banded. More rarely, embolisation or vasopressin may be used. Surgery is almost never indicated nowadays except in desperate situations.

2D
This is a complication of long-standing GORD. Barrett's oesophagus may be present. Smooth tapering and absence of shouldering differentiate this from malignancy.

3C
Patients present with severe epigastric pain, retching and mild haematemesis. The clinical differential diagnoses include duodenal perforation, acute pancreatitis, myocardial infarction and oesophageal perforation. Endoscopy confirms the diagnosis, which is self-limiting.

4F
Increased duodenogastric reflux results in bile-induced damage to the pyloric area. CLO test for *H. pylori* should be done.

5H
The mucosa may appear deceptively normal (though a bit stretched) and biopsies may be negative. Patients usually present late and hence this carries a very poor prognosis.

6I
This may be an incidental finding but can cause upper gastrointestinal bleed, which draws attention. Prognosis, though variable, is a lot better than adenocarcinoma. Even advanced cases respond well to imatinib.

7B
This causes profound weight loss and rapidly progressive dysphagia. Staging investigations such as endoscopic US, computed tomography scan and laparoscopy are important before embarking on major resections. Prognosis still remains poor.

8A
This is becoming increasingly important after its association with malignancy was confirmed. The incidence of adenocarcinoma at the lower end of the oesophagus is presently increasing. Barrett's oesophagus showing dysplastic changes needs regular surveillance. There is still some debate about its management but most agree that severe dysplastic changes would be a strong candidate for surgery. Invasive carcinoma may be found in almost half of these cases.

9E
A small hiatus hernia may be an incidental finding. Some are associated with features of reflux oesophagitis. This can rarely present with complications such as incarceration, necrosis and perforation.

→ 2. Endoscopic complications

1C, 2A, 3B, 4E, 5D

12 Tissue diagnosis

Multiple choice questions

→ Specimens for histology

1. Which of the following statements regarding specimens for histology are false?

A They must always be sent fixed in formalin.
B They can be obtained by fine-needle aspiration cytology (FNAC).
C They are classified as biopsies and resections.
D Frozen section histology has many disadvantages.
E Both macroscopic and microscopic findings are reported.

→ Cytology

2. Which of the following statements are true with regard to cytology?

A It gives as much information as histology.
B In some instances, an invasive method has to be used to obtain material.
C A negative cytology has no value.
D There is risk to laboratory personnel associated with cytology and histology.

→ Principles of microscopic diagnosis

3. With regard to microscopic diagnosis, which of the following statements are true?

A Malignancy is diagnosed histologically by invasion, architectural changes and cytological features.
B Dysplasia indicates microscopic features of cancer.
C False-positive diagnosis can occur.
D Tissue assessment helps in prognosis.

→ Inflammation and cytology

4. Which of the following statements is untrue?

A Inflammatory conditions are characterised by the predominant cell type.
B Cytology has some advantages over histology.
C In an ulcerated tissue, ideally cytology and biopsy should be taken from the centre of the lesion.
D Additional techniques may be necessary to elucidate the diagnosis.
E Special stains may sometimes be necessary.

→ Immunohistochemistry

5. Which of the following statements are true with regard to immunohistochemistry?

A This is just a special staining method.
B It relies on the use of a specific antibody.
C It helps to determine cell type and differentiation.
D It has a role in the determination of treatment and prognosis.

→ Special techniques

6. Which of the following statements is false?

A Electron microscopy is routinely used in histology.
B Polymerase chain reaction (PCR) is a useful investigation to detect microorganisms.
C Study of chromosomes (cytogenetics) can be done using fluorescence in-situ hybridisation (FISH).
D Autopsy can only be done with the coroner's permission.

Answers: Multiple choice questions

➜ Specimens for histology

1. A, B

All specimens need not be sent fixed in formalin (10 per cent formaldehyde). Samples for routine histology are sent fixed. Fresh tissue samples are sent for frozen section, when microbiological assessment is necessary as in suspected tuberculosis. In such a situation, a part of an excised lymph node is sent fresh and the remainder is fixed in formalin.

Fine-needle aspiration cytology only gives cytology; compared with histology, it has a limited value. Cytology gives an idea about the cell type. FNAC is an invasive method and is helpful in breast and thyroid lumps and in lymphadenopathy. In certain situations, FNAC needs to be carried out under CT or ultrasound guidance.

While biopsy means any tissue sample, histology specimens are classified as biopsies and resections. Types of biopsy include punch biopsy, as in skin lesions, and core biopsy as in Tru-Cut of breast lump or a prostatic nodule. Biopsy following a resection is usually also therapeutic as in small ulcerated skin lesions.

The speed of a diagnosis after frozen section is outweighed by many disadvantages: the patient will not have a preoperative diagnosis and so cannot make an informed choice with regard to the definitive treatment; the tissue is not fixed and so there is a risk of infection to laboratory staff; the quality is inferior, thereby compromising diagnostic accuracy; the procedure is time-consuming.

Any specimen sent for histology is first sliced up into parts depending upon the size, fixed in formalin, and after about 24 h a description of the macroscopic appearance is reported. Slices for microscopic examination are then reported. Report from a malignant specimen will include resection margins, tumour, lymph nodal status and neighbouring non-neoplastic tissue.

➜ Cytology

2. B. C, D

Cytology does not give as much information as histology. It is a study of cells and gives an idea about the presence of malignancy. Therefore, in a breast lump, cancer can be established by FNAC. A Tru-Cut biopsy gives histological tissue which helps to grade the tumour, may show the presence of perivascular and lymphovascular invasion, and gives an idea of the oestrogen receptor status. There is always a risk for transmissable infection, such as hepatitis B or tuberculosis, particularly when fresh tissue is being sent.

In some instances, cells for cytology can be obtained only by invasive techniques, e.g. CT guidance for mediastinal lymph nodes, transbronchial fine-needle aspiration for mediastinal masses or fine-needle aspiration of liver, pancreas and kidney. A negative cytology has no value. Absence of cancer cells from an FNAC may mean that the incorrect tissue has been needled.

➜ Principles of microscopic diagnosis

3. A, B, C, D

Features confirming a histological diagnosis of malignancy are invasion of neighbouring tissue, blood vessels and lymphatics; architectural changes; atypical mitotic figures; and nuclear abnormalities of hyperchromatism and pleomorphism.

Dysplasia is a term used to indicate microscopic features of cancer. It is graded as mild, moderate and severe. Severe dysplasia is regarded by most as indicating carcinoma in situ, e.g. colorectal carcinoma in inflammatory bowel disease, oesophageal carcinoma in Barrett's oesophagus or cervical intraepithelial neoplasia.

False-positive diagnosis can occur from contamination or interchanging of tissue, pitfalls in interpretation which are best avoided by good clinical details. A history of previous radiotherapy must be disclosed to the pathologist, as radiotherapy changes may mimic cancer.

Prognosis can be determined by tissue assessment. Stage is the important prognostic factor according to the UICC (Union Internationale contre le Cancer). Grade is determined microscopically: low-grade, well-differentiated tumours have a good prognosis as opposed to poorly differentiated, high-grade tumours. Vascular and perineural invasion with positive resection margins carry a poor prognosis.

Inflammation and cytology

4. C

The type of cell does determine the type of inflammation. Polymorphonuclear leucocytosis indicates acute inflammation. Presence of lymphocytes and plasma cells are seen in chronic inflammation. Eosinophilia indicates parasitic infestation. Granulomas, a collection of epithelioid histiocytes, are seen in mycobacterial infection (tuberculosis and leprosy), fungal infection and as a foreign body reaction.

Cytology does have some advantages over histology: a wider area may be sampled; it is less invasive, fast and cheap; and non-medical staff can be trained in its interpretation.

When taking a piece of tissue for biopsy (incision biopsy), it should be taken from the periphery with some apparently normal tissue. This enables interpretation of invasiveness and architectural changes. A sample from the centre of an ulcer may only show necrosis and non-viable tissue.

In a minority of difficult situations, further specimens may need to be obtained from deeper levels with extra blocks, as in linitis plastica. Special stains and immunohistochemistry are additional techniques available.

Special stains are used when routine ones do not provide the answer. For example, the periodic acid-Schiff (PAS) stain demonstrates glycogen and mucin; a diastase PAS (D-PAS) stain shows up mucin in adenocarcinoma. Iron accumulation, as in haemochromatosis, is demonstrated by Perls' Prussian blue stain. Fibrosis is shown up by reticulin stain while Congo red shows up amyloidosis.

Immunohistochemistry

5. A, B, C, D

This technique is a special staining method. It detects a specific antigen using a specific antibody which is labelled with a dye and, when bound to its target antigen, is seen as a coloured stain. It determines cell type and differentiation and site of origin. The method has a role in the selection of treatment and in the prediction of prognosis. It also has a role in infections. There are antibodies to many infective agents such as cytomegalovirus (CMV), Epstein–Barr virus (EBV), herpes virus and hepatitis B.

Special techniques

6. A, D

Electron microscopy is time-consuming, labour-intensive and expensive and is used selectively. PCR amplifies DNA. The amplified DNA is detected using techniques such as electrophoresis. The technique is used to detect chromosomal abnormalities and microorganisms. The study of chromosomes, called cytogenetics, is done using the FISH technique. Autopsy does not always require the coroner's permission; it can be done for the purpose of medical education and audit with the consent of the next of kin.

PART 3

Perioperative care

13 Preoperative preparation 113

14 Anaesthesia and pain relief 118

15 Care in the operating room 122

16 The high-risk surgical patient 124

17 Nutrition and fluid therapy 127

18 Basic surgical skills and anastomosis 135

19 Laparoscopic and robotic surgery 137

20 Postoperative care 144

13 Preoperative preparation

Multiple choice questions

➜ Preoperative patient preparation

1. Which of the following are true of preoperative patient preparation?

A It includes a thorough history-taking and medical examination.
B The patient's medical state is optimised
C It is to anticipate and plan for management of perioperative problems.
D Good communication is required.
E It involves taking informed consent.

➜ Preoperative investigations

2. Which of the following statements regarding preoperative investigations are true?

A Chest X-ray is routinely requested in all patients over 60 years old.
B A ventricular ejection fraction of less than 35 per cent indicates a high risk of cardiac complications.
C A body mass index (BMI) <15 is associated with significant hospital mortality.
D ECG is usually required in patients above 65 years.
E HIV testing requires patient consent.

➜ Preoperative management

3. Which of the following statements regarding preoperative management of specific medical problems are true?

A Patients with a diastolic pressure above 95 mmHg should have their elective operations postponed.
B Elective surgery should be delayed until at least 1 year after a myocardial infarction (MI).
C There is no need to control tachyarrhythmias preoperatively.
D Preoperative transfusion should be considered if the Hb level <10 g/dL.
E In patients with malnutrition, preoperative nutrition therapy should be started 2 weeks prior to surgery.

➜ Surgery in obese patients

4. Which of the following is a problem associated with surgery in obese patients?

A Myocardial infarction
B Aspiration
C Deep vein thrombosis (DVT)/embolism
D Pressure sore
E Pain control.

➜ Surgery in the jaundiced patient

5. Which of the following is a problem associated with surgery in the jaundiced patient?

A Clotting disorders
B Hepatorenal syndrome
C Infection
D Poor wound healing
E Myocardial infarction.

➜ Surgery in the diabetic patient

6. Which of the following is a surgical risk in a diabetic patient?

A Infection
B Myocardial infarction
C Pressure sore
D Poor wound healing
E Pain control.

➜ DVT risks

7. Which of the following is a risk factor for thrombosis?

A Young age
B Pregnancy
C Smoking
D Trauma
E Malignancy.

➜ Consent for surgery

8. Regarding consent for surgery, which of the following are true?

A Children below the age of 16 years cannot give consent.
B A social worker can give consent for a child under a care order.
C All minor complications with an incidence above 1 per cent should be discussed.
D Consent is not required for life-saving surgery in a competent patient.
E Two senior doctors need to sign the form explaining reasons for the actions if an adult is deemed not competent to consent.

Extended matching questions

➜ 1. Potential operative and postoperative risk factors

A Difficult intubation
B Aspiration
C Poor wound healing
D Postoperative infection
E Increased need for postoperative admission to an intensive treatment unit (ITU)
F DVT/pulmonary embolism (PE)
G MI.

Choose and match the correct diagnosis with each of the scenarios below:

1 A 76-year-old female is scheduled to have an elective operation on her bowels. She is known to have severe and long-standing chronic obstructive pulmonary disease (COPD).

2 A 66-year-old male needs to have an urgent abdominal operation. He has had type 2 diabetes for the past 15 years and the control has been erratic.

3 A 72-year-old male has had an MI 2 months ago. He has now been diagnosed to have cancer of the caecum which requires urgent surgery.

4 A 70-year-old woman with long-standing rheumatoid arthritis and an unstable cervical spine needs to have an emergency laparotomy for a perforated peptic ulcer.

5 A 60-year-old obese female is scheduled to have an abdominal operation. She has a history of previous DVT and has not been mobile for the last 2 months.

6 An 86-year-old male is scheduled to have an operation for his bowel carcinoma. He is malnourished and jaundiced.

7 A 45-year-old obese male known to have a hiatus hernia presents with symptoms and signs of small-bowel obstruction, for which he is due to have an operation.

➜ 2. Perioperative medications/interventions

A Antihypertensives
B Steroids
C Diabetic medications – minor surgery
D Warfarin for AF
E Smoking

F Preoperative nutritional support
G Insulin – major surgery
H Anticonvulsants.

Choose and match the correct condition with each of the interventions below:

1 Sliding scale and IV fluids.

2 Should be continued perioperatively and be changed to IV forms if starvation is prolonged.

3 This is stopped 3–4 days prior to surgery and restarted on the evening after the surgery.

4 The medications can be given up to the time of surgery and then selectively as required in the immediate postoperative period. The previous dose will need to be recommenced once the patient recovers from surgery.

5 This should be given for at least 2 weeks preoperatively to have any real benefit.

6 This should be stopped at least a month prior to elective surgery.

7 The dose on the morning of surgery should be omitted and medications recommenced once the patient has started eating.

8 Patients who have been receiving this on a regular basis (and have received this within the past 2 months) will require increased doses to avoid a crisis.

Answers: Multiple choice questions

➜ Preoperative patient preparation

1. A, B, C, D, E

A consultant surgeon leads a large team of people involved in safely seeing a patient through their individual operating experience. A trainee is a key member of that team. The trainee hence has various responsibilities and duties that are essential for a safe patient journey.

Recording information accurately, completely and legibly is of paramount importance. The medical file is a long-lasting record of all aspects of patient care, including the history, examination findings, investigations, diagnosis, treatment and the progress/problems encountered from admission to discharge. It is a legally admissible document and would be a reflection of the quality of care delivered by the team.

Good preoperative planning to optimise medical problems before surgery minimises risk and maximises benefits. All medical problems should be identified, assessed and addressed before an elective operation. In an emergency setting, there should be a balance between potential harm caused by delay against benefits of treating medical problems prior to surgery.

Anticipating adverse events allows many of them to be avoided. Inevitably, things do not turn out as expected – comprehensive planning will allow contingency plans to be made for immediate implementation.

Good communication with the patient and amongst the members of the team is vital. This is especially important in the increasing 'shift work' culture imposed by the European Working Time Directive and during handover before weekends/to the on-call team.

➜ Preoperative investigations

2. B, C, D, E

Investigations should only be ordered when clinically indicated. Most hospitals have protocols to guide preoperative investigation requests. The request forms need to be filled out legibly and completely, giving relevant clinical details. The results should be checked promptly, recorded and appropriate actions instituted.

A preoperative full blood count (FBC) is needed in all operations where significant blood loss is expected, in menorrhagia and in the case of any other known chronic blood loss and elderly patients.

Urea and electrolytes (U&E) are normally required in all patients over 65, in patients who may lose a significant amount of blood in theatre, those with a history of cardiac, pulmonary or renal problems and in patients on regular diuretics.

Liver function tests (LFTs) are indicated in patients with jaundice, cirrhosis, known or suspected hepatitis, malignancy, portal hypertension, poor nutritional reserves or clotting problems. Clotting screen is indicated in any patient on anticoagulants, with compromised liver function or evidence of bleeding diathesis.

Arterial blood gases (ABGs) are occasionally required for detailed assessment of chronic respiratory conditions. Electrocardiogram (ECG) is indicated in all patients over 65, those with a history of cardiovascular, pulmonary or anaesthetic problems and before major operations where significant blood losses are expected.

Chest X-ray is not usually required unless the patient has a significant cardiac history or respiratory problems. Dipstick analysis of urine is usually carried out routinely preoperatively. It can detect urinary infection, biliuria, glycosuria and inappropriate osmolality.

→ Preoperative management

3. A, E

Patients with systolic pressures of 160 mmHg or above should have elective surgery deferred. Newly diagnosed hypertension may require investigations to look for an underlying cause.

Recent MI is a strong contraindication to elective anaesthesia. There is significant mortality from anaesthesia within 3 months of infarction. Elective surgery should ideally be delayed until at least 6 months have elapsed. Fast atrial fibrillation (AF) must be controlled before surgery. Second- and third-degree blocks may require pacing preoperatively.

Preoperative transfusion should be considered if the preoperative Hb < 8 g/dL. Preoperative antibiotic cover is usually necessary in patients with prosthetic or leaky cardiac valves. Significant lower respiratory tract infections should be treated before surgery except when it is life-threatening.

→ Surgery in obese patients

4. A, B, C, D

The other problems of surgery in the obese include difficult intubation, cardiovascular accident (CVA), respiratory compromise, poor wound healing, infection and mechanical problems such as lifting, transferring and operating table weight limits.

→ Surgery in the jaundiced patient

5. A, B, C, D

Infective causes of jaundice may pose a risk to members of staff potentially exposed to body fluids.

→ Surgery in the diabetic patient

6. A, B, C, D

Diabetic patients are at high risk of complications. A careful preoperative assessment of their cardiovascular, peripheral vascular and neurological status should always be made. Other complications that occur more often in diabetics include CVA, renal problems and problems with fluid and electrolyte balance.

→ DVT risks

7. B, C, D, E

There are well defined risk factors for DVT including age > 40 years, burns, major surgery, hip and other joint surgery, paraplegia, lower limb amputation and family history or previous personal history.

→ Consent for surgery

8. B, C, E

The person obtaining the consent must be fully conversant with planned surgery, including possible complications and alternatives. There should be a structured approach to obtaining consent. Firstly, the patient's demographic details should be checked. Secondly, the planned operation should be outlined and confirmed with the patient. Alternative treatments and all complications that are significant or have an incidence of at least 1 per cent or more should be discussed. Finally, it is important to ensure that the patient has understood what has been discussed and has no more questions, before being asked to sign.

Answers: Extended matching questions

→ 1. Potential operative and postoperative risk factors

1E, 2D, 3G, 4A, 5F, 6C, 7B

→ 2. Perioperative medications/interventions

1G, 2H, 3D, 4A, 5F, 6E, 7C, 8B

14 Anaesthesia and pain relief

Multiple choice questions

For the following questions, choose the single best answer.

➜ The anaesthetic triad

1. Which of the following is not part of the anaesthetic triad used during surgery?

A Unconsciousness
B Pain relief
C Amnesia
D Muscle relaxation.

➜ Laryngeal mask airway

2. What is the most significant disadvantage of the laryngeal mask airway (LMA) over an endotracheal tube?

A Failure to provide a competent airway
B Risk of pulmonary aspiration
C Unreliable placement
D Enhanced risk of tube obstruction
E Failure to allow tracheal suction.

➜ Correct placement of an endotracheal tube

3. What is the most reliable way to ascertain correct placement of an endotracheal tube?

A Detection of a pressure waveform on inflation
B Direct visualization
C Detection of breath sounds on auscultation
D Measurement of end-tidal carbon dioxide concentration
E Movement of the chest wall on manual inflation.

➜ Suxamethonium (succinylcholine)

4. What is the most frequent complaint made by patients in whom suxamethonium (succinylcholine) has been used?

A Pain at the site of injection
B Prolonged action in those with pseudocholinesterase deficiency
C Diplopia
D An increase in body temperature
E Diffuse muscle pains.

➜ Lidocaine vs bupivacaine

5. Lidocaine can be injected intravenously, but what is the main reason why bupivacaine should not be injected into a vein during local anaesthesia?

A It lasts longer.
B It is often used with adrenaline.
C It can cause methaemoglobinaemia.
D It may cause convulsions.
E It is cardiotoxic.

➜ Bier's block

6. A Bier's block is a useful technique to provide anaesthesia for upper limb surgery. Which is the best local anaesthetic to use?

A Prilocaine
B Lidocaine
C Levobupivacaine
D Bupivacaine
E Amethocaine.

7. **What is the extra risk involved when a Bier's block is used for lower-limb surgery?**
   A The difficulty in adequately exsanguinating the limb
   B The cuff is more likely to deflate.
   C Because adrenaline cannot be used
   D That failure is likely to be more frequent
   E That toxicity is more likely.

→ Assessment of pain

8. **Patients vary greatly in their requirement for postoperative analgesia. What is the best way to assess adequacy of pain relief?**
   A Measure the degree of tachycardia.
   B Ask the patient to measure the pain.
   C Assess the level of hypertension.
   D Look for tachypnoea.
   E Examine for wound splinting.

9. **Which of the following is associated with too much analgesia?**
   A Hypocarbia
   B Agitation
   C Depression of conscious level
   D Deep vein thrombosis
   E Small tidal volumes.

→ Chronic pain control

10. **Which of the following should be avoided for pain control in malignant conditions?**
   A Remifentanil
   B Fentanyl
   C Pethidine
   D Codeine
   E Methadone.

11. **Which of the following is not an alternative strategy for the treatment of chronic pain?**
   A Tamoxifen
   B Radiotherapy
   C Corticosteroids
   D Antidepressants
   E Tramadol.

Answers: Multiple choice questions

→ The anaesthetic triad

1. C

The anaesthetic triad consists of unconsciousness, pain relief and muscle relaxation in varying degrees for all procedures. Amnesia may occur but it is not actually sought. It is an interesting debating point as to whether it would be reasonable to offer amnesia without the other components since some may believe that it does not matter what the patient experiences as long as they do not remember it.

→ Laryngeal mask airway

2. B

An unprotected airway with risk of aspiration is the main problem of the LMA over an endotracheal tube. Unreliable placement and tube obstruction should be no different if both are used correctly.

→ Correct placement of an endotracheal tube

3. D

Unrecognised incorrect placement of an endotracheal tube can have disastrous consequences, and often a failure to accept the possibility that the tube is not in the trachea is a cause of delay. It has now become a standard within Western practice to verify correct tube placement by seeing a trace on the capnograph – carbon dioxide monitor. Unfortunately, being able to hear breath sounds, seeing the chest moving and actually visualizing the tube going through the vocal cords with a Mackintosh laryngoscope are not sufficiently reliable.

➜ Suxamethonium (succinylcholine)

4. E

Suxamethonium is a short-acting muscle relaxant of the depolarising class. Its use is associated with muscle fasciculations shortly before relaxation occurs. Muscle tone returns after 3–4 min in most cases. Suxamethonium is metabolised by pseudocholinesterase and its effect is prolonged in those with an inherited or acquired deficiency in this enzyme. Examples of acquired deficiency include pregnancy and liver diseases. Patients would not complain of being paralysed for a long time because it would be necessary to keep them anaesthetised until normal muscle power has returned. Diplopia can occur with any muscle relaxant because of the sensitivity of the orbital muscles of the eye. Patients who have had suxamethonium are unlikely to complain of diplopia, however, because they will still be anaesthetised when the effect of suxamethonium has worn off.

Suxamethonium is a known trigger for malignant hyperpyrexia which can be associated with an increase in body temperature, but again the patient would not complain of this. Interestingly, other drugs used during anaesthesia can also increase body temperature, most importantly atropine. A surprisingly large number of patients do complain of generalized muscle aches and pains, usually in the postural muscles and most often in young and fit males. This is thought to be related to the muscle fasciculations.

➜ Lidocaine vs bupivacaine

5. E

Lidocaine and bupivacaine are both local anaesthetics used for local infiltration, field blocks and spinal and epidural blocks. Bupivacaine should not be used for IV regional anaesthesia (Bier's block). Bupivacaine is considerably more cardiotoxic than other local anaesthetics.

➜ Bier's block

6. A

Although other local anaesthetics can be used for Bier's block, prilocaine is advocated as the safest and best agent to use. As stated above, bupivacaine should not be used.

7. E

➜ Assessment of pain

8. B

Although all the other answers are features of inadequate pain relief, they are subjective measures. The best way of assessing the adequacy of pain relief is to ask the patient about the quality of pain relief, or, more formally, to ask them to complete an analogue score where a mark is placed on a 10 cm line, with 'no pain' at one end and 'the worst pain ever' at the other.

9. C

Too much pain relief, usually associated with opioid use, will result in hypercarbia, slow respiratory rate, often with large tidal volumes, and a depression of conscious level.

➜ Chronic pain control

10. A

Remifentanil is an ultra-short-acting opioid which is often used as part of a total intravenous anaesthetic (TIVA) regimen. It is very short-acting and is not used in chronic pain circles. Any of the other agents could be used and are often used in varying preparations – skin patches, oral as a syrup, subcutaneous or intravenous.

11. E

Many agents other than well known analgesics are used as adjunctive therapy in patients with chronic pain – particularly when related to cancer. Tramadol is an agent on the second rung of the WHO pain ladder – it is an intermediate-strength opioid and, as such, would have been tried before adjunctive therapy.

15 Care in the operating room

Multiple choice questions

→ Diathermy

1. Which of the following statements with regard to diathermy are false?

A Shave the patient's hair over the site for the diathermy plate the day before the operation.
B Ensure good contact between the patient and the plate.
C Check the plate if the patient is moved during surgery.
D Place the plate as close to the operative site as possible.
E Make sure that the patient is not touching any earthed metal objects.

→ Use of a tourniquet

2. Which of the following statements regarding use of a tourniquet are true?

A The theatre charge nurse has overall responsibility in its use.
B Distal neurovascular status must be checked before and after its use.
C The tourniquet must be placed as proximally as possible.
D The tourniquet must be placed snugly enough so as not to slide during the operation.
E Always note the time of inflation and deflation.

→ Set-up on the operating table

3. In a transfer and patient set-up on the operating table, which of the following statements are true?

A Although the operating table is padded, make sure that pressure areas have additional padding.
B Limbs not involved in surgery should be especially protected to prevent nerve damage.
C Eyelids should be taped to protect the corneas.
D Extra precautions are needed if the patient is to be held in a lateral position.
E All of the above.

→ Scrubbing

4. In scrubbing, which of the following statements are false?

A If the surgeon has a suspected infected lesion, it is sprayed with iodine and covered with a sterile dressing before gloving.
B The first scrub of the day should take about 5 min from start to drying.
C A sterile scrubbing brush and nail cleaner are used for 1–2 min at the first scrub provided the surgeon stays within the theatre suite in between cases.
D After applying disinfectant, the arms are washed from distal to proximal with hands up and elbows flexed.
E Drying, using a towel for each side, should start with the fingers and work across the hand and up the arm.

→ Skin preparation

5. In skin preparation prior to operation, which of the following statements are true?

A In preparing open wounds, aqueous solutions are used.
B For intact skin, alcohol-based solutions may be used.
C Prepare the skin from the incision site outwards.
D Heavily contaminated areas are prepared last, with the swab being discarded.
E All of the above.

Answers: Multiple choice questions

→ Diathermy

1. A

The site where the diathermy plate is to be applied should be shaved after the patient has been anaesthetised. Earlier shaving should not be done because it encourages skin colonisation by organisms.

→ Use of a tourniquet

2. B, C, D, E

Surgeons always have overall responsibility regarding the use of the tourniquet. They must make sure that all precautions have been followed and that circulation and sensation have returned after deflation.

→ Set-up on the operating table

3. E

→ Scrubbing

4. A

A surgeon should not scrub if there is an open wound or a suspected infected lesion.

→ Skin preparation

5. E

16 The high-risk surgical patient

Multiple choice questions

High-risk patient

1. Which of the following groups constitute 'high-risk' patients?

A Elderly
B Ethnic minority
C Significant co-morbidities
D Emergency surgery
E Complex major surgery.

Preventable factors of mortality in high-risk patients

2. Which of the following are preventable factors of mortality in high-risk patients?

A Pain
B Insufficient patient monitoring
C Lack of early intervention as complications develop
D Advanced age
E Inadequate critical care facilities.

Risk scoring systems

3. Regarding risk scoring systems, which of the following statements are true?

A ASA does not provide an objective assessment of the risk of death.
B POSSUM works best for individuals, not population.
C MET measures exercise tolerance.
D PARSONNET is used in neurosurgery.
E Anaerobic threshold is time-consuming and needs measuring several days prior to surgery.

Preoperative management of high-risk patients

4. Regarding preoperative management of the high-risk patient, which of the following statements are true?

A A course of antibiotics should always be given in patients with chronic sputum production.
B Stopping smoking prior to surgery is of little benefit.
C Oral medications can still be given with a little water in patients who are nil-by-mouth.
D A course of steroids prior to surgery may be necessary in patients with chronic obstructive airways disease.
E Preoperative physiotherapy has no role.

Goal-directed therapy

5. Regarding goal-directed therapy (GDT), which of the following statements are true?

A It is a term used to describe the perioperative administration of intravenous (IV) fluids and inotropic agents to achieve a predefined 'optimal' goal for oxygen delivery to the tissues.
B This aims to reduce cardiac and renal output.
C This has no effect on patient survival if used for short periods after surgery.
D Observations have shown that patients who survive have higher cardiac output, oxygen delivery and oxygen consumption than those who did not.
E GDT uses a minimally invasive cardiac monitoring technique.

Management strategies in high-risk patients

6. Which of the following statements are true about specific management strategies for high-risk patients?

A Prophylactic beta-receptor antagonist agents have been used to decrease perioperative myocardial infarction.
B Oesophageal Doppler-guided fluid therapy is an accurate estimation of the patient's fluid needs.

C Sustained use of goal-directed therapy in patients with established critical illness is beneficial.
D Better fluid management can reduce post-operative ileus after abdominal surgery.
E Early return to enteric feeding is not associated with reduced hospital stay.

Extended matching questions

1. Interventions/assessment in the high-risk surgical patient

A Arterial pressure monitoring
B Cardiac output monitoring
C Goal-directed therapy
D Non-invasive ventilation
E Prophylactic perioperative beta-blockade
F Oesophageal Doppler

Choose and match the correct intervention with each of the scenarios given below:

1 This is used in patients considered to be at risk of perioperative myocardial ischaemia.

2 This is invaluable in critically ill patients who require IV fluid replacements or vasoactive infusions to stabilise their circulatory status.

3 This is used to measure cardiac output to guide IV fluid administration.

4 This refers to treatment aimed at achieving predefined levels of oxygen delivery to tissues. This improves cardiac output, renal output, complication rates and patient survival.

5 This facilitates immediate recognition of haemodynamic changes, especially in an unstable patient, and enables repeated blood sampling for arterial blood gases.

6 This is delivered via a tight-fitting mask and is helpful in postoperative respiratory management. The main benefits are the absence of need for a general anaesthetic and intubation.

Answers: Multiple choice questions

High-risk patient

1. A, C, D, E

Every surgical procedure involves some risk of significant postoperative complications or death. In most cases, this risk is well below 1 per cent. However there is a subgroup comprising 10–15 per cent of in-patient surgical procedures, in which serious complications and death are more frequent. This represents the high-risk group. In the UK 1.3 million hospital in-patients undergo general surgical procedures each year, of whom 166 000 can be identified as at high risk for complications or death.

Some of the patient-related factors which make them high risk include ischaemic heart disease, chronic obstructive pulmonary disease, diabetes, advancing age, poor exercise tolerance and poor nutritional tolerance. The surgical factors include emergency surgery, major or complex surgery, body cavity surgery, large anticipated blood loss and large insensible fluid loss.

Preventable factors of mortality in high-risk patients

2. A, B, C, E

Dehydration and hypothermia are also preventable factors that increase perioperative risk.

→ Risk scoring systems

3. A, C, E

POSSUM and PARSONNET systems were designed for populations of patients and are much less reliable when applied to individuals. PARSONNET is used in cardiac surgery.

Preoperative assessment of risk should include a history that focuses on cardiac and respiratory problems. Exercise tolerance gives a good guide to cardiac reserve, age and BMI are useful indicators, as are alcohol and tobacco intake and information on medications regularly taken.

→ Preoperative management of high-risk patients

4. C, D

A course of preoperative antibiotics is tempting in patients with chronic sputum production but should be given careful consideration. Indiscriminate antibiotic use may simply result in the selection of resistant bacteria without any therapeutic benefit, and, worse still, may complicate the treatment of any subsequent pneumonia. Smoking cessation should be encouraged wherever possible with the offer of counselling and other practical support. Preoperative physiotherapy is helpful for patients with chronic sputum production.

→ Goal-directed therapy

5. A, D, E

Goal-directed therapy aims to improve cardiac output, renal output, complication rates and patient survival. Significant reductions in complication rate can be achieved with up to 8 h of postoperative GDT using a minimally invasive cardiac output monitoring technique. It is important to note that sustained use of GDT in patients with established critical illness is not beneficial and, in fact, may be harmful.

→ Management strategies in high-risk patients

6. A, B, D

Sustained use of GDT in patients with established critical illness is not beneficial and, in fact, may be harmful. Early return to enteric feeding is associated with reduced hospital stay and is part of the Enhanced Recovery Programme (ERP).

Answers: Extended matching questions

→ 1. Interventions/assessment in the high-risk surgical patient

1E, 2B, 3F, 4C, 5A, 6D

17 Nutrition and fluid therapy

Multiple choice questions

➜ Starvation

1. **Which of the following statements regarding starvation are true?**

A Cerebral energy metabolism requirement is 100 g/day of glucose.
B Glycogenolysis comes into play in the first 2–3 days.
C Mobilisation of fat is dependent on a fall in circulating insulin levels.
D Intravenous dextrose has a protein-sparing effect.
E Ketone bodies cannot substitute for glucose for cerebral energy metabolism.

➜ Total parenteral nutrition

2. **A 67-year-old female is referred for consideration of total parenteral nutrition (TPN) following a total colostomy. Which of the following biochemical and clinical markers are suggestive of malnutrition?**

A Albumin
B Urea
C Transthyretin
D Skin fold thickness
E Weight loss.

➜ Serum proteins and disease

3. **Which of the following is a cause of hypoproteinaemia?**

A Burns
B Syndrome of inappropriate antidiuretic hormone hypersecretion (SIADH)
C Liver disease
D Analbuminaemia
E AIDS.

➜ Ketoacidosis

4. **Which of the following is a major cause of ketoacidosis?**

A Alcoholism
B Diabetic ketoacidosis (DKA)
C Inborn errors of metabolism
D Starvation
E Insulin therapy.

➜ Fluid compartments

5. **Which of the following statements regarding water homeostasis are true?**

A The total body water (TBW) content in an adult male is 70 per cent of body weight.
B Two-thirds of TBW is intracellular.
C An average adult has approx. 3 L of plasma.
D TBW is highest in elderly women.
E Water moves freely across cell membranes.

➜ Malabsorption

6. **Which of the following statements are untrue?**

A The small bowel receives approximately 7–8 L of fluid/day.
B Malabsorption is inevitable if 30 per cent of the small intestine is removed.
C The jejunum is vital in the absorption of nutrients.
D Vitamin B12 and bile salts are absorbed in the ileum.
E The enterohepatic circulation of bile salts is essential to maintain the bile salt pool.

➜ Starvation

7. **Which of the following statements regarding starvation are true?**

A Fats are initially mobilized to meet energy requirements.
B Muscle glycogen can be directly utilized.
C After a short fast, insulin level falls.

D After a short fast, adaptive ketogenesis occurs.
E Gluconeogenesis only takes place in the liver.

Intravenous fluids

8. Which of the following statements regarding 0.9 per cent normal saline are true?
A It has the same sodium concentration as plasma.
B It has equimolar concentration of sodium and chloride.
C It is low in potassium.
D It does not contain dextrose.
E It is the best fluid to be used in hypovolaemia.

Gastrointestinal secretions

9. Which of the following statements are true of gastrointestinal (GI) secretions?
A Pancreatic fluid is rich in bicarbonate.
B The chloride content of gastric fluid is around 110 mmol/L.
C Gastric fluid has the highest quantity of potassium.
D Gastric outlet obstruction is associated with hypochloraemic alkalosis.
E Most intestinal losses are replaced with normal saline and potassium.

Bowel resections

10. Which of the following statements regarding bowel resections are true?
A Diarrhoea is unusual, following ileal resection.
B The sodium content of high output fistulas is about 90 mmol/L.
C It is appropriate for patients with high output from jejunostomy to drink plenty of water.
D Peptic ulceration is a complication of short-bowel syndrome.
E Oxalate stones are commoner following bowel resection.

Pre-analytical errors

11. The following results were obtained on an elderly gentleman seen in A&E with melaena: Na, 133 mmol/L; K, 10 mmol/L; creatinine, 153 µmol/L; urea, 12.7 mmol/L; corrected Ca, 0.82 mmol/L; aspartate transaminase (AST), 32 IU; alanine transaminase (ALT), 40 IU; alkaline phosphatase (ALP), undetectable. What is the cause?
A K^+ overdosage
B Renal failure
C Contaminated blood
D Liver failure
E All of the above.

Hypovolaemia

12. Which of the following are associated with hypovolaemia?
A Tachycardia
B Uraemia
C Decreased urinary sodium excretion
D Hypotension
E Increased urine output.

Diarrhoea and electrolyte imbalances

13. A 15-year-old girl was admitted with abdominal pain and severe diarrhoea after return from holiday in Kenya. She is hypokalaemic with a metabolic acidosis. Her investigations are as follows:
- **Blood: Na, 147 mmol/L; K, 2.0 mmol/L; Cl, 115 mmol/L; HCO3, 13 mmol/L**
- **Diarrhoeal fluid: Na, 77 mmol/L; osmolality, 248; K, 50 mmol/L**

What condition are these features consistent with?
A Carcinoid syndrome
B Tropical sprue
C Zollinger–Ellison syndrome
D Secretory diarrhoea
E Coeliac disease.

Acidosis

14. A 6-year-old child has been unwell with abdominal pain and vomiting for 2 days. He has been unable to take any food and has been drinking sips of milk. On examination, the child is irritable and dehydrated. The following results were obtained: Na, 143 mmol/L; K, 3.0 mmol/L; Cl, 90 mmol/L;

bicarbonate, 16 mmol/L; glucose, 7.5 mmol/L; urea, 7.6 mmol/L; creatinine, 119 μmol/L; beta-OH-butyrate, 6 mmol/L (<0.3). What condition does this metabolic picture suggest?

A DKA
B Starvation ketosis
C Lactic acidosis
D Severe sepsis
E Malnutrition.

Metabolic consequences of vomiting

15. In case of small-bowel obstruction and vomiting, which of the following statements are true?

A The urea and creatinine can rise.
B There is a rise in urine osmolality.
C There is increased urinary Na excretion.
D Hyperchloraemia is a common feature.
E ADH rises.

Acid–base balance

16. Which of the following statements regarding acid–base balance are true?

A Na and K are the major cations.
B Bicarbonate is the major anion.
C A decreased anion gap can occur in myeloma.
D A raised anion gap can occur in DKA.
E A raised anion gap can occur in ethanol intoxication.

Extended matching questions

1. Risk of refeeding syndrome

A High probability of refeeding syndrome
B Intermediate probability of refeeding syndrome
C Low probability of refeeding syndrome

Choose and match the probabilities with the following clinical scenarios (the above options can be used more than once):

1 A 27-year-old asylum seeker who is fit and well is on a hunger strike for 2 days protesting his deportation order. He has only consumed sips of sweet tea during this time. His BMI is 25 kg/m^2.

2 A young woman with anorexia underwent a laparotomy for bleeding duodenal ulcer. Her BMI is 14.7 kg/ m^2.

3 A chronic alcoholic with a BMI of 26 kg/m^2 is admitted with bleeding varices.

4 A 46-year-old male with oesophageal cancer has lost 12 kg in the preceding 4 weeks prior to admission with dysphagia.

5 A 64-year-old male with coeliac disease and BMI of 19 kg/m^2 presents with generalized weakness and hypokalaemia.

2. Fluid and electrolyte abnormalities

A Pancreatitis
B SIADH
C Fluid overload
D Multiple myeloma

Choose and match the conditions above with the clinical scenarios described below:

1 An 87-year-old woman is admitted to hospital following a vertebral fracture. Blood tests following operative repair to stabilise the fracture are as follows: Na, 123 mmol/L; K, 3.9 mmol/L; total protein, 102 g/L; albumin, 30 g/L; creatinine 134μmol/L.

2 A 25-year-old man under care of lipidologists, presents with vomiting and non-specific abdominal symptoms. His blood tests are as follows: total cholesterol, 6.0 mmol/L; triglycerides, 66 mmol/L; AST/ALT/amylase, unable to be analysed.

3 A 62-year-old man who underwent a laparotomy for pancreatitis shows the following profile: Na, 124 mmol/L; K, 4.5 mmol/L; serum osmolality, 250 mmol/L; urine Na, < 5.0 mmol/L.

4 An 82-year-old man with a bronchial tumour has the following results: Na. 130 mmol/L; K, 3.3 mmol/L; urine Na, 30 mmol/L.

→ 3. Metabolic presentations in young and old patients

A Transcellular shift
B Inborn error of metabolism
C Pituitary tumour
D Response to illness

Choose and match the conditions above with the clinical scenarios described below:

1 A male infant developed seizures following circumcision. His blood results are as follows: glucose, 2.2 mmol/L; ammonia 256 nmol/L.

2 A young diabetic is recovering after undergoing an endoscopic retrograde cholangiopancreatography (ERCP) for jaundice. He is on sliding scale insulin and K^+ IVI. His blood results are as follows: glucose, 7.2 mmol/L; K^+, 3.5 mmol/L; PO_4, 0.30 mmol/L.

3 A 68-year-old man is in ITU following a craniotomy for a subdural haematoma. He has low T3, T4 and low hypothalamic hormones.

4 A 56-year-old man presents with visual disturbance and low Na of 110.

Answers: Multiple choice questions

→ Starvation

1. A, C, D

During starvation, the body faces a need to generate glucose. This is achieved in the first 24 h by mobilizing glycogen stores. Thereafter, gluconeogenesis is achieved from amino acids, glycerol and lactate. Ketone bodies can serve as a substitute for glucose for cerebral energy metabolism.

→ Total parenteral nutrition

2. C, E

The best way of assessing nutritional supplementation is an estimation of weight loss.
The Malnutrition Universal Screening Tool (MUST) for adults is widely used and takes into consideration body mass index (BMI), recent weight loss and presence or absence of acute disease. Anthropometric measurements such as skin-fold thickness and midarm circumference are indirect measures and are subject to huge variation – they are not helpful in an in-patient setting. Albumin is prone to variation with dilutional state (e.g. IV fluids), liver disease etc. Further it has a long half-life of about 20 days and levels could still be normal despite nutritional inadequacy. Urea is also prone to dilutional effect, type of protein consumed and presence of GI bleed.

Transthyretin is also called prealbumin and has a shorter half-life, making it a good marker, but the assay is not routinely available.

Serum proteins and disease

3. A, B, C, D, E

The term plasma proteins describe a very large number of different proteins, such as albumin, globulin, acute phase proteins, Apo lipoproteins, immunoglobulins and clotting factors. Albumin is the most abundant protein and is produced in the liver. Hypoproteinaemia can occur in dilutional states such as water overload, specimen from drip arm or SIADH. Loss can also occur via the skin in burns and large exudative lesions and in protein-losing enteropathy. Analbuminaemia is a benign condition in which patients lack albumin. There is often a compensatory increase in other proteins.

Ketoacidosis

4. A, B, C, D

Ketoacidosis is a metabolic response of the body to low insulin:glucagon ratio when there is low glucose. This triggers release of free fatty acids as an alternative source of energy. During ketogenesis, there is consumption of bicarbonate ions, which results in metabolic acidosis with an increased anion gap.

Fluid compartments

5. B, C, E

Total body water is approximately 60 per cent of total body weight. Infants have a relatively higher proportion of TBW while elderly women have a lower proportion. There is variation with sex and age. In an average male of 70 kg, TBW is 42 L, intracellular water is 23 L and plasma volume is 3 L. The remainder of 16 L is interstitial fluid. Water moves freely across cell membranes in response to changes in tonicity of adjoining compartments. Na and K^+ are influenced by the Na/K-ATPase pump.

Malabsorption

6. B, C

Only 200–300 cm of small intestine is needed to meet the nutritional needs of an individual. Thus, up to 50 per cent of the small bowel could be resected without permanent effects. The ileum has the slowest intestinal transit time and the highest absorptivity of nutrients. It is thus critical for the conservation of fluid and electrolytes. Depletion of the bile salt pool results in fat malabsorption and thus reduced absorption of the fat-soluble vitamins A, D, E and K.

Starvation

7. C, D

Following an overnight fast, insulin level declines and counter-regulatory hormones such as glucagons and cortisol begin to rise. In early starvation, glycogenolysis occurs in the liver (breakdown of liver glycogen). Additional stores of glycogen are present in the muscle as well. Glycogen here is converted to lactate which is metabolised in the liver to useful glucose. Continued fasting (>24 h) results in gluconeogenesis from breakdown of amino acids. Subsequently, fats are mobilized.

Intravenous fluids

8. B, D

Normal saline has 154 mmol/L of sodium and chloride. It contains no dextrose or K^+. The solute load (Na^+) is excessive compared with plasma. Hartmann's solution resembles plasma more closely, but for a higher quantity of lactate, and is the preferred replacement fluid in hypovolaemia.

Dextrose solutions are considered when pure water replacement is considered without electrolyte load, e.g. in hypernatraemic dehydration.

Gastrointestinal secretions

9. A, B, D, E

Fluid replacement therapy is best managed by assessing deficit from GI tract (if appropriate) urine, faeces and insensible losses. Duodenal, pancreatic, biliary secretions are similar in their sodium and chloride content (140 and 100 mmol/L, respectively), pancreatic fluid has a high bicarbonate content and loss of these results in metabolic acidosis. Saliva has a high K^+ content (25 mmol/L) and gastric juice has a high chloride content (around 110 mmol/L).

Bowel resections

10. B, D, E

Following ileal resection, large volumes of bile salt-laden fluid reach the colon, predisposing to diarrhoea. When >200 cm of the bowel is resected, a jejunostomy becomes essential. Net absorbers have over 100 cm of intact jejunum and absorb most of the fluid and electrolytes. Net secretors only have a short portion of intact jejunum and lose water through their stoma. They often require parenteral supplementation, as drinking large amounts of oral hypotonic solutions could worsen the situation. Peptic ulceration due to excessive gastric acid secretion and renal stones due to increased oxalate absorption from the colon are not uncommon.

Pre-analytical errors

11. C

Ethylenediaminetetra-acetic acid (EDTA, used for full blood count) contamination of blood is a cause of hyperkalaemia. The low serum calcium and ALP activity are further clues. EDTA chelates calcium and Mg. EDTA is often found as K^+ salt in full blood count bottles. Hyperkalaemia is also a common association with old, stale or haemolysed blood samples. K^+ overload (by supplements or drugs) will not cause changes in calcium or ALP levels.

Hypovolaemia

12. A, B, C, D

Intravascular volume depletion is associated with characteristic clinical and biochemical features. Clinically tachycardia, hypotension, reduced skin turgor, increased capillary refill time and reduced urine output are typical. Biochemically there is a tendency for healthy kidneys to attempt correction by retaining Na^+ so that intravascular volume increase. This results in elimination of <10 mmol/L of urinary sodium.

Diarrhoea and electrolyte imbalances

13. D

This is consistent with secretory diarrhoea (possibly due to parasitic infestation). The electrolytes suggest hypokalaemia and metabolic acidosis (low bicarbonate), which is due to loss of these metabolites via diarrhoeal fluid. The Na is mildly elevated as a result of dehydration. The hyperchloraemia is typical of the kidney's compensatory mechanism to the loss of bicarbonate.

The stool shows excretion of electrolytes. The stool osmolality is measured at 248 but calculated osmolality is 2(Na) + K and is 204.

This difference in osmolality of 42 mmol/L is due to unmeasured osmotically active substances (such as glucose) which are seen in secretory diarrhoea. It is caused by toxins such as *Vibrio cholerae* and *E. coli.* Hormonal causes such as Zollinger–Ellison and vasoactive intestinal polypeptides could cause a similar picture but are not consistent with clinical details provided.

Acidosis

14. B

Starvation ketosis is commoner in children due to low glycogen stores. The child is able to maintain normoglycaemia due to effective gluconeogenesis. The slightly high glucose could also be due to the effect of counter-regulatory hormones, such as cortisol and glucagon, that are released during stress. Mounting a ketone response is appropriate in this situation as the brain and muscles are able to utilize this as a source of energy. The associated metabolic acidosis shows an anion gap of 40 mmol/L (a third of this is accounted for by glucose and beta-OH-butyrate) and thus other ketone bodies such as acetoacetate may be responsible.

Metabolic consequences of vomiting

15. A, B, E

Water and Na loss results in a reduction in intravascular volume. This will elevate the urea and creatinine. This also triggers release of ADH, which increases urinary osmolality. There is renal reabsorption of Na, and fractional excretion of Na is reduced to <1 per cent. The plasma chloride can give a clue to the cause of loss. Hypochloraemia is common in vomiting and hyperchloraemia is seen in diarrhoea.

Acid–base balance

16. A, C, D, E

Anion gap is a measure of anions other than chloride and bicarbonate and is calculated as: $(Na + K) - (Cl + HCO_3)$. The major cations in the body are Na (140 mmol/L) and K (4 mmol/L). Ca and Mg are the other cations.

The major anions are chloride (100 mmol/L) and HCO_3 (27 mmol/L). Proteins and phosphate are among the other anions. Normal anion gap is around 8–16. It is elevated in metabolic acidosis, such as DKA, lactic acidosis, renal failure, salicylate and ethanol intoxication. It can be reduced when there are paraproteinaemia states.

Answers: Extended matching questions

1. Risk of refeeding syndrome

1C

Refeeding syndrome occurs due to severe fluid and electrolyte shifts and their associated complications in malnourished patients undergoing feeding by the oral, enteral or parenteral route. Underlying malnutrition, low BMI, pre-existing abnormalities and electrolyte abnormalities increase risk. These are absent in the case above.

2A

BMI < 16 kg/m^2, unintentional weight loss greater than 15 per cent in recent months and no nutritional intake for more than 10 days are, individually, high-risk features for the development of refeeding syndrome.

3B

Caution must be exercised in patients with alcohol-induced liver disease, especially if associated with BMI < 18.5 kg/m^2 or unintentional weight loss of 10 per cent of their body weight in the last 3–6 months or if they are on chemotherapeutic agents, insulin or diuretics.

4A

Cachexia and underlying malnutrition contribute to high risk.

5A

Low levels of potassium, magnesium and phosphate prior to feeding put patients at high risk. However, it is not always necessary to correct the electrolyte imbalance before feeding. Electrolytes can be supplemented during feeding.

In starvation:

↑ Glucogenolysis ⇒ ↑gluconeogenisis ⇒ protein catabolism ⇒ negative nitrogen balance

In refeeding:

↑ Availability of glucose ⇒ insulin release ⇒ stimulation of ATPase pump ⇒ K^+ and PO_4 move intracellarly ⇒ clinical symptoms of refeeding syndrome

2. Fluid and electrolyte abnormalities

1D

Abnormal proteins in melanoma or paraproteinaemia can cause spurious hyponatraemia. The serum osmolality will, in fact, be normal in these cases.

2A

Hypertriglyceridaemia causes spurious hyponatraemia like the abnormal proteins. This is because they occupy a large part of the plasma, displacing water.

3C

Overzealous fluid replacement is the commonest cause of postoperative hyponatraemia. A low urinary sodium is an appropriate response in this case (<10 mmol/L).

4B

SIADH could be due to ectopic ADH production by the bronchial tumour, resulting in excessive excretion of Na^+ via the kidneys despite the presence of hyponatraemia.

3. Metabolic presentations in young and old patients

1B

Hypoglycaemia is a commoner feature in neonates, however in this infant it is associated with hyperammonaemia following stress (circumcision). One must consider a differential diagnosis of an inborn error of metabolism such as a urea cycle defect, amino acid disorder or a fatty acid disorder.

2A

Insulin causes transcellular shifts in electrolytes. It moves potassium and phosphate into the cells. Very low phosphate can cause muscle weakness, including respiratory paralysis.

3D

In the chronic phase of critical illness, the hypothalamic-pituitary-target axis slows down.

4C

A pituitary tumour can cause chiasmal compression, leading to visual disturbances and associated hyponatraemia.

18 Basic surgical skills and anastomosis

Multiple choice questions

Tissue apposition

1. Which of the following statements are true?

A Skin wound edges should not be closed tightly.
B Glues have a place in the approximation of tissues.
C Bowel anastomosis is always done in single layer.
D Vascular anastomosis is always done with non-absorbable sutures.
E All arteriotomies must be closed with a vein patch.

Sutures

2. Which of the following statements are false?

A Polymeric synthetic suture materials cause minimal inflammatory reaction.
B Monofilament non-absorbable sutures are easy to use in tying secure knots.
C The integrity of polypropylene sutures in holding tissues together can last indefinitely.
D Braided suture material can be a nidus for infection.
E Absorption is more predictable and complete with absorbable sutures.

Needles

3. Which of the following statements are true?

A Cutting needles are used for skin and aponeurosis.
B Hand needles are ideal for skin closure.
C Round-bodied needles are used for closure of laparotomy wounds.
D Needles with a loop-suture should be used for laparotomy closure.
E In arterial suturing, double-ended needle sutures are used.

Anastomosis

4. Which of the following statements are false?

A Large-bowel anastomosis must be done only by one-layer technique.
B The bowel ends being anastomosed must be well mobilised so as not to create tension in the anastomosis.
C Synthetic polymers are to be used for intestinal anastomosis.
D In vascular anastomosis the needle must pass from within outwards.
E Polypropylene-like sutures with indefinite integrity must be used for vascular anastomosis.

Answers: Multiple choice questions

Tissue apposition

1. A, B, D

Wounds should be closed with no tension, with a minimal gap between the edges to allow for the swelling that inevitably occurs as a result of the inflammatory process of normal healing. Tissue glues, the cyanoacrylates, can be used for skin closure. Their use requires perfect haemostasis and they are ideally used in children for a laceration on the forehead. They are relatively expensive. Fibrin tissue glues work on the conversion of fibrinogen by thrombin to fibrin. They are extensively used: for haemostasis in the liver and spleen, for dural tears, in ear, nose and throat and ophthalmic surgery and to prevent postoperative adhesions in cardiac and general surgery. In upper gastrointestinal haemorrhage, fibrin glues in combination with collagen are an effective method of stopping bleeding endoscopically.

Bowel anastomosis can be done in one or two layers depending upon the choice of the individual surgeon. One method is the single-layer interrupted extramucosal anastomosis. This causes the least tissue necrosis or luminal narrowing. When done in two layers, the inner continuous all-layer suture is supplemented by inverting the seromuscular, second layer of sutures on the outside.

All vascular anastomosis must be done using non-absorbable sutures as the integrity of the material needs to be permanent. It should be monofilament. The size of the suture depends upon the calibre of the vessel and the closure has to be precise and watertight.

All arteriotomies need not be closed with a vein patch. While doing a femoral embolectomy, if a transverse incision is made it can be closed in the direction of the incision. However, if a longitudinal incision is used, it is preferable to close it with a vein patch to prevent narrowing of the lumen; in carotid endarterectomy, the arteriotomy is always closed with a synthetic patch.

→ Sutures

2. B

Polymeric synthetic suture materials cause minimal inflammatory reaction and are of predictable strength. In their monofilament form, they require more skill in tying knots. The braided form of the material can cause bacterial colonisation, resulting in a suture knot sinus. As the integrity of polypropylene sutures in holding tissues together can last indefinitely, they are used in vascular anastomosis.

→ Needles

3. A, C, D, E

Hand needles should not be used because surgery should be carried out using the no-touch technique. Moreover, hand needles increase the danger of needlestick injuries.

→ Anastomosis

4. A

Large-bowel anastomosis can be done by either one- or two-layer technique. When done in two layers, the inner layer is an all-layer continuous suture and the outer is an interrupted seromuscular suture. When done in a single layer, extramucosal interrupted anastomosis is carried out. The suture material is 2/0–3/0 synthetic polymer using inverting sutures.

In vascular suturing, the needle must always pass from within outwards to avoid creating an intimal flap and to fix any atherosclerotic plaque. Polypropylene-like sutures which have an indefinite integrity must always be used.

19 Laparoscopic and robotic surgery

Multiple choice questions

➜ Minimal access surgery

1. **Which of the following are advantages of minimal access surgery?**
   - A Decrease in wound size
   - B Decreased postoperative pain
   - C Shorter operating time
   - D Improved vision
   - E Reduced operating theatre costs.

2. **Which of the following are limitations of minimal access surgery?**
   - A Technically more demanding
   - B Loss of tactile feedback
   - C Extraction of large specimens
   - D Poor vision
   - E Difficulty with haemostasis.

➜ Pneumoperitoneum

3. **What are the desired characteristics of the gas used to provide pneumoperitoneum in laparoscopic surgery?**
   - A It should be a supporter of combustion.
   - B It should be highly soluble in blood.
   - C It should be rapidly excreted from the body.
   - D There should be a low risk of embolism.
   - E It should have a low diffusion coefficient.

4. **Which of the following are gases used to provide pneumoperitoneum?**
   - A Methane
   - B Carbon dioxide
   - C Helium
   - D Nitrous oxide
   - E Argon.

5. **Which of the following are complications associated with pneumoperitoneum?**
   - A Hyperthermia
   - B Acidosis
   - C Cardiac arrhythmias
   - D Gas embolism
   - E Reduced cardiac return.

6. **Which of the following statements regarding pneumoperitoneum are true?**
   - A A Tuohy needle can be used to achieve access to the peritoneal cavity.
   - B The usual intraperitoneal pressure maintained during surgery is 25 mmHg.
   - C The temperature of the gas used is maintained at normal body temperature.
   - D Nitrous oxide is preferable to carbon dioxide in patients with cardiac disease.
   - E The gases used for pneumoperitoneum have high water content.

7. **Which of the following are complications associated with creating pneumoperitoneum?**
   - A Bleeding
   - B Bowel injuries
   - C Gas dissection within the abdominal wall
   - D Puncture of blood vessels
   - E Omental tears.

➜ Laparoscopic surgery

8. **Which of the following are energy sources used in laparoscopic surgery?**
   - A Monopolar diathermy
   - B Bipolar diathermy/combinations (Ligasure)
   - C Laser
   - D Ultrasonic energy (harmonic scalpel)
   - E Vapour pulse coagulation (VPC).

9. **What parameters are taken into account while using laparoscopic simulators to assess laparoscopic skills competencies?**
   - A Time taken to do the task
   - B Age
   - C Left/right side dominance
   - D Number of errors
   - E Depth (3D) perception.

Robotic surgery

10. Which of the following are advantages of robotic surgery to the surgeon?

A Better visualisation (higher magnification) and stereoscopic views
B Greater precision due to elimination of hand tremor
C Improved manoeuvring due to 'robotic wrist' with seven degrees of freedom
D Ergonomic environment
E Reduced costs.

11. Which of the following statements regarding robotic surgery are true?

A AESOP is a robotic camera system.
B ZEUS and the Da Vinci are tele-robotic manipulators.
C SOCRATES is a combination of telebiotics and telementoring systems.
D Specialities that use microsurgery will particularly benefit.
E It has a short learning curve.

12. What are the benefits of robotic surgery over laparoscopic surgery?

A Better ergonomic operating positions
B Reduces the need for assistants
C Guidance from experienced surgeons not physically present in the operating theatre
D Shorter operating time
E Shorter learning curve.

13. What are the current drawbacks of robotic surgery?

A Increased costs
B Prolonged learning curve
C Haemostasis
D Socioeconomic implications
E Increased operating time.

Trochar site bleeding

14. How can bleeding from a trochar site be controlled?

A By applying upwards and lateral pressure with the trochar itself
B By using a percutaneous monofilament suture loop
C By suturing
D Applying pressure from a Foley catheter balloon
E Diathermy.

Electrosurgery in laparoscopic surgery

15. Which of the following statements are true in relation to the risks of electrosurgery in laparoscopic surgery?

A The majority occur following the use of monopolar diathermy.
B The incidence is about 1 to 2 cases per 1000 operations.
C The electrical injuries are usually recognised at the time of occurrence.
D The injuries are usually minor.
E Bipolar diathermy is equally dangerous.

16. What are the main causes of electrosurgical injuries in laparoscopic surgery?

A Inadvertent touching or grasping of tissue during current application
B Direct coupling
C Insulation breaks
D Direct sparking
E Current passage to bowel from recently coagulated tissue.

Natural orifice transluminal surgery

17. Which of the following can be used as the entry point in natural orifice transluminal surgery (NOTES)?

A Mouth
B Vagina
C Umbilicus
D Anus
E Retroperitoneum.

Extended matching questions

1. Laparoscopy complications

A Bowel perforation
B Major vessel injury
C Port-site bleeding
D Deep vein thrombosis (DVT)/pulmonary embolism (PE)
E Referred pain
F Port-site hernia
G Port-site recurrence

Choose and match the correct diagnosis with each of the scenarios given below:

1 A 64-year-old male who has had a laparoscopic resection of his colonic cancer presents with a lump on his abdominal wall over one of the port-site scars. This is painless and hard. There is no cough impulse and it is not reducible.

2 A 36-year-old female who had a laparoscopic cholecystectomy 2 days ago is brought to A&E with increasing abdominal pain and distension. On examination she is very unwell and the abdomen shows signs of peritonitis.

3 A 32-year-old female had an uneventful diagnostic laparoscopy 4 h previously. The nurses observe that the dressings are getting soaked with blood despite repeated changing. The woman is tachycardic but otherwise okay. The abdomen is soft and not distended.

4 A 40-year-old female who underwent a laparoscopic cholecystectomy the previous day complains of pain over her right shoulder. She is otherwise stable and her abdomen is soft and non-tender.

5 A 55-year-old male who underwent a laparoscopic cholecystectomy 2 years ago presents with a slowly increasing lump over the substernal scar. This gets more prominent on sitting and coughing. It is causing him local discomfort. Clinical examination reveals a 2 cm soft lump over the area. It is reducible and has a cough impulse.

6 A 70-year-old obese female who had a laparoscopic cholecystectomy a week ago is readmitted with chest pain and shortness of breath. A CT pulmonary angiogram confirms the diagnosis.

7 A 34-year-old slim female was scheduled to have a diagnostic laparoscopy for her unexplained pelvic pain. The woman collapsed soon after the introduction of the trochar. The laparoscopist could not visualise any structures in the peritoneal cavity as the view had a 'red-out'. The abdomen was distended and the end of the telescope was covered with blood despite repeated cleaning.

2. Laparoscopic/robotic nomenclatures

A Master-slave unit
B Hasson
C CCD
D NOTES
E VATS
F Verres

Choose and match the correct intervention with each of the scenarios given below:

1 This helps to provide excellent image quality. It detects different levels of brightness and adjusts for the best image possible.

2 This needle is used to create a pneumoperitoneum by the closed method.

3 This enables thoracic surgery to be done under video assistance.

4 These are the two parts of robotic surgery such as the Da Vinci robotic system with the preset arms controlled by a surgeon via a remote console and binocular viewer.

5 This trochar is useful when creating a pneumoperitoneum in patients who have had previous abdominal operations.

6 This may be the future of minimally invasive surgery, whereby the peritoneal cavity is entered via a natural orifice such as the mouth, rectum or vagina.

Answers: Multiple choice questions

➜ Minimal access surgery

1. A, B, D

The other advantages are reduction in wound pain and wound-related problems, such as wound dehiscence, bleeding, herniation and nerve entrapment. It reduces postoperative adhesions due to less tissue trauma. It also aids early postoperative mobility and decreased heat loss. It is hence one of the important components of an Enhanced Recovery Programme (ERP), which is gaining popularity to reduce postoperative hospital stay.

2. A, B, C, E

The other limitations are reliance on remote vision and operating, dependence on hand-eye feedback and reliance on new techniques. The set-up costs and some operating costs can also be higher, although some of this is recovered by reduced length of hospital stay.

➜ Pneumoperitoneum

3. B, C, D

The gas used to provide pneumoperitoneum should not be combustible or a supporter of combustion, as this will cause fire with the use of diathermy. It should have a high diffusion coefficient to minimise risks of embolism. They should have low water content.

4. B, C, D, E

The most common gas used is carbon dioxide. Methane cannot be used, as it is combustible.

5. B, C, D, E

The other complications include hypothermia and referred shoulder-tip pain.

6. A, D

A Verres needle is used in the closed method of creating pneumoperitoneum. The most common method employed by general surgeons is the 'open method', where the layers of the abdominal wall are incised under direct vision. This avoids the morbidity related to a blind puncture. A Hasson trochar or a similar blunt-tip trochar is employed in the open technique. The usual intraperitoneal pressure employed is between 12 and 14 mmHg and rarely exceeds 15 mmHg. Increased pressures risk affecting tissue microcirculation similar to compartment syndrome. The temperature of the gas used to provide pneumoperitoneum is 21°C and hence can cause hypothermia.

7. A, B, C, D, E

The procedure for creating a pneumoperitoneum can be associated with potential major risks, and hence utmost care needs to be employed. Risks can be reduced by avoiding a blind puncture and taking extra care in difficult cases, such as those who have had previous operations. Gas dissection within the abdominal wall can be avoided by confirming, without doubt, placement in the peritoneal cavity before starting insufflation and closely observing correlation between pressures generated and the volumes of gas insufflated. Injury to major vessels is life-threatening and should be promptly recognised. The abdomen is opened without delay and expert help sought, if needed, to repair the damage.

➜ Laparoscopic surgery

8. A, B, C, D, E

The monopolar diathermy is the most common source. This has potential risks and hence needs to be used with the utmost caution. It is safer but presently more expensive methods, such as bipolar diathermy and ultrasonic energy sources, are being more widely used and are likely to become the mainstay in future.

9. A, C, D, E

The other parameters include completing the task successfully and the paths taken by instruments during the activities.

➜ Robotic surgery

10. A, B, C, D

A robot is a mechanical device that performs automated physical tasks according to direct human supervision, a predefined programme or a set of general guidelines using artificial intelligence techniques. This has been primarily employed in the form of automated camera systems and tele-manipulator systems, thus creating a human-machine interface. These systems are, however, still not widely available apart from being expensive.

11. A, B, C, D

These systems offer advantages to the surgeons by reducing the need for assistants and providing better ergonomic operating positions. They also enable experienced guidance to be provided by surgeons not physically present in the operating theatre. The learning curve, not surprisingly, is long.

12. A, B, C

It is believed that robotic surgery will be more widely used in future but their use is currently limited by cost and availability.

13. A, B, C, D, E

Despite drawbacks, robotic surgery still has potential advantages and is expected to be more widely used in future.

➜ Trochar site bleeding

14. A, B, C, D, E

Considerable bleeding can occur if the falciform ligament is impaled with the substernal trochar or if one of the epigastric arteries is injured. This is best avoided by taking care during trochar insertion. Control of the bleeding should always be ensured.

➜ Electrosurgery in laparoscopic surgery

15. A, B

The injuries can be potentially serious. They are often not recognised at the time of operation and patients may present 3–7 days after injury with complaints of fever and abdominal pain. Bipolar diathermy is safer than monopolar diathermy and is preferred, especially in anatomically crowded areas.

16. A, B, C, D, E

Electrosurgical injuries can be caused by various mechanisms. Awareness of this will help to minimise injuries. The important safety measures include attainment of a perfect visual image, avoiding excessive current application, meticulous attention to insulation and using alternative safer energy sources.

→ Natural orifice transluminal surgery

17. A, B, D

This is also called 'scarless' or 'incisionless' surgery. It is a technique whereby the peritoneal cavity is entered endoscopically via a natural orifice and the surgery carried out using specialised endoscopic technology and techniques. NOTES cholecystectomy and appendicectomy have been successfully carried out. Minimising potential contamination of the peritoneum and the ability to carry out a safe closure of the peritoneal entry site are the main technical challenges.

Answers: Extended matching questions

→ 1. Laparoscopy complications

1G

Port-site recurrence is a potential problem after laparoscopic surgery for malignancies. The incidence is fortunately low due to increased awareness and taking precautions such as using wound protectors and endobags for specimen retrieval.

2A

Bowel perforation is a potential complication after laparoscopic surgery. This could be due to diathermy injury, which is frequently out of sight and not recognised. Graspers can also crush the bowel with subsequent necrosis and perforation. This should hence be suspected in any patient presenting with signs of peritonitis a few days after the operation.

3C

Port-site bleeding can either present with overt wound bleeding or signs of shock due to internal bleed. The bleeding from epigastric arteries or the vessels in the falciform ligament can cause significant bleeding.

4E

Referred pain to the shoulders is not uncommon after laparoscopic surgery. This is referred from the diaphragm and should subside within a couple of days.

5F

Port-site hernia is known to occur in 1–2 per cent of patients. It is hence important that all port incisions of 1 cm or more are sutured. Lateral ports made using bladeless trochars, which are muscle splitting, and not cutting, may be associated with a lower risk of hernia formation.

6D

DVT and PE are still potential risks after laparoscopic surgery. Hence all patients should receive appropriate DVT prophylaxis.

7B

This is a major complication and is life-threatening. It requires immediate recognition and opening up of the abdomen. The injury can be caused by both the Verres needle and the trochar. The utmost care should hence be exercised during their use.

→ 2. Laparoscopic/robotic nomenclatures

1C

Advances in optic technology including high-definition images have greatly contributed to developments in laparoscopic surgery.

2F

This is presently less widely used by general surgeons, as most are resorting to 'open technique'.

3E

This refers to video-assisted thoracic surgery to enable some thoracic operations to be done under video guidance.

4A

This creates a human-machine interface, with the operator being the 'master' and the robot the 'slave'. This provides several benefits for the surgeon, such as higher magnification with better stereoscopic views, elimination of hand tremors, greater precision, improved manoeuvring due to the 'robotic wrist', which allows seven degrees of freedom, ability to carry out complex and large external movements in a limited space, and a better ergonomic environment.

5B

The blunt tip and direct visualisation make this safer.

6D

Minimising potential contamination of the peritoneum and the ability to carry out a safe closure of the peritoneal entry site are the main technical challenges.

20 Postoperative care

Multiple choice questions

The immediate postoperative period

1. Which of the following statements are false?

A Infusion and certain monitoring systems can cause complications.
B Abdominal surgical wounds may compromise postoperative respiratory function.
C The commonest cause of postoperative hypotension is bleeding or insufficient fluid administration.
D Postoperative deep vein thrombosis (DVT) is classically diagnosed by Homan's sign.
E Oliguria is defined as urinary output of less than 0.5 mL/kg per h.

Postoperative shortness of breath

2. Which of the following is not a cause of acute shortness of breath on the first postoperative day?

A Atelectasis
B Pulmonary embolism
C Myocardial infarction
D Chest infection
E Pneumothorax.

Postoperative hypotension

3. After an anterior resection, which of the following conditions are causes of postoperative hypotension within the first 12–24 h?

A Postoperative bleeding
B Myocardial infarction
C Epidural anaesthesia or excessive morphine
D Inadequate fluid replacement
E Leakage of bowel anastomosis.

Deep vein thrombosis

4. Which of the following statements are true with regard to deep vein thrombosis (DVT)?

A Obese patients are more prone to DVT
B Clinical diagnosis is very obvious
C Hip and knee replacement surgery are high risk
D Confirmation is by venography and/or duplex Doppler ultrasound (US)
E Optimum hydration is essential to prevent DVT.

Postoperative vomiting

5. Which of the following statements with regard to postoperative vomiting are false?

A Inadequate analgesia can be a cause of postoperative vomiting.
B All abdominal operations must routinely have a nasogastric tube inserted preoperatively.
C Metoclopramide and cyclazine can help.
D Pulmonary aspiration may inadvertently occur.
E Wound dehiscence is a distinct possibility.

Postoperative oliguria

6. Which of the following statements with regard to postoperative oliguria are false?

A The commonest cause is inadequate fluid replacement.
B Oliguria is defined as <1 mL urine/kg of body weight per h.
C Patients undergoing an operation for obstructive jaundice are particularly susceptible.
D Renal US is carried out to look for hydronephrosis from blocked ureters.
E Inotropic support may be necessary.

Extended matching questions

1. Postoperative pyrexia

A Atelectasis
B Urinary tract infection
C Subphrenic abscess
D Wound infection

Choose and match the correct diagnosis with each of the scenarios below:

1 A 75-year-old patient underwent a right hemicolectomy. On the second postoperative day he developed a pyrexia of 39°C. He was tachypnoeic, centrally cyanosed, with his ala nasi moving with every attempt at breathing. The chest wall movement was restricted on the right with reduced breath sounds on that side.

2 A 50-year-old patient underwent closure of a perforated duodenal ulcer laparoscopically 5 days ago. He is unwell with a fever of 40°C, with rigors and pain in his right shoulder tip. He is hypoxic. There is oedema of the skin in the right upper quadrant and no air entry in the right lung base.

3 Following an emergency Hartmann's operation for perforated diverticulitis, a 70-year-old female patient recovered after a stormy postoperative period. On the 10th postoperative day she complained of pain in the wound. She had a temperature and the wound looked red and inflamed.

4 After an abdominoperineal resection, a 70-year-old man recovered well. On the day he was due to go home, 10 days later, he developed pyrexia with rigors. He complained of frequency of micturition and burning pain during voiding.

2. Postoperative confusion

A Electrolyte disorder
B Pneumonia
C Septic shock
D Alcohol withdrawal

Choose and match the correct diagnosis with each of the scenarios below:

1 A 70-year-old patient underwent a transurethral resection of his prostate 2 days ago. He is now very drowsy and rousable with difficulty. His catheter still shows some light haematuria and he has oliguria. There is some pitting oedema of his ankles and sacrum. His serum sodium is 120 mmol/L.

2 A known patient of chronic pancreatitis aged 75 had a hemiarthroplasty for a fractured neck of femur. Three days into the postoperative period, he became incoherent and garrulous. His breathing was normal. His electrolytes were normal, as was his chest X-ray.

3 A 70-year-old patient underwent an endoscopic retrograde cholangiopancreatography (ERCP) and endoscopic papillotomy for a stone in the common bile duct (CBD). He was due to go home on the second postoperative day when he became confused and disorientated. He has a temperature of 39°C, a white cell count (WCC) of 16 000, a serum amylase of 3500 IU and a hyperdynamic circulation.

4 An 80-year-old man, who suffers from chronic obstructive airways disease (COAD), had an emergency laparotomy for intestinal obstruction for gangrenous bowel from ischaemic colitis. He underwent a left hemicolectomy with end colostomy and a Hartmann's closure of the

distal stump. From the second postoperative day, he has been very confused, with laboured breathing and an oxygen saturation of 89 per cent on the pulse oximeter. His chest wall is not moving, with severely reduced air entry in both lungs.

→ 3. Postoperative renal failure

A Hepatorenal syndrome
B Nephrotoxin
C Septic shock
D Postrenal iatrogenic cause

Choose and match the correct diagnosis with each of the scenarios below:

1 A 60-year-old man underwent a right hemicolectomy for carcinoma of the caecum. The operation was straightforward and uneventful. In the past, at the age of 30, he underwent a left nephrectomy for trauma from a motorcycle accident. He put out only 50 mL of urine in the immediate postoperative period. Serum electrolytes show features of incipient renal failure. A catheter inserted into the bladder shows anuria.

2 A 25-year-old male patient was involved in a serious motorcycle accident resulting in polytrauma. He sustained fracture shaft of femur, fracture-dislocation of elbow, renal contusion and blunt abdominal trauma. The injuries have been appropriately treated – open reduction and fixation of the orthopaedic injuries and conservative management of soft tissue injuries. He was put on antibiotics – cefuroxime, metronidazole and gentamicin. On the fifth postoperative day he has been transferred to the ward from the ITU. While on the ward, over 2 days his urinary output has dropped, he is acidotic and his serum electrolytes show features of early renal failure.

3 A 55-year-old male patient underwent a Whipple's operation for periampullary carcinoma. The operation was straightforward. On the third postoperative day, he is back on the ward from the HDU. His urinary output during the last 24 h has been 700 mL. His CVP is 8 cmH_2O and his blood pressure is 130/80 mmHg. His electrolytes show a raised urea and creatinine.

4 A 60-year-old woman underwent an emergency Hartmann's operation for perforated diverticulitis with faecal peritonitis. In the ITU on the second postoperative day, her urinary output has been 20 mL/h. Her central venous pressure (CVP) is 10 cmH_2O and her BP is 130/60 mmHg. She is acidotic with biochemical features of renal failure.

Answers: Multiple choice questions

→ The immediate postoperative period

1. D

Monitoring equipment can cause complications. It is important to make sure that the monitoring equipment has not caused any complications. Air embolism may occur when more than 15 mL of air is accidentally introduced, causing hypotension, tachycardia and distended jugular venous pressure. Thrombophlebitis arising from the nature of fluid infused may occur. This is manifested by pain, redness and induration around the site of needle entry. Those who have an arterial line must be closely inspected for finger necrosis.

Abdominal incisions splint the diaphragm postoperatively, thereby causing the patient to breathe ineffectively because of pain. This results in retention of secretions and encourages postoperative atelectasis. Adequate relief of pain, including epidural analgesia, administration of oxygen and regular physiotherapy, should minimise the chances of this complication.

The most common cause of postoperative hypotension is postoperative bleeding or inadequate fluid replacement; other causes are myocardial infarction and excess of analgesics, particularly epidural analgesia. Monitoring of the CVP would help in finding the cause of hypotension.

Homan's sign (John Homan, 1877–1954, professor of clinical surgery, Harvard Medical School) is extremely unreliable in the diagnosis of DVT. Being aware of the risk factors will help to identify such a complication. Pain, swelling, tenderness, warmth and shiny skin in the calf in a patient with pyrexia are typical of DVT. The diagnosis is confirmed by duplex Doppler (Christian Johann Doppler, 1803–1853, professor of experimental physics, Vienna, enunciated the principle in 1842) ultrasound or venogram.

Oliguria is defined as urinary output of less than 0.5 mL/kg per h. This is a direct result of hypotension causing reduced renal perfusion. Once the patient is adequately perfused, as seen by a normal CVP and blood pressure, various other causes of renal failure should be sought and appropriately treated.

→ Postoperative shortness of breath

2. B

The commonest cause of early postoperative shortness of breath is atelectasis. The patient is usually cyanosed, with the accessory muscles of respiration working to combat the hypoxia. Clinical examination and a chest X-ray confirm the diagnosis. Treatment is prompt, vigorous physiotherapy. Pulmonary embolism is a late cause around the 10th postoperative day. Myocardial infarction, chest infection and pneumothorax are the other causes that are prone to occur in those with cardiac and respiratory pathology preoperatively.

→ Postoperative hypotension

3. A, B, C, D

The commonest cause of low blood pressure in the early postoperative period is bleeding or inadequate fluid replacement. An epidural anaesthetic or too much morphine can be other causes. If the patient suffered from myocardial ischaemia preoperatively, then myocardial infarction must be borne in mind. Anastomotic leakage occurs usually around the fifth postoperative day.

→ Deep vein thrombosis

4. A, C, D, E

The clinical diagnosis in DVT is often not obvious. Most patients show no clinical signs, which classically are calf pain, swelling, warmth, redness and pyrexia. Clinical awareness and duplex Doppler US on the slightest suspicion are the hallmark of an early diagnosis.

→ Postoperative vomiting

5. B

Abdominal operations do not routinely require a nasogastric tube unless the operation has been on the oesophagus or stomach. If acute dilatation of the stomach is suspected, a nasogastric tube is inserted to keep the stomach decompressed and prevent aspiration pneumonia.

→ Postoperative Oliguria

6. B

Oliguria is defined as urine output of <0.5 mL/kg body weight per h. The commonest cause is inadequate fluid replacement. Hence the initial treatment should be a fluid challenge of 250 mL of fluid infused in 1 h. The urine output, jugular venous pressure and CVP are monitored very closely.

Answers: Extended matching questions

→ 1. Postoperative pyrexia

1A

This patient has the classical features of atelectasis – hypoxia with reduced chest wall movement, cyanosis, use of accessory muscles of respiration and reduced air entry in the right lung. On auscultation, bronchial breathing may be heard. A chest X-ray may be helpful. Blood gases are done. The patient is treated by oxygen, vigorous physiotherapy and antibiotics. If the patient does not improve, bedside flexible bronchoscopic aspiration by an anaesthetist will be necessary.

2C

This patient has the typical features of a subphrenic abscess with pain in the shoulder tip, overlying skin oedema, pyrexia towards the end of the first week and signs of pleural effusion on the right side. Following laparoscopic closure, peritoneal lavage might not have been very thorough. Confirmation is done by ultrasound or CT scan followed by CT-guided drainage of the abscess and insertion of a catheter. Rarely, open extraperitoneal drainage may be necessary.

3D

An operation after perforated diverticulitis with faecal peritonitis has a high chance of developing septic complications. Here the patient has come through the immediate postoperative period and has developed late sepsis. The features are those of a wound infection. This needs to be drained with the wound left open to granulate. The patient should be on an antibiotic.

4B

Following abdominoperineal resection, the catheter has been removed and the patient is ready to go home. The symptoms are typical of urinary tract infection from catheterisation. Urine and blood are sent for culture, an ultrasound is done to make sure that the patient is emptying his bladder satisfactorily and he is put on an appropriate antibiotic, which might need to be changed after the culture reports are available.

→ 2. Postoperative confusion

1A

Patients undergoing transurethral resection of prostate may suffer from dilutional hyponatraemia from a condition called TURP (transurethral resection of the prostate) syndrome. This occurs particularly when large resections are undertaken over a prolonged operating time. The irrigating fluid (1.5 per cent glycine) is absorbed through the large venous channels that are opened up during resection. The patient has hypertension, is confused, restless, has visual disturbances and, in extreme cases, seizures and collapse.

The patient needs ITU monitoring. Treatment is supportive in the form of fluid restriction and frusemide. In case of seizures, 3–5 per cent hypertonic saline (250–500 mL) is infused through the CVP line (infusion through a peripheral line will cause thrombophlebitis). This is controversial, as some feel that fluid restriction is all that is needed. Keeping the irrigating fluid below 20 cm above the operating table, using an irrigating resectoscope and IV normal saline for 12 h postoperatively may help to prevent this complication.

2D

Having been treated for his fractured neck of femur, this patient is confused. He has normal biochemical parameters. He is known to suffer from chronic pancreatitis, the commonest cause of which is alcohol abuse. A history of alcoholism should be obtained from him or his relatives. Advice from the physician should be sought with regard to the best form of treatment. Disulfiram (antabuse), an antioxidant, may be used.

3C

This patient would have been jaundiced and septic because of his stone in the CBD. Following ERCP and endoscopic papillotomy he has been confused. His WCC shows that he is septic, in addition to having acute pancreatitis with a raised amylase, which may be a direct complication of ERCP. It is also possible that he is still jaundiced after the procedure. His hyperdynamic circulation (bounding pulse, raised pulse pressure) denotes septic shock.

He needs to be treated in the ITU with close monitoring, antibiotics and mannitol intravenously to prevent hepatorenal syndrome. His acute pancreatitis should be properly stratified and appropriately treated.

4B

Elderly patients undergoing emergency laparotomy, particularly those with co-morbid disease such as COAD, are prone to postoperative bronchopneumonia. Tachypnoea, cyanosis and confusion are the hallmarks of this condition. Diminution of chest wall movements, dullness on percussion and lack of air entry are the clinical signs. The diagnosis is confirmed by a chest X-ray. Prompt and aggressive treatment is instituted with the help of an anaesthetist. The patient may require respiratory support. In extreme cases, acute respiratory distress syndrome (ARDS) may result.

3. Postoperative renal failure

1D

This patient, who has only one kidney on the right side, has had a right hemicolectomy. He has developed virtual anuria immediately after the operation. Although the operation was 'straightforward and uneventful', iatrogenic damage to the right ureter resulting in postrenal renal failure should be considered unless otherwise proven. It is a sad fact that iatrogenic damage to structures at operation occur mostly during 'relatively easy' operations. The 50 mL of urine passed would have been the urine produced before the right ureter was tied off. Classically it is the right ureter that is in danger during this operation.

The patient needs an urgent ultrasound of his kidney to show any hydronephrosis, followed by an urgent IVU to determine renal function from his solitary kidney. Once this mishap is proven, the patient needs urgent exploration by a urologist who would consider some sort of ureteric repair or reimplantation (see Skinner R, Watson D. Renal failure. In: Goldhill DR, Stuart Withington P, eds. *Textbook of Intensive Care*, Chapman and Hall, 1997, Ch. 52).

2B

This young patient is susceptible to renal failure for two reasons: use of gentamicin and myoglobinuria, both of which act as nephrotoxins. In multiple trauma, rhabdomyolysis occurs, releasing myoglobin from damaged muscle. Myoglobin precipitates in the renal tubules, causing acute tubular necrosis. Diagnosis is confirmed by raised plasma creatine kinase and myoglobinuria. Treatment is to maintain hydration and encourage alkaline diuresis. In addition, gentamicin levels are measured to ensure there is no drug toxicity and advice is sought from the microbiologist.

3A

This patient with periampullary carcinoma would have been suffering from obstructive jaundice and incipient liver failure preoperatively. Such patients are susceptible to renal failure from hepatorenal syndrome. Liver failure causes systemic vasodilatation, resulting in the secretion of vasoconstrictors, catecholamines and angiotensin-producing intrarenal vasoconstriction. This causes a decrease in the production of intrarenal prostaglandins (which is normally responsible for intrarenal vasodilatation), resulting in poor renal perfusion and causing renal failure. It may be precipitated by hypovolaemia, sepsis and nephrotoxins.

This problem is best prevented by good preoperative and intraoperative hydration, preventing infection with prophylactic antibiotics and maintaining diuresis with peri- and postoperative mannitol. To minimise the chances of hepatorenal syndrome, some surgeons alleviate the jaundice by inserting a CBD stent preoperatively and leaving it in for a few days, thus reducing the level of serum bilirubin. However, other surgeons prefer not to do so because stent insertion may introduce infection and, by reducing the girth of the CBD, makes the choledochojejunal anastomosis more difficult.

4C

This patient has septic shock, causing renal failure. This is of renal origin as infection is nephrotoxic. Treatment is mainly supportive: care in the ITU, use of appropriate antibiotics, avoidance of nephrotoxic drugs, maintenance of optimum hydration closely monitored by CVP and use of diuretics. The use of dopamine is controversial.

PART 4 Trauma

21 Introduction to trauma 153

22 Trauma epidemiology 156

23 Head injury 160

24 Neck and spine 166

25 Trauma to the face and mouth 171

26 Trauma to the chest and abdomen 176

27 Extremity trauma 185

28 Burns 195

29 Plastic and reconstructive surgery 205

30 Disaster surgery 212

21 Introduction to trauma

Multiple choice questions

➜ Trauma

1. **In trauma, which of the following statements are true?**

A It is the third most common cause of death overall.
B It is the leading cause of death and disability below 40 years of age.
C In children, one must always be alert to the potential of non-accidental injury (NAI).
D The 'imperative of time' dictates the priority of treatment.
E The pressure of time shapes trauma management.

➜ Assessment of trauma

2. **Which of the following statements are false?**

A The mechanism of injury and the injury produced are the keystones in management.
B It is as essential to identify overt (obvious) injuries as it is to identify the covert (hidden) injury.
C Penetrating injuries usually involve the use of weapons.
D Blunt injuries are the outcome of acceleration/deceleration, such as falls or road traffic accidents (RTAs).
E Knife injury over a limb is easy to evaluate.

➜ Firearm injury

3. **In firearm injuries, which of the following statements are true?**

A Low-velocity bullet wounds behave like knife injuries.
B High-velocity bullets cause cavitation.
C A permanent cavity is one that remains after the initial impact.
D A temporary cavity is one that lasts momentarily and is not apparent during clinical examination.
E A permanent cavity gives an idea of the extent of damage.

➜ Blunt injury

4. **Which of the following statements regarding blunt injury are false?**

A The mechanisms are direct or indirect.
B In indirect injury, associated injuries may be present and should be sought.
C Overt injury should lead the clinician to look for a covert injury as well.
D Proper exposure is essential so as not to miss other injuries.
E In chest injuries damage to abdominal organs is rare.

➜ Covert injury

5. **Regarding covert injuries, which of the following statements are true?**

A Adopt a deductive approach.
B Adopt a look-everywhere approach.
C Adopt a focused approach.
D Positively exclude a critical diagnosis.
E Screen patients where clinical signs are obvious.

➜ Non-accidental injury

6. **In relation to NAI in children, which of the following statements are false?**

A History is inconsistent with the injury sustained.
B There is a changing history.
C There are likely to be injuries of differing ages or duration.
D There is likely to be aggressive behaviour from the carers.
E In multiple fractures, osteogenesis imperfecta may be first diagnosis.

Polytrauma

7. Which of the following statements are true with regard to a polytrauma patient?

A A drop in body temperature occurs.
B There is a generalised immune response.
C The patient has compensatory mechanisms to blood loss.
D The early management is protocol-driven.
E A protocol-driven system should never be transgressed.

Answers: Multiple choice questions

Trauma

1. A, B, C, D, E

The term 'imperative of time' means determining which injuries need to be dealt with immediately and those that can wait. For example, an obstructed airway, tension pneumothorax, an extradural haematoma or an ischaemic limb can be dealt with by various grades of urgency. The order of ABCD (airways, breathing, circulation and disability) enunciated by the ATLS (Advanced Trauma Life Support) protocol precisely helps in a polytrauma situation when time is at a premium.

Assessment of trauma

2. E

In civilian practice the two commonest groups of mechanisms of injury are blunt and penetrating. Blunt wounds are caused by falls, at sport or in RTAs, whereas penetrating wounds are caused by knives or low-velocity firearms. Knife injuries over a limb are not always easy to evaluate because penetration of a neighbouring joint may not always be obvious.

Firearm injury

3. A, B, C, D

High-velocity bullet injury crushes the tissues in its pathway and produces a cavity. Two types of cavity can be produced: a permanent cavity that remains after the initial impact and a temporary cavity that is not apparent and can extend well beyond the site of injury. A permanent cavity gives no idea about the extent of underlying damage. This necessitates wide wound exploration and may require radical wound excision.

Blunt injury

4. E

Anatomically the abdominal contents extend into the chest. Therefore, in blunt trauma to the lower chest, liver and splenic injuries are common. In direct blunt trauma, the injury is concentrated at the site of impact and the effects on the soft tissues are at the injured site. In indirect injury, damage away from the site of injury should be sought. For example in fracture of the shaft of the ulna caused by indirect trauma from fall on an outstretched hand (overt injury), there may be a covert injury of a dislocated upper end of head of radius (Monteggia fracture dislocation).

Covert injury

5. A, B, C, D

Ideally screening of at-risk patients should be carried out before clinical signs are obvious. This can be done by the deductive approach, such as looking for a flexion spinal injury and damage to the pancreas and duodenum in a child with a lap seatbelt in the back seat of a car involved in a head-on collision. Another example is to look for a posterior cruciate ligament tear and/or posterior dislocation of hip in a dashboard injury.

A look-everywhere approach is essential in an unconscious patient to exclude ankle fracture, scaphoid fracture, peripheral nerve injuries and ruptured diaphragm. This approach is summarised by the term 'secondary survey' in the ATLS protocol.

A focused exclusion approach is mandatory in life-threatening injuries, such as performing a CT scan in suspected extradural haematoma or a focused abdominal sonography in trauma (FAST) or echocardiography in cardiac tamponade.

➜ Non-accidental injury

6. E

The carers of an allegedly abused child would usually cite brittle-bone disease (osteogenesis imperfecta) as the cause of multiple fractures. This should not be accepted as the cause and the clinician should admit the patient for further, thorough evaluation and care as a team.

➜ Polytrauma

7. A, B, C, D

As a part of the patient's metabolic response to trauma, there is a drop in body temperature. This may be due to exposure, inactivity, hypovolaemia and loss of vasomotor control. Heat loss should be prevented. The patient has compensatory mechanisms to blood loss to maintain perfusion of vital organs; hypotension in itself is therefore not a problem. In most cases, early management is usually protocol-driven, which allows for easier and quicker decision-making. Moreover, their use protects the patient and the doctor, the latter from litigation. The surgical plan will be recorded in the patient's notes, but a good method is to record all the details on a whiteboard in the theatre, outlining the proposed overall management. Whilst protocols denote good practice, the team leader may not always decide to adhere slavishly to a protocol in the best interest of the patient. For example, in a bullet injury of the popliteal fossa, deliberations between the vascular and orthopaedic surgeons will tailor the need of that particular individual patient.

22 Trauma epidemiology

Multiple choice questions

➜ Epidemiology

1. **Which of the following statements regarding trauma are true?**

A Trauma is the second commonest cause of death worldwide in the population aged 1–40 years.
B Road traffic accident injuries are the commonest cause of injury-related death worldwide.
C Falls are the commonest cause of injury-related death worldwide.
D A 10 per cent increase in vehicle speed leads to a 20 per cent rise in case fatality risk.
E Ejection from the vehicle at the time of accident saves a significant number of people from more serious injury.
F Seatbelts and airbags can actually cause injuries.
G The Advanced Trauma Life Support initiative (ATLS) required that a primary survey is performed before resuscitation is started.
H The secondary survey is designed to ensure that no new injuries have developed in what is an emergent situation.

➜ Assessment and management of the polytraumatised patient

2. **Which of the following statements regarding the immediate management of a polytraumatised patient are true?**

A When the patient enters the resuscitation room the first priority is to listen to the history given by the rescue team.
B The patient should be asked a simple question such as 'What is your name?'
C ABC (airway, breathing, circulation) is the primary survey.
D Airway management should be accompanied by cervical spine control.
E Oxygen should be administered with great care in polytraumatised patients who might suffer from chronic bronchitis.
F The physical signs of a tension pneumothorax are difficult to pick up in the resuscitation room and so it is best diagnosed by an immediate chest X-ray.

3. **A 25-year-old motorcyclist comes in on a spine board with cervical spine control. He was found at the roadside unconscious following a collision with an oncoming car. The airway is clear but his breathing is clearly laboured with a respiratory rate of 40/min. His pulse is 110/min and his blood pressure is 90/60. It appears that the wing mirror of the car has penetrated his chest and there is a wound on the right side which is bubbling. He is not responding to verbal command but is muttering incoherently. He will not open his eyes.**

(a) **List the following tasks in their order of priority:**

A Insert a chest drain.
B Give 100 per cent oxygen.
C Put a flap valve dressing over the bubbling wound.
D Insert two wide-bore cannulae.
E Take an arterial blood gas (ABG) sample.
F Start checking for other injuries.
G Give intravenous (IV) fluids.
H Start a blood transfusion.

During the secondary survey, you discover blood in one ear. The abdomen is silent and distending. The pelvis feels stable, but there is a wound over the left tibia which is obviously angulated. After the first bolus of fluid, the blood pressure rises to 100/70 mmHg (from 90/0) and the pulse falls to 105/min (from 110). A second bolus produces a further improvement, as does a third. The blood pressure is maintained. The chest drain is swinging normally and has drained 100 mL of blood. The patient's conscious state has improved to the extent that he will open his eyes to command. The left foot is dusky-coloured. No pulses can be felt in the foot and there is no capillary refill.

(b) List in order the priorities of your next actions:

A Take the patient to theatre immediately for a laparotomy.
B Get X-rays of the cervical spine, chest and pelvis.
C Get a CT of the chest and abdomen and head.
D Take the patient to theatre for debridement of the tibial wound.
E Ask for an arteriogram of the left leg.
F Put in a urinary catheter.

4. **A child of 3 years is brought into the A&E department having fallen from a first floor balcony. He is unconscious and breathing rapidly (60/min) but blood pressure and pulse are within normal limits. Primary survey reveals a bruise on the forehead and that pupils are equal and responding to light. Air entry is good into both lungs. The abdomen appears distended and is silent. The pelvis is stable. The legs appear normal. It is not possible to gain IV access.**

Put the following actions into order of priority:

A The child should be moved to the ward and put on hourly neurological observation.
B Intraosseous needles should be inserted.
C Blood gases should be taken.
D Blood should be sent for cross-match.
E An ultrasound scan or CT scan of the abdomen should be obtained.
F The child should be taken straight to the operating theatre for a laparotomy.

5. **A 70-year-old female falls and sustains a fractured neck of femur. She is admitted to hospital at 7.30pm. She is a known hypertensive who is on diuretics and lives alone. You find her blood pressure is 160/100 mmHg and her pulse is 70/min. She is fully alert and orientated and has no other injuries.**

Choose the best option:

A Set her up for operation as soon as possible that evening.
B Wait until the blood results are back and then discuss the situation with the anaesthetist planning to optimise her for surgery on the morning list.
C Leave all planning until the morning as it is now 'out of hours'.
D Insist that you operate that night, however long you have to wait.

Answers: Multiple choice questions

→ Epidemiology

1. B, F

Trauma is the commonest cause of death worldwide in the population aged 1–40. Within that group, road traffic accidents are the commonest cause of death with falls running second. Energy is important in predicting severity of injury. As the energy involved in an accident is proportional to the square of the velocity, an increase in speed of as little as 10 per cent leads to a 40 per cent increase in mortality.

Seatbelts reduce the risk of injury by nearly 50 per cent and also prevent ejection, which is associated with a much higher mortality rate. Both seatbelts and airbags prevent large numbers of deaths and injuries. However, they also cause injuries (a far fewer number), characteristically in the abdomen and thorax.

The ATLS is a system for providing the safest and quickest possible diagnosis and treatment for any patient who has sustained polytrauma. The primary survey is carried out at the same time as the initial resuscitation. The secondary survey is aimed at checking all other parts of the body and systems once the primary survey has identified immediate life-threatening problems.

→ Assessment and management of the polytraumatised patient

2. A, B, C, D

When the patient first enters the resuscitation room it is important that the handover is taken from the ambulance (rescue) crew who can give vital information on the energy involved in the accident, the time since the accident occurred and the likely major injuries, all crucial pieces of information. The patient should then be asked a simple question such as 'What is your name?' because if they can respond, then you have effectively completed the primary ABC survey. In order to speak coherently, a patient must have a clear airway, be able to breathe and have adequate perfusion of the brain. The cervical spine needs protecting as soon as resuscitation starts, and so control should be started at the same time as the airway is checked. All trauma patients (without fail) should receive 100 per cent oxygen at high rate (15 L/min) via a rebreathing mask. The signs of a tension pneumothorax can be difficult to see and hear in the resuscitation room, but the diagnosis should never be made by X-ray as the condition can progress so quickly that the patient may be dead before the picture is available.

3. (a) B → C → D → G → E → A → F

The fact that the patient is muttering, albeit incoherently, suggests that his airway is clear, although it should still be checked anyway. The next priority is breathing, so the first action here is to give 100 per cent oxygen. The patient clearly has a sucking wound so a flap valve dressing should be put over this as soon as possible, as this will improve his ventilatory effort. A chest drain will be needed but this is not the next priority, as you have dealt with the critical respiratory crisis. The next priority is therefore circulation. He needs two wide-bore cannulae, but his blood pressure and pulse suggest that he is already in hypovolaemic shock and so IV fluids should be given as soon as the cannulae are in place. Blood should be sent for cross-match but there is no place for giving blood yet until we see how his pulse and blood pressure respond to the initial fluids. Blood gases will be needed as soon as possible, and then, once the hypovolaemic shock has been stabilised, a chest drain will be needed. Only when AB and C have been sorted should you proceed on to the secondary survey.

3. (b) B → F → E → C → D → A

The patient has responded well to a fluid bolus so, although he may have lost a lot of blood, it does not appear that he is currently bleeding hard. There is therefore no need to take him to theatre immediately. His conscious state is also improving, suggesting that he is perfusing oxygenated blood. There is therefore time to carry out some investigations. He needs the standard set of X-rays (cervical spine, chest and pelvis) and these should be performed before the urinary catheter is put in, just in case there is a pelvic fracture which has torn the urethra. The left leg has got some sort of vascular damage so the next priority is defining the level and extent of that damage with an arteriogram. The left tibia is an open fracture and so needs cleaning in theatre once the arteriogram has been performed. However, it would be wise to get a CT of the head, abdomen and chest to determine the full extent of the abdominal and thoracic damage so that, if necessary, more than one surgical team can work on him under the same anaesthetic.

4. B → D → E → F → C → A

Children have a higher respiratory rate than adults but this respiratory rate is higher than it should be. In young children the only sign of hypovolaemic shock may be an increase in respiration rate as fall in blood pressure and rise in pulse are very late changes in children (when blood loss exceeds 30 per cent). In the absence of any abnormal findings in the chest, it must be assumed that this child is developing severe hypovolaemic shock. The first priority is therefore some form of access to give fluids. This will be via intraosseous needle if IV access cannot be obtained. Blood should also be sent immediately for cross-match as it may be needed imminently. Either ultrasound (FAST scan) or a CT scan of the abdomen (combined with a CT of the head) is vital for planning the next stage of treatment. This is likely to be a laparotomy as this child is showing the cardinal signs (in this age group) of hypovolaemic shock.

5. B

Patients with a fractured neck of femur should be operated on as soon as possible, firstly to relieve their pain and secondly to keep their stay in hospital as short as possible so that they can maintain independence. However, elderly patients usually have more than one thing wrong with them and it is best practice to ensure that the patient's condition is optimised before surgery is undertaken, to minimise the anaesthetic risk. This planning needs to start immediately, but surgery should only be undertaken when it is complete. It is unlikely that the work-up will be completed before 10pm when all surgery should cease apart from that involving life and limb. The surgery should therefore be planned for first thing in the morning.

23 Head injury

Multiple choice questions

Cerebral physiology

1. What is normal cerebral blood flow?

A 10mL/100 g per min
B 25 mL/100 g per min
C 55 mL/100 g per min
D 100 mL/100 g per min
E 5.5 mL/100 g per min.

2. Cerebral autoregulation maintains normal cerebral blood flow in what range of mean arterial blood pressures?

A 50–150 mmHg
B 50–100mmHg
C 25–50 mmHg
D 80–200 mmHg
E 100–250 mmHg.

3. How is cerebral perfusion pressure defined?

A Systolic arterial blood pressure minus diastolic blood pressure
B Systolic arterial blood pressure minus venous pressure
C Mean arterial blood pressure minus venous pressure
D Mean arterial blood pressure minus intracranial pressure (ICP)
E Venous pressure minus ICP.

4. Which of the following compensatory mechanisms maintain normal ICP in the face of an increasing intracranial mass lesion in adults?

A Reduction in venous blood volume
B Increase in skull volume
C Sunsetting eyes
D Reduction in cerebrospinal fluid (CSF) volume
E Increase in CSF production.

Head injury

5. Which of the following statements regarding Glasgow Coma Scale (GCS) are true?

A The maximum score is 15.
B The minimum score is 0.
C A GCS of 10 means the patient is in coma.
D Eye opening to command/speech is scored as 2.
E A GCS of 6 means the patient is in coma.

6. When does primary brain injury occur?

A At the moment of impact
B In the first hour after injury
C In the first 4 h after injury
D Only if the patient is in coma
E In the first 24 h after injury.

7. Which of the following can cause secondary brain injury?

A Hypoxia
B Hypotension
C Raised ICP
D Reduced cerebral perfusion
E Pyrexia.

8. What is the incidence of traumatic brain injury in the UK?

A 450 cases per 100 000 population
B 100 cases per 100 000 population
C 20–40 cases per 100 000 population
D 20–40 cases per 1 000 000 population
E 5 cases per 100 000 population.

Clinical management of head injury

9. Which of the following clinical signs are evidence of a base of skull fracture?

A CSF rhinorrhoea
B CSF otorrhoea

C Battle's sign
D Periorbital bruising
E Haemotympanum.

10. Which of the following statements regarding extradural haematoma are true?

A It is often caused by a skull fracture with laceration of the middle meningeal artery.
B It commonly occurs at the pterion.
C There is often a lucid interval.
D Treatment is with a burrhole.
E Prognosis is poor.

11. Which of the following statements regarding acute subdural haematoma are true?

A It is a collection of blood between the dura and arachnoid membranes.
B It can be caused by laceration of the brain.
C It can be due to disruption of a cortical blood vessel.
D It has a good prognosis.
E It has a biconvex shape on CT scans.

12. Patients with severe head injury often develop a low blood sodium level (hyponatraemia). Which of the following are causes?

A The syndrome of inappropriate secretion of antidiuretic hormone (ADH)
B Uncontrolled diabetes insipidus
C Secretion of atrial natriuretic factor
D Uncontrolled diabetes mellitus
E Excess production of cortisol.

13. In what percentage of patients with head injury do late seizures (i.e. >1 week after head injury) occur?

A 20 per cent
B 5 per cent
C 50 per cent
D 90 per cent
E Never, unless they had an early seizure.

14. Which of the following statements regarding third nerve palsy in head injury are true?

A It causes a fixed, dilated pupil.
B It may cause the eye to deviate upwards.
C It is caused by pressure on the third nerve by a herniated uncus.
D It usually occurs on the opposite side to the haematoma.
E It is never bilateral.

Extended matching questions

→ 1. Head injury

A Extradural haematoma
B Subdural haematoma
C Petrous temporal skull fracture

Choose and match the conditions above with the clinical scenarios described below:

1 A 45-year-old man is involved in a road traffic accident. He is deeply unconscious at the scene. Examination shows him to be GCS 7 with a fixed dilated right pupil. He is intubated for transfer to A&E.

2 A 30-year-old man is involved in a fight. He is punched and falls to the ground, striking his head on the kerb. He is briefly knocked out but recovers quickly. In A&E he is GCS 15. He has blood and clear fluid leaking from his right ear. Examination shows a Battle's sign.

3 A 25-year-old man fell 15 feet from a tree. There was a brief loss of consciousness witnessed by his friends. When the ambulance arrived he was GCS 15. In A&E he was noted to have a right

temporal scalp laceration. One hour later his GCS score dropped to 13. Thirty minutes later he was noted to be GCS 8 with a fixed dilated right pupil.

Answers: Multiple choice questions

→ Cerebral physiology

1. C

The brain does not have large stores of glucose or oxygen and is dependent on cerebral blood flow to deliver these essential substrates. Cerebral blood flow is therefore tightly regulated. A normal cerebral blood flow is 55 mL/100 g per min, equating to approximately 770 mL/min of blood flow. Brain function will quickly cease if cerebral blood flow falls below 20 per cent of normal.

2. A

Cerebral autoregulation maintains normal cerebral blood flow between mean arterial blood pressures of 50 and 150 mmHg. Cerebral autoregulation is the mechanism whereby cerebral blood flow is maintained in the face of variations in arterial blood pressure. Three main mechanisms are involved:

- Smooth muscle in the walls of the arterioles in the brain respond to stretch in the vessel wall and alter the diameter of the blood vessel accordingly. Constriction reduces flow and dilatation increases flow.
- The concentration of O_2 and CO_2 (but principally CO_2) causes alteration in the diameter of the arterioles, e.g. increased CO_2 causes dilatation and increased blood flow.
- Concentrations of metabolites such as K^+ and H^+ cause variations in the blood vessel diameter. Increased concentrations of these metabolites cause vasodilatation and increased blood flow.

Autoregulation is often abnormal or lost completely in severe brain injury. In this case, cerebral blood flow may be 'pressure-passive', i.e. cerebral blood flow increases as the blood pressure increases and falls as the blood pressure falls.

Reducing CO_2 levels (hyperventilation) can be used therapeutically. It causes cerebral vasoconstriction (if autoregulation is still present) and reduces cerebral blood volume and therefore reduces ICP. Unfortunately, the cerebral vasoconstriction thus caused can result in brain ischaemia so it should be used with caution.

3. D

Perfusion pressure generally equates to mean arterial pressure minus venous pressure but cerebral perfusion pressure is defined as mean arterial BP minus ICP. ICP is usually the same as cerebral venous pressure but is easier to measure.

4. A, D

Compensatory mechanisms that maintain normal ICP in the face of an increasing intracranial mass lesion in adults include reduction in venous blood volume and reduction in CSF volume. This is the doctrine of Monro–Kellie. It states that the head is a closed box that cannot expand. It contains brain, blood and CSF. An expanding mass lesion will initially cause reduction in venous blood volume and CSF volume and therefore pressure will remain constant. As the mass lesion increases, it may compress the brain. Arterial volume is maintained until the late stages. At a certain point the mass lesion will overcome the compensatory mechanisms and ICP will start to rise. At this point, small increases in volume will cause large increases in pressure. This can be shown as a pressure–volume curve.

This is why neurosurgical patients can rapidly deteriorate having been apparently stable and why it is so important to take seriously small deteriorations in function or level of consciousness.

Head injury

5. A, E

The GCS is a three-point scale used to describe the level of consciousness in patients with head injury. The highest score is 15 (normal) and the lowest score is 3 (deep coma). The patient is assessed on ability to open eyes, motor responses and vocalisation. A patient of GCS 8 (with no eye opening) or less is considered to be in coma.

6. A

Primary brain injury describes the injury that happens at the moment of impact or injury.

7. A, B, C, D, E

Secondary brain injury can occur at any time after the primary injury and is often caused by hypoxia, hypotension, raised ICP, expanding mass lesions, seizures and increased temperature.

8. C

The incidence of traumatic brain injury in the UK is well documented at 20–40 cases per 100 000 population. Many of these cases are in young men. Head injury is a significant cause of permanent disability in young men.

Clinical management of head injury

9. A, B, C, D, E

A base of skull fracture in the anterior cranial fossa may cause leakage of CSF through the nose via fractures in the frontal or ethmoid sinuses. This can predispose to meningitis or brain abscess.

Base of skull fractures affecting the petrous temporal bone can cause deafness in the ipsilateral ear due to damage to the cochlea or its nerve, ipsilateral lower motor neuron facial weakness due to laceration or compression of the facial nerve, or CSF otorrhoea if the tympanic membrane is ruptured. If the tympanic membrane is intact, blood and CSF may be seen behind the bulging eardrum. If the tympanic membrane is intact, CSF may track down the Eustachian tube into the back of the throat and from there may be seen as rhinorrhoea.

Battle's sign is a patch of bruising behind the ear, indicating a fracture of the petrous temporal bone. Periorbital bruising (often known as racoon eyes), which may be associated with subconjunctival haemorrhages with no obvious posterior margin, is often seen in fractures of the anterior skull base.

Prophylactic antibiotics are not indicated for CSF leaks as their use has not been shown to reduce the risk of meningitis, but they have been shown to increase the incidence of multiply resistant organisms in the CSF if meningitis occurs.

10. A, B, C

Extradural haematomas are usually associated with a skull fracture, often in the region of the pterion, as this is where the middle meningeal artery runs. The edges of the fracture rupture the middle meningeal artery, which then bleeds into the potential space between the skull and the dura. The dura is stripped off the internal aspect of the skull as the haematoma increases in size. There is often no underlying brain injury and these patients classically have a 'lucid interval' but then slowly deteriorate in the hours following the injury. The prognosis is good if the haematoma can be evacuated promptly.

CT scan shows a biconvex haematoma which does not cross suture lines. The treatment of choice is craniotomy. Burrhole evacuation is not recommended as the bleeding vessel cannot be controlled and the blood clot is often solid and cannot be evacuated through a small burrhole.

11. A, B, C

Acute subdural haematoma has a poorer prognosis than an extradural haematoma because it is usually associated with underlying brain injury. The cause of the haematoma is often laceration of a cortical vessel in association with severe cortical contusions. This often affects the tips of the frontal or temporal lobes ('burst temporal lobe'). In some cases the blood comes from torn cortical bridging veins around the superior sagittal sinus. Multiple bleeding points are not unusual. The blood collects under the dura, usually between dura and arachnoid membranes, although in some cases the arachnoid membrane is also breached.

On CT scan the haematoma is less well defined than an extradural haematoma and does not have a biconvex shape.

12. A, C

Hyponatraemia is often caused by syndrome of inappropriate ADH secretion (SIADH) or excess secretion of atrial natriuretic factor (ANF). It is important to distinguish between the two. SIADH is caused by the kidneys holding on to water due to the action of excess ADH on the renal tubules. The total body sodium is normal but total body water is increased. Sodium is low due to a dilutional effect and water restriction can be used to treat this condition.

Excess secretion of ANF causes sodium to be lost by the kidneys, and therefore total body sodium will be low and total body water will also be low as water follows the sodium into the urine. The patient is dehydrated and CVP measurements will show a low CVP. Excess salt excretion by the kidneys can be shown by collecting 24 h urine samples. Treatment is salt and water replacement.

Diabetes insipidus is caused by lack of secretion of ADH and causes a high urine output and dehydration as the kidneys are unable to concentrate the urine. The sodium will rise (hypernatraemia). Diabetes mellitus (raised blood glucose) is common in severely injured patients but is not a cause of hyponatraemia. Increased cortisol secretion will occur as part of the stress response to injury but will not cause hyponatraemia.

13. B

Late seizures occur in 5 per cent of patients with head injury and for that reason patients with severe head injury are not allowed to drive for some time after injury. Patients must be told to inform the DVLA. Seizures can usually be controlled with anticonvulsants.

14. A, C

The third cranial nerve leaves the midbrain in the interpeduncular fossa. Expanding haematomas cause the uncus of the temporal lobe to be pushed across and through the tentorial hiatus where it compresses the third nerve on the same side as the lesion. This causes a dilated pupil which will then become fixed. This is usually on the same side as the lesion. As the pressure and shift increase, the opposite third nerve will be affected and both pupils will become fixed and dilated. A third nerve palsy causes the eye to lie in a 'down and out' position.

Answers: Extended matching questions

→ 1. Head injury

1B

Subdural haematomas are serious injuries often associated with severe underlying brain injury. The patient is usually unconscious from the time of injury. It is important to avoid secondary brain injury, and airway management (i.e. intubation and ventilation) is essential in an unconscious patient to avoid hypoxia or hypercarbia. Hypotension must also be treated.

2C

Base of skull fractures affecting the petrous temporal bone can cause otorrhoea. The patient may also have a facial nerve palsy or deafness on the same side. Battle's sign is an area of bruising behind the ear. The patient will have an increased risk of meningitis but should not be started on prophylactic antibiotics as these have not been shown to reduce the risk of meningitis.

3A

Extradural haematomas often present with a lucid interval following the injury when the patient can appear very well. The patient must have had an underlying skull fracture which lacerated the middle meningeal artery or one of its branches. The extradural collects over time. Initially the compensatory mechanisms described in the Monro–Kellie doctrine maintain ICP, but eventually brain shift occurs with raised ICP and the patient starts to deteriorate. When this starts to happen, further deterioration can happen quickly.

The patient should be intubated and ventilated and an urgent CT scan should be performed. Mannitol may be given. Urgent referral to the neurosurgeon is essential.

24 Neck and spine

Multiple choice questions

➜ Anatomy of spine injury

1. **Which of the following statements regarding spine injury are true?**

A Cervical spine cord injuries are common.
B Pre-hospital care has slightly reduced their incidence.
C A factor which reduces length of stay and improves outcome is referral to specialist spinal centres.
D The size of the spinal canal makes the cervical spine especially susceptible to injury.
E The stability of the cervical spine is mainly provided by the bony anatomy.
F The cervicothoracic junction is especially susceptible to injury because it is a transition zone from the mobile to the rigid segment of the spinal cord.
G All three columns of the spinal column must be injured for the spine to be unstable.
H The spinal cord ends at L5/S1.
I The cervical roots exit above the vertebral body of the same name, while the thoracic and lumbar roots exit below.
J The secondary spinal injury is usually a result of the unstable spine moving during rescue and treatment of the patient.

➜ Case study: injury after fall

2. **A patient is admitted unconscious with a head injury following a 4-metre fall from the roof of a building. His blood pressure is 80/60 mmHg, pulse 45/min, and he has well-perfused extremities.**

(a) What is the likelihood of him having a significant spinal injury?
A <20 per cent
B >20 per cent
C >50 per cent.

(b) What is the safest and most reliable way to clear the cervical spine?
A Cervical spine series of plain X-rays
B Flexion and extension views
C Magnetic resonance imaging (MRI)
D Keep him on a spine board until he recovers consciousness.

(c) What fluids need to be given?
A No fluids are needed at this stage.
B Two litres of saline should be given stat and then further litres until the systolic pressure comes above 110 mmHg.
C Put a central venous pressure line, and a urinary catheter. Fluids should be titrated against preload pressure and urine output.

The patient wakes up and cannot move his legs. Examination reveals a step between T10 and T11 which is painful.

(d) Which of the following tests give the best idea of prognosis?
A Perianal sensation
B Bulbocavernosus reflex
C A loss of power proprioception on one side with loss of temperature and pain sensation on the other side.

Examination of the lower limbs of the patient reveals sensation present in the lower limbs but no motor power.

(e) What Frankel Grade is this patient?
A A
B B
C C
D D
E E.

Visualisation in neck and spine injury

3. **Which of the following statements regarding visualisation are false?**
   A Provided that the cervicothoracic junction is visualised, plain X-rays are adequate to identify almost 100 per cent of significant spinal injuries.
   B CT scan is best at demonstrating soft-tissue haematoma in the cord.
   C MRI is best for reconstructions which help understand the nature of the bone injury.

Cervical spine injury

4. **A patient is found to have an unstable cervical spine injury, with bifacet dislocation. He has a partial neurological deficit (Frankel C).**

   (a) What investigation is needed?
   A Tomograms
   B CT
   C MRI.

   (b) What is the optimum treatment?
   A Stiff collar
   B Traction via a halo
   C Open reduction and internal fixation with bone graft plates and screws.

   (c) The neurology now starts to deteriorate. What is your management plan now?
   A Stiff collar
   B Traction via a halo
   C Open reduction and internal fixation with bone graft plates and screws.

Extended matching questions

1. Fractures, dislocations and subluxations

A Anterior craniocervical dislocation
B Atlantoaxial instability
C Teardrop fracture.
D Type A thoracic fracture
E Type B thoracic fracture
F Wedge fracture
G Type C thoracic fracture
H SCIWORA
I Hangman's fracture
J Type 1 odontoid peg fracture
K Posterior craniocervical dislocation
L Facet dislocation
M Chance fracture
N Type 2 odontoid peg fracture
O Type 3 odontoid peg fracture
P Jefferson's
Q Burst fracture

Choose and match the correct fracture/dislocation/subluxation for each of the scenarios given below:

1 A patient presents having fallen on their head from a height. The atlas is fractured and expanded.

2 A patient presents having fallen on their head from a height. The C4 vertebra is fractured and expanded.

3 A patient is found to have a Power ratio of more than one. What fracture/dislocation/subluxation is this?

4 A child spontaneously develops a wry neck with a cock robin appearance.

5 A patient is noted on MRI to have an isolated rupture of the transverse ligament.

6 CT of the patient's cervical spine reveals a transverse fracture through the neck of the odontoid peg.

7 A patient sustains a rotational unstable fracture of the thoracic spine.

8 A patient has a fracture, which is effectively a spondylolisthesis of C2 on C3.

9 A patient has a hyperflexion injury. The X-ray shows that the vertical height of C4 vertebra is 50 per cent less at the front than the back.

10 A patient has a hyperextension injury. X-ray shows a small chip of bone off the front of a vertebral body next to the disc space.

11 A patient has a hyperflexion injury combined with axial loading. X-ray shows C3 subluxed forward on C4.

12 A patient sustains a flexion distraction injury at the thoracolumbar junction following a high-speed road traffic accident where they were wearing a seatbelt.

13 An elderly female patient slips and lands on her bottom. She now has severe thoracic spine pain and a kyphus at T6.

14 A child sustains a high-speed flexion injury. There is a neurological deficit but no abnormality visible on X-ray.

Answers: Multiple choice questions

→ Anatomy of spine injury

1. C, F, I

Cervical spine cord injuries are really very rare (< 50 per million per annum). Their incidence has not changed despite the introduction of stringent protocols for pre-hospital care, but the outcome does seem to have improved. However, the single factor which has been shown to make the largest difference to length of stay in hospital, and indeed to eventual outcome, is referral to a specialist spinal injuries unit.

The spinal canal in the cervical region is very spacious, so relatively large displacements of the vertebra of the cervical spine can occur without compromise to the spinal cord itself. The cervical spine is very mobile in several planes and so there is very little bony stability. Instead, the stability is provided by the ligaments connecting the motion segments. In contrast, the thoracic spine is relatively rigid. The transition between mobile and stiff segments in any mechanical structure is the area most vulnerable to extreme loads, and so the cervicothoracic junction (the area most difficult to visualise) is also the very area most likely to be fractured or dislocated.

The anatomy of the spinal column provides stability through three columns: the anterior (the front of the vertebral body and intervertebral discs), the middle (the back of the vertebral body and the anterior longitudinal ligaments) and the posterior (the spines with their interspinous ligaments and the facet joints with their pedicles). Disruption of one column does not produce instability, but disruption of all three does. Where there is disruption of two columns, the spine is usually stable but not always.

At birth the spinal cord extends the length of the spinal canal, but by adulthood the conus medullaris (the end of the spinal cord) stops at T12/L1. From then on the spinal roots (cauda equina) pass down to exit below their vertebral bodies. In the cervical spine, the spinal roots exit above the vertebral body with the same number. But there are eight cervical roots and only seven cervical vertebrae so C8 exits below C7 vertebra and the T1 root exits below T1 vertebra.

Primary spinal injury is the neurological deficit apparent immediately after the injury caused by disruption of the anatomy of the spinal canal with damage to the spinal cord. The secondary injury is usually a result of haemorrhage and oedema, causing further ischaemia to the spinal cord. It can best be minimised by making sure that the patient remains well perfused and oxygenated. If the spine injury involves displacement through fracture or dislocation then this too should be reduced as soon as possible to minimise any further ischaemia caused by pressure on the cord or its blood supply. Failure to properly immobilise the spinal cord is probably not a common cause of secondary injury.

→ Case study: injury after fall

2. (a) B

The likelihood of a significant cervical injury accompanying a head or facial injury is around 30 per cent.

2. (b) C

As the patient is unconscious, it can be difficult to 'clear' the cervical spine. Plain X-rays will not be adequate and flexion and extension views carry an unquantified risk of causing further damage. The patient should certainly not be left on a spine board any longer than absolutely necessary because of the risk of causing bed sores. An MRI would be the safest and most reliable way of ruling out an unstable spine injury.

2. (c) C

The vital signs are highly suggestive of neurogenic shock with a low blood pressure, a bradycardia and a well-perfused periphery. Fluids should be given with great care here because of the risk of flooding the patient. Thus titration of fluids to ensure adequate perfusion while minimising the risk of overloading a circulation which may lack sympathetic tone would be best.

2. (d) A, C

The bulbocavernosus reflex returns in 24–48 h after spinal transection. It is no indicator of prognosis. It merely indicates that the period of spinal shock has ended and that tests of prognosis can now be reliably performed. Return of perianal sensation indicates a good prognosis. A loss of power proprioception on one side with loss of temperature and pain sensation on the other side is the Brown-Sequard syndrome and also carries a good prognosis.

2. (e) B

The American Spinal Injury Association measures muscle power using the MRC grading system (0–5), and sensation in each dermatome. These are then combined into the Frankel grade. A is absent sensory and motor. B is sensory present, motor absent (this patient). Grade C is sensory present with motor function which is not good enough to be useful (MRC grade less than 3). Grade D is sensory present with useful but not normal motor function. Grade E is normal function.

→ Visualisation in neck and spine injury

3. A, B, C

Plain X-rays will only diagnose 85 per cent of significant spinal injuries and even that is only true provided there is good visualisation of the cervicothoracic junction. If the cervicothoracic junction cannot be visualised with conventional films then a 'swimmer's view' may need to be taken. CT is best for diagnosing bony injury in the spine and can also prove valuable in understanding the nature and extent of the injury using reconstructions. MRI is always much better for soft-tissue injuries, so will show up oedema and haematoma of the cord.

→ Cervical spine injury

4. (a) C; (b) C; (c) C

An unstable cervical spine fracture can either be treated in traction via a halo or by open reduction and internal fixation. Either way it is best to get an MRI to make sure that there is not a prolapsed intervertebral disc which might compress the cord when reduction is achieved. The best treatment is open reduction as the patient can then be mobilised safely, minimising the risks of other complications, such as bed sores, developing. The indications for surgery are relative if the neurology is stable, but if the neurology is deteriorating then the indication for surgery is absolute – surgery offers the only option.

Answers: Extended matching questions

→ 1. Fractures, dislocations and subluxations

1P, 2Q, 3A, 4B, 5B, 6N, 7M, 8I, 9F, 10C, 11L, 12M, 13F, 14H

The classic fracture from landing on the top of the head is the C2 burst fracture, otherwise known as a Jefferson's fracture, which can be stable or unstable. At any other level it is simply a 'burst' fracture. The fragments can be displaced into the spinal canal, causing cord damage. These fragments will need to be removed at open reduction and stabilisation. Craniocervical dislocation is usually fatal. The Power ratio measures the degree of subluxation of the occiput on the axis. A ratio of more than 1 indicates anterior translation, and a ratio of less than 0.75 indicates a posterior one. The ratio is the distance from the front of the foramen magnum (occiput edge) to the front edge of the back of the atlas over the distance between the back edge of the front of the axis (front of spinal canal) to the front of the back edge of the foramen magnum.

A child with a cock robin neck may just have sternomastoid spasm but can also have a spontaneous onset of atlantoaxial instability. Halter traction should lead to reduction. Traumatic atlantoaxial instability may produce an isolated rupture of the transverse ligament.

There are three types of odontoid peg fracture: type 1 is through the tip of the peg; type 2 (the case here) is through the neck; while type 3 extends down into the vertebral body of the axis.

Thoracic spine fractures are also classified into three types: type A is an anterior crush type and stable; type B also has disruption of the posterior elements and is more unstable; while type C is the rotatory fracture, which is very unstable indeed.

The Hangman's fracture is effectively a spondylolisthesis of C2 on C3 caused by traumatic hyperextension. Hyperextension pulls off a small fragment of bone on the front of the vertebral body. This is known as a teardrop fracture. Its mild appearance belies a severe and unstable fracture. If the hyperflexion is combined with axial compression then either one (uni-) or both (bi-) facets may dislocate and lock over the front of the facet below, locking into position. There is often damage to the intervertebral disc and also neurological damage. Before reduction is undertaken, an MRI should be performed to make sure there is not a prolapsed intervertebral disc.

The thoracolumbar junction is especially susceptible to injury, and the introduction of seatbelts has produced a characteristic flexion/distraction injury at this level called the Chance fracture.

Osteoporotic flexion wedge fractures are common in the elderly following minor trauma. They are usually stable but the pain and deformity can be helped with vertebroplasty performed under image intensifier control.

SCIWORA is a spinal cord injury without objective radiological abnormality. This occurs in young children with a hyperelastic spine where the deformity at the time of trauma produces haematoma of the cord (visible on MRI) without any apparent musculoskeletal damage.

25 Trauma to the face and mouth

Multiple choice questions

➜ Le Fort II maxillary fractures

1. What are the common findings in patients with Le Fort II fractures?

A Malocclusion
B Inferior alveolar nerve paraesthesia
C Infraorbital nerve paraesthesia
D Palatal mobility
E Exophthalmos.

➜ Zygomatic fractures

2. What are the common signs and symptoms of a fractured zygoma?

A Battle's sign
B Infraorbital paraesthesia
C VII nerve palsy
D Supraorbital paraesthesia
E Subconjunctival haemorrhage.

➜ Mandibular fractures

3. The action of which of the following muscles can displace bilateral fractures of the mandible in the canine region posteriorly?

A Thyrohyoid, genioglossus and geniohyoid muscles
B Anterior belly of digastric, geniohyoid and genioglossus muscles
C Mylohyoid, genioglossus and styloglossus muscles
D Mylohyoid, masseter and geniohyoid muscles
E Masseter, medial pterygoid and styloglossus muscles.

➜ Maxillofacial injuries

4. Which of the following statements regarding maxillofacial injuries are true?

A Orthopantomogram (OPT) radiographs are ideal to image middle-third fractures.
B The condyle is the most commonly fractured site in the mandible.
C The orbital roof is the weakest area of the orbital cavity.
D Nasal fractures are best treated at 3 weeks post-injury.
E Retrobulbar haemorrhage is a potential complication of fractures of the zygoma.

➜ Epidemiology of facial fractures

5. What is the most commonly fractured facial bone?

A Mandible
B Zygoma
C Nasal bones
D Maxilla
E Orbital floor.

➜ Epistaxis

6. Which of the following may be associated with epistaxis?

A Fractured zygomatic arch
B Fractured anterior wall of frontal sinus
C Orbital blow-out injury
D Le Fort II fracture of maxilla
E Fractured mandible.

➜ Avulsed teeth

7. Which of the following has an impact on successful reimplantation of avulsed permanent teeth?

A The aetiological cause of the injury
B The transport medium used
C The use of steroids in the peri-implant period
D The presence of dental caries in the crown of the tooth
E The length of time between avulsion and reimplantation.

Immediate management

8. In a patient who has sustained a severe facial injury, which of the following statements are true?

A The patient should be nursed in a supine position.
B Inhaled blood and debris can cause airway obstruction.
C An immediate danger to life may be blood loss.
D Surgical cricothyroidotomy may be necessary to establish an airway.
E Cervical spine injury should always be considered.

Extended matching questions

1. Maxillofacial trauma

A Orbital blow-out injury
B Epiphora
C Supraorbital paraesthesia
D Lower motor neuron VII nerve palsy
E Bilateral mandibular condylar fracture

Choose and match the correct diagnosis/symptoms with each of the clinical scenarios given below:

1 A 40-year-old male is involved in a severe road traffic accident (RTA). As a result of the accident he sustains a head injury with a Glasgow Coma Scale of 13/15 on admission to hospital. This improves over the next 12 h. Clinical examination demonstrates a positive Battle's sign on the right, and an associated cerebrospinal fluid otorrhoea on the same side. There are no soft-tissue facial injuries.

2 A 30-year-old female suffers a fracture of the left nasorbital region. Radiographs and CT scan demonstrate significant disruption of the medial and inferior orbital rims, frontal process of the maxilla and nasal bones.

3 A 46-year-old male sustains a blow to the face with a blunt object. Clinical examination demonstrates bilateral periorbital ecchymosis, epistaxis and cosmetic flattening in the region of the glabella. CT scans suggest a fracture of the anterior wall of the frontal sinus.

4 An 18-year-old female suffers a blow to the point of her chin after falling from a horse. Clinically her maxilla is stable, but she demonstrates a marked anterior open bite, with premature contacts of her posterior teeth.

5 A 45-year-old male presents 7 days following a blow to the face. He complains of numbness of the left cheek and occasional altered blood from the left nostril. There is no clinical flattening of the zygoma on that side.

2. Maxillofacial trauma

A Ptosis of the upper eyelid and forehead paraesthesia
B Sialocele of the parotid gland
C Mental paraesthesia
D Increasing proptosis, marked subconjunctival oedema, loss of direct light reflex with preservation of the consensual light reflex
E Palatal mobility.

Choose and match the correct diagnosis/signs with each of the clinical scenarios given below:

1 A 40-year-old male sustains a blow to the right cheekbone. Shortly after the accident he complains of eye pain and decreased vision on the affected side.

2 An unrestrained 55-year-old female passenger strikes her face on the dashboard of a car in a RTA. Clinical examination demonstrates bilateral epistaxis, bilateral infraorbital paraesthesia and significant oedema. The dental occlusion is deranged, and there is no clinical evidence of a fracture of the mandible.

3 A 28-year-old male undergoes repair of a 7 cm vertical, penetrating cheek laceration, extending from just below the zygomatic arch to the lower border of the mandible. Resorbable sutures are used for the deep tissue planes, and monofilament nylon for skin closure.

4 An 18-year-old male suffers a fractured mandible as the result of an alleged civil assault.

5 A 60-year-old female suffers a severe injury to the bony orbit on the left side. Radiographic examination suggests medial displacement of the greater wing of the sphenoid, with evidence of reduction in the dimensions of the superior orbital fissure.

Answers: Multiple choice questions

Le Fort II maxillary fractures

1. A, C, D

Le Fort II fractures of the maxilla are pyramidal in shape. The fracture involves the orbit, running through the bridge of the nose and the ethmoids. It continues to the medial part of the infraorbital rim, and often through the infraorbital foramen. It continues posteriorly through the lateral of the maxillary antrum to the pterygoid plates. Infraorbital paraesthesia is a common sign, and malocclusion is evident, unless the fracture is undisplaced. Palatal mobility is seen in all maxillary fractures, unless the fracture is impacted.

Zygomatic fractures

2. B, E

The common signs and symptoms of a fractured zygoma are cosmetic flattening, diplopia on upward gaze, ocular tethering, infraorbital paraesthesia and subconjunctival haemorrhage. In addition, limitation of mandibular lateral movements can be see if a displaced zygomatic arch impinges on the coronoid process of the mandible.

Mandibular fractures

3. B

The muscles attached to the anterior mandible which can cause posterior displacement in a bilateral parasymphyseal mandibular fracture are the anterior belly of digastric, geniohyoid and genioglossus.

Maxillofacial injuries

4. B, E

The most appropriate way to image middle-third fractures with plain radiographs are with occipitomental views, and lateral facial bone views. An OPT radiograph is better for imaging the mandible. The orbital floor, followed by the medial orbital wall, is the weakest area of the orbital cavity. Isolated orbital roof fractures are rare. Injuries of the orbital roof occur more commonly with associated frontal bone fractures. Nasal fractures should be treated after the associated soft-tissue swelling has subsided, so that any degree of deformity can be better assessed. Ideally, the fractures are best treated at 7–14 days; after this period the bony fragments become less mobile and more problematic to treat.

→ Epidemiology of facial fractures

5. C

The nasal bones are the most commonly fractured facial bones. This is then followed by the zygomatic bones and the mandible. In studies, the zygoma is marginally more commonly fractured than the mandible, but this difference is probably insignificant.

→ Epistaxis

6. B, C, D

Epistaxis is a common clinical sign in facial injuries. Any fracture that involves the nasal cavity or antra can result in epistaxis. In this manner fractures of the orbital floor, zygoma (but not the zygomatic arch), maxilla and anterior wall of frontal sinus can all result in epistaxis.

→ Avulsed teeth

7. B, E

The successful reimplantation of permanent teeth is dependent on several factors. Ideally the tooth should be adequately reimplanted as soon as possible after the injury. Any delay after 60 min post-avulsion is associated with a poor prognosis. Any period of delay should see the avulsed tooth transported in some form of clean, physiological transport medium. In the absence of any medical transport media, the patient's own saliva, or milk, are acceptable alternatives. Successful reimplantation also requires 7–14 days' rigid dental fixation, and therefore any reimplanted tooth should be splinted by the patient's dental surgeon as soon as possible.

→ Immediate management

8. B, C, D, E

Patients who have sustained severe facial injuries should never be transported in the supine position. To avoid complications during transfer, patients should always be nursed in the semi-prone position, with their head supported on their bent arm, never lying on their back.

Damaged teeth, blood and secretions can then fall out of the mouth, and gravity pulls the tongue forward. Due consideration must always be given to the possibility of both cervical spine and head injuries in patients who have sustained facial injuries.

Answers: Extended matching questions

→ 1. Maxillofacial trauma

1D

Battle's sign indicates a possible base of skull fracture involving the middle cranial fossa. CSF leakage from the ear confirms a base of skull fracture. The facial nerve can be injured as it passes through the facial canal by bony fracture/disruption. Facial nerve palsy is otherwise relatively rare, even in the more severe facial injuries, unless associated with deep, penetrating injuries of the parotid region.

2B

Epiphora may result from any soft-tissue injury to the canalicular apparatus, from soft-tissue eyelid injury. Less frequently it can result from bony fracture in the nasomaxillary region where the lacrimal passages are damaged. This can result in epiphora or sometimes a mucocele of the lacrimal sac, necessitating a dacrocystorhinostomy.

3C

Fractures of the frontal sinus may involve the supraorbital (and supratrochlear) foramina, where these nerves exit from the superior aspect of the orbit over the orbital rim. If involved, supraorbital paraesthesia is a characteristic sign.

4E

Anterior open-bite deformity can characteristically be caused by fractures of the maxilla, or more commonly by bilateral, displaced fractures of the mandibular condyles. In the absence of clinical signs of a maxillary fracture, this acquired deformity points toward a bilateral fracture of the mandibular condyles.

5A

Orbital blow-out injuries classically result from blunt injuries to the globe. The signs and symptoms are infraorbital paraesthesia, diplopia on upward gaze and often a history of epistaxis, as the injury results in haemorrhage into the maxillary antrum. In addition, the herniation of periorbital soft tissue into the maxillary antrum can result in enophthalmos, although this sign can often be masked in the initial stages post-injury from oedema accompanying the injury.

2. Maxillofacial trauma

1D

Retrobulbar haemorrhage is a rare, but important, complication of zygomatic body fractures and orbital disruption. It may occur as a result of the actual injury, or sometimes as a result of surgical treatment of a zygomatico-orbital injury. If progressive and untreated, it will lead to retinal ischaemia and subsequent blindness. Symptoms of pain and decreasing visual acuity/blindness should alert the surgeon to the possibility of retrobulbar haemorrhage. Clinical signs include proptosis, marked subconjunctival oedema and haemorrhage, a tense globe, a dilating pupil, ophthalmoplegia and a loss of the direct light reflex with preservation of the consensual light reflex. In progressing cases, medical measures may slow retinal ischaemia, but urgent surgical decompression is the necessary treatment.

2E

Palatal mobility is the classic sign of a fractured maxilla. Deranged occlusion, in the absence of a fractured mandible and dentoalveolar injuries, is pathognomonic of a fractured maxilla. Palatal mobility alone does not help in clinically differentiating between a Le Fort I, II or III fracture, which relies on other clinical signs and radiographic features.

3B

A parotid sialocele is caused by obstruction to the outflow of saliva from the parotid gland. The parotid duct may be severed in penetrating soft-tissue injuries of the cheek, and failure to recognize this result at the time of initial repair can result in salivary fistulas, parotid cysts and sialocele. Tight closure of the severed duct is more likely to result in total obstruction of the duct drainage, and subsequent cyst/sialocele formation.

4C

The inferior alveolar nerve is commonly involved by fractures of the mandible, especially those in the angle of the mandible and those in the body of the mandible (posterior to, or involving, the mental foramen). The insult to the nerve may be a simple neuropraxia, an axontmesis or, in the more severe, displaced fractures, a complete neurotmesis.

5A

Superior orbital fissure syndrome results from compression of the structures passing through the superior orbital fissure. There can be variation in clinical presentation, according to which structures are involved. In the complete syndrome, all nerves passing through the fissure may be involved – lacrimal, frontal, trochlear, nasociliary, oculomotor and abducent nerves. Ptosis, due to IIIrd nerve palsy and supraorbital/supratrochlear palsy, due to injury to the frontal branch of the ophthalmic division of Vth nerve, are usually evident in this syndrome.

26 Trauma to the chest and abdomen

Multiple choice questions

Chest and abdominal injury

1. **Which of the following statements are false?**
   - A 40 per cent of deaths from trauma are due to torso injury.
   - B Good history and understanding of the mechanism of injury will help predict the type of injury.
   - C Junctional zones help in the overall management.
   - D Multiorgan failure is the commonest cause of death in trauma.
   - E The vast majority of chest injuries can be managed closed.
   - F Early preventable deaths due to trauma are often the result of lack of delay in airway control.

2. **Which of the following statements are false?**
   - A 80 per cent of chest injuries can be managed non-operatively.
   - B In the unstable patient, chest X-ray is the first investigation of choice.
   - C A chest drain can be both diagnostic and therapeutic.
   - D A penetrating chest injury always requires a thoracotomy.
   - E In a chest injury, auscultation from the front only can be misleading.

Life-threatening injury

3. **Which of the following are not immediately life-threatening injuries?**
   - A Tension pneumothorax
   - B Cardiac tamponade
   - C Flail chest
   - D Open pneumothorax
   - E Massive haemothorax
   - F Liver injury
   - G Airway obstruction.

4. **Which of the following are not potentially life-threatening injuries?**
   - A Aortic injuries
   - B Tracheobronchial injuries
   - C Myocardial contusion
   - D Rupture of the diaphragm
   - E Oesophageal injuries
   - F Pulmonary contusion
   - G Hollow viscus injury.

Investigations

5. **Which of the following statements regarding focused abdominal sonography in trauma (FAST) are false?**
   - A It is accurate when there is >100 mL of free blood in a cavity.
   - B The technique focuses on pericardial, splenic, hepatic and pelvic areas.
   - C It is operator-dependent.
   - D It is a useful tool to diagnose hollow viscus injury.
   - E It can be used in penetrating injury.

6. **Which of the following statements are untrue?**
   - A All patients with multiple injuries must have a contrast-enhanced computerised scan (CECT) of the abdomen for accurate evaluation.
   - B In the stable patient with intra-abdominal injury, CECT is the 'gold standard' of investigations.
   - C Diagnostic laparoscopy has a screening role in the stable patient.
   - D Video-assisted thoracoscopy (VATS) is an accurate method of evaluating diaphragmatic injury.
   - E Diagnostic peritoneal lavage (DPL) as an investigation has largely been superseded by FAST.
   - F A negative DPL is often more helpful.

Extended matching questions

1. Chest trauma

A Tension pneumothorax
B Cardiac tamponade
C Flail chest
D Open pneumothorax
E Massive haemothorax

Choose and match the correct diagnosis with each of the scenarios below:

1 A 40-year-old van driver has been brought to the accident and emergency (A&E) department with severe shortness of breath. He was involved in a road traffic accident (RTA) when there was a head-on collision while not wearing a seatbelt. There is bruising over his sternum and a penetrating injury caused by a part of the broken steering wheel. His neck veins are distended with a systolic pressure of 80 mmHg and pulse rate of 130/min. The trachea is in the midline, but breath sounds are difficult to discern because there is a lot of noise in the A&E department. The pulse oximeter shows an oxygen saturation of 92 per cent.

2 A 25-year-old motorcyclist has been brought to the A&E department in a panicky state as he is unable to breathe properly and is intensely hypoxic (oxygen saturation of 90 per cent). The trachea is shifted to the right, the left hemithorax does not move and there is hyperresonance over the left chest wall. The noise in the A&E department makes listening to breath sounds difficult.

3 Following an injury at a building site where a piece of heavy masonry fell on his chest, a 35-year-old man has been sent to the A&E department with severe pain in his chest and marked bruising of the chest wall on the left. On examination his blood pressure is 80/50 mmHg, the left chest is dull on percussion and there is no air entry.

4 A 22-year-old rugby player has been brought to the A&E department with severe left-sided chest pain following blunt injury sustained in a match about 2 h ago. He is very tachypnoeic and extremely tender over the central part of his left hemithorax. The skin over the ribs looks badly bruised and the chest wall is unstable when he coughs or tries to take a deep breath.

5 A 15-year-old boy has been brought into the A&E department having been stabbed on the left side of his axilla. He is gasping for breath and his pulse oximeter shows a saturation of 90 per cent. There is an open wound in the region of the fifth left interspace through which a sucking sound can be heard.

2. Investigations

A FAST
B DPL
C CECT
D Diagnostic laparoscopy (DL)

Choose and match the correct diagnosis with each of the scenarios below:

1 A 30-year-old patient has been admitted following blunt abdominal and lower chest trauma. He has been resuscitated according to the ATLS protocol and is stable with a pulse rate of 110/min and blood pressure of 130/80 mmHg. He has considerable bruising over his abdomen and lower chest and there is a clinical suspicion of an intra-abdominal bleed. What imaging investigation should be done at this stage in the A&E department?

2 Following blunt abdominal trauma, after a boxing match, a 22-year-old male has been brought into the A&E department complaining of right-sided abdominal pain which is radiating to the right shoulder tip. He is stable haemodynamically and tachypnoeic with bruising around his umbilicus (Cullen's sign). Clinically liver laceration is suspected. A FAST shows fluid (blood) in the subhepatic pouch. Which imaging technique should be used next to confirm the diagnosis?

3 A 70-year-old patient has been brought into the A&E department having been brutally assaulted in his upper and lower abdomen. After resuscitation according to the ATLS protocol, his pulse is 110/min and blood pressure is 110/80 mmHg. He looks pale and is tender all over his abdomen. He has a history of chronic obstructive airways disease (COAD) and angina. Although clinically haemoperitoneum is suspected, a laparotomy would be considered only on confirmation of the clinical suspicion in view of his co-morbid disease. Unfortunately FAST is not available and CECT is not immediately available. What investigation would you consider?

4 A 25-year-old male patient has been brought in with a stab injury to his central abdomen. Although in severe pain around the injured site, he is stable haemodynamically. At this stage an intraperitoneal injury needs to be excluded. FAST is normal. What screening procedure might you consider?

→ 3. Abdominal injury

A Liver injury
B Pancreatic injury
C Splenic injury
D Renal injury
E Diaphragmatic injury
F Abdominal compartment syndrome

Choose and match the correct diagnosis with each of the scenarios below:

1 A fit 35-year-old man who was working on a building site sustained severe blunt upper abdominal trauma. He had a splenectomy for ruptured spleen and partial hepatectomy for torn liver. On the third postoperative day, while still in the ITU, he became oliguric, had cardiorespiratory compromise, type 2 respiratory failure and gross abdominal distension.

2 A 30-year-old man sustained an injury at a building site when a heavy piece of masonry fell on his lower abdomen. He is tachypnoeic and in hypovolaemic shock, with a pulse of 130/min and a blood pressure of 80/60 mmHg. He has been resuscitated by the ATLS protocol and is stable after 4 h – pulse of 100/min, blood pressure of 130/90 mmHg and CVP of 4 cmH_2O. He continues to be short of breath with an oxygen saturation of 92 per cent. He has an indwelling catheter, two IV cannulae with crystalloids and blood, and a nasogastric tube. A chest X-ray shows the tip of the nasogastric tube next to the heart in the left chest.

3 A 17-year-old boy sustained a kick in the right side of his abdomen and loin while playing rugby. After a brief period of rest, he finished his game. In the changing room when he passed urine it was haematuria. He was brought to the A&E department. He was stable with a pulse of 90/min and blood pressure of 110/80 mmHg. On examination he had bruising over the right lumbar region and right loin with some obliteration of the loin curve.

4 A 50-year-old man was brought to the A&E department having been viciously assaulted by being kicked in his upper abdomen and lower right chest. He is in very severe pain, short of breath with tachycardia. His pulse is 110/min, BP is 90/70 mmHg and clinically he has fracture of his right fifth to ninth ribs. Abdominal examination shows Cullen's sign with marked tenderness and bruising in the right upper quadrant. Following resuscitation by the ATLS protocol, his blood pressure comes up to 120/90 mmHg and his pulse rate is 100/min. His CVP is 5 cmH_2O.

5 Following a severe RTA, a 35-year-old female passenger in the back seat of a car had to be extricated. She has been brought in with generalised abdominal pain across the site of the seatbelt. She is breathless and complaining of pain in the left upper quadrant and left shoulder which had impacted against the front seat. Her pulse is 110/min and blood pressure is 100/60 mmHg. She is very tender over the left upper quadrant and clinically there is no shoulder injury. She has fracture of her left 9th, 10th and 11th ribs.

6 A 10-year-old girl has been brought to the A&E department complaining of upper abdominal pain of 10 days' duration. She has not been feeling well, with nausea and occasional vomiting, and a feeling of listlessness and she has been off school. On examination she has a distended upper abdomen where there is a suggestion of a smooth firm mass in the epigastrium where the skin is bruised. When asked about the skin bruising, she said that it occured 10 days ago when she fell off her bicycle.

Answers: Multiple choice questions

➜ Chest and abdominal injury

1. D

Torso injury accounts for 40 per cent of deaths from trauma. The reason for this is major haemorrhage, most of these being the result of failure to appreciate the extent of the bleeding. Half the deaths from trauma occur in the pre-hospital situation, 30 per cent during the first few hours and the remaining 20 per cent are late deaths. With improvements in pre-hospital care, more severely injured patients are reaching the hospital so that almost 50 per cent of deaths occur in the early in-hospital situation.

A good history and understanding the mechanism of the injury help to predict the actual damage in the patient. This history is often obtained from the paramedical staff and sometimes those at the scene of the accident. For example, unrestrained vehicle passengers suffer injury to face, chest and knees; pedestrians suffer injury to the lower legs and pelvis and then the head due to impact with the ground; those wearing only lap seatbelts (as opposed to full lap and diagonal belts) are prone to acute flexion injury over the belt with vertebral injury; duodenal and pancreatic injuries result from the compression between the steering wheel or a seatbelt and the vertebral column.

In a patient with multiple trauma, the injury usually traverses anatomical zones in the body, a knowledge of which is essential for proper management. Each side of the traditional anatomical zones, referred to as junctional zones, may be damaged. The junctional zones are: between the neck and the chest, between the chest and the abdomen, and between the abdomen and the pelvis. Such injuries are extremely challenging and require a multidisciplinary approach by the orthopaedic surgeon, the neurosurgeon, the cardiothoracic surgeon, the general surgeon and the urologist. Retroperitoneal injuries may be masked and a high index of suspicion must be entertained.

Multiorgan failure accounts for a minority of 7 per cent of deaths. This is usually from a combination of hypothermia, acidosis, coagulopathy and systemic inflammatory response syndrome.

Thoracic injuries account for 25 per cent of all trauma. About 80 per cent of chest injuries can be managed non-operatively by the closed method. Most patients require appropriate resuscitation and intercostal drainage. An open pneumothorax should not be closed until an intercostal drain has been inserted.

Immediately following trauma, the commonest cause of preventable death is due to failure of attention to airway control – hence the 'A' of ABCD in the Advanced Trauma Life Support (ATLS) protocol takes the highest priority. Foreign bodies such as dentures, teeth, blood and secretions are the contributory factors. Maxillofacial trauma with delayed nasopharyngeal oedema and injury to thyroid and cricoid cartilages call for expert airway control with intubation and control of cervical spine.

2. D

Life-threatening injury

3. F
4. G

Investigations

5. D, E
6. A

Answers: Extended matching questions

1. Chest trauma

1B

This van driver is a shocked patient with distended neck veins following direct blunt and penetrating chest injury. Any patient with a penetrating injury near the heart who is shocked is deemed to have pericardial tamponade unless otherwise proven. The classic triad consists of low systolic pressure, raised jugular venous pressure (JVP) and muffled heart sounds (Beck's triad). The last sign may not be reliable as it may be difficult to interpret because of noise in the busy surroundings of an A&E department. The neck veins may not be engorged if there is serious bleeding elsewhere.

A chest X-ray, FAST, echocardiography and a rising central venous pressure (CVP) may help if the diagnosis is in doubt. Pericardiocentesis under ECG control is the emergency treatment. Withdrawal of 10–15 mL of blood will result in marked improvement and is a life-saving emergency measure before a formal thoracotomy is carried out by a cardiac surgeon. However, if the patient has lost a large amount of blood elsewhere, the JVP and CVP may not be elevated.

2A

This motorcyclist has a left tension pneumothorax. He has intense hypoxia, is tachypnoeic, has a deviated trachea, hyperresonant percussion note and probably no breath sounds, which may be difficult to hear in a busy A&E department. This is an absolute emergency which needs to be dealt with immediately by inserting a large-bore needle into the second intercostal space in the midclavicular line. This allows one to buy time for some 20 min or so during which the definitive procedure of insertion of an intercostal drain in the fifth intercostal space in the anterior axillary line is carried out.

The usual causes are penetrating or blunt chest trauma with lung injury, causing air leak or iatrogenic lung puncture while inserting a CVP line through the subclavian route. This occurs when air leaks through a one-way valve from the lung. Air is forced into the chest cavity without any route of escape, causing complete lung collapse. There is a decrease in the venous return, causing engorgement of neck veins. The differential diagnosis is cardiac tamponade.

3E

This patient's type of injury typically will produce a massive haemothorax, the bleeding occurring from intercostal vessels or the internal mammary artery. The patient suffers from haemorrhagic shock with collapsed neck veins, absence of breath sounds and dullness on percussion on the left side.

Massive haemothorax is defined as an initial drainage of more than 1.5 L of blood or more than 200 mL of blood per h over 3–4 h. Urgent vigorous resuscitation for the haemorrhagic shock followed by insertion of an intercostal drain is carried out. This is followed by an urgent thoracotomy by a cardiothoracic surgeon.

4C

This rugby player, having sustained a blunt injury to the left side of his chest, has an unstable segment of chest wall on the left side. This is typical of a flail chest. A flail chest is defined as a segment of the chest wall that is discontinuous with the rest of the thoracic cage. It occurs when there are more than 3 ribs fractured at more than two sites. On inspiration the loose segment of chest wall moves inwards and on expiration it moves outwards – paradoxical respiration. This is a clinical diagnosis made on observation when the patient breathes or coughs. Hypoxia is primarily caused by the inevitable underlying lung contusion and lack of chest wall movement due to pain; paradoxical respiration contributes a minor part in the hypoxia.

Pneumothorax or haemothorax is a complication. The treatment is mechanical ventilation to help internally splint the flail segment. Intercostal nerve block to relieve pain is a good alternative to opiates. Some surgeons perform internal operative fixation in selected cases to stabilise the chest.

5D

This young boy has an open pneumothorax or a sucking chest wound. The wound should be immediately closed with a plastic Opsite dressing taped only on three sides to create a valve so that the air can escape out and not cause a tension pneumothorax. A formal intercostal drain (using as large a drain as possible) is inserted. The drain may be attached to a low-pressure suction. An early referral to a cardiothoracic surgeon is mandatory as a thoracotomy might be needed.

2. Investigations

1A

As this patient is stable, one needs to find out if there is any haemopericardium or haemoperitoneum. FAST is the next investigation of choice. It is a non-invasive technique, without any radiation, used to assess the chest (particularly cardiac tamponade) and abdomen for the presence of blood or fluid. The technique looks at the cardiac, splenic, hepatic and pelvic areas. It is a rapid, reproducible bedside technique and can easily be done while resuscitation is being carried out.

FAST will detect free fluid or blood when it is in excess of 100 mL. It is operator-dependent and unreliable in an obese patient or if the bowel is full of gas. It will not detect injury to hollow viscus.

2C

This young boxer clinically has the classical features of liver injury from blunt abdominal trauma: right-sided abdominal injury with pain in the right shoulder tip and positive Cullen's sign because of blood tracking along the ligamentum teres to the umbilicus. The majority of liver injuries are managed conservatively. But it is important to ascertain the exact damage for future reference, particularly as the patient is stable at present. A CECT is the investigation of choice.

3B

This elderly patient, who has been assaulted, has co-morbid disease. Although he may have haemoperitoneum and laparotomy may be necessary, it is best not to do so without a firm diagnosis. As FAST is unavailable and CECT is not readily available, a DPL is used. In good hands, DPL has 97–98 per cent sensitivity rate for blood and a 1 per cent complication rate. In a patient with chest injury who has an intercostal drain, egress of lavage fluid through the chest drain indicates diaphragmatic injury. In general, a negative DPL is often more helpful because the presence of blood in the peritoneal cavity does not always require a laparotomy. Hence, in this particular patient, DPL would be very useful.

4D
In stable patients with penetrating trauma to the abdomen, DL is a useful method to detect any intraperitoneal trauma, injury to the diaphragm or any injury requiring a laparotomy. It is useful to prevent an unnecessary laparotomy in penetrating abdominal trauma although the investigation should not be used as a substitute for open laparotomy.

3. Abdominal injury

1F
Patients who have undergone major surgery following trauma are prone to the complication of abdominal compartment syndrome (ACS). This is a major cause of mortality and morbidity in the patient with multiple injuries. Quite often it is not recognised. All the clinical features result from raised intra-abdominal pressure, which compresses the individual organs, thereby causing deterioration of their individual functions. Renal failure, decreased cardiac output from reduction in preload and increase in afterload, respiratory embarrassment from raising of the diaphragm and reduction in visceral perfusion account for this complication.

Measurement of intra-abdominal pressure by measuring the intravesical pressure through the indwelling catheter will help in making a diagnosis.

An intra-abdominal pressure of more than 25 mmHg is sinister and the patient requires immediate abdominal decompression. Some surgeons following major surgery after severe abdominal trauma would leave the abdomen open, covered with a plastic mesh. Definitive surgery is carried out later. The condition has a high mortality of about 60 per cent.

2E
This patient has suffered a blunt injury to his abdomen and pelvis, resulting in a compression force. This nature of injury should alert one to the possibility of a diaphragmatic injury. On the chest X-ray, the tip of the nasogastric tube next to the heart confirms the injury. As the patient is stable, VATS is the investigation of choice. A DL is also useful if only to exclude intra-abdominal injury. Surgical repair is carried out in all cases. The abdominal route is preferred so that injury to abdominal organs is excluded and repaired if necessary.

3D
This young man has right renal injury as a result of blunt abdominal and loin trauma. He is stable. After instituting ATLS resuscitation policy, an emergency intravenous urogram (IVU) is carried out (see Fig. 26.1). This is mainly done to make sure that the other kidney is normal. A renal ultrasound is done to gauge the size of the perirenal haematoma and repeated if necessary in a few days' time to make sure that it is reducing in size. Some may do a CECT scan. But as the same information can be obtained from an US scan, unnecessary radiation is avoided particularly as the patient is 17 years old.

The vast majority of renal injuries are treated conservatively (see Fig. 26.2). Every time the patient passes urine, some of it is saved in a transparent jar and the time of passing urine is noted (see Fig. 26.3). This would give an idea if the haematuria is getting better. In selected cases, if the haematuria does not improve while the patient is still stable, there is a place for selective renal angiogram with a view to renal artery embolisation. Haematuria following minor trauma should alert the surgeon to the possibility of injury to a pathological kidney, such as a congenital hydronephrosis or horseshoe kidney.

4A
This badly assaulted patient's injuries are mostly on the right lower chest and abdomen. He has Cullen's sign which is a telltale finding of liver injury because blood from the torn liver tracks to the umbilicus through the ligamentum teres. Liver is damaged typically as a result of blunt trauma. This patient is resuscitated according to the ATLS protocol. He is now reasonably stable. A CECT scan is carried out to determine the exact degree of liver injury and exclude other solid organ damage.

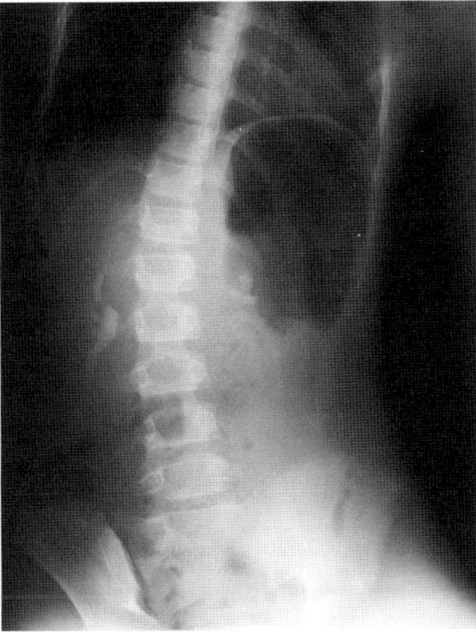

Figure 26.1 Emergency intravenous urogram in 17-year-old boy kicked in the right side of his abdomen and loin while playing rugby, showing: marked scoliosis with concavity to the right; elevated left dome of diaphragm; loss of left psoas shadow; extravasation of contrast on the left side; and normal excretion from right kidney. These findings are typical of a left renal injury with a peri-renal haematoma.

If the patient remains stable, liver injuries are treated conservatively, as most of them are. If the patient becomes unstable, laparotomy is undertaken. Liver injury can be graded by various systems. The principles of surgery in liver injury can be summarised by the four Ps – push,

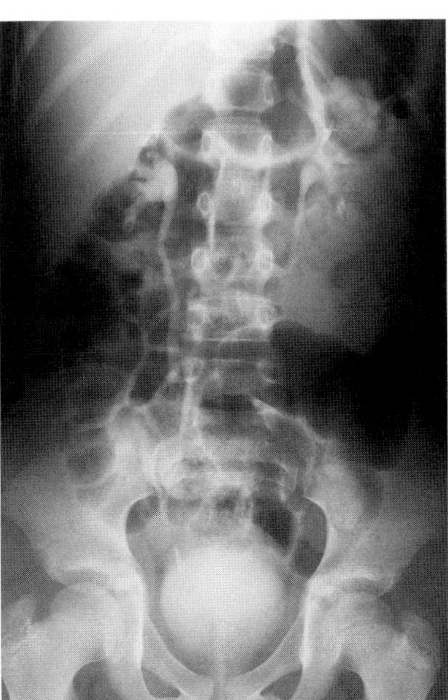

Figure 26.2 Intravenous urogram of the same patient 6 months later showing both kidneys perfectly functioning after conservative management of the injury.

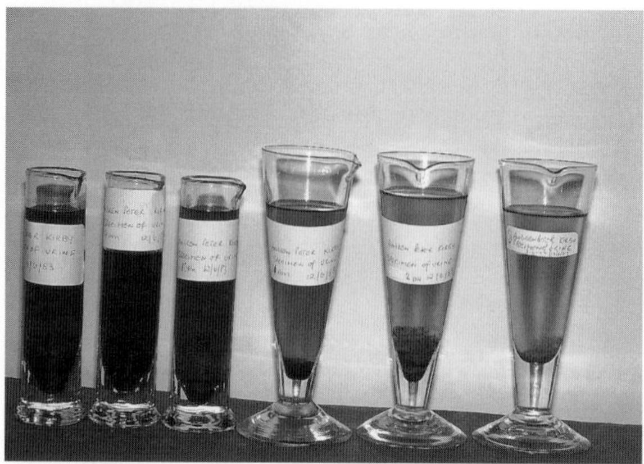

Figure 26.3 Serial specimens of urine collected from a patient with renal injury during conservative management showing that the urine is becoming clear.

Pringle's method, plug, pack. In very severe injuries, after packing the damaged liver, the patient should be transferred to a tertiary hepatobiliary unit.

5C

This female back-seat passenger in a car has had blunt trauma over the left lower chest and abdomen. She has fractured left lower ribs and referred pain to her shoulder tip due to diaphragmatic irritation from blood under the left dome from a ruptured spleen. A CECT scan will confirm the diagnosis. The patient is observed if she continues to be stable. Otherwise a laparotomy is done at which a splenectomy or splenorrhaphy or splenic preservation by placing it in a mesh bag is attempted.

6B

This 10-year-old girl has the classical manifestation of a traumatic pseudocyst of the pancreas. The commonest cause of acute pancreatitis in a child is from blunt trauma to the abdomen from a cycle handlebar injury. This girl sustained such an injury 10 days ago. At the time she suffered from traumatic acute pancreatitis which obviously was not clinically bad enough to seek hospital help. Over the ensuing 10 days she has developed a mass in the epigastrium typical of a pseudocyst.

This should be confirmed by ultrasound scan, which would show a cyst behind the stomach. Depending upon the size and the patient's symptoms, it should be managed accordingly. A cyst larger than 6 cm will need to be drained. A cystogastrostomy is done by the endoscopic route.

27 Extremity trauma

Multiple choice questions

Commonly missed injuries

1. **Which of the following important injuries are commonly missed, because some X-rays may look normal?**

A Fractured neck of femur
B Fractured patella
C Posterior dislocation of the shoulder
D Perilunate dislocation
E Colles' fracture
F Broken ribs
G Compartment syndrome
H Slipped upper femoral epiphysis
I Talar neck fracture

Compartment syndrome

2. **Which of the following statements regarding compartment syndrome are true?**

A It is detected by a loss of distal pulses and sensation.
B It produces pain out of all proportion to the injury.
C It is more common in closed fractures than open ones.
D It only occurs close to a fracture.
E It is a result of raised pressure in a compartment collapsing the veins.
F It is a clinical diagnosis.
G It is treated by a fasciotomy.

Classification of fractures

3. **Which of the following statements regarding the Gustillo and Anderson classification of fractures is true?**

A It applies only to the soft tissues.
B It relies primarily on the length of any laceration.
C It is influenced primarily by the energy involved.
D It takes account of whether or not there is soft-tissue cover of fractured bone.
E It takes account of contamination.
F It takes account of the body part involved.

Growth plate injuries

4. **Which of the following statements about growth plate injuries are true?**

A Fractures which pass along the line of the physis (Salter–Harris type 1) commonly cause growth arrest.
B Fractures which pass along the epiphyseal plate and then deviate off into the metaphysis (Salter–Harris type 2) are the commonest and rarely cause growth arrest.
C Fractures which track along the epiphyseal plate and then deviate into the joint (Salter–Harris type 3) may cause arthritis secondary to joint incongruity.
D Fractures which pass across the epiphyseal plate from the metaphysis to the epiphysis (Salter–Harris type 4) are unlikely to cause problems.
E Fractures which compress the growth plate (Salter–Harris type 5) are difficult to diagnose and cause growth arrest.

Treatment of fractures

5. **Which of the following statements regarding the treatment of fractures are true?**

A All fractures should be reduced.
B Reduction of a fracture means jamming the fragments together.
C All fractures should be stabilised.
D Relative stability means that some movement at the fracture site is going to occur.

E Absolute stability is obtained by getting exact reduction and then compressing the fragments of the fracture together.
F Absolute stability leads to secondary bone healing.
G Absolute stability should not be attempted if, in achieving it, the blood supply to the bone will be compromised.

6. Which of the following statements regarding the holding of fractures is true?

A Plaster of Paris has the advantage that it does not damage circulation.
B Treating a fracture in traction leads to delayed healing.
C Plates and screws allow absolute stability to be obtained.
D Intramedullary nails should always be used in growing bones.
E External fixators are especially useful where there is loss of soft tissue.
F Arthroplasty should not be used to treat a fracture.

Extended matching questions

→ 1. Imaging in trauma

A Plain X-rays
B Fluoroscopy
C Magnetic resonance imaging (MRI)
D Ultrasound
E Bone scan
F Computed tomography (CT) scan

Choose and match the optimal imaging modality with each of the scenarios given below:

1 A patient presents after a game of squash with pain in the back of the calf which was sudden in onset and accompanied by a sharp cracking noise.

2 A displaced intra-articular distal radial fracture is being reduced under general anaesthetic and held with K-wires introduced percutaneously.

3 A patient who had a breast cancer excised 5 years previously presents with weight loss and a pathological fracture of the femur. You want to know if there are any other secondaries.

4 A road traffic accident victim presents with a multi-fragment and displaced fracture of the pelvis, which now needs reconstruction.

5 A footballer has twisted his ankle in a tackle. The ankle is very tender over the medial and lateral malleolus.

6 A rugby player is tackled and feels a crack in his knee. Since then, every time he turns with his weight on that leg it is liable to give way under him, and also locks on occasions.

2. Types of fracture

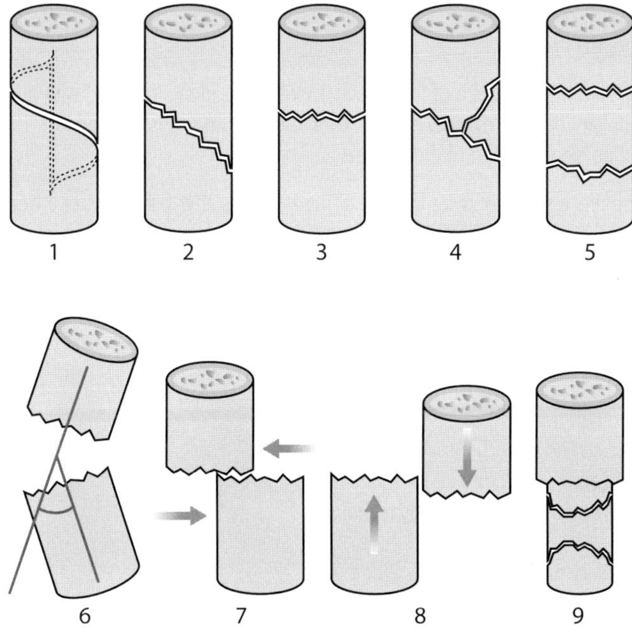

Figure 27.1

Choose and match the diagrams of fractures in Fig. 27.1 with each of the descriptions given below. Decide whether each is stable or unstable.

A Rotated
B Shortened
C Translated
D Angulated
E Segmental
F Wedge
G Transverse
H Oblique
I Spiral

3. Types of fracture union

A Malunion
B Non-union
C Infected non-union
D Delayed union

Choose and match the correct diagnosis with each of the scenarios given below:

1 A patient breaks his femur. It is treated in traction and then with a plaster brace, because he refuses surgery. Over a period of 8 weeks the femur bends into 15° of varus, producing a prominent lump on the outside of the thigh. Four months after the fracture it is painless, and he can walk on it.

2 An elderly patient falls and breaks the lower end of their femur. It is fixed with a blade plate but at review 3 months after the accident, the fracture is still visible on X-ray. Some weeks after that the plate breaks and the fracture falls apart. A new plate is put in but this plate also breaks some months later.

3 A young man has a fracture of the tibia in a football accident. It is fixed with a locking intramedullary nail. At review 3 months later, the fracture site is red and hot. There is a lot of pain and no sign of union of the fracture.

4 A child suffers a supracondylar fracture of the humerus after falling out of a tree. It is treated in a plaster. At 6 weeks, the plaster is removed but it is clear that the fracture is still mobile, although some callus is visible on X-ray.

→ 4. Methods of holding fractures

A Dynamic hip screw
B Balanced traction
C Collar-and-cuff traction
D Plates and screws
E Plaster of Paris
F Kirschner (K) wires – the Kapandji technique
G Analgesia
H Intramedullary nail
I Hemiarthroplasty
J External fixator

In each of the following scenarios, choose the optimum method of stabilisation:

1 An elderly woman falls and sustains an oblique fracture of the midshaft of the humerus.

2 An elderly man with carcinoma of the lung and metastases presents with a pathological fracture through the upper third of the femur. Up until now he was reasonably well.

3 A young motorcyclist sustains a fracture of the tibia where the skin and muscle have been ripped off over a distance of 10 cm.

4 A teenager falls and suffers a transverse displaced midshaft fracture of both the radius and the ulna.

5 An elderly woman falls and sustains a distal radial fracture which is very angulated and so is reduced to a better position. The reduction is good and the position is fairly stable.

6 The woman in Scenario 5 has the fracture reduced but it will not stay in position.

7 A child is involved in a road traffic accident and sustains a fracture across the midshaft of the femur.

8 A footballer breaks his ankle in a tackle and now has a fracture of both the tibia and the fibula. The talus has shifted laterally in the mortice joint.

9 An elderly patient falls and sustains a displaced subcapital fractured neck of femur.

10 An elderly patient falls and sustains a displaced pertrochanteric fractured neck of femur.

11 A young man falls and sustains three broken ribs.

Answers: Multiple choice questions

→ Commonly missed injuries

1. C, D, G, H, I

All the conditions which are commonly missed are rare and also difficult to diagnose. Posterior dislocation of the shoulder is much rarer than an anterior dislocation and easily missed on X-ray as it looks almost normal on the anteroposterior (AP) X-ray.

Perilunate dislocations are much rarer than a scaphoid fracture and are very difficult to see on X-ray unless you know how to look for the change in relationship of the bones of the carpus

Compartment syndrome is very rare and has no reliable investigation for proving or excluding its presence. It can only reliably be diagnosed by having a high coefficient of suspicion.

Slipped upper femoral epiphysis is like a posterior dislocation of the shoulder and looks fairly normal on an X-ray. Only a frog's-leg lateral view shows the true extent of the slip.

Talar neck fracture is like the scaphoid fracture. It can be difficult to see on X-ray and yet can have dire consequences, as the fracture may divide the blood supply from the talar head and lead to avascular necrosis of the talar body.

→ Compartment syndrome

2. B, C, E, F, G

Compartment syndrome is a surgical emergency. Although it is normally associated with a closed fracture, it can result from any blunt trauma and the bone does not need to be fractured. In fact, it is more common in closed fractures than open ones. It occurs most commonly in the deep flexor compartment of the calf and in the flexor compartment of the forearm but can occur anywhere that the muscles are held in an inextensible fascial sac, e.g. peroneal and anterior tibial compartments and small muscles of the hand and foot. It results from swelling (usually bruising) increasing the pressure inside an inextensible fascial compartment. The thin-walled veins containing blood at low pressure collapse in on themselves and no longer drain blood from the compartment, but the high-pressure, stiff-walled arteries continue to pump blood into the compartment. A vicious cycle is therefore set up where the pressure in the compartment continues to rise, and this prevents the blood from draining out. The distal pulses and even sensation may be unimpaired, because the arteries still pump blood, and if the distal nerve does not pass through that compartment it will be unaffected.

If a compartment syndrome develops in the deep posterior compartment of the leg then neither the anterior nor the posterior tibial nerve will be affected and so sensation in the foot will be grossly normal. Once the pressure in the affected compartment has reached mean systolic pressure, all circulation ceases because blood cannot enter or leave the capillary bed of the compartment and ischaemia begins. It is very difficult to measure the intracompartmental pressure and so the diagnosis is a clinical one.

The patient experiences pain out of all proportion to the injury, and if the muscles are stretched (passive extension), the patient experiences extreme pain. The pressure in the compartment needs to be released within hours if permanent damage is to be avoided. The initial treatment is to release any external factor which might be causing compression, such as a plaster or bandage. If there is not immediate relief of symptoms then the compartments involved need to be opened surgically (fasciotomy) and then left open until the swelling has reduced.

→ Classification of fractures

3. A, D, E

The Gustillo and Anderson classification is designed for open fractures and applies only to the state of the soft tissues. It takes little account of the length of any lacerations, as its primary concern is the energy that has been imparted to the soft tissues and hence their disruption.

It also takes account of whether there is soft-tissue cover of the fracture and whether there is contamination, as both these factors are important in determining treatment and predicting outcome. It does not take any account of the body part involved, despite the fact that blood supply and soft-tissue cover vary greatly in different parts of the body.

→ Growth plate injuries

4. B, C, E

Fractures involving the growth plate are classified according to shape and prognosis using the Salter–Harris classification:

- Salter–Harris 1 is rare and is a translational fracture (sideways slip) which passes all the way along the epiphyseal plate. The metaphysis is the weakest side and the blood supply enters from the epiphysis, so this fracture does not damage the growth potential of the plate.
- Salter–Harris 2 is similar to 1, but the fracture line exits and breaks off a fragment of the metaphysis. This fracture is by far the most common and luckily has a good prognosis as, once again, it is tracking along the safe (metaphyseal) side of the epiphyseal plate.
- Salter–Harris 3 is similar to 2 but the angulation of the fracture line is into the epiphysis and then on into the joint line. If it creates a step in the joint, there is a significant risk of the onset of premature traumatic osteoarthritis, so this fracture needs careful management.
- Salter–Harris 4 fractures cross from the metaphysis to the epiphysis. If there is any displacement then, when healing occurs, a bar of bone bridges across the epiphyseal plate from the metaphysis to the epiphysis. This will cause growth arrest.
- Salter-Harris 5 is a crush fracture of the epiphyseal plate. This may not be obvious on X-ray and is a rare fracture. But growth arrest is common as the growth plate has been destroyed.

→ Treatment of fractures

5. D, E, G

There are two stages in treating a fracture. The first of these is reduction, or putting the fragments back together so that the shape and alignment of the bone are correct. This is not always necessary. If the fracture is undisplaced or the displacement does not matter, the reduction is not needed.

The second stage is 'stabilisation'. Not all fractures need extra stabilisation. Some are so impacted that they are quite stable already. Others, like broken ribs cannot easily be reduced or stabilised. Nevertheless they will heal. Relative stability means that some movement at the fracture site is inevitable. This may be because the fracture is in multiple fragments or there may even be fragments missing. Relatively stable fractures heal by secondary bone union with callus formation.

Absolute stability is only possible when the bone fragments can be reduced perfectly and then compressed together. It leads to primary bone healing, which is in effect the same as bone remodelling. The risk of attempting to obtain absolute bone stability in a complex fracture is that the fragments of bone may get stripped from their bone supply and so fail to unite.

6. C, E

Plaster of Paris allows a fracture to be stabilised (relatively) without the need for open surgery. However, if a closed plaster is put on, swelling in the early stages may lead to circulatory compromise of the limb. This is why all initial plasters should be split.

The alternative, non-operative way of treating a fracture is to apply traction and use the tension created in the soft tissues to stabilise it. This stability is relative and so secondary bone healing (callus formation) occurs. This is the fastest form of fracture healing.

Fixation with plates and screws is one form of open reduction and internal fixation (ORIF). It enables, on occasions, absolute stability to be obtained. In these circumstances the patient can mobilise, leave hospital and return to many activities of daily living long before the fracture has united.

Intramedullary nails are another form of internal fixation, but as they have to be introduced through the ends of bones, they inevitably will have to cross epiphyseal plates. They should therefore not be used in children in case they damage the growth plate.

External fixators can bridge across damaged tissue and so are especially useful when there is soft-tissue damage or loss and the use of a plate or nail would give an unacceptable risk of infection.

Arthroplasty is an important tool in the armamentarium of a trauma surgeon for giving quick recovery in a fracture which has damaged a joint beyond the possibility of reconstruction (through loss of blood supply to fragments etc.).

Answers: Extended matching questions

1. Imaging in trauma

1D

Sudden onset of pain in the calf during a game of squash may be a rupture of the Achilles tendon. Soft tissues are usually best visualised with ultrasound, especially if dynamic imaging is needed.

2B

When fractures are being reduced under anaesthetic, it may be necessary to get a set of images of the bone fragments. Fluoroscopy (image intensifier) is the best way of achieving this while keeping the radiation dose to a minimum.

3E

If metastases are suspected, a radioisotope bone scan allows the whole skeleton to be screened for increased lytic activity.

4F

In complex fractures, a three-dimensional reconstruction of the fracture will be helpful in planning the reconstruction. CT scan allows this.

5A

A footballer who has gone over on his ankle may have fractured the malleolus. Plain X-rays are the best way of imaging this type of injury.

6C

The rugby player has an internal derangement of the knee, either a ruptured anterior cruciate ligament or a torn meniscus, or both. MRI is the best imaging modality for this type of soft-tissue injury.

2. Types of fracture

1I

This is a spiral fracture caused by a rotatory force. It is an unstable fracture. If it is seen in the femur of young children, it is commonly the result of non-accidental injury.

2H

This is an oblique fracture probably caused by a bending force. It, too, is unstable and will slide out of position if weight is taken on this broken bone.

3G

This is a transverse fracture, caused by three-point loading (a force is applied across the fracture point, while the two ends are fixed). This injury occurs in the tibia of footballers when another player lands on their leg. It can be a relatively stable fracture, if a perfect reduction is obtained, as axial loading merely compresses it.

4F

A wedge or butterfly fragment fracture occurs when the bone receives a sharp and heavy blow. The bone bends and the wedge fragment blows out on the other side. This is classically the injury seen in a pedestrian hit on the tibia by the bumper of a car.

5E

This is a segmental or comminuted fracture. It is in many pieces. It is a high-energy injury and is very unstable. The central fragments can sometimes lose their blood supply, so non-union may be a problem.

6D

This fracture is angulated, and so is likely to need reduction before fixation, otherwise a malunion will result.

7C

This fracture is displaced. One fragment has moved in relation to the other. Once again it is likely to need reduction before fixation, otherwise a malunion will result.

8B

This fracture is so displaced that the two fragments have slid past each other. If this is not reduced, the fracture will still heal, but the limb will heal much shorter than before.

9A

This fracture has rotated. Normally this is accompanied by a spiral fracture, in which case the fragments are usually displaced and shortened. On X-ray the diameter of the cortices may not match as the bones are often oval in cross-section.

→ 3. Types of fracture union

1A

If a fracture heals in a poor position, this is called malunion. This femur has shifted into varus, producing an unsightly bump on the lateral side. The deformity is likely to interfere with the mechanics of the knee and the ankle.

If fractures are fixed internally, the fragments are held rigidly together. The result is that secondary bone healing (callus formation) is not stimulated. If primary healing is delayed for any reason, for example the blood supply has been damaged during internal fixation, then the 'race against time' of the bone healing before the implant fails will be lost and the fracture will bend unless new fixation is applied.

2B

This fracture is not showing any signs of healing at all, so is probably heading towards non-union unless something is done. It may be that the fracture site has completely lost its blood supply, but something more than simply re-fixing the fracture will be needed. It is normal to put bone graft in at this time.

3C

The fact that the fracture is red and hot suggests there is inflammation. This could be a result of rapid bone healing, but the X-ray shows no sign of union. The likely diagnosis here then is infected non-union.

4D

There is some callus on the X-ray but the fracture is not yet united. In a child, an upper limb fracture should have united in 4–6 weeks, so this is delayed union.

4. Methods of holding fractures

1C

The oblique fracture of the humerus is an unstable fracture pattern but the upper limb can be rested (unlike a lower limb which must take weight). It is therefore possible to use the weight of the patient's arm to provide traction using a collar and cuff. If the result is not union in a perfect position, this does not matter too much in the humerus, as it does not show, or affect function.

2H

The intramedullary nail is valuable in treating long bone fractures, including pathological fractures. Combined with locking screws it can provide adequate 'relative' stability to allow immediate weight-bearing, while minimising vascular compromise.

3J

An external fixator provides an optimum way of stabilising an open fracture with such severe soft-tissue damage that it would not be safe to try to apply internal fixation. The fixator is cumbersome and the tracks of the pins or wires used to fix the bones to the fixator can become infected.

4D

The AO system provides a set of interchangeable plates and screws to enable fixation of fractures with maximum stability and minimum damage to soft tissues. In simple fractures, it is possible to obtain compression and 'absolute stability' so that the patient can make full use of that limb (including weight-bearing) immediately after fixation. The anatomical fix obtainable with plates and screws is ideal for forearm fractures where a perfect reduction is needed if full pronation and supination are to be achieved. Optimal fixation requires careful planning, and infection is a risk even in the best-equipped and organised operating theatre.

5E

Plaster of Paris provides good protection to an injured limb, and if it is applied carefully, then it can provide relative stability, which may be adequate for a fracture which is not too unstable, such as a simple Colles' fracture. It is a safe and cheap method of stabilising a fracture but carries the complication that, if there is significant swelling within a closed plaster, serious ischaemia may result.

6F

Kirschner (K) wires can be inserted percutaneously (the Kapandji technique). When used with plaster of Paris, they will help to control a very unstable fracture either by providing a buttress or by impaling it without the need to open the fracture.

7B

Balanced traction is the method of pulling on a fracture with weights while balancing that force with the patient's weight by tilting the bed. It is a very safe way of treating a fracture but is very resource-intensive in hospital beds, as the patient is confined to a bed until the fracture has healed. However, fractures in children heal very fast, and internal fixation has significant disadvantages in these cases, as it may damage growth of the bone, so balanced traction is still routinely used to manage femoral fractures in children.

8D

Fractures which enter a joint pose special problems as any incongruity in the joint surface is likely to lead to premature arthritis. In cases like the ankle fracture in the footballer, open reduction and fixation with plates and screws offers the best opportunity for obtaining an accurate and stable reduction.

9I

Arthroplasty is the treatment of choice in patients with unreconstructable intra-articular fractures. Reconstruction may be impossible either because of bone necrosis (articular fractures have a parlous blood supply) or because of actual bone or cartilage loss. The intracapsular fracture of the neck of femur destroys the blood supply to the femoral head, so it needs replacing with a hemi-arthroplasty.

10A

The pertrochanteric fracture has no problem with blood supply but needs great strength to allow early weight-bearing. The dynamic hip screw is effectively a combination of an intramedullary nail fitted up the femoral neck which connects to a heavy plate screwed to the side of the femur. The nail in the neck is able to slide into a slot in the nail so that the fracture ends can be compressed together. This improves stability and stimulates bone healing.

11G

Some fractures simply cannot be stabilised in any meaningful way. One example is a rib fracture, which tends to be splinted by the neighbouring ribs and which cannot be stabilised without impairing breathing. The only assistance that can be given to the patient is analgesia.

28 Burns

Multiple choice questions

➜ Burns: general

1. **Which of the following statements regarding burns in children in the UK are true?**

A The majority are electrical or chemical.
B The majority are most commonly scalds.
C Hot water thermostat setting at 60°C helps to improve safety in homes.
D Intravenous (IV) resuscitation in children is required for burns greater than 5 per cent of total body surface area (TBSA) and less than 10 per cent.
E Non-accidental injury is common in children's burns.

2. **Regarding burn injury in adults in the UK, which of the following statements are true?**

A Electrical and chemical burns are common.
B Scalds in the home are more common than flame burns.
C Alcohol problems are rare in relation to burn injury.
D Effective care requires multidisciplinary input.
E Intravenous fluids are required for burns of 15 per cent TBSA or more.

➜ Respiratory problems in burns

3. **Which of the following statements regarding respiratory problems in burns are true?**

A Burn injury to this function may be lethal.
B Injury can be due to inhalation of hot or poisonous gases.
C Burn injury is more common in the supraglottic than in the lower airway.
D Haemoglobin combines with carbon monoxide less easily than with oxygen.
E Hydrogen cyanide interferes with mitochondrial respiration.

➜ Smoke inhalation

4. **Which of the following statements regarding smoke inhalation are true?**

A Inhaled smoke particles can cause a chemical alveolitis and subsequent increased gaseous exchange.
B Inhaled smoke particles may be suspected with a specific situation in an enclosed space.
C Early elective intubation is contraindicated.
D Symptoms can take 24 h or up to 5 days to develop.
E The result of carbon monoxide poisoning is a metabolic alkalosis best treated by low inspired oxygen.

➜ Extent of burns

5. **Which of the following statements are true in relation to burns and TBSA?**

A Epidermal destruction can occur when a surface temperature of 70°C is applied for 1 s.
B A child's head comprises a smaller percentage of TBSA than that of an adult.
C According to the Lund and Browder chart, an adult with burns involving both sides of one upper limb as well as the hand has been burned on 15 per cent of TBSA.
D The 'rule of nines' is an accurate guide to the size of a burn outside the hospital environment.

E In small burns the patient's whole hand is 1 per cent of TBSA and is a useful guide to assess a burn.

6. Which of the following statements regarding burn depth are true?

A The depth of a burn together with percentage of TBSA and smoke inhalation are key parameters in the assessment and management of a burn.

B Alkalis, including cement, usually result in superficial burns.

C Fat burns are deeper than electrical contact burns.

D Capillary filling is not present in superficial burns.

E Deep dermal burns take a maximum of 2 weeks to heal without surgery.

Consequences of burns

7. Which of the following statements regarding the consequences of burns are true?

A As a result of a burn, complement causes degranulation of mast cells and, subsequently, neutrophils.

B Mast cells do not release primary cytokines.

C As a result of a burn, an increase in vascular permeability occurs.

D Following a burn, water only moves from intravascular to the extravascular space.

E In burns affecting more than 15 per cent TBSA in an adult, fluid loss results in shock and the volume lost as fluids is directly proportional to the area of burn.

8. Which of the following statements regarding burn complications are true?

A Cell-mediated immunity is increased in major burns.

B Infections with bacteria and fungi are rare in large burns.

C Malabsorption from gut damage is a known complication in a burned patient.

D Circumferential full-thickness burns of a limb can result in ischaemia.

E A change in voice is an important clinical sign in a burned patient.

Treatment of burns

9. Which of the following statements regarding the treatment of burns are true?

A Cooling of a scald for a minimum of 10 min is of no value in giving analgesia or slowing the injury associated with a fresh burn.

B Other non-burn injuries may coexist with a burn.

C Major determinants of burn outcome are percentage of TBSA, depth and the presence of any inhalation injury.

D Criteria for acute admission to a burns unit do not exist or are unnecessary.

E A significant hand burn should not be admitted to a burns unit and can easily be managed as an outpatient.

Burn depth

10. Which of the following statements are true?

A The depth of a burn can initially be assessed from the offending temperature, time of application and nature of the causative agent.

B Electric contact burns are almost certainly full-thickness.

C Deep, partial-thickness burns involve destruction of the whole dermis.

D Sensation is totally absent in a full-thickness burn.

E Tangential shaving may be a useful diagnostic and management tool in partial-thickness burns.

Fluid management

11. Which of the following statements are true?

A Oral fluids containing no salt are essential when given as fluid replacement in burns.

B Fluids required can be calculated from a standard formula.

C Hyponatraemia can be avoided in oral fluid management by rehydrating with a solution such as Dioralite.

D Urine output gives a major clue as to adequacy of fluid replacement.

E Three types of fluid can be used for IV fluid replacement in burns: Ringer's lactate, hypertonic saline or colloids.

12. **Which of the following statements are true?**
A The simplest and most commonly used crystalloid is Ringer's lactate.
B Hypertonic saline produces an excess of intracellular water shifting to the extracellular space.
C Human albumin solution is a colloid which reduces protein leak out of cells, thereby helping to reduce oedema.
D The Parkland formula is the most widely used formula in the UK and calculates the fluid replacement in the first 24 h.
E Using the Parkland formula, the fluid requirement in the first 24 h for a man of 70 kg with a burn involving both upper limbs, including the hands, is 4800 mL.

13. **Which of the following statements are true?**
A In resuscitation, a urine output of 0.5 mL/kg body weight per h does not mean that the rate of infusion should be altered
B In resuscitation, a urine output of 1 mL/kg body weight per h indicates the fluid rate infusion is too low
C In resuscitation, hypoperfusion is recognised by cool extremities
D Urine output in excess of 2 mL/kg body weight per h is associated with a low haematocrit.
E In large burns, monitoring tissue perfusion by a central line may be required even though there is increased infection risk.

Escharotomy

14. **Which of the following statements are true?**
A Escharotomy is associated with non-circumferential superficial burns.
B Significant blood loss is not a feature to be considered when escharotomy is contemplated.
C Damage to major nerves will not be the result of incorrect escharotomy incisions.
D Escharotomy of the hand and fingers is best done outside of a main operating theatre.
E In the lower limb, for escharotomy, the incision should be anterior to the ankle medially.

Dressings

15. **Which of the following statements are true?**
A Superficial burns can be treated by a variety of simple dressings, such as Vaseline gauze, or by the exposure method, particularly for small burns of the face, when the climate is hot and intensive nursing support is readily available.
B Deep dermal burns, or those that are nearly deep dermal, require dressings in order to reduce pain, reduce or treat infection, reduce scarring, and operations.
C Hydrocolloid dressings such as Duoderm can be left on for 14 days.
D Silver sulphadiazine (1 per cent) can be used effectively as a broad spectrum-antibiotic but not for methicillin-resistant *Staphylococcus aureus* (MRSA).
E An optimal healing environment can make a difference to the outcome in borderline-depth burns.

16. **Which of the following statements are true?**
A Biological dressings and synthetic ones such as Biobrane do not need to be changed and are useful in deep and mixed-depth burns.
B Amniotic membranes are ideal dressings for one-stop management of superficial burns but not for deep burns.
C A fenestrated silicone sheet such as Mepitel can be used in superficial burns and is non-permeable.
D Honey or boiled potato peel are unusual dressings for superficial burns but can be effective.

E *Pseudomonas aeruginosa* is not treatable by 1 per cent silver sulphadiazine cream.

Burn management

17. Which of the following statements are true?

A Analgesia is a vital part of burn management.
B For large burns over 10 per cent TBSA, intramuscular (IM) injections of opiates are best.
C Removing the burn tissue and achieving healing reduce pain and are also effective in stopping the catabolic drive.
D In adults with burns covering 15 per cent TBSA or more, extra feeding is required.
E The greatest nitrogen losses in burns occurs between 20 and 25 days.

Infection control

18. Which of the following statements are true?

A Infection control requires attention to handwashing and cross-contamination prevention.
B A rise or fall in white cell count and a decreasing clinical status are signs of infection.
C Swabs taken from the burn and sputum are of no use in building a picture of the patient's flora.
D Antibiotics given should be ideally based on cultures and on discussion with a microbiologist.
E Catheter tips are a possible source of an infection.

Allied therapies

19. Which of the following statements regarding allied therapy in burn patients are true?

A Success or failure of both physical and psychological care of the burn patient is dependent on intensive nursing and physiotherapy management.
B Physiotherapy can be best done after 2–3 weeks.
C Post traumatic stress disorder can occur as a result of burns.
D Psychological help may be required for relatives of the burned patient.
E Elevation of hands that have sustained burns is not indicated.

Treatment of blisters and burn depth

20. Which of the following statements are true?

A The management of blisters – leaving them intact or removing them – remains debatable.
B Initial cleaning of a burn wound with chlorhexidine solution is contraindicated.
C If a burn has not healed within 3 weeks, it is worth avoiding debridement and skin grafting
D Any burn of indeterminate depth should be reassessed after 2 weeks.
E Deep dermal burns need tangential shaving and split-skin grafting while all but the smallest full thickness burns need surgical excision and grafting if possible.

Surgical management

21. Which of the following statements regarding surgical management of burns are true?

A The anaesthetist is of great assistance and essential in the management of a major burn.
B Blood loss is not a feature of surgery in major burns.
C Blood loss may be reduced by use of a tourniquet or by application of a skin graft or topical or subcutaneous diluted solution of adrenaline.
D A core temperature below 36°C may affect blood clotting.
E Synthetic dermis, including Integra or homografts, may provide temporary stable cover following excision of larger burns.

Role of physiotherapy, escharotomy and eyelid care

22. Which of the following statements are true?

A Physiotherapy and splintage are important in maintaining range of movement and reducing joint contracture

B It is not necessary to splint the hand after skin grafting.

C Supervised movement by physiotherapists under direct vision of any affected joints should begin after about 2 weeks.

D Escharotomy of the circumferential burn of the upper trunk should help respiratory function.

E Early care must be taken when eyelids are burned.

Surgical management

23. Which of the following statements are true?

A Early surgery is indicated in the hands and axilla.

B Contractures are best treated with split-skin grafts.

C Tissue expansion is useful in treating alopecia caused by a burn.

D A Z-plasty is a useful technique for reconstruction of broad areas of burn scarring causing restricted movement.

E Full-thickness grafts or vascularised tissue, as in a free flap, are generally unnecessary in burn scar management when good vascularised tissue is available in the treated burn scar.

Scar management

24. Which of the following statements regarding scar management of burns are true?

A Hypertrophy of a burn scar can be treated by the use of pressure garments worn for a month.

B Intralesional steroid injection or silicon patches may be useful in small areas of burn scar hypertrophy.

C Pharmacological treatment of itchy burn scars is not important.

D Use of Integra to resurface a healed full-thickness burn scar can improve scar quality.

E Flamazine cream should not be used as a topical agent in pregnant or nursing mothers.

Electrical burns

25. Which of the following statements are true?

A Low-tension electrical burn injury is most likely to be found in accidents in the home.

B Underlying heart muscle damage is likely in low-tension injuries.

C Large amounts of damage to subcutaneous tissues and muscle are associated with high-tension electrical burns.

D Myoglobinuria is a serious complication of low-tension burns.

E Severe alkalosis is common in large electrical burns.

Chemical and radiation burns

26. Which of the following statements are true?

A Copious water lavage is the best first-aid measure for phosphorus burns.

B Elemental sodium burns should not be treated by water lavage.

C Damage from alkalis is usually less than with acids.

D Hydrofluoric acid burns can be associated with hypercalcaemia.

E Local radiation burns causing ulceration need excision and split-skin graft repair

Answers: Multiple choice questions

→ Burns: general

1. B, C

The majority of burns in children are scalds with kettles, pans, hot drinks and bath water. Legislation, health promotion and appliance design, together with education of patients regarding smoke alarms and hot water thermostats kept at 60°C, have reduced the incidence of burns. IV fluids in children is required when the TBSA is 10 per cent or more.

2. A, D, E

Most electrical and chemical burns occur in adults, while scalds are less common than flame burns. The presence of alcohol, drug abuse, epilepsy and mental disorder is not uncommon in those who have suffered burn injury. A multidisciplined approach must be available for effective care. IV fluids in adults is required when 15 per cent or more of TBSA is affected.

→ Respiratory problems in burns

3. A, B, E

Burns can damage the airway and lungs with life-threatening consequences. This can occur when the face or neck are burned, when the fire causing the burn is in an enclosed space, or when hot gases or poisonous vapours are inhaled. Burn injury is more common in the lower airway than in the supraglottic airway. Carbon monoxide has an affinity 240 times greater than oxygen for combining with haemoglobin and thus blocks the transport of oxygen. Blood gas measurement can be done to confirm the diagnosis. A concentration of carbon monoxide above 10 per cent is dangerous; 60 per cent is likely to be lethal. Hydrogen cyanide is a metabolic toxin produced in house fires, which interferes with mitochondrial respiration.

→ Smoke inhalation

4. B, D

Inhaled smoke particles can cause a chemical irritation or alveolitis. This results in interference with gaseous exchange. Early elective intubation is important and is definitely not contraindicated. Symptoms may not be immediately evident and can take up to 5 days to develop. Carbon monoxide poisoning causes a metabolic acidosis and is treated by inhalation of pure oxygen.

→ Extent of burns

5. A, E

The first indication of burn depth comes from the history of temperature and time of application at that temperature. Burn area can be measured by a series of formulae plotted on a chart. The 'rule of nines' offers a rough guide to area but is probably useful outside the hospital environment. It should be remembered that the size of a child's head is proportionally larger than in an adult. The Lund and Browder chart is widely used in UK burn units and measures a whole arm and hand (both sides) as 8 per cent of TBSA. In small burns it may be useful to use the patient's whole hand–palm as 1 per cent of TBSA.

6. A

The key factors in the assessment and management of a burn are smoke inhalation, depth and percentage of TBSA affected. If oral fluids are to be used, salt must be added to counter salt loss in the stressed situation. The likely depth of any burn can be derived from the causative agent. Thus fat usually causes deep dermal burns, while full-thickness burns are more certain in electric contact injuries. The burns caused by alkalis such as cement usually produce deep dermal or full-thickness burns. Any burn that heals spontaneously within 3 weeks is superficial; deep dermal burns will take longer. Sensation and capillary filling are features of a superficial burn.

Consequences of burns

7. A, C, E

As a result of a burn, complement is produced which degranulates mast cells and leucocytes. Mast cells act on leucocytes and produce primary cytokines. There is a movement of water and salt from the intra- to the extravascular compartment due to an increase in vascular permeability. The resulting shock is related to this fluid loss and in an adult becomes significant when TBSA affected is 15 per cent or more.

8. C, D, E

In the burned patient there is a reduction in cellular immunity, and one should be on the lookout for infections with bacteria and even fungi. Damage in the gut lining tissues may cause malabsorption. Ischaemic changes are a definite risk for full-thickness circumferential burns of the limbs as a result of swelling and a tourniquet effect. For the same reason, circumferential full-thickness burns of the chest may cause respiratory impairment. Warning signs of burns to the respiratory system include stridor or change in voice.

Treatment of burns

9. B, C

Cooling of a fresh burn for 10 min by lowering the temperature of the agent causing the burn and the local tissues will help to reduce burn injury – this may sometimes be done by using cold water but not for every burn. Non-burn injuries may coexist with burns and should not be overlooked. Criteria for admission to each burns unit exist and advice on this and any burn is readily available. A significant hand burn should always be admitted even though the percentage of TBSA may be small.

Burn depth

10. A, B, D, E

Most burns can be assessed from the history, the temperature, the time of application, and the nature of the causative agent. Electrical contact usually results in full-thickness burns. In deep, partial-thickness burns some dermal tissue remains. Sensation is absent in full thickness burns as all nerve endings have been destroyed. Tangential shaving using a skin grafting knife is a useful management and diagnostic operation in partial thickness burns – the presence of punctate bleeding after one or two shaves confirms this type of injury.

Fluid management

11. B, C, D, E

It is important to give salt and water in oral fluids given for resuscitation instead of water alone, to take account of salt loss. Dioralite is useful in the treatment of hyponatraemia. The output of urine gives a good indication of fluid requirements. Various formulae are available to calculate fluid requirements which may be given as Ringer's lactate, hypertonic saline or colloid.

12. A, C, D

Ringer's lactate is the most commonly used, and cheap, burn crystalloid fluid, while albumin is a colloid that can reduce oedema by preventing protein leak from the tissue cells. Hypertonic saline also reduces oedema by producing hyperosmolarity and hypernatraemia – this reduces the shift of intracellular water to the extracellular space. The Parkland formula calculates the fluid to be replaced in the first 24 h, with half of this volume to be given in the first 8 h: TBSA percentage $\times$ weight (kg) $\times$ 4 $=$ volume (mL). For a 70 kg patient with two times 8 per cent TBSA burn, the fluids required would be 4480 mL.

13. C, D, E

Adequacy of fluid replacement can be assessed from measuring urine output, haematocrit and clinical status. For adults, a urine output of 0.5–1.0 mL/kg body weight per h is normal. If it is lower than this and the haematocrit is higher than normal, more fluid should be given – there may be signs of restlessness, tachycardia and cool extremities. It is important that patients are not overresuscitated and a urine output in excess of 2 mL/kg per h means the rate of infusion should be reduced. Care should be taken in patients with acute or chronic cardiac problems and the use of a central line should be considered even though there may be an increased risk of introducing infection.

Escharotomy

14. None of the answers is correct

Escharotomy is indicated for circumferential burns of limbs or trunk – deep dermal or greater. A tourniquet effect occurs due to the increasing pressure and swelling that result. This procedure should be done early to aid respiration and prevent limb ischaemia and can be associated with a significant blood loss. Adequate blood should be available for transfusion. Care should be taken in performing an escharotomy to avoid damage to major structures, including nerves. In the lower limb it is also important to make the incision posterior to the ankle to avoid damage to the saphenous vein.

Dressings

15. A, B, E

Superficial burns can be dressed or left exposed. Most heal irrespective of the dressing unless they are contaminated or become infected. Cleaning the contaminated wound under general anaesthetic is prudent and application of silver sulphadiazine cream for 2–3 days may be helpful if it is heavily contaminated. Vaseline gauze is a commonly used dressing. Duoderm, a colloid dressing, is useful in mixed depth burns but should be changed every 3–5 days. Silver sulphadiazine (1 per cent) is effective in cases of MRSA. It is important to remember that the optimal healing environment will provide the best chance of healing quickly and well, especially when the depth is mixed or uncertain.

16. B, D

Biobrane and amnion can be used for dressings for superficial but not deep dermal or deep burns. Honey or banana has also been used around the world. Mepitel is a permeable fenestrated silicone sheet that can also be used. Silver sulphadiazine 1 per cent is effective against *Pseudomonas* infection.

Burn management

17. A, C, D

Analgesia is a vital part of burn management. Oral paracetamol is useful in small burns, especially if they are superficial. Intravenous opiates are indicated for larger burns – not IM as absorption is uncontrolled and dangerous. Administration of this and other agents such as general anaesthesia, ketamine or midazolam may require an anaesthetist. There are catabolic changes as long as the burn wound remains unhealed, and rapid excision of the burn and stable wound coverage are the most significant factors in reversing this. Extra feeding must be given and this should be by nasogastric tube in burns covering 15 per cent TBSA or more; 20 per cent of kilocalories should be provided by proteins. The greatest nitrogen losses occur between 5 and 10 days.

Infection control

18. A, B, D, E

Control of infection begins with policies on handwashing and other cross-contamination prevention measures. A rise in white blood cell count, thrombocytosis and an increase in catabolism are warnings of infection. Swabs taken from the burn wound and sputum can help in establishing the flora picture. The role of a bacteriologist and advice are of great importance in the decision on antibiotics. Catheter tips can be a source of infection.

Allied therapies

19. A, C, D

Intensive nursing, physiotherapy, and psychological management of a burned patient are of importance. Psychological support may help the relatives and prevent post traumatic stress. Physiotherapy should be started early and in the case of hand burns this should be on day 1 and reinforced daily. All burns of the hands cause swelling and elevation and splintage will improve the outcome.

Treatment of blisters and burn depth

20. A, E

Eyelids must be treated before exposure keratitis arises – full-thickness grafts, transposition flaps or Z-plasties may be indicated.

Surgical management

21. A, C, D, E

An anaesthetist must be available for dressing or debridement of a major burn. As blood loss can be a feature of large burn debridement, facilities for blood transfusion and blood must be available. The application of limb tourniquet, topical or subcutaneous adrenaline solution – diluted 1:500 000 – will help to control or reduce bleeding. Blood-clotting irregularities can occur when the core temperature of the patient falls below 36°C; thus the operating room must be kept warm. In large burns the use of Integra or homograft can be a useful temporary way of dressing a large burn that has been excised.

Role of physiotherapy, escharotomy and eyelid care

22. A, D, E

Physiotherapy and splintage both help considerably in preventing joint contractures. A hand splint is used in hands treated by split-skin grafts. Supervised physiotherapy for any affected joints should occur on day 1 so that early recovery can be aided. In full-thickness burns or deep dermal circumferential burns of the upper trunk, escharotomy will help to improve respiration. It is important to provide early care, including surgery if necessary, if eyelids are burned.

Surgical management

23. A, C, E

Early excision and grafting are indicated in burns of the axilla and hands. Contractures are usually best treated by grafts with Z-plasties being used for narrow, not broad, scar contractures. Tissue expansion may be useful in treating alopecia of the scalp caused by burns. Full-thickness grafts are useful in situations where blood supply is good; and free flaps are useful where it is poor or absent in the latter.

Scar management

24. B, D, E

Pressure garments may be effective in reducing burn scar hypertrophy but require to be fitted and worn for at least 6 months and would be ineffective if only used for 1 month. Intralesional injection of steroid or application of a silicon patch or sheet may be useful for smaller hypertrophic areas. It is important to treat any itchy areas with appropriate pharmacological agents, as patient scratching may cause distress and increase the chance of introducing infection and delayed healing. The use of Integra may improve the quality of burn scars. Flamazine cream, although useful, should not be used in nursing or pregnant women.

Electrical burns

25. A, C

Low-tension electrical burns are associated with electrical burns in the home due to the fact that appliances are 'low tension'. Heart damage is not a feature of low-tension burns but can be in high-tension burns which are associated with large amounts of subcutaneous and muscle damage, resulting in myoglobinuria and renal damage. Acidosis is found in large burns and may require treatment with boluses of bicarbonate.

Chemical and radiation burns

26. B

With phosphorus and elemental sodium burns, washing with copious water is contraindicated. Alkali burns are generally deeper than acid burns and act for a longer time. Hydrofluoric acid burns are associated with hypocalcaemia – hence treatment is with 10 per cent calcium gluconate. Radiation burns cause tissue damage that is associated with blood vessel necrosis – split-skin grafts will not take on avascular tissue so vascularised flaps or free flap reconstructions are required.

29 Plastic and reconstructive surgery

Multiple choice questions

→ Plastic surgery – general

1. **Which of the following statements are true?**
   - A The word 'plastic' is derived from the French word 'plastique'.
   - B Plastic surgery is a new speciality.
   - C Plastic surgery involves techniques to restore form and function in tissues damaged by injury, cancer or congenital abnormalities.
   - D Sir Harold Gillies did his reconstructive work after the Second World War.
   - E Some of the work of Gillies was portrayed by Harry Monks.

→ Skin characteristics

2. **Which of the following statements are true?**
   - A The surface of the skin is an important biological layer for homeostasis.
   - B Epidermis regenerates from deeper follicular elements.
   - C Epidermal keratinocytes cannot be cultured and thus are of no value in wound management.
   - D The depth of skin varies in different parts of the body.
   - E In the absence of skin, a wound heals by secondary intention with fibrosis and contracture.

→ Skin grafts

3. **Which of the following statements regarding blood supply and grafts are true?**
   - A Skin blood supply comes from muscle and fascial perforating vessels.
   - B Direct cutaneous vessels can also contribute to the blood supply of the skin.
   - C A graft has a separate blood supply which enables it to survive on an avascular wound.
   - D A full-thickness graft has the whole dermis attached with fat trimmed off.
   - E A composite graft is a full-thickness graft to which other structures such as hair may be added by suturing on.

4. **Which of the following statements regarding grafts are true?**
   - A Imbibition is not a process associated with survival of split-skin grafts in the first 48 h.
   - B Gentle handling and the best postoperative care help to ensure the successful take of a full-thickness graft.
   - C Grafts will take on exposed tendons and cortical bone.
   - D Contraction occurs in all grafts used in tissue repair but is dependent on amount of dermis taken with the graft.
   - E The more dermis in the graft, the more is the contraction.

5. **Which of the following statements regarding grafts are true?**
   - A Split-skin grafts are sometimes known as Thiersch grafts.
   - B Full-thickness grafts are useful in small areas such as fingers, eyelids, or on the face.
   - C John Wolfe, an Aberdeen orthopaedic surgeon, described a composite graft in 1902.
   - D Split-skin grafts produce a superior cosmetic result compared with full-thickness grafts.
   - E Scars placed in 'the lines of election' or lines of minimal tension produce the best cosmetic results.

6. **Which of the following statements regarding split-skin grafts are true?**
A Split-skin grafts can be cut at varying thicknesses using handheld or electrical dermatomes.
B The best donor site for getting a split-skin graft in children or females is the thigh.
C Other useful donor sites for split-skin grafts are the buttocks and the scalp.
D The size and number of bleeding points in the donor tissue for split-skin grafts do not identify the thickness of the graft.
E The take of a split-skin graft is affected by a number of factors, including the presence of group A beta-haemolytic *Streptococcus*.

7. **Which of the following statements regarding mesh grafts are true?**
A Mesh grafting enables expansion of a split-skin graft to be done.
B Mesh grafting prevents release of exudates from under a split-skin graft.
C The possible donor site for a full-thickness graft is from behind the ear.
D Condition for take of a full-thickness graft are not as critical as for a split-skin graft.
E Large full-thickness grafts when used in the face and over good facial muscle do not produce a satisfactory cosmetic result.

Flaps

8. **Which of the following statements regarding flaps are true?**
A Flaps introduce blood supply into an area for reconstruction.
B Classification of flaps can be made on the basis of their blood supply.
C In a random pattern flap, the maximum length:breadth ratio that is safe is 2:1.
D Delay is a technique that can further lengthen a random flap.
E Axial flaps, based on known blood vessels, enable longer flaps to be moved over longer distances.

9. **Which of the following statements regarding flaps are true?**
A Islanding of a random flap can safely and usefully be done.
B Inclusion of fascial tissue in a skin flap does not make for greater safety.
C The design of a transposition flap demands knowledge of a pivot point.
D The transposition flap length equals the length of the defect to be covered – assuming the breadth:length ratio is no greater than permitted.
E Following the use of a transposition flap, skin grafting of the donor defect is a likely necessity though direct closure may be just possible.

10. **Which of the following statements regarding flaps are true?**
A Z-plasties are triangular transposition flaps.
B Z-plasties are able to lengthen very broad contracture scars.
C A bilobed flap is useful to close a small convex defect in the nose tip.
D Rhomboid flaps are useful in the repair of defects of the fingertips.
E Rotation flaps are used for buttock or scalp defect repairs.

11. **Which of the following statements regarding flaps are true?**
A Burrow's triangles are not of significance in the use of bipedicle flaps.
B Multiple Y to V releases are one of the most effective means of managing moderate isolated burn scars over flexion creases.
C V to Y flaps are ineffective in the management of fingertip injuries.
D The key to successful random flap use is to pull available local spare lax skin into the defect so that the closed scar lies in a good line of election.
E A disadvantage of using local flaps may be a poor cosmetic result.

12. **Which of the following statements regarding myocutaneous and fasciocutaneous flaps are true?**
A Myocutaneous and fasciocutaneous flaps are unreliable in plastic surgery repairs.
B The above flaps require complex equipment to be available.

C Knowledge of blood supply in the area of use is essential when these flaps are used.
D These flaps can be used without skin if required.
E Survival of the skin when used in these flaps as skin island flaps depends on small perforating vessels.

13. Which of the following statements regarding free flaps are true?
A Free flaps are the best way of reconstructing major composite loss of tissue.
B Surgical expertise and equipment in microsurgery are essential for the use of free flaps.
C Debridement of the area of reconstruction is necessary for the use of free flaps.
D Major donor site morbidity is a possible disadvantage in free-flap surgery.
E It usually takes more time to perform the surgery associated with a microsurgical procedure unless the surgeon is experienced.

14. Which of the following statements regarding complications with flaps are true?
A A pale and cold flap is a sign that the venous supply is compromised.
B Too much tension of flap inset can cause flap failure in every type of flap, including free flaps.
C Poor knowledge of anatomy and the blood supply to flap tissue will be a cause of flap failure.
D Medicinal leeches can be useful as a last resort in flaps which have an arterial input problem.
E Well-controlled analgesia to reduce catecholamine output is good advice in the management of major tissue transfers.

15. Which of the following statements regarding flaps are true?
A Burrow's triangles are associated with the use of Z-plasties.
B A defect of the lower eyelid may be repaired using a 'bucket handle' flap.
C An inner canthal defect can be repaired using a transposition flap from the glabellar area.
D A bilobed flap is an example of an axial pattern flap.
E A disadvantage of the use of local flaps used in tumour surgery may be compromise to excision.

➜ Reconstructive options

16. Which of the following statements are true?
A A large scalp defect – say as much as 75 per cent in area and involving skull excision – can be best repaired using a rhomboid flap.
B A defect in the heel may be repaired using an islanded pedicled instep flap.
C The definitive repair covering for an Achilles tendon scar problem is a split-skin graft.
D Repair of an ankle defect involving the skin can be accomplished by using a fasciocutaneous flap.
E Position of perforating vessels can be identified using a Doppler apparatus.

➜ Types of flaps

17. Which of the following statements are true?
A Nerves and tendons cannot be transferred as free, non-vascularised grafts.
B The fibula can be used in jaw reconstruction as a free flap.
C The radial forearm flap is a musculocutaneous flap.
D The latissimus dorsi and transverse rectus abdominis flaps can be used as free flaps or pedicled flaps in breast reconstruction.
E The jejunum is a useful means of free flap repair for oesophageal defects.

➜ Major tissue repair options

18. Which of the following statements are true?
A Success in repair of major tissue defects requires a team approach and meticulous planning.

B In the absence of trained staff or equipment, free flap surgery can still be a good option.

C Free flap success is dependent on the availability of a suitable flap, good artery and venous connecting vessels in the recipient site, and no infection or local tissue induration.

D Microsurgery is best done using the increased magnification provided by loupes.

E The ischaemic time for safe transfer of free flaps is 10 h.

Answers: Multiple choice questions

Plastic surgery – general

1. C

The word 'plastic' is derived from the Greek *plassein*, meaning to shape or mould. It is an old speciality with descriptions in ancient Egypt hieroglyphics and in India in the 6th century where Sushruta described the forehead flap to reconstruct noses. Plastic surgery deals with the repair of defects caused by trauma, after surgery of tumours, or through accidents of birth. Sir Harold Gillies was a pioneering plastic surgeon who became famous after the First World War. Much of his work was illustrated in paintings by Henry Tonks.

Skin characteristics

2. A, B, D, E

Skin is important for sensation and temperature control – it is an important homeostatic tissue. Its depth varies in different parts of the body and regenerates from follicular elements of the dermis. Keratinocytes can be cultured and can be used in wound care. If wounds have no dermis in their base, healing occurs by secondary intention from the sides.

Skin grafts

3. A, B, D

Skin blood supply comes from direct cutaneous vessels and perforators from underlying fascia and, where present, from underlying muscle. A skin graft is part of epidermis and dermis which has been detached as a 'shaving' – it requires the bed or receiving area to be vascularised so that ingress of capillaries into the graft can occur and revascularise it. A similar situation exists for successful take of either a full-thickness graft or a composite graft. The former consists of epidermis and the whole of the dermis from which fat has been removed; the latter is a full-thickness graft which contains hair follicles, cartilage or other adnexal tissues deliberately taken as part of the complete graft and not secondarily sutured on, e.g. hair transplants or reconstruction of deficient nasal rim.

4. B, D

Imbibition is the means whereby a split-skin graft is nourished during the first 48 h of life in its recipient site. Gentle handling is important to create the best conditions for take of a full-thickness graft. Grafts do not take on bare tendon or cortical bone because these do not produce granulations or vascular support. Graft contraction depends on the amount of dermis in the graft and is thus greatest in split-skin grafts and least in full-thickness grafts.

5. A, B, E

Thiersch was a professor of surgery in Leipzig, Germany, who described free skin grafting in 1874. Full-thickness grafts were described by John Wolfe, a Glasgow ophthalmic surgeon in 1875, to reconstruct an eyelid. Full-thickness grafts are useful in the repair of face and eyelids and produce a better cosmetic result than split-skin grafts. Incisions and resulting scars are best placed in lines of minimal tension to get the best cosmetic result but do not always correspond to Langer's lines.

6. A, C, E
Split-skin grafts can be cut by using a handheld, hand-powered dermatome or one powered by electricity. The best donor site for taking a split-skin graft in a child or in females is the buttock, where any problems in healing and the risk of poor scars can be hidden. Other useful donor sites are the thighs and the shaved scalp. It is possible to determine the depth of split skin taken from the bleeding nature of the donor site – larger-spaced punctate bleeding points indicate a thicker graft. Graft take depends on a number of factors, including presence of infection, notably group A beta-haemolytic streptococci, shearing forces and a good blood supply in the recipient area. Grafts will not take on avascular tissue.

7. A, C
Mesh grafting of split-skin grafts is a useful technique to expand a smaller graft. The holes in the graft also enable escape of exudates. The retroauricular tissue provides a useful donor site for full-thickness grafts – other sites include the supraclavicular neck or hairless groin skin. The take of split-skin grafts is easier than for full-thickness grafts because there is less tissue depth requiring to be vascularised. If the conditions are good, the cosmetic results are superior for a full-thickness graft and the presence of active muscle underneath a full-thickness graft of the face will improve, not worsen, the result.

Flaps

8. A, B, D, E
Flaps can be classified according to the types of blood supply and, in contrast to grafts, introduce their own blood supply to the recipient area. Flaps can thus be used to reconstruct areas with no, or poor, vascularity. For a random flap, the maximum safe breadth:length ratio is 1:1.5; extending more can be done if the extra portion is 'delayed' or temporarily raised and replaced for a few weeks before the whole flap and delayed portion are used in the reconstruction. When the main vascular supply is confidently known, a longer flap can also be used at a greater distance. This is an example of an axial pattern flap such as the groin flap.

9. C, E
A random flap cannot be islanded because the blood supply is not known precisely; this is not the case for an axial pattern flap, which can be islanded. Inclusion of underlying muscle or fascia with a skin flap increases the flap blood supply if perforators are included. In the design of a transposition flap, it is important to take note of the pivot point as this determines the length of the flap to be used. This point is situated at the base of the flap on the side furthest away from the defect to be covered. The length of this type of flap will be longer than the length of the defect. Usually the donor defect will have to be grafted in part, though in some cases a direct closure may be possible if this is in a very lax area of skin.

10. A, C, E
Z-plasties are triangular transposition flaps which are useful in lengthening narrow, not broad, contracture bands. For tip-of-the-nose defects of about 1 cm in diameter, a bilobed flap is a good alternative to a retroauricular full-thickness graft. The rhomboid flap is not a flap for use in fingertips but can be in the temple or back. Rotation flaps are mostly used in moderately sized scalp defects or in the buttocks.

11. A, B, D
Burrow's triangles do not play any part in the design or use of bipedicle flaps. Multiple Y to V flaps are useful in treating burn scars over flexure creases, and V to Y flaps are useful in repair of fingertip defects. A good cosmetic result in random flaps can be obtained when attention in design

is made to the lines of election in the located area. The cosmetic result of a flap is better than a graft because it is thicker, has a better blood supply and retains colour and texture better.

12. C, D, E

Myocutaneous and fasciocutaneous flaps have very reliable blood supply, and complex equipment and highly trained surgeons are not required. However, it is important to have a good knowledge of anatomy and blood supply for these flaps. Skin survival depends on the perforators, especially if islanded, but the fascia and muscle can be used as flaps without the overlying skin.

13. A, B, C, D

Free flap reconstruction is the best method for composite tissue loss but requires expertise and microsurgical instruments. Careful debridement of the area for reconstruction is essential for success but major donor site morbidity when chosen carefully as part of a team management is not a problem. The operative time for microsurgical procedures is usually longer than for other types of reconstruction but depends on the experience of the operator and assistants.

14. B, C, E

A pale, cold flap has arterial input problem while a blue distended flap has a venous problem. Tension can affect all types of flap adversely, as can failure to know both the anatomy and blood supply to the flap being used. Medicinal leeches are useful in situations where the venous output has been compromised but are of no value if there is an arterial problem. Each leech can only be used once on an individual patient. It is important that appropriate analgesia is given in major tissue transfers so that catecholamine production is reduced.

15. B, C, E

Z-plasties do not need to make use of Burrow's triangles. The bucket handle flap is used in reconstruction of the lower eyelid. A glabellar transposition flap can be used to repair a defect of the inner canthus. The bilobed flap is not an axial pattern flap as it is not based on known vessels – if anything, it is a modified rotation or transposition flap. Compromising tumour excision to fit the design of a local flap should not be done but it is a risk. Excision of any tumour should always be the first priority, with the repair of the resulting defect by a flap designed to fit the defect created and not vice versa.

→ Reconstructive options

16. B, D, E

A large scalp defect with bone tissue removed cannot be repaired by a rhomboid flap but would require reconstruction with a free flap. Heel ulcers are difficult due to their site but can be treated by employing a pedicled instep flap. Achilles tendon wounds are not permanently and properly repaired by using split-skin grafts because of durability, vascularity and mobility problems – a flap repair is better. Wounds of the ankle and lower third of the leg can be repaired using fasciocutaneous or free flaps. Doppler apparatus is an easy and good way to identify perforating vessels on the skin surface.

→ Types of flaps

17. B, D, E

Nerve and tendons can be used as free grafts – the sural nerve and, when available, the palmaris longus tendons are useful sources of donor tissue. The fibula is a useful source of free flap for bone to reconstruct the jaw The radial forearm flap is a good example of an axial pattern flap as it is designed around well-known vessels. Latissimus dorsi or transverse rectus abdominis flaps can be used as free flaps or pedicled muscle or musculocutaneous flaps in breast reconstruction. For oesophageal defects, free jejunum grafts offer a good way for reconstruction.

→ Major tissue repair options

18. A, C

For major tissue reconstructions, meticulous planning and teamwork is essential for success. If this is to be done using a microvascular procedure, the use of loupes is not satisfactory and the best results are obtained using proper staff and apparatus. Good vessels in both donor flap and recipient area, the lack of tissue induration, lack of tension and lack of infection in the area of reconstruction are also important for successful repair. The ischaemic time is dependent on the presence or absence of muscle tissue in the free flap – it is less in the case of the former. A 1–2 h period is safe for muscle-containing free flaps – longer times of up to 6 h are permissible only in skin or/and fascia flaps.

30 Disaster surgery

Multiple choice questions

Natural disasters

1. **Which of the following are characteristics of a natural disaster?**

A Civil administration is usually disrupted.
B The armed services will be needed to restore order and reconstruct.
C Shelter for large numbers will be one of the first priorities.
D They occur over a short period of the time.
E Most countries have organisations prepared to handle these disasters.

2. **Which of the following statements regarding action priorities in a natural disaster are true?**

A Assessment of the extent of damage is undertaken once rescue operations are underway.
B Experienced senior staff should stay back from the disaster area to carry out planning.
C Local volunteers should not be involved, only trained staff.
D The first priority is to prevent further damage or harm to staff from occurring.

Triage

3. **Which of the following statements regarding triage are true?**

A Triage means treating the most seriously injured first.
B Triage is carried out where the casualties are found.
C Triage is carried out at the same time as simple emergency life-saving procedures.
D Triage does not mean that a patient's triage category cannot be reviewed.
E Triage is best recorded with an appropriately coloured label attached to the patient.

Transport of patients

4. **Which of the following statements regarding transport of patients is true?**

A It should be delayed until the patient is stabilised.
B It should be carried out using the fastest form of transport.
C Casualties must be accompanied by trained staff.
D Patients should not be sent out with drip sets and fluids if these are needed at the scene of the accident.

Emergency care in the field hospital

5. **Which of the following statements regarding emergency care in the field hospital are true?**

A Major surgery should only be considered if the patient will not survive transfer to a major centre.
B Measures to control haemorrhage should be undertaken in the field.
C Amputation of devitalised limbs and for gas gangrene should be undertaken in the field.
D Replantation of limbs should be attempted.
E Open fractures should be cleaned in the field.
F Repair of damaged major vessels should be attempted, if this is needed to save a limb.
G Repair of damaged nerves should be attempted.

Debridement of contaminated wounds

6. Which of the following statements regarding debridement are true?

A The term now means letting out pus.
B It can be done through a short incision.
C All doubtful tissue should be removed.
D It may require repeated exploration.
E It frequently involves leaving the wound open.
F It does not involve definitive treatment.

Tetanus

7. Which of the following statements regarding tetanus are true?

A It is caused by the organism *Clostridium perfringens*.
B It causes damage by releasing an exotoxin.
C It thrives in anaerobic conditions.
D The spores are found in soil.
E Heavily contaminated wounds require anti-tetanus globulin as well as tetanus toxoid.
F Penicillin V is ineffective against the organism.
G Patients developing tetanus can be managed using sedation and do not require paralysing and ventilating.

Necrotising fasciitis

8. Which of the following statements regarding necrotising fasciitis are true?

A This is primarily caused by beta-haemolytic *Streptococcus*.
B It can also be caused by infection with several different organisms.
C Necrosis is associated with thrombosis of the microvasculature.
D It spreads steadily and skip lesions are not found.
E The mortality rate is over 50 per cent.
F Surgery should not be undertaken while the patient is toxic.
G Hyperbaric oxygen reduces the mortality.

Gas gangrene

9. Which of the following statements regarding gas gangrene are true?

A It may be caused by coliforms.
B A variety of toxins are produced.
C It thrives only in well-perfused tissues.
D It is more likely to occur if wounds are left open.
E The gas produced is oxygen from haemolysed red cells.
F The toxin released causes malignant hypertension.
G The absence of crepitus excludes the diagnosis.

Blast injuries

10. Which of the following statements regarding blast injuries are true?

A Casualties hidden behind walls or other obstructions are protected from blast injury.
B Blasts mainly affect fluid-filled cavities in the body.
C Penetrating wounds from fragments are deep and their borders difficult to define.
D Contamination of a wound is not an issue as the heat sterilises any fragments.
E Patients are usually deaf so communication is a problem.

Case study – crush syndrome and hypothermia

11. A patient is trapped under a collapsed building for 18 h. When he is finally freed, he is confused, his pulse is faint but regular and his right arm and leg are cold, pale and pulseless. He does not appear to be able to feel or move either of them. The core temperature of the patient is 27°C.

(a) Which two of the following are likely causes of his confusion?

A Hypothermia
B Head injury

C Hypovolaemia secondary to crush syndrome
D Septicaemia
E Social isolation
F Atrial fibrillation
G Hypoxia
H Uraemia
I Liver failure
J Alcohol.

(b) **Which three of the following techniques are most appropriate for his rewarming?**

A Hot oral fluids
B Blankets and a warm environment
C Heated humidified oxygen for the patient to breathe
D Large volumes of warmed IV fluids
E Extracorporeal bypass.

(c) **What organ is most at risk as the limbs start to reperfuse?**

A Brain – due to hypoxic shunting to the crushed limbs
B Liver – due to blood breakdown products
C Lung – due to multiple microemboli
D Kidney – due to release of muscle degradation products
E Heart – due to sludging of blood and high 'end load'.

Answers: Multiple choice questions

Natural disasters

1. A, B, C

The specific characteristics of a natural disaster are that the very services needed to maintain civil order and bring help to those in need are equally affected by the disaster and so will be crippled. The armed forces will be needed to maintain law and order and to provide the skilled manpower for transport of food, water, shelter and medicines. These are going to be the early priorities. Natural disasters such as flooding can develop over an extended period and are not always a single event. Disasters attract attention and support in the short term but there is a natural fatigue within the media and the public, which frequently results in interest being lost long before the consequences of the disaster have been repaired. The countries most susceptible to natural disasters are often those least prepared for them in terms of planning and infrastructure. Even those countries who should, and can, plan for disaster usually find that the size and complexity of major disasters overwhelm the best-laid plans.

2. B, D

Assessment of the extent of damage must take place before and during the initial rescue efforts, not afterwards. Experienced staff will need to go into the field as only they can tell what is needed. However, other senior staff will need to stay back to organise the strategy and logistics of the rescue effort. It is tempting only to allow trained specialist staff to deal with a disaster but in the early hours and days they may not have arrived and local knowledge and initiative are going to be key to sustainable recovery in the long term.

Triage

3. B, C, D, E

Triage does not necessarily mean treating the most seriously injured first. They may have to be left to die, because devoting all your resources to a small number of them might result in a far greater loss of life amongst the many for whom quick and simple interventions could be life-saving. Triage is carried out simultaneously with simple life-saving procedures which should not be allowed to delay the process of triage. There is nothing to prevent a patient having their triage category changed when they are reassessed at a later time. Some patients may deteriorate and others improve during the minutes and hours after the disaster. The triage category of a patient is best recorded on a coloured label attached to their wrist or hung around their neck, so that any other medical worker can see at once that they have been triaged and what it is felt needs to be done.

Transport of patients

4. A, B, C, D

Patients should be stabilised before they are transferred, as assessment and treatment of a patient during transfer (whether in a helicopter or in an ambulance) is very difficult indeed. All tubes and lines (IV access, chest drains etc.) should be set up and carefully tied in before the journey starts. The patient will also need to go with all the equipment that they need. Journeys always take longer than expected so the patient should be prepared for the worst possible scenario, and adequate supplies provided to cover the journey, however delayed; otherwise there is little point in starting the journey. If the patient is being monitored and lines are being used, then the patient will need to be accompanied by a trained member of staff, despite the fact that this will remove skills from the disaster zone. Each patient should go with enough fluids and medication to enable their evacuation to be completed safely.

Emergency care in the field hospital

5. A, B, C, E, F

Major surgery should not be undertaken in the field, unless there is a threat to life of limb which can be averted by surgery (damage limitation). This might be to control catastrophic haemorrhage or amputation of a devitalised and potentially gangrenous limb. Open fractures also need cleaning in the field as otherwise contamination will rapidly turn to rampant infection. If a rapid repair of a major vessel can be undertaken and this will save a limb, this too should be attempted. Replantation and other long and complex operations should not be undertaken as they tie up resources, which cannot then be used for maximum gain, nor should nerve repairs be attempted. They can better be undertaken later in a definitive environment.

Debridement of contaminated wounds

6. C, D, E, F

The 'old' meaning of this word was to release pus, but it has now come to be used to describe the process of cleaning and tidying of a wound, removing foreign material, contaminated and non-viable tissue. It requires a long incision to be sure that all of the affected tissue can be clearly seen and adequately dealt with. It is the single most powerful tool for preventing a contaminated wound from becoming infected, and most especially for preventing tetanus and gangrene. All tissue of doubtful viability should be removed, and the wound should be left open and packed. The process should be repeated at 24–48 h intervals until it is certain that all non-viable tissue has been removed and that the wound is clean. This is not definitive treatment – that should be left to be done by specialist teams in an appropriately equipped unit.

Tetanus

7. B, C, D, E

The organism is *Clostridium tetani* (*C. perfringens* produces gas gangrene). The organism is a Gram-positive cocci which produces an exotoxin (tetanospasmin). The spores are found in soil, and it thrives in anaerobic or dead tissue. If a wound is heavily contaminated then it is advisable to give anti-globulin as well as tetanus toxoid to protect the patient. The organism is very sensitive to penicillin V but antibiotics cannot substitute for good debridement. Once patients develop full-blown tetanus they will have difficulty breathing for themselves, and if spasms become severe, they will need to be paralysed and ventilated.

→ Necrotising fasciitis

8. A, B, C, E, G

The main causative agent is beta-haemolytic *Streptococcus*, but the condition can also result from infection with several different species of organism. Necrosis spreads rapidly because release of toxins causes thrombosis of the microvasculature, but surprisingly there may also be skip lesions with new areas developing remote from the original site. The mortality rate is over 70 per cent, and there should be no delay in surgery to remove dead tissue if the patient is to have a chance of surviving. Hyperbaric oxygen may help to prevent spread of the infection but is no substitute for early aggressive surgery.

→ Gas gangrene

9. A, B

Gas gangrene is usually caused by *Clostridium perfringens* but can also be caused by coliforms. It only thrives in dead or very poorly perfused tissues which create an anaerobic environment. If a wound is left open, it is more difficult for an anaerobic environment to develop. The gas produced is mainly hydrogen sulphide. Oxygen is completely absent. The organism produces a variety of toxins, some of which cause shock, and so the patient's blood pressure falls. Although the condition is called 'gas' gangrene and the gas in soft tissues does produce crepitus, absence of crepitus does not exclude the diagnosis.

→ Blast injuries

10. C, E

Obstructions do not protect victims as the blast spreads around fixed objects as it is a sound wave. Damage within the body is focused on air-filled cavities such as lungs, bowel and, indeed, eardrums (so they are frequently deaf). The blast may be accompanied by fragments which are moving very fast and so can penetrate deeply, leaving a large track of damaged soft tissue behind it, whose borders may be ill-defined. The fragments may be heavily contaminated and are certainly not sterile.

→ Case study – crush syndrome and hypothermia

11. (a) A, C

This patient is likely to have a 'crush injury' and to be hypothermic. The likely causes of his confusion are therefore hypothermia and hypovolaemia. It will be too soon for this confusion to be caused by infection, uraemia or liver failure. Social isolation does not cause confusion and his pulse is regular so it is unlikely that he is in atrial fibrillation. There is no suggestion of a head injury or that alcohol could be involved, so these explanations should not be invoked until the other more likely causes have been explored.

11. (b) B, C, D

Rewarming should be undertaken with care. Warmed fluids orally should not be used. A warm environment and blankets will allow the core temperature to rise slowly and steadily. Heated humidified air is a powerful technique for warming the core (when it is available). Large volumes of warmed IV fluids can be used to treat the hypovolaemic shock caused by the crush syndrome, as well raising core temperature. Extracorporeal bypass is very difficult to use but is said to be helpful in very severely hypothermic patients, but is unlikely to be appropriate here.

11. (c) D

As the patient rewarms and the limbs start to reperfuse, there is a real risk of myoglobin (released from damaged muscle) which will block the kidneys unless a rapid diuresis is started as soon as possible. No other organ is primarily at risk in the same way after crush syndrome.

PART 5

Elective orthopaedics

31 Elective orthopaedics: musculoskeletal examination 219

32 Sports medicine 224

33 The spine 233

34 The upper limb 238

35 The hip and knee 246

36 The foot and ankle 252

37 Infection and tumours 257

38 Paediatric orthopaedics 264

31 Elective orthopaedics: musculoskeletal examination

Multiple choice questions

➜ Musculoskeletal history

1. Introducing yourself to a patient includes:

A Giving your own name
B Checking the patient's name
C Explaining what is to happen
D Obtaining the patient's consent to proceed.
E Washing your hands
F Obtaining adequate exposure
G Checking for tenderness.

➜ Musculoskeletal examination

2. Which of the following statements about the Apley system of examination are true?

A It is a four-stage system.
B The 'look' stage only starts once the patient has been undressed.
C It requires exposure only of the affected limb and one joint above and below.
D It starts with checking the skin for scars, wounds and redness.
E It then moves to bone-checking for deformity.
F It requires that the distal neurovascular status is checked in all cases.

3. Which of the following statements regarding the 'feel' stage of the Apley system of examination are true?

A The 'feel' stage is the second stage of the Apley system.
B It is wise to ask the patient if anywhere is tender before starting 'feeling'.
C When feeling, the same triad is used as in looking.
D Distal neurovascular status must be checked in all musculoskeletal examinations.
E Examiners should not watch their hands when feeling.

4. Which of the following statements regarding the 'move' stage of the Apley system of examination are true?

A 'Move' is the third stage of the Apley system of examination.
B You should move the limb first.
C Stability includes checking power of muscles, stability of joints and special tests.
D Abduction is a movement away from the midline.
E Muscle power is measured on a 6-level scale.

➜ Spine examination

5. Which of the following statements are true?

A Asking the patient to bend forward accentuates the rib hump of idiopathic scoliosis.
B The thoracic spine normally has a lordosis.
C A hairy tuft at the base of the spine is diagnostic of Down's syndrome.
D The Lasègue straight-leg raise test specifically tests the range of movement in the hip joint.
E Palpation of the spinous processes allows you to feel a spondylolisthesis.

➜ Hand and wrist examination

6. Which of the following statements are true?

A Dupuytren's contracture is seen as tight bands in the skin, usually pulling down the fingers on the ulnar side of the hand

B Wasting of the thenar eminence is diagnostic of an ulnar nerve palsy.
C Two point discrimination provides an accurate way of detecting sensory loss in the hand.
D Allen's test should always be performed before performing surgery in the hand.
E Transection of flexor digitorum superficialis can be tested by holding the patient's finger firmly and asking them to flex the distal interphalangeal joint alone.
F A useful test for median nerve compression in the carpal tunnel is to tap over the flexor retinaculum and see if the patient feels lightning pains in the fingers.

→ Elbow and shoulder examination

7. Which of the following statements are true?

A The physiological carrying angle of the elbow is the degree of flexion a patient finds most comfortable.
B Tenderness over the common flexor origin is diagnostic of tennis elbow.
C The rotator cuff in the shoulder runs under the tip of the acromion.
D In dislocation of the shoulder the humeral head usually moves anteriorly.
E Jobe's empty can test is specific for rotator cuff impingement.
F The shoulder apprehension test is diagnostic of the shoulder being out of joint.

→ Hip examination

8. Which of the following statements are true?

A Fixed abduction deformity is characteristic of osteoarthritis of the hip.
B Leg-length discrepancy can be divided into true and apparent.
C Patients with weak abductor muscles bob up and down as they walk.
D Asking the patient to stand on one leg with their hands resting on yours is called the Trendelenburg test.
E Rotation of the hip is best tested with the hip flexed to 45° and the knee flexed to 90°.

→ Knee examination

9. Which of the following statements are true?

A A small effusion in the knee is most easily seen on the medial side when a stroke test is performed.
B The lag test checks for loss of extension in the knee joint.
C The integrity of the collateral ligaments is tested with the knee in full extension.
D A patient with a posterior cruciate ligament disruption will have a positive draw test.
E A patient who has previously dislocated their patella will have a positive apprehension test.

→ The foot and ankle

10. Which of the following statements are true?

A Pes cavus is associated with Marfan's syndrome.
B Loss of sensation in a glove-and-stocking distribution is associated with diabetes.
C Inversion and eversion occur at the ankle joint.
D The windlass test distinguishes physiological from spastic flat foot.
E Patients with a ruptured tendo Achilles can still stand on their toes.

Answers: Multiple choice questions

→ Musculoskeletal history

1. A, B, C, D

Introduction consists of giving your own name and checking the patient's name. You should then explain what you are proposing to do before obtaining the patient's permission to proceed.

Musculoskeletal examination

2. D, F

The Apley system is a triad (three parts) comprising 'look', 'feel', 'move'. Looking actually starts as the patient comes through the door (checking for limp, pain and walking aids) and when you introduce yourself (check the eyes for a Horner's syndrome) and shake hands (be very gentle if the patient obviously has rheumatoid arthritis). Exposure consists of removing covering clothes from one joint above and one below the affected area as well as the opposite side, so that a comparison can be made between normal and abnormal. The Apley system starts with looking at the skin. This is often best done with the patient standing, walking around the patient to make sure that no view (especially the back) is missed. Soft tissues are the next to be checked, looking for both swelling and wasting. Finally the bones are checked for deformity.

3. A, B, C, D, E

Feeling is the second stage of the Apley system of 'look', 'feel', 'move', the same system as used for 'looking'. It is wise to ask a patient if there is any area that is especially tender; leave this until last and then work very carefully. Distal neurovascular status must be tested and recorded in all examinations. It is best to watch the patient's face, not your hands, when palpating as it is on the patient's face that the first signs of discomfort will be found.

4. A, C, D, E

Move is the third stage of the Apley system of the examination. Patients should first be invited to move their own limb – be 'active' – as this will demonstrate any limits of pain. The examiner then follows with 'passive' movement, watching the patient's face carefully for signs of discomfort especially when moving beyond the limits of active movement. Each joint should be put through the full range of movement: flexion (forward), extension (backwards), adduction (towards the midline) and abduction (away from the midline). The 'stability' checks include checking muscle power, ligament stability and special tests. Muscle power is usually measured on the MRC scale, which goes from zero to 5 (6 grades).

Spine examination

5. A, E

Examination of the spine – cervical, thoracic and lumbar – follows the same system as elsewhere. A tuft at the base of the spine is diagnostic of spina bifida occulta (the mildest form of this condition). The spine should be straight in the sagittal plane. However, looked at from the side, the cervical spine is concave (lordosis), the thoracic spine convex (kyphosis), and the lumbar spine again has a lordosis. Palpation of the spinous processes allows you to feel the characteristic gap and step caused by the forward slip of one vertebral body on the one below (spondylolisthesis). Asking the patient to bend forward accentuates the rib hump caused by the rotation of idiopathic scoliosis. The Lasègue straight-leg test specifically excludes pain arising from the hip joint, and from tight hamstrings focusing on pain produced by tugging on the sciatic nerve roots (sciatica).

Hand and wrist examination

6. A, C, D, F

Dupuytren's contracture is immediately visible when first inspecting the hand. The skin is contracted by tight bands and the little and ring finger are pulled down into flexion. In the soft tissues, wasting of the thenar eminence is diagnostic of damage to the median nerve. Abnormal sensation in the hand can be quickly excluded using the stroke test, using the opposite hand for comparison, but for accurate delineation of extent and severity of sensory loss, two-point discrimination needs to be tested with a paper clip. Allen's test ensures that the palmar arch is supplied by both the radial and ulnar nerves. It is always important to check this before operating on the hand as it is crucial to know about the blood supply and any reserve if an artery has to be divided. Flexor digitorum superficialis splits and crosses flexor digitorum profundus to insert into the distal end of the middle phalanx. The distal interphalangeal joint is therefore only flexed by profundus. When testing for carpal tunnel syndrome, Tinel's test is useful. The tip of a finger is used to 'tap' over the flexor retinaculum. Shooting or lightning pains running into the fingers in the distribution of the median nerve are diagnostic of nerve compression.

→ Elbow and shoulder examination

7. C, D, E

The physiological carrying angle is the angle of valgus which the forearm makes with the upper arm when the patient stands with the elbow straight, arms at the sides and hands pointing forwards, and may be altered if there is malunion of a supracondylar fracture. Tennis elbow is painful inflammation of the common extensor origin on the lateral side of the elbow. Golfer's elbow is the rarer equivalent in the common flexor origin. In the shoulder, the rotator cuff passes under the acromion to insert into the rim of the glenoid and it is the formation of a beak of bone on the tip of the acromion which can lead to the painful rotator cuff syndrome. Jobe's test is specific for impingement as it places the supraspinatus tendon under the acromion and then presses the most likely part to be inflamed up on to the beak of bone causing the problem.

When the shoulder dislocates, it is paradoxical that the humeral head usually moves anteriorly. The apprehension test is useful for diagnosing a patient who has, in the past, had an anterior dislocation. It cannot be used when the shoulder is out of joint.

→ Hip examination

8. B, D, E

Osteoarthritis of the hip is the commonest condition affecting the hip, which moves into a position of comfort, flexed and adducted. This creates an apparently 'short' leg (because of the deformity) even when there is no difference in the 'real' leg lengths as measured by checking the bone lengths. Patients with weak abductor muscles (after polio or surgery on the hip) have to throw their body sideways over that hip when they take weight through it, so they sway but do not bob. The test for weak abductors is the Trendelenburg. One way of doing it is to ask patients to stand on each leg in turn while resting their hands on yours. If the abductors are weak, then as they take weight on that leg they will be forced to press down on your hand on the opposite side to prevent themselves from toppling over.

When testing range of rotation of the hip, it is best to put it into the middle of its range of flexion (45°) and then to put the knee at 90° so that the lower leg can be used as a protractor to measure the range of internal and external rotation.

→ Knee examination

9. A, D, E

When testing for a knee effusion, the most sensitive test is the 'stroke test'. Any fluid in the medial side of the knee is stroked out and up into the large synovial pouch under the quadriceps. This fluid is then squeezed down, inflating the dimple on the medial side of the knee. The lag test is a sensitive test for weakness in the extensor mechanism (quadriceps) of the knee. A check is first made that the patient can passively extend the knee fully. They are then asked to perform the same manoeuvre actively. A difference between passive range of movement and active indicates a positive lag test.

When testing the collateral ligaments, it is necessary to flex the knee slightly, as otherwise the posterior structures of the knee lock it and mask any instability. A disruption of either cruciate ligament will produce a positive draw sign. The difference is that a posterior ligament draw starts from an abnormal position 'sagged' and moves to a normal one, while the patient with a disrupted anterior cruciate has the tibia in a normal position at rest, but it is then possible to draw the knee forward to an abnormal position from there.

Dislocation of the patella can be difficult to diagnose as it normally relocates spontaneously. However, from then on any manual attempt to dislocate the patella laterally will cause apprehension in the patient.

➜ The foot and ankle

10. B, D, E

Pes cavus is a high arched foot and is associated with spinal and neurological disorders. Marfan's syndrome produces hyperlaxity and so tends to produce a flat foot. Loss of sensation in the foot resulting from nerve root entrapment will be in the distribution of a dermatome, but diabetes produces a glove-and-stocking distribution of sensory loss. Dorsiflexion and plantarflexion occur at the ankle joint, while inversion and inversion occur at the subtalar joint. When you ask a patient to stand on tiptoes, the arch of the foot should increase. This is the windlass test. If the arch does not appear/increase then the patient has a peroneal spastic flat foot (often caused by a tarsal coalition). It is a paradox that patients with a complete rupture of the tendo Achilles can usually still stand on their toes using their toe flexors as plantarflexors of the ankle.

32 Sports medicine

Multiple choice questions

Case study – shin injury

1. A cricketer complains of pain in his shin which has been present for several months but which got worse today after a prolonged bout of fast bowling. The shin is slightly red, a little swollen and tender to touch.

(a) What class of injury is this likely to belong to?

A Acute extrinsic
B Acute intrinsic
C Chronic.

(b) What is the physical treatment plan?

A Immediate intensive physiotherapy
B Plaster of Paris immobilisation
C Continue sport, by controlling symptoms with analgesics
D Steroid injection
E Find alternative exercise plan which does not load the tibia.

(c) Give two reasons why non-steroidal anti-inflammatories might be helpful.

A To reduce pain
B To reduce oedema
C To enable immediate return to sport before the injury is healed
D To prevent the problem spreading to the other leg.

Soft-tissue haematoma

2. Which of the following statements regarding soft-tissue haematomas are true?

A Most resolve spontaneously.
B If a cyst develops, surgical excision may be needed.
C The changes can become malignant.
D The bruised muscle may sometimes be replaced with cartilage.

Tendon injuries

3. Which of the following statements regarding tendon repair are true?

A The strength of a damaged tendon decreases for some time after injury and only returns back to normal after 6 months.
B Tendons heal by degeneration of the distal portion followed by regrowth from the proximal end.
C Paratendinitis has a poor prognosis.
D Tendinosis can be painless.
E Tendons consist of type 1 fibres.

Case study – ligament injury

4. A sportsman presents having sprained his thumb. There is slight painless laxity in the ulna collateral ligament. What grade of ligament injury is this?

A Grade 0
B Grade 1
C Grade 2
D You cannot tell until you have compared it with the other side.

Bursae

5. What are the characteristics of bursae?

A They are normal structures designed to reduce friction.
B They are lined with synovial membrane and connected to the joint beneath.
C They are able to become inflamed and infected.
D They have no nerve supply.

Bone healing

6. Which of the following statements are true?

A The first phase of bone healing is the laying down of bone in the fracture cleft.

B Callus is mature bone laid down around the fracture area.
C Remodelling of the bone goes on for many months after the fracture.
D Stress on bone stimulates more bone to be laid down.

Stress fractures

7. Stress fractures:

A Are most common in high intensity high load sports
B Produce highly localised pain
C Are difficult to see on X-ray
D Show up well on magnetic resonance imaging (MRI)
E Heal quickly.

Ankle injury

8. Why is the anatomical reduction of an ankle fracture so important?

A To enable return of a full range of movement
B To allow full strength in the ankle
C To improve proprioception
D To avoid premature onset of osteoarthritis
E To avoid the onset of premature osteoporosis.

Injuries to the plantarflexor mechanism of the ankle

9. Which of the following statements regarding plantarflexor mechanism injury are true?

A Musculotendinous junction tears of the Achilles tendon do not require surgery.
B Re-rupture of the Achilles tendon within 1 year of injury occurs in less than 10 per cent of cases however they are treated.
C Simmond's test involves squeezing the calf and looking to see if the foot moves.
D Surgical repair of the ruptured tendo Achilles carries a significant risk of causing nerve damage.

Case studies – shoulder injury

10. A 20-year-old man sustains a dislocation of the shoulder playing rugby.

(a) What would you tell him is the chance of this shoulder dislocating again?

A <50 per cent
B >50 per cent
C >80 per cent.

(b) The man asks what is the chance of the other shoulder dislocating. What answer would you give him?

A <50 per cent
B >50 per cent
C >80 per cent.

11. A 25-year-old suffers a tear of the rotator cuff in a bad fall. You offer to repair it. What would you offer him as the chances of the repair being successful?

A <50 per cent
B >50 per cent
C >80 per cent.

12. A rugby player fell onto his shoulder some weeks ago. He now presents with a painful lump about 4 cm in diameter on the top of his shoulder. What has he injured?

A Common extensor origin
B The acromioclavicular joint
C The head of the humerus
D The sternoclavicular joint
E The rotator cuff.

Case studies – elbow injury

13. A sportsman complains of pain over the lateral side of his elbow. What is the source of the problem?

A Common extensor origin
B Acromioclavicular joint
C The radiohumeral joint
D The radioulnar joint
E The ulnar nerve.

14. A weight-lifter complains of numbness and tingling in his fingers. What has he injured?

A Common extensor origin
B Acromioclavicular joint
C The ulnar nerve
D The median nerve
E The brachial plexus.

Extended matching questions

→ 1. Knee injury

1 A skier twists with his body turning outwards (the tibia rotates inwards) as he falls. The binding fails to release and he feels a crack in his knee. Nothing seems to be out of place, but it swells immediately and he has to be brought down off the mountain on a stretcher.

2 A joy rider, who is not wearing a seatbelt, is finally arrested when he loses control of the car and crashes into a wall. He has facial injuries from the windscreen and a fractured sternum from the steering wheel. His right knee is also painful and swollen.

3 An elderly woman hurrying to church trips on the steps and falls on to her left knee. It is now painful and swollen and she cannot walk.

4 A window cleaner who plays football at weekends complains that from time to time his leg will not straighten and he has to jiggle it until it frees up.

5 A teenage girl develops knee pain following a trivial injury. It is at its worst when she sits for any length of time and when trying to go down stairs.

6 A teenage long jumper injures his knee by landing with it hyperextended. He now has chronic knee pain, especially when he tries to straighten it.

7 A footballer is involved in a heavy tackle where another player falls across the outside of his knee. He feels something give way and is carried off the pitch.

8 A rugby player is tackled and his knee twists. He feels severe pain and notices something out of place in this knee. However, as he rolls over to try to stand up, whatever it was clicks back into place.

(a) Choose and match each of the above scenarios with the structure that is likely to be damaged or the injury likely to be sustained:

A Osteochondritis dissecans
B Tibial plateau fracture
C Torn meniscus with bucket handle tear
D Dislocated patella
E Hoffa's syndrome
F Medial collateral ligament tear
G Torn posterior cruciate ligament
H Femoral condyle fracture
I Snapping pes anserinus
J Torn anterior cruciate ligament
K Fractured patella
L Chondromalacia patellae

(b) Choose a test or investigation from the following that is most appropriate to confirm each of the diagnoses in (a):

A Lachmann's test
B Posterior sag test
C MacMurray's test
D Tenderness on palpation of the synovium around the patella
E Standard X-rays of the knee
F MRI of the knee

G Tenderness to palpation over the anterior fat pad
H Stressing the knee into valgus in slight flexion
I Injection of local anaesthetic
J Apley grind test
K Patella apprehension test
L Anterior draw test
M Tunnel views of the knee

2. Ankle injury

1 A patient with a high-arched foot complains of the spontaneous onset of a snapping sensation in the outside of her ankle.

2 An elderly woman notices a sudden collapse of the longitudinal arch of her foot with her heel falling into valgus.

3 A long-distance runner develops pain, swelling, tenderness and crepitus over the front of the lower third of the tibia.

4 A squash player feels a sharp blow in the back of the ankle, although it appears that nothing hit him.

5 A middle-aged active patient develops unilateral heel pain without any trauma. It is worst after sitting still for any length of time.

(a) Choose and match each of the above scenarios with the injury that is likely to be sustained:

A Rupture of the tibialis posterior tendon
B Tendinitis of the tibialis anterior
C Subluxation of the peroneal tendons
D Rupture of the Achilles tendon
E Plantar fasciitis

(b) Choose the most appropriate treatment for each of the diagnoses:

A Non-steroidal anti-inflammatories and rest
B Surgical repair of the tendon sheath
C Modified footwear with insoles
D Heel cups ± local steroid injection
E Serial plaster splints

3. Foot injury

A Morton's neuroma
B March fracture
C Metatarsalgia
D Turf toe
E Freiberg's disease
F Heel bumps

Choose and match a suitable diagnosis for each of the scenarios given below:

1 A cricketer develops pain around the metatarsophalangeal joint of his big toe after a bout of fast bowling.

2 A cyclist falls from his bicycle and injures his forefoot. There is no bone injury but he develops pain and numbness in 2 toes.

3 A long-distance runner does much of her training barefooted. She starts to develop pain under the front of her foot at the base of the 2nd, 3rd and 4th toes.

4 An adolescent with pain in the forefoot is found to have avascular necrosis of the 2nd metatarsal head.

5 An adolescent who is growing fast develops a hot and tender area over the heel apparently associated with the apohyseal growth plate where the Achilles tendon inserts into the calcaneum.

6 A long-distance runner spontaneously develops a painful crack (undisplaced) across the neck of the 2nd metatarsal.

Answers: Multiple choice questions

→ Case study – shin injury

1. (a) C

This is a chronic injury. There is no history of a direct blow (acute extrinsic) or of a sudden failure (acute intrinsic), and it has continued for some time.

1. (b) E

The diagnosis is likely to be some form of shin splint, either a tendinitis or a stress fracture. There is no evidence of a full-blown fracture with potential instability (although there may be a stress fracture), so there is no need for plaster immobilisation. There is also no value in physiotherapy, which may actually exacerbate this problem. Although professional athletes do it all the time, there is no place for using medication to suppress symptoms so that an athlete can continue sport. Equally a steroid injection is not indicated until other methods have been tried. The best management plan is to keep the athlete active but advise them to choose a sport which rests the tibia and the muscles around it. This is likely to be swimming, cycling or a rowing machine.

1. (c) A, B

Non-steroidals will reduce pain and swelling, but as discussed in the previous answer they should not normally be used to suppress symptoms so that sport can be re-started before the problem has healed.

→ Soft-tissue haematoma

2. A, B, D

Most haematomata in soft tissues resolve spontaneously, but if they are very large (usually in the thigh) then a cyst may form, and in rare cases this cyst may need excising. This is, however, a course of last resort. The changes do not become malignant but the cartilage, and even bone which forms (myositis ossificans), can look quite like a malignant sarcoma on X-ray.

→ Tendon injuries

3. A, D, E

Tendons are made up of tightly packed type 1 collagen. Tendons heal by fibroblasts laying down new collagen. It is nerves that heal by distal degeneration (Wallerian). As a tendon heals from a partial tear, there is a period when it is actually weaker than before (for 7–10 days) before it starts to build up strength. Paratendinitis (inflammation of the membrane around the tendon) has a good prognosis with a period of rest. Tendinosis (degeneration of the tendon itself) can be completely symptomless before it presents with a catastrophic failure.

Case study – ligament injury

4. D

The laxity of ligaments is very variable between different people, so before diagnosing a lax ligament as a disruption, it is always worth comparing the laxity with the other (normal) side. Grade 0 is no pain or laxity. Grade 1 is pain on stressing without increased laxity. Grade 2 is a partial disruption, pain and increased laxity with an end-point. Grade 3 is a complete disruption. There is usually tenderness but there is always significant laxity with no firm end-point.

Bursae

5. A, C

Bursae are normal structures which are found wherever structures under load are likely to rub on each other. They are lined in synovium but do not normally connect with the joint beneath. They can become inflamed and painful, and so they obviously have a nerve supply.

Bone healing

6. C, D

The first phase of bone healing is organisation of the haematoma and the laying down of fibrin, so no bone is involved initially. This scar tissue may then form cartilage, which in turn is replaced by bone. Callus is immature bone, which is then replaced by mature bone in the final stages of healing. The Heuter–Volkmann principle states that bone is laid down in response to stress, so loading a fracture does stimulate healing, provided that the load is not excessive.

Stress fractures

7. C, D

Stress fractures are common in low-intensity, low-load sports which involve very large numbers of repetitions, e.g. long-distance running. The pain is not at all well localised, and the partial fractures can be very difficult to see on X-ray. However, MRI has proved useful for visualising the fracture. They are depressingly slow to heal.

Ankle injury

8. D

The proper reduction of an ankle fracture is crucial because the fracture is intra-articular. If the fragments heal more than 2 mm out of place, there will be such high peak loads on the articular cartilage that premature arthritis will result.

Injuries to the plantarflexor mechanism of the ankle

9. A, B, C, D

The musculotendinous junction of the tendo Achilles has a good blood supply (unlike the body of the tendon), and so it will heal quickly and does not require any assistance from surgery. The tendon itself has a poor healing potential, and opinion is divided as to whether surgical repair should be used to assist serial plastering. Either way, the re-rupture rate is less than 10 per cent. However, return to normal activities may be slightly quicker after surgery. Against that there is a small but significant risk of nerve damage while performing the repair. The classic test for a rupture of the tendo Achilles is to squeeze the calf. If the foot plantarflexes then the tendon is intact. This is Simmond's test.

→ Case studies – shoulder injury

10. (a) B; (b) A

There is a 60 per cent chance of a further dislocation and a 10 per cent chance of the other shoulder dislocating.

11. C

In the young patient, the cuff still has some ability to repair so the prognosis is good. In the elderly, however, the prognosis is poor.

12. B

The acromioclavicular joint is typically injured by a fall on to the point of the shoulder. The result is inflammation then early aggressive arthritis which produces a painful lump just where the shoulder straps of a rucksack press on to the shoulder. The only possible treatment is to excise the joint, but this may not cure the pain.

→ Case studies – elbow injury

13. A

This is likely to be 'tennis elbow' irritability of the common extensor origin. The condition is difficult to treat but may be helped by local steroid injection.

14. D

Weight-lifters commonly injure the median nerve at the wrist (carpal tunnel syndrome). If non-operative measures do not work, then surgical release will be needed.

Answers: Extended matching questions

→ 1. Knee injury

(a) Structure/injury – 1J, 2G, 3K, 4C, 5L, 6E, 7F, 8D

(b) Test/investigation – 1A, 2B, 3E, 4F, 5D, 6G, 7H, 8K

Scenario 1

A twisting injury of the flexed knee when the foot is locked onto the ground tears the anterior cruciate ligament. This is an acute intrinsic injury. It may then go on to tear the medial meniscus and the medial collateral ligament (the so-called unhappy triad of O'Donoghue). The anterior cruciate ligament has a blood supply (unlike the meniscus) and so the knee swells immediately with blood. The injured person is usually unable to carry on. A torn meniscus sometimes allows a sportsperson to play on and may not swell until some hours later. The diagnosis of a disrupted anterior cruciate ligament is made by finding that the patient has a positive anterior draw test, or a positive Lachmann's test, both of which test for abnormal subluxation of the tibia forward on the femur.

Scenario 2

When a joy rider crashes without a seatbelt, the knee is driven back by impact with the dashboard. This posterior displacement of the flexed tibia on the femur ruptures the posterior cruciate ligament. Patients with a ruptured posterior cruciate ligament have a positive anterior draw test (just like a patient with a ruptured anterior cruciate). However, the draw is forward from a posterior sag position. It is therefore the posterior sag which is diagnostic.

Scenario 3

This injury is a classic acute extrinsic injury. She has taken a direct blow on the front of the knee and so the most likely injury is a fracture of the patella. It can be diagnosed by X-ray.

Scenario 4
This history is classic locking. There is most likely a torn meniscus. If the tear is bucket-handled in shape then sometimes the bucket handle will fold over and lock in the knee joint. The patient then has to wiggle the knee to relocate the torn fragment before they can move the knee again. There is no reliable test on physical examination (MacMurray's test is not reliable) and it is best diagnosed by MRI.

Scenario 5
Anterior knee pain or chondromalacia patellae develops in adolescents (usually women) often after a trivial injury. It is most painful after long periods of sitting or on descending stairs. It can be very disabling and is quite resistant to analgesia. It almost always resolves spontaneously. There is no test which helps with the diagnosis, but palpation of the synovium around the patella is tender.

Scenario 6
A hyperextension injury of the knee crushes the fat pad in the front of the knee. The fat pad then becomes swollen and painful. This is called Hoffa's syndrome and usually settles spontaneously but may require arthroscopic resection of the fat pad. Examination reveals tenderness of the fat pad.

Scenario 7
This is a classic acute intrinsic injury. The medial collateral ligament will have been torn by the valgus force. Stressing the knee into valgus with the knee slightly flexed (to release the posterior stabilisers) will be diagnostic.

Scenario 8
This is one of the commoner acute intrinsic injuries to the knee. The patella has dislocated but then spontaneously relocated (as it so often does). The knee will be painful and swollen initially and so will be difficult to examine, but once the initial inflammation has settled, the patient will be left with a patella apprehension sign. Any attempt to push the patella laterally as you passively flex the knee will be resisted by the patient, who will have a sense of impending doom (the apprehension).

→ 2. Ankle injury

(a) Injury – 1C, 2A, 3B, 4D, 5E

(b) Treatment – 1B, 2C, 3A, 4E, 5D

Scenario 1
This problem commonly arises from the peroneal tendons subluxing over the lateral malleolus. This is most likely if the patient has suffered some kind of injury which has ruptured the sheath that holds the tendons in place. The only useful treatment is surgical repair of the sheath.

Scenario 2
This is a typical presentation of a ruptured tibialis posterior tendon. Surgical repair is a last resort, and many are managed using modified footwear with insoles to support the fallen arch.

Scenario 3
Long-distance runners may develop tendinitis of the tibialis anterior. There will be pain, swelling and tenderness over the tibialis anterior. There may also be palpable crepitus. The treatment is anti-inflammatories accompanied by rest to let the tendinitis settle.

Scenario 4
Rupture of the tendo Achilles occurs quite suddenly in middle-aged men performing strenuous sport. There is often a sharp crack and patients feel as if they have been hit on the back of the

heel. Treatment is serial plasters or surgical repair with serial plasters. There is no clear evidence as to which treatment is best.

Scenario 5

Plantar fasciitis may develop after local trauma or it may arise spontaneously. It is a self-limiting condition but may be helped with heel cup supports; some clinicians inject steroids into the tender area.

→ 3. Foot injury

1D

This is a tear of the metatarsophalangeal joint capsule due to forcible hyperextension of the big toe. Its common name is turf toe. Treatment is rest and analgesia

2A

This is a neuroma forming in the interdigital nerve (Morton's neuroma), in this case probably secondary to trauma. The treatment is excision of the neuroma but this will almost certainly leave the patient with permanent numbness in that nerve distribution.

3C

Repetitive bruising of the metatarsal heads will produce metatarsalgia. This can also occur in patients with rheumatoid arthritis. It is best treated with modified footwear to reduce the load on the tender metatarsal heads.

4E

Spontaneous avascular necrosis of the second metatarsal head is known as Freiberg's disease. It is best treated symptomatically, but the necrotic head and remaining fragments can be excised.

5F

These are heel bumps, caused by shoes rubbing. Changing footwear can improve things.

6B

The March fracture is another stress fracture and is best managed by prolonged rest from the sport that caused it.

33 The spine

Multiple choice questions

Epidemiology, anatomy and physiology of back pain

1. **Which of the following statements regarding back pain are true?**

A The chances of anyone having back pain at some time in their life is around 50 per cent.
B Over 80 per cent of episodes of back pain settle within 6 weeks.
C The radicular artery of Adamkiewicz is the main blood supply to the lower spinal cord.
D Onset of back pain after the age of 55 is a 'red flag' sign.
E 'Yellow flags' are worrying but less critical than 'red flags'.

Case study – sudden onset of urinary incontinence

2. **A 30-year-old nurse lifting in the ward experiences sudden pain in her back. She goes to Sister's office to sit down. The pain eases but now she notices that she has difficulty standing and walking (her legs feel weak and wobbly, and she has been incontinent of urine).**

(a) What is the rare but very dangerous diagnosis which needs excluding?

A Collapsed vertebral body secondary to occult myeloma
B Central disc prolapse
C Transverse myelitis
D Dissecting aneurysm blocking off the blood supply to the spinal cord.

(b) What physical tests (when present) would help to exclude this diagnosis?

A Testing for weakness of extensor hallucis longus
B Unilateral loss of ankle reflex
C Saddle anaesthesia
D Loss of anal tone
E Increase in pain.

(c) What action needs to be taken?

A Analgesia and bed rest
B Immediate lumbar spine X-ray
C Lumbar puncture
D Urgent referral to a neurologist
E Immediate referral to a spine surgeon.

Imaging in back disorders

3. **Which of the following statements about imaging are true?**

A Plain X-rays of the spine should only be taken if there is a history of trauma.
B Magnetic resonance imaging (MRI) is the best way of visualising the disc and nerve roots.
C CT scan is best for looking for patients with multiple vertebral body collapses secondary to myeloma.
D Bone densitometry is needed to diagnose osteoporosis.
E Bone scintigraphy is a simpler method for measuring bone density.

Case study – collapsed vertebrae

4. **A 70-year-old man who has smoked all his life now presents feeling unwell and with weight loss. He also has**

backache which wakes him at night. Chest X-ray is normal but plain X-ray of the spine shows several collapsed vertebrae. Blood tests have already been sent.

(a) What investigation is likely to be most useful for identifying the cause of the collapses?

A Computed tomography (CT)-guided biopsy
B Barium enema
C CT of lung
D Barium meal and follow-through
E Intravenous pyelogram.

(b) The man's lesion is thought to be an adenocarcinoma of unknown origin (probably bowel). What treatment options are available?

A Radiotherapy
B Chemotherapy
C Harrington rods to the spine
D Steroids
E Embolisation of tumours

➜ Case study – pain which wakes at night

5. A 65-year-old man who has lived all his life in Britain presents with severe and constant back pain at L3, which does not radiate down the legs. It wakes him at night and he has night sweats. X-rays show destruction of the disc space at L2/L3 with invasion of the destruction into the adjacent vertebral bodies. What would you expect to find on needle biopsy?

A Tumour cells (metastases)
B Primary chondrosarcoma cells
C *Mycobacterium tuberculosis*
D *Escherichia coli*
E Sterile avascular necrosis.

➜ Case study – sciatica

6. A 40-year-old labourer presents with backache radiating down the left leg to the foot. His left foot drags and on examination he has weakness in extensor hallucis longus. There is also diminished sensation over the dorsum of the foot and the lateral side of the calf. What is the likely diagnosis?

A Prolapse of the L5/S1 disc pressing on the S1 nerve root
B Prolapse of the L5/S1 disc pressing on the L5 nerve root
C Facet joint arthritis
D Infective discitis
E Neuroma of a nerve root.

➜ Claudication

7. How can spinal claudication be distinguished from vascular claudication?

A Only vascular claudication is initiated by exercise.
B Spinal claudication is worse in extension vascular in flexion.
C Distal pulses are present only in spinal claudication.
D Spinal claudication progresses in less than 50 per cent; vascular progresses in more than 50 per cent of cases.
E Spinal claudication can be treated by spinal decompression.

➜ Case study – low back pain

8. A young rower complains of sudden onset of low back pain when weight-lifting. There is no radiation of the pain and there is no neurological deficit. There is considerable lordosis of the lumbar spine with a step palpable at L5/S1. What is the most likely diagnosis?

A Prolapsed intervertebral disc
B Spondylolisthesis
C Collapsed vertebra
D Muscle strain.

➜ Case study – rib hump in teenager

9. A 13-year-old female presents with a rib hump. She has had no problems previously. Abdominal reflexes are equal and normal.

(a) What is the likely diagnosis?

A Neuromuscular scoliosis
B Lipoma

C Steroid-induced rib hump
D Idiopathic scoliosis
E Undescended scapular.

(b) What test can be used to measure the severity of the problem?
A Lung function test
B Cobb's angle on a spine X-ray
C Rib X-rays with intercostal measurement
D Self-esteem questionnaire
E Coronal section MRI chest.

(c) What method can be used to predict the prognosis (likely progression of the curve)?
A Age of the patient
B Risser's sign
C Further growth potential as calculated from parental height
D Degree of curvature
E Plasma calcium.

Answers: Multiple choice questions

➜ Epidemiology, anatomy and physiology of back pain

1. B, C, D

The chance of someone having back pain at some time in their life is between 60 and 80 per cent, but over 80 per cent of episodes settle spontaneously within 6 weeks of onset without the need for any aggressive investigation or treatment. The blood supply to the spinal cord is mainly by the radicular arteries, but the lower spinal cord is supplied by the anterior spinal artery which is mainly filled from the radicular artery of Adamkiewicz. 'Red flag' signs are those which are associated with a non-benign prognosis. New onset of backache after the age of 55 is one of these. 'Yellow flag' signs are those which warn that the back pain is not likely to be amenable to conventional surgical treatment but is more likely to be psychological in origin.

➜ Case study – sudden onset of urinary incontinence

2. (a) B

The scenario described could be the presentation of a central disc prolapse (cauda equina syndrome). It is unlikely to be occult malignancy or an aneurysm as the patient is too young and transverse myelitis is not usually painful.

2. (b) C, D

There are no completely reliable signs of central disc prolapse but saddle anaesthesia and loss of anal tone (when present) are reliable signs. Absence of pain does not exclude a central disc, and unilateral signs are usually related to a single nerve root trapped in the lateral foramen (a lateral protrusion).

2. (c) E

There is evidence that the sooner the compression is released, the better the chance of recovery and so an immediate referral to a spine surgeon for MRI (to confirm the diagnosis) followed by decompression surgery is important.

➜ Imaging in back disorders

3. B, D

Plain X-rays of the spine are needed whenever there is back pain with 'red flag' signs. This includes trauma, but also includes patients under 20 or over 55, those with a history of cancer, and anyone with a history of night pain, fever and/or weight loss. The best way to image the soft tissues of the spine, including the disc, the theca and the nerve roots, is by MRI, but the best way to image bone contours is with CT. However, the radiation dose needed to search for lesions of multiple myeloma using X-rays would be large and bone scintigraphy would be a better screening method. Osteoporosis cannot be diagnosed reliably on plain X-ray or by scintigraphy, and so bone densitometry should be used.

→ Case study – collapsed vertebrae

4. (a) A

A CT-guided biopsy will give a tissue diagnosis and this in turn will point to a possible source. Most tumours in the spine are secondaries (98 per cent) and the commonest secondaries are breast (20 per cent), lung (15 per cent), prostate, renal, gastrointestinal and thyroid (all under 10 per cent), so there is little point in starting with lung, bowel or kidney tests until more information is available.

4. (b) B, D, E

Adenocarcinomas are radio-resistant so chemotherapy will offer the best palliation. There is no indication for internal fixation with rods. Steroids might help the pain and embolisation should probably only be attempted if surgery is planned to decompress the spine or remove the tumour.

→ Case study – pain which wakes at night

5. D

The lesion is around the disc. This effectively excludes tumour osteonecrosis or TB, so the most likely diagnosis is *E. coli* discitis.

→ Case study – sciatica

6. B

The fact that the pain radiates down to the foot suggests that it is radicular rather than referred, so facet joint arthritis and discitis are unlikely to be the cause. The motor supply to extensor hallucis longus is pure L5, and the dermatomal distribution of L5 is the dorsum of the foot and lateral side of the calf. So this is L5 radiculopathy. A neuroma is rare and is not always painful.

→ Claudication

7. B, C, D, E

In both spinal and vascular claudication, pain is initiated by exercise, but as a general rule vascular claudicants get pain going uphill (when the leg muscles require more oxygen) while spinal claudicants get worse pain going downhill (when the spinal canal narrows in extension). Spinal claudication only progresses in around 20 per cent of cases and if it does, spinal decompression can offer significant relief of symptoms.

→ Case study – low back pain

8. (a) B

The most likely diagnosis in this age group is spondylolisthesis and this does produce a step in the spine as well as a lordosis. A young, fit person would be most unlikely to collapse a vertebra without very major trauma. He or she could have prolapsed a disc but then there would likely be pain radiating down the leg (sciatica). A muscle strain would not produce a step in the spine.

→ Case study – rib hump in teenager

9. (a) D

This is the normal age and gender for idiopathic scoliosis. The normal abdominal reflexes make neuromuscular scoliosis unlikely. She has not been on steroids and lipomas are rare in this age group. An undescended scapula would have been picked up long before 13.

9. (b) B

The severity of an idiopathic scoliosis curve is measured with Cobb's angle. This is a measure of the maximum angle of the curvature of the spine on an anteroposterior X-ray. Lung function is commonly affected in neuromuscular scoliosis but rarely affected in idiopathic adolescent scoliosis. Self-esteem may indeed be damaged but there is no validated measure in these cases.

9. (c) B

The likely progression of the curve depends on how much more growth is anticipated and the rate at which it is occurring. Rapid growth with a 'long way to go' is associated with a likely rapid and severe deterioration of the curve, so the younger the patient presenting, both chronologically and skeletally, the more likely that the curve will become severe, especially if the parents are very tall and therefore a considerable amount of further growth is likely. Risser's sign is the method to determine skeletal maturity from the closure of epiphyseal growth plates in the pelvis and therefore predicts how much more growth (and deformity) potential there is in the skeleton. Obviously the more severe the deformity when the patient first presents, the more severe the deformity is likely to be when growth ends and the deformity stops progressing.

34 The upper limb

Multiple choice questions

→ Rotator cuff

1. **Which muscles control the rotator cuff?**

A Supraspinatus
B Teres major
C Teres minor
D Infraspinatus
E Pectoralis minor
F Subscapularis.

→ Shoulder replacement

2. **What benefits are offered by a shoulder replacement?**

A Pain relief is guaranteed.
B Range of movement will improve dramatically.
C An absence of the rotator cuff makes no difference.
D An arthrodesis would give a much worse range of movement.
E A partial shoulder replacement is also an option.

→ Case studies – shoulder dislocation

3. **A young woman notices that her shoulder comes out of joint sometimes when she is asleep. She is able to put it back by jiggling her shoulder carefully.**

(a) What type of dislocation is this most likely to be?

A Habitual
B Traumatic anterior
C Traumatic posterior
D Atraumatic subluxation.

(b) What is the best treatment?

A Physiotherapy and re-education
B Physiotherapy first but if that fails then surgical repair of the Bankart lesion
C Physiotherapy first but if that fails then reefing of the capsule.

4. **A child develops a habit (party trick) of subluxing her shoulder backwards.**

(a) What type of dislocation is this most likely to be?

A Habitual
B Traumatic anterior
C Traumatic posterior
D Atraumatic subluxation.

(b) What is the best treatment?

A Physiotherapy and re-education
B Physiotherapy first but if that fails then surgical repair of the Bankart lesion
C Physiotherapy first but if that fails then reefing of the capsule.

5. **A rugby player puts his shoulder out falling in a scrum.**

(a) What type of dislocation is this most likely to be?

A Habitual
B Traumatic anterior
C Traumatic posterior
D Atraumatic subluxation.

(b) What is the best treatment?

A Physiotherapy and re-education
B Physiotherapy first but if that fails then surgical repair of the Bankart lesion
C Physiotherapy first but if that fails then reefing of the capsule.

→ Rheumatoid arthritis

6. **Which of the following deformities are seen in a patient with chronic and severe rheumatoid arthritis?**

A Swan neck deformity
B Boutonnière deformity

C Heberden's nodes
D Extensor tendon rupture
E Trigger finger
F Dupuytren's contracture
G Radial deviation of the metacarpophalangeal (MCP) joints
H Subluxation and dislocation of the MCP joints
I Ulnar deviation of the wrist
J Prominent ulnar head
K Extensor tenosynovitis.

7. **Which of the following treatments give reliable results in rheumatoid arthritis of the hand?**

A Synovectomy
B Excision of the distal ulna
C Prosthetic replacement of the wrist
D Prosthetic replacement of the MCP and interphalangeal joints
E Arthrodesis of the wrist
F Tendon repair
G Tendon transfer

Extended matching questions

→ 1. Shoulder injury

1 A patient presents with gradual onset of pain in the shoulder. This is especially severe when she tries to lift her arm from her side. However, if the arm is lifted by the examiner, the pain is much less severe, and once the arm is right up, it is no longer painful.

2 An elderly patient presents with a painless but weak shoulder. It has got worse over the years. He can only abduct it with a trick movement hunching his shoulder. Otherwise there seems to be very little power of abduction.

3 A patient develops severe and sudden onset of pain in the shoulder after a minor trauma. All movements are restricted. She cannot sleep for the pain.

4 A young man injures his shoulder playing rugby. It feels as if it came out of place but went back in again. It was swollen and painful for some weeks but is now better. However, when the examiner lifts the arm up and back he becomes very apprehensive and asks them to stop.

5 A patient who sustained a severe intra-articular fracture of the right shoulder as a young man now presents with increasing pain stiffness and weakness of the shoulder.

6 A middle-aged woman gets sudden onset of pain in her shoulder after no trauma. She is tender anterolaterally and the pain is so severe that she cannot sleep. She is able to rotate the shoulder externally without much pain, but other movements are painful, especially active ones. X-ray shows calcification floating between the acromion and the humeral head.

7 An elderly woman running for church trips and lands on her shoulder. The shoulder is swollen and painful with a graze over the deltoid. All movements are restricted.

8 A builder trips while carrying a girder and wrenches his shoulder. He presents with severe pain in the shoulder which limits movement and power.

9 A patient with rheumatoid arthritis complains of increasing pain, stiffness and weakness in the shoulder.

(a) Choose and match each of the above scenarios with the likely diagnosis:

A Chronic rotator cuff tear
B Acute massive rotator cuff tear
C Dislocating shoulder
D Rotator cuff impingement
E Frozen shoulder

F Arthritis of the glenohumeral joint
G Fracture head of humerus
H Calcifying tendinitis
I Osteoarthritis

(b) For each scenario, choose the most appropriate treatment:

A Steroid injection
B Physiotherapy
C Shoulder replacement
D Subacromial decompression
E Advice and commiseration; no active treatment
F Analgesia and gentle physiotherapy
G Collar and cuff.
H Rotator cuff repair

2. Elbow injury

1 A patient attends with pain over the lateral side of the elbow following a weekend redecorating the house.

2 A patient with rheumatoid arthritis attends with pain in the elbow mainly on pronation and supination.

3 A patient with rheumatoid arthritis attends with pain and weakness in the elbow and significant bone destruction.

4 A young patient who gives no history of elbow problems now presents with sudden and repeated locking of the elbow joint.

5 A patient who broke their elbow many years ago now presents with pain and numbness down the medial side of the forearm into the little finger.

6 A patient who broke their elbow many years ago now presents with pain, weakness and stiffness in the elbow. He does heavy manual labour.

7 A patient presents with a red hot lump over the back of the elbow.

8 A patient has a chronic hot swollen and painful elbow and a low-grade fever.

(a) Choose and match each of the above scenarios with the likely diagnosis:

A Tennis elbow
B Arthritis of the radiohumeral joint
C Arthritis of the elbow
D Olecranon bursitis
E Ulnar nerve entrapment
F Tuberculosis
G Osteochondritis dissecans

(b) For each scenario, choose the test or investigation that is likely to be most useful for diagnosis:

A Forced palmar flexion and pronation
B Injection of local anaesthetic
C X-ray
D Aspiration and culture

E Electrical conduction studies
F Arthroscopy
G Formal clinical examination

(c) **For each scenario, choose the treatment most likely to be of benefit in the first instance:**

A Synovectomy and excision of the radial head
B Total elbow replacement.
C RICE
D Time
E Arthrodesis
F Nerve decompression with possible transposition
G Intra-articular arthroscopy
H Appropriate antibiotics

3. Hand grip

A Pinch
B Power
C Hook
D Key
E Chuck

Choose and match the correct type of grip with each of the following activities:

1 Holding a pen

2 Holding a hammer

3 Picking up loose change

4 Carrying a suitcase

5 Holding a credit card as you put it into a cash machine

4. Hand injury

A Rupture of the extensor hood
B Malunion of an oblique fracture of the proximal phalanx
C Pilonidal sinus
D Flexor tendon sheath infection
E Disjunction of the palmar arch on the ulnar side
F Nerve damage

Choose and match the correct diagnosis with each of the following scenarios:

1 A patient complains that when they make a fist one finger crosses and tangles with the rest.

2 An examiner notices that as a pen is stroked across the palm of this patient's hand, it runs smoothly, whereas on the other hand it sticks.

3 The patient clenches their fist while the radial artery is occluded with pressure. When they open their hand it does not 'pink up'.

4 The patient, who is a hairdresser, has a chronic sinus in the interdigital cleft.

5 The patient got a thorn in their finger when gardening. Now the finger is red and swollen. Even passive flexion is painful, and pressing on the palmar side of the finger is very sore.

6 A patient with rheumatoid arthritis has a peculiar shaped finger with flexion of the proximal interphalangeal joint and hyperextension of the distal interphalangeal joint.

➜ 5. Other conditions in the hand

A de Quervain's tenosynovitis
B Nerve compression in Guyon's canal
C Ganglion
D Dupuytren's contracture
E Keinbock's disease
F Trigger finger
G Carpal tunnel syndrome

Choose and match the correct condition with each of the following descriptions:

1 An autosomal dominant common in Anglo-Saxons but also associated with the use of vibrating tools and alcoholic cirrhosis.

2 A hand which looks completely normal until the patient makes a fist.

3 Inflammation of the tendon sheaths of abductor pollicis, and extensor pollicis.

4 Painful wakening at night; having to hold the hand down out of bed; clumsiness in the fingers.

5 Wasting of the hypothenar eminence.

6 Spontaneous avascular necrosis of the lunate bone diagnosed on MRI.

7 A lump on the palmar side of the wrist which is attached to the joint capsule below but not to the skin.

Answers: Multiple choice questions

➜ Rotator cuff

1. A, C, D, F
There are four muscles which insert into the rotator cuff and control it: supraspinatus, infraspinatus, subscapularis and teres minor.

➜ Shoulder replacement

2. A, E
Shoulder replacement gives reliable pain relief but often does not increase shoulder range of movement. Indeed, the pain relief provided by a glenohumeral arthrodesis often results in a better range of movement than a replacement, as the full range of movement available in the scapulothoracic joint can now be used. The absence of the rotator cuff makes shoulder replacement much less reliable unless the cuff can be repaired at the same time (which is unlikely). If the glenoid is well preserved, a partial (hemi) joint replacement will also give good results.

➜ Case studies – shoulder dislocation

3. (a) D; (b) A
There is no trauma involved and this is likely to be an atraumatic subluxation (just a partial dislocation), as otherwise she would not find it so easy to get back into position. Physiotherapy and re-education appear to give a reasonable chance of success.

4. (a) A; (b) A

This is a habitual dislocation. There is no history of dislocation. Once again, physiotherapy and re-education should be sufficient as the child will grow out of it if they stop doing it.

5. (a) B; (b) B, C

The most common form of traumatic dislocation is the anterior dislocation. If the dislocation does not settle and recurs, then surgery to repair the Bankart lesion and reefing of the capsule will provide good results in over 90 per cent of cases.

→ Rheumatoid arthritis

6. A, B, D, E, H, J, K

There are a large number of deformities associated with rheumatoid arthritis. However, Heberden's nodes are associated with osteoarthritis. Dupuytren's contracture is a separate condition altogether. The deviation of the MCP joints is ulnar, not radial, whereas in the wrist the deviation is radial.

7. A, B, D, E, G

Synovectomy gives good pain relief and improves function. Excision of the distal ulna also helps but may produce some wrist instability. Prosthetic replacement of the wrist is not currently proving as valuable in terms of pain relief and function as arthrodesis. However, prosthetic replacement of the MCP and interphalangeal joints is proving valuable. Tendon repairs tend not to work well but tendon transfer using healthy tendons gives better results.

Answers: Extended matching questions

→ 1. Shoulder injury

(a) Diagnoses – 1D, 2A, 3E, 4C, 5I, 6H, 7G, 8B, 9F

(b) Treatments – 1D, 2E, 3F, 4B, 5C, 6A, 7G, 8H, 9C

Disability in the shoulder can consist of stiffness, pain and/or weakness or a mixture of the three. It is the pattern of these three, the age and gender of the patient, and the cause of the onset of symptoms (traumatic or gradual) which give a clue to the diagnosis in most of the conditions.

The patient (Scenario 4) who feels his shouler has 'come out' and gone back in and who is apprehensive when it is abducted, extended and externally rotated shows the classic pattern of a shoulder that has dislocated anteriorly. In the first instance, the treatment is physiotherapy to build the strength of the muscles around the shoulder. Repeated dislocations will need a surgical repair of the labrum and of the capsule.

The woman who has fallen onto her shoulder (Scenario 7) will have suffered a fracture through osteoporotic bone. If the fracture is extra-articular then it can be managed in a collar and cuff. If, however, it is intra-articular or grossly displaced (so that the blood supply to the humeral head is damaged), a hemiarthroplasty may be the only option. If the intra-articular fracture is left (as used to happen), then traumatic osteoarthritis is inevitable in the years to come. This will present with gradual onset of pain, stiffness and weakness, and the best treatment is probably a shoulder replacement. Arthritis in the shoulder also develops in patients with rheumatoid arthritis, and they too respond well to a shoulder replacement.

The patient presenting with a painless but weak shoulder (Scenario 2) where the problem has developed over the years has almost certainly got a massive tear of the rotator cuff. The cuff has a poor blood supply and so any attempt at repair is doomed to failure. It may therefore be best to simply explain the diagnosis and commiserate with them. If, however, the tear is post-traumatic and in a younger patient, then a rotator cuff repair should be attempted, as there is some blood supply in the younger patient and the disability is not acceptable to the patient.

The presentation of severe pain and stiffness after minor trauma (Scenario 3) is characteristic of a frozen shoulder. This is very slow to resolve and it is doubtful whether anything helps reduce the months of pain and stiffness, but most clinicians would offer analgesia and gentle physiotherapy.

Severe pain and stiffness developing rapidly without any trauma at all (Scenario 3) could be a frozen shoulder but could also be calcifying tendinitis of the supraspinatus tendon. Frozen shoulder produces global pain and loss of movement, including pain on external rotation. Calcific tendinitis usually does not affect external rotation. On X-ray a calcific cloud will be visible in the supraspinatus tendon between the acromion and the humeral head.

Painful arc syndrome is the finding that the patient cannot actively abduct their arm from their side beyond a certain point (the start of the painful arc) because it becomes very painful (Scenario 1). If, however, examiner lifts the arm for the patient through this painful arc, they are quite suddenly able to abduct the final bit without much pain. This is characteristic of rotator cuff impingement under the acromion. This condition can be diagnosed with an injection of local anaesthetic into the impinging area, and some attempt treatment with a steroid injection. However, trimming of the downward-pointing tip of the acromion (subacromial decompression) should relieve the impingement and therefore the pain.

→ 2. Elbow injury

(a) 1A, 2B, 3C, 4G, 5E, 6C, 7D, 8F

Tennis elbow does not only develop after playing tennis but can start after any heavy activity. In rheumatoid arthritis, the elbow is frequently attacked first in the radiohumeral joint. However, it then goes on to affect the rest of the elbow. Sudden onset of locking in the elbow without a history of trauma is the typical presentation of osteochondritis dissecans (a fragment of the articular surface breaking off spontaneously). Fractures into the elbow will go on to aggressive traumatic arthritis if it is not possible to get anatomical reduction of the joint surfaces. A red and hot lump over the extensor surface of the elbow is likely to be olecranon bursitis, whereas a hot and painful elbow joint with a low-grade fever is more likely to be infection, and in the elbow tuberculosis must be in the differential diagnosis.

(b) 1A, 2B, 3C, 4C, 5E, 6C, 7G, 8D

Forced palmarflexion with pronation puts specific load onto the common extensor origin and is diagnostic of tennis elbow. Radiohumeral pain can be diagnosed by injecting local anaesthetic into this joint and demonstrating pain relief. Plain X-ray is the most useful diagnostic test in rheumatoid and osteoarthritis as well as osteochondritis dissecans. Arthritis in the elbow can lead to irritation and compression of the ulnar nerve where it passes behind the elbow joint. Electrical conduction studies should confirm the diagnosis. Olecranon bursitis can be diagnosed by good clinical examination. Tuberculosis has a predilection for the elbow joint. It produces an indolent septic arthritis.

(c) 1C, 2A, 3B, 4G, 5F, 6E, 7D, 8H

The treatment for tennis elbow and olecranon bursitis is RICE (rest, ice, compression, and elevation). Local steroid injection may also be used. If a patient with rheumatoid arthritis has isolated radiohumeral arthritis, as demonstrated by pain on pronation and supination relieved by injection of local anaesthetic, then synovectomy and excision of the radial head should give good pain relief without creating too much instability in the elbow joint. However, if the whole elbow joint is involved, a total elbow replacement is indicated. If the patient performs heavy labour, an arthrodesis will last better than an elbow replacement. Osteochondritis dissecans can be managed by arthroscopic removal of the loose fragment in the first instance. Patients with signs of ulnar nerve entrapment will need release and transposition of the ulnar nerve. Tuberculosis of the elbow joint will need the appropriate antibiotics (check the organisms sensitivity) to be given for a considerable time to ensure that the infection is eradicated. Even then, a fibrous ankylosis of the joint may be the end-point.

3. Hand grip

1E, 2B, 3A, 4C, 5D

4. Hand injury

1B, 2F, 3E, 4C, 5D, 6A

5. Other conditions in the hand

1D, 2F, 3A, 4G, 5B, 6E, 7C

35 The hip and knee

Multiple choice questions

➜ Anatomy and physiology of the hip

1. Which of the following are involved in blood supply to the adult femoral head?

A Artery of the ligamentum teres
B Retinacular branches of the medial circumflex femoral artery
C Capsular branches of superior gluteal artery.

2. Which of the following structures are involved in static stability of the hip joint?

A Capsule
B Labrum
C Gemelli
D Pectineus
E Iliopsoas
F Ligamentum teres
G Anterior inferior iliac spine
H Cup and socket shape of hip joint
I Abductor muscles
J Hamstrings
K Gluteals.

3. Which of the following structures are involved in supporting the pelvis when standing on one leg?

A Capsule
B Labrum
C Gemelli
D Pectineus
E Iliopsoas
F Ligamentum teres
G Anterior inferior iliac spine
H Cup and socket shape of hip joint
I Abductor muscles
J Hamstrings
K Gluteals.

➜ Radiological features in osteoarthritis

4. Which of the following are radiological features of osteoarthritis of the hip?

A Subchondral sclerosis
B Multiple microfractures
C Subchondral cysts
D Coarsening of the trabecular pattern
E Narrowing of the joint space
F Osteophyte formation
G Periarticular osteoporosis.

➜ Total hip replacement

5. If you had to explain to a patient the complications of total hip replacement, which of the following would you mention?

A Infection
B Deep vein thrombosis
C Renal failure
D Urinary tract infection
E Nerve damage
F Synergistic gangrene
G Chest infection
H Stroke
I Dislocation
J Fracture
K Severe bleeding requiring transfusion
L Death from any cause less than 1 per cent
M Leg length inequality more than 10 cm
N Compartment syndrome.

➜ Knee stability

6. Which of the following are dynamic stabilisers of the knee?

A Biceps femoris
B Anterior cruciate ligament
C Posterior cruciate ligament

D Sartorius
E Gracilis
F Semitendinosus
G Medial meniscus
H Lateral meniscus
I Quadriceps femoris
J Adductor longus.

Arthroscopy of the knee

7. Which of the following are indications for arthroscopy of the knee?

A Diagnose and treat torn meniscus
B Check for avascular necrosis
C Repair ruptured patella tendon
D Remove loose bodies
E Repair cruciate ligament rupture
F Decompress Osgood–Schlatter disease
G Relieve a joint effusion.

Extended matching questions

1. Aetiology of hip problems

A Idiopathic osteoarthritis
B Avascular necrosis
C Secondary osteoarthritis

Choose and match the correct condition with each of the following factors:

1 Alcohol or treatment with high-dose steroids

2 Genetic predisposition or femoro-acetabular impingement

3 Slipped upper femoral epiphysis

4 Perthes' disease

2. Management of hip conditions

A Surface hip replacement
B Hemiarthroplasty
C Conventional stemmed hip replacement
D Core graft to hip
E Arthrodesis
F Osteotomy

Choose and match the correct treatment with each of the following scenarios:

1 A patient presents with reduction of movement of the hip. X-ray merely shows a slight increase in sclerosis but no loss of joint space. Magnetic resonance imaging (MRI) shows several areas of dead bone.

2 A young patient who is a manual labourer has a painful and stiff hip secondary to an acetabular fracture.

3 An adolescent with Perthes' disease has a small area of collapse immediately in the main load-bearing area of the femoral head.

4 A patient in her early 50s has severe osteoarthritis of the hip, limiting walking and preventing sleep.

5 A patient of 80 has severe osteoarthritis of the hip, limiting walking and preventing sleep.

6 A 75-year-old patient has a severely displaced subcapital fractured neck of femur.

→ 3. Hip replacement

A Aseptic loosening
B Dislocation
C Periprosthetic fracture
D Infected implant

Choose and match the correct diagnosis with each of the following scenarios:

1 On getting out of bed, a patient who had a hip replacement 4 days previously felt a severe pain in his new hip.

2 A patient with a total hip replacement performed some 6 months before complains that the pain in the hip never really settled. X-ray shows a lucent line appearing around the cement of the femoral component.

3 A patient who had a hip replacement 15 years ago now complains of increasing pain in the hip, which is also starting to clunk.

4 A patients who had a hip replacement some years before stumbled on some steps and now has severe pain in what was a painless hip.

→ 4. Management of knee conditions

A Total knee replacement
B High tibial osteotomy
C Unicompartmental knee replacement
D Arthrodesis of the knee

Choose and match the correct treatment with each of the following scenarios:

1 A 20-year-old patient has medial compartment osteoarthritis after an intra-articular fracture. He has severe pain, a good range of movement and a significant varus deformity.

2 A 65-year-old patient has idiopathic unicompartmental osteoarthritis.

3 A 65-year-old patient has tricompartmental idiopathic arthritis of the knee.

4 A 70-year-old has an infected knee replacement which has been revised and has become infected again.

Answers: Multiple choice questions

→ Anatomy and physiology of the hip

1. B

The blood supply to the femoral head is parlous. In the adult, very little comes through the ligamentum teres, the bulk comes in the retinacular branches of the medial circumflex artery. This is an important fact because these arteries are closely attached to the periosteum within the joint capsule and so are disrupted in an intra-articular fractured neck of femur.

2. A, B, F, H

The static supports of the hip cannot include muscles (these are dynamic). The anatomical shape of the hip (ball and socket is an important stabiliser, as is the cartilaginous labrum (lip) around the margin of the acetabulum. A strong fibrous capsule encloses the whole hip joint. The ligamentum teres also provides some stability.

3. H, I

The abductor muscles provide the leverage power which supports the pelvis against the fulcrum of the cup and socket of the hip joint. Both must be present and working normally for a patient to be able to stand on one leg easily.

Radiological features in osteoarthritis

4. A, C, E, F

There are four characteristic features of idiopathic osteoarthritis of the hip: subchondral sclerosis and cysts, narrowing of the joint space and osteophyte formation. Periarticular osteoporosis is usually seen in inflammatory arthritis and coarsening of the trabeculae is found in Paget's disease. Microfractures cannot be seen on X-ray.

Total hip replacement

5. A, B, E, I, J, K, L

It is normal to mention all severe complications and any other complications with more common than 1 per cent incidence when obtaining consent from a patient. Infection occurs in 1–2 per cent of cases in good units. Deep vein thrombosis (with significant clinical problems) probably occurs in around 5 per cent. Renal failure is not associated with hip replacement, nor are urinary tract infection, synergistic gangrene, chest infection, compartment syndrome or stroke, although these are all possible but rare complications of any major surgery. Damage to nerves around the hip, especially the sciatic nerve, occurs in 1–5 per cent of cases and so should be mentioned, as should the possibility of significant blood loss requiring transfusion (5–10 per cent). Dislocation occurs in around 5 per cent, especially in the early stages, and fracture is a rare but serious complication of inserting the implant (<1 per cent). Death is a possibility in any major surgery but the incidence is well below 1 per cent. Leg-length inequality is a common problem but is rarely more than 2 cm; 10 cm would be most unlikely.

Knee stability

6. A, D, E, F, I

The dynamic stabilisers of a joint are the muscles which act across that joint. In this case, the biceps stabilise the posterolateral side, while the semimembranosus, semitendinosis, gracilis and sartorius act on the posteromedial side. Quadriceps femoris stabilises from the front.

Arthroscopy of the knee

7. A, D, E

Most intra-articular conditions in the knee can now be managed by an expert arthroscopist. So, a torn meniscus can be diagnosed, trimmed or repaired, while loose bodies can be removed from the knee. Even cruciate ligament repairs can be performed through the arthroscope. There is little point in draining a joint effusion through the scope, as this can be done more simply by needle aspiration. Extra-articular problems such as a ruptured patella tendon are best treated open while Osgood–Schlatter disease (swelling and inflammation of the tibial tubercle in adolescents) does not need any kind of surgery.

Answers: Extended matching questions

1. Aetiology of hip problems

1B, 2A, 3C, 4C

Both alcohol and treatment with steroids are associated with an increased incidence of avascular necrosis. Both slipped upper femoral epiphysis (SUFE) and Perthes' disease in childhood lead to an increased risk of secondary osteoarthritis later in life probably because of damage to the congruity of the joint surfaces. Idiopathic osteoarthritis of the hip is thought to have a significant genetic component but it has also been suggested that femoro-acetabular impingement is a predisposing factor.

2. Management of hip conditions

1D

The presentation is characteristic of avascular necrosis in the early stages. The treatment of choice is forage, drilling out a core of bone and replacing it with a vascularised graft.

2E

Young patients with severe arthritis of the hip who are involved in heavy manual labour should not have a total hip replacement as it will fail rapidly. The best option is an arthrodesis (fusion) of the hip. This can always be unpicked and replaced with total hip replacement later in life.

3F

A patient with a local area of collapse from Perthes' disease needs that damaged area moving out of the load-bearing area and replacing with healthy cartilage. The method of doing this is a rotation osteotomy.

4A

A young patient with hip arthritis and low demand (not a heavy manual labourer) could be offered a surface replacement as this removes the minimum of bone and therefore may give more options for revision in the future.

5C

An older patient might be better offered a conventional standard total hip, which is relatively easy to perform and with reliable results which will last the lifetime of the patient.

6B

An elderly patient with a grossly displaced subcapital fracture will certainly have a dead femoral head and so will require a hemiarthroplasty.

3. Hip replacement

1B

Dislocation is most common in patients when they first start to mobilise and the capsule has not yet re-formed around the hip. If the hip is put straight back, it may not cause further trouble.

2D

Pain persisting for 6 months after a hip replacement may be a low-grade infection and so needs investigating, especially if there are radiological signs of premature loosening.

3A

If the hip is starting to give pain and even clunk after 15 years then it has come to the end of its natural life span. This is aseptic loosening.

4C

If patients trip or fall with a total hip replacement, extreme loads can be placed on the bone around the joint replacement (stress raisers) and the bone can fracture.

4. Management of knee conditions

1B, 2C, 3A, 4D

In the very young, high-activity patient, a knee replacement should be avoided as it is unlikely to withstand the loads put on it for very long. If there is a good range of movement, then a high tibial osteotomy will retain that range of movement while unloading the arthritic side of the joint. It can do this by changing the alignment of the knee so that the bulk of the load goes through the unaffected side. If, however, the knee was painful and the range of movement was minimal then an arthrodesis would be a better option. Arthrodesis is also the only option, apart from amputation, if a total knee replacement has failed and a revision cannot be performed (such as in uncontrollable infection).

A patient who has more than 20 years' life expectancy and in whom there is only arthritis in one compartment (either the medial or the lateral) should be considered for a unicompartmental knee replacement, although these operations are tricky to perform compared with a conventional total knee replacement. For the elderly patient with conventional tricompartmental osteoarthritis, a standard total knee replacement is the operation of choice.

36 The foot and ankle

Multiple choice questions

➜ Foot – general

1. Which of the following statements are true?

A The talus is narrower posteriorly so that as the foot comes into dorsiflexion the talus locks in the mortice between the medial malleolus on the tibia and the lateral malleolus on the fibula. The foot then rotates externally.

B The subtalar joint is responsible for inversion and eversion of the hindfoot.

C The third metatarsal head is recessed to act as a 'keystone' in the transverse arch.

D The windlass test is performed to check the integrity of the flexor muscles in the sole of the foot.

E The skin on the dorsum of the foot is mainly supplied by the superficial peroneal nerve.

➜ Midfoot and hindfoot

2. Which of the following statements are true?

A Surgery to deal with deformity in the knee should only be undertaken once problems of pain, stiffness and deformity in the foot have been resolved.

B Surgery in the foot should be undertaken early and aggressively, not once all non-operative possibilities have been exhausted.

C Ankle replacement is a good option for arthritis of the tibiotalar joint in the low-demand patient, providing there is not severe deformity.

D Arthrodesis is the treatment of choice for an ankle joint which has severe arthritis and which is painful in a high-demand patient.

E Osteophyte removal is a good alternative in the painful ankle where it can be shown that impingement is causing pain and there is no significant osteoarthritis.

F When only one joint of the hindfoot complex is involved, it is nevertheless best to perform a triple fusion because all the joints are interrelated.

G Rupture of tibialis posterior leads to a valgus flatfoot, which is painful.

H Pes cavus is a common presentation of a neurological condition such as Charcot–Marie–Tooth or of diastomatomyelia.

I Osteomyelitis in the diabetic foot does not usually spread and so can be treated with minimal local interference.

J Charcot joints tend to be painful, with X-ray changes minimal compared with the pain experienced by the patient.

Extended matching questions

➜ 1. Diagnosis in foot problems

1 A child is born with one foot plantarflexed, inverted and supinated. The position can almost be corrected but reverts to its original position as soon as the foot is released

2 A teenager presents with pain in the foot. On examination there is a flatfoot which does not form an arch when he stands up on tiptoe.

3 A child aged 10 is brought along by her mother because her dancing teacher says that she is flatfooted. She is not in pain and when she stands on tiptoe, an arch forms.

4 A child with cerebral palsy is toe-walking. She is referred to you for help in getting her to walk on the soles of her feet (plantigrade).

5 A middle-aged woman whose work involves being smartly dressed presents with a painful red lump over the medial side of the big toe metatarsophalangeal joint. She is very distressed by the unsightliness of this bump and the fact that she can no longer wear high-heeled shoes comfortably for more than a few minutes.

6 A middle-aged runner complains of increasing pain in his right big toe which he broke many years ago. The first metatarsophalangeal joint is red dorsally and has a very limited range of painful movement. The patient wants to be able to continue running.

7 A teenager with a family history of a progressive neurological disorder affecting the lower limbs presents with problems in his feet. The arches are very high and the toes bent up so that they rub on his shoes. However, the toes can still be straightened out.

8 A teenager presents with pain at the base of the second toe. X-rays show a highly abnormal head of the second metatarsal with flattening of its head.

9 A young woman who likes wearing tight, fashionable shoes complains of increasing pain and numbness in her foot localised around the base of the third and fourth toes, and especially in the cleft.

(a) Choose and match each of these scenarios with the likely diagnosis:

A Hallux valgus
B Claw toes
C Hammer toes
D Curly toes
E Mallet toes
F Morton's neuroma
G Talipes equinovarus
H Physiological flatfoot
I Hallux rigidus
J Tarsal coalition
K Tight tendo Achilles
L Freiberg's disease

(b) For each scenario, choose the initial management:

A A careful review by physiotherapy to assess the whole lower limb, then release of tight structures, if appropriate
B Soft-tissue surgery to release tight structures and transfer tendons
C Removal of the prominent bone (osteophyte) and fusion of the joint
D Reassurance that this is not abnormal and no treatment is needed or appropriate
E An osteotomy to narrow the forefoot, straighten the toe and remove the prominent lump
F Reassurance that this will usually improve with time
G Serial splints
H Non-operative measures, then surgery if the problem does not settle.

Answers: Multiple choice questions

➜ Foot – general

1. A, B, E

The talus is narrower posteriorly, allowing increased rotatory mobility to the plantarflexed foot. In dorsiflexion, the talus jams tightly in the mortice, externally rotating the fibula and the foot and locking it into position.

Dorsiflexion and plantarflexion occur almost exclusively in the ankle (tibiotalar) joint, while inversion and eversion occur in the subtalar joint. The midfoot has a longitudinal and a transverse arch.

The second (not the third) metatarsal head is recessed to act as a keystone to this transverse arch.

The 'windlass' test consists of asking the patient to stand on tiptoe. This tightens the plantar fascia (not the muscles), and if this and the arch of the foot are intact, the longitudinal arch becomes more pronounced.

The skin on dorsum of the foot is supplied by the superficial peroneal nerve, with the sural nerve supplying the little toe and its base, and the saphenous nerve supplying the medial side of the foot.

➜ Midfoot and hindfoot

2. C, D, E, G, H

Deformities in the knee produce highly abnormal forces in the foot, which will compromise any attempts to put things right in the foot. It is therefore important to sort out any problems in the knee before embarking on corrections in the foot.

The foot does not respond well to surgery and even when it does, it takes a long time to recover. Therefore, all non-operative options should be explored before surgery is considered.

Ankle replacement is now giving good long-term reproducible results in patients who do not put high load on their ankles and in whom there is not severe deformity. However, arthrodesis remains the operation of choice for the patient with significant deformity or who is going to make significant demands on the limb (builders etc.)

In ankles where a prominent osteophyte can be seen, which is impinging (local anaesthetic injection relieves the pain), simple osteophyte removal may produce a significant improvement in pain and range of movement. This will not work if there is significant arthritis.

It used to be thought that fusion of only one joint in the hindfoot merely produced a rapid deterioration in the other joints. This is now known not to be the case, so single fusion of affected joints is a viable option for a stiff and painful hindfoot.

Rupture of the tibialis posterior tendor is most common in middle-aged overweight women and leads to a painful and rapidly progressive flatfoot with a valgus hindfoot. Modified footwear can only offer limited symptomatic support, so repair of the tendon or a tendon transfer to reconstitute the arch should be considered.

The development of pes cavus in a teenager is an ominous sign and is usually the presentation of a progressive neurological disorder such as Charcot–Marie–Tooth. Alternatively a spina bifida occulta may leave a bar of bone or scar tissue across the spinal canal which traps the cauda equina as the teenager grows. This is called a diastomatomyelia. Release of the bar does not always lead to full recovery.

Osteomyelitis in the diabetic foot may be indolent in its presentation but there is nothing indolent in its spread, which may be much faster and more extensive than superficial clinical examination would suggest. Surgical treatment needs to be aggressive to find and remove all necrotic and infected tissue, otherwise treatment will merely consist of a sequence of ever-higher amputations.

The Charcot joint is now most commonly seen in diabetics. The pain is minimal but the foot is swollen and the X-ray shows joint destruction out of all proportion to what the minimal pain would suggest. The differential diagnosis is infection and only biopsy will be able to reliably differentiate the two. Charcot foot needs supportive treatment while fusion takes place.

Answers: Extended matching questions

→ 1. Diagnosis in foot problems

(a) Diagnoses – 1G, 2J, 3H, 4K, 5A, 6I, 7B, 8L, 9F

(b) Treatments – 1G, 2H, 3D, 4A, 5E, 6C, 7B, 8F, 9H

Scenario 1

One of the commoner deformities found at birth is clubfoot, or talipes equinovarus. Here the foot is plantarflexed, inverted, adducted and supinated. If the deformity is rigid, there may be a severe underlying problem and surgery will be the only option. If, however, the foot is correctable then the deformity may, in part, be positional in the uterus, and serial splinting may give a good result without the need to resort to surgery.

Scenario 2

A flat foot which does not form an arch when the patient stands on tiptoes (windlass test) indicates that there is a severe abnormality such as a tarsal coalition in the foot. In the first instance, treatment is non-operative as some of these will settle. However, if it does not settle, a formal fusion may be needed to prevent repeated stress fractures and arthritis in the non-union of the tarsal coalition.

Scenario 3

Many children are told that they are flatfooted simply because they have a 'physiological' flatfoot. This can be differentiated from a pathological flatfoot because it is painless, and because when he stands on tiptoe the arch re-forms (windlass test). Orthotics are of no value here, especially as there is nothing wrong with the child, so reassurance that this is a normal variant is all that is appropriate.

Scenario 4

Children with cerebral palsy frequently toe-walk, partly because they often have a tight tendo Achilles, but also because the loads transmitted through to the tibia help them to stand and walk. They may have fixed-flexion deformities of both knee and hip, and so need considerable strength to remain standing. Their problems may be compounded by weak or uncoordinated knee and hip extensors, so standing on tiptoe helps them prevent the knee from collapsing under them. If the tendo Achilles is lengthened without thinking about this, the child may be able to stand plantigrade but the knee will then collapse. It is therefore important that there is a careful physiotherapy assessment of the child's gait before any surgery is undertaken 'non nocere'.

Scenario 5

Bunions result from pressure between a wide forefoot and a narrow shoe. Rubbing on the medial side of the first metatarsal head creates red thickened skin, a bursa and an osteophyte over the underlying bone. The big toe is forced laterally (hallux valgus) and may cause overlap of the second and third toes. In the very early stages, then, careful choice of footwear may delay progress, but once the deformity has developed, it is progressive and surgery is the only option. The number of operations described suggest that none are completely successful. But the principle behind most is the same. An osteotomy of the first metatarsal is performed to narrow the forefoot and correct the metatarsus primus varus. At the same time the big toe is straightened on the metatarsal head to remove the hallux valgus. Finally the bunion itself is removed.

Scenario 6

Arthritis in the first metatarsophalangeal joint is common, especially after previous trauma. The joint becomes stiff and painful especially at toe-off. Modified footwear can help, but in a patient who wishes to continue playing sport, a fusion of the joint should be considered.

Scenario 7

Teenagers developing pes cavus must be suspected of developing a neurological disorder such as Charcot–Marie–Tooth or of having some kind of entrapment of the spinal roots (diastomatomyelia). If the deformity is passively correctable, there is a possibility that soft-tissue releases and tendon transfer will correct or slow the progression of the disorder. However, if the correction cannot be corrected passively, only bone surgery (such as an arthrodesis) is likely to offer any benefit.

Scenario 8

Freiberg's disease is a spontaneous osteonecrosis of the second metatarsal head, which develops in young people and may be a surprising finding on X-ray. It usually settles spontaneously, so does not require any active treatment, but if it fails to do so then debridement of the joint may be helpful.

Scenario 9

Transverse pressure on the forefoot, especially that caused by tight shoes, may trap an interdigital nerve between the metatarsal heads. This is especially common between the 3rd and 4th metatarsal heads and is known as Morton's neuroma. If a change of footwear does not result in an improvement, surgery to excise the swollen and traumatised nerve can improve the symptoms but will obviously leave a numb interdigital cleft.

37 Infection and tumours

Multiple choice questions

➜ Rheumatoid arthritis

1. Which of the following statements regarding rheumatoid arthritis are true?

A It is much commoner in women than in men.
B A negative rheumatoid factor excludes this diagnosis.
C The disease appears to be based on a T-cell autoimmune response.
D The disease usually attacks large joints, such as the hip.
E Joints are destroyed by an inflammatory pannus.

2. Which of the following are extra-articular manifestations of rheumatoid arthritis?

A Retinal detachment
B Subcutaneous nodules
C Myocardial infarction secondary to atherosclerosis
D Renal failure secondary to nephritis
E Sarcoidosis
F Heberden's nodes
G Early malignancies in affected tissues
H Asthma.

3. Which of the following are characteristic features of rheumatoid arthritis of the hands?

A Ulnar deviation of the wrist
B Spontaneous ruptures of the flexor tendons
C Ulnar deviation and subluxation of the metacarpophalangeal joints
D W-deformity of the thumb
E Carpal tunnel syndrome
F Hyperflexion of the proximal interphalangeal joint with hyperextension of the distal interphalangeal joint
G Hyperextension of the proximal interphalangeal joint with hyperflexion of the distal interphalangeal joint
H Dupuytren's contracture.

➜ Gout and pseudogout

4. Which of the following statements regarding gout are true?

A Gout leads to pyrophosphate deposition.
B Gout and septic arthritis are similar and can coexist in the same joint.
C Gout is associated with renal calculi.
D The key to the treatment of gout is to lower the plasma urate levels as quickly as possible.
E Gout is the commonest cause of acute monoarthropathy in the elderly.
F The metatarsophalangeal joint is the first joint to be attacked in most cases of gout.
G Pyrophosphate crystals are positively birefringent under polarised light.

➜ Bone tumours

5. Which of the following statements about bone tumours are true?

A Patients with a past history of malignancy who present with backache have metastases until otherwise proven.
B The extent of metastases can best be demonstrated on a bone scan.
C All patients with suspected bone tumours should have plain X-rays.
D Pathological fractures through metastases should be fixed but patients should not be given radiotherapy as this will prevent healing.
E Biopsy should be performed at the same time as staging to minimise delay.

F The biopsy track should be kept well away from any possible future surgical approach
G Local en bloc excision of primary bone and soft-tissue tumours has no worse a survival rate than primary amputation.
H Metastases from the prostate are notoriously vascular and so should be embolised if at all possible before any surgical approach is attempted.
I In patients with pathological fracture through metastases, the normal rule that the medical condition should be optimised is ignored.

Extended matching questions

1. Treatment of rheumatoid arthritis

A Joint replacement
B Arthrodesis
C Tendon transfer
D Supportive splint
E Local bone excision
F Fusion
G Synovectomy

Choose and match the correct treatment with each of the following scenarios:

1 A patient with rheumatoid arthritis presents with an unstable wrist which compromises hand function. She does not wish to consider surgery. What could she be offered apart from systemic treatment for her disease?

2 A patient with rheumatoid arthritis presents with a painful prominent lump on the back of her wrist on the medial side. What could be offered surgically?

3 A patient with rheumatoid arthritis presents with painful tenosynovitis resistant to medical treatment.

4 A patient with rheumatoid arthritis presents with an unstable cervical spine which is starting to cause neurological compromise.

5 A patient with rheumatoid arthritis presents with a painful elbow on pronation and supination localised over the proximal radial head.

6 A patient with rheumatoid arthritis presents with a rupture of extensor pollicis longus.

7 A patient with rheumatoid arthritis presents with a painful and very stiff ankle.

8 A patient with rheumatoid arthritis presents with a mobile but painful elbow in all ranges of movement.

2. Diagnosis in arthritis

A Tuberculosis
B Juvenile rheumatoid arthritis
C Infected implant
D Osteomyelitis
E Ankylosing spondylitis
F Psoriatic arthropathy
G Yersinia arthritis
H Avascular necrosis
I Septic arthritis

Choose and match the correct condition with each of the following scenarios:

1 A middle-aged man presents with his wife who says that he is walking in a strange way with bent legs and a curved back (question mark position). He has had some years of backache, which is at its worst in the mornings.

2 A medical student returns from his elective in the tropics where he had the usual attack of mild diarrhoea but no malaria or other tropical illnesses. He has now developed a painful and swollen knee. He also has pain in the sole of his foot, which makes him limp.

3 A patient who has had scaly rashes on the extensor surfaces of his elbows develops backache. An X-ray of the spine shows massive osteophyte formation.

4 A young teenager, who is very small for her age, presents with pain and stiffness in her knees. The examiner notices that she can only open her mouth a little.

5 A patient who has positive anti-Sm antibodies presents with severe pain in the hip after a course of steroids for his systemic lupus erythematosus. X-rays are unremarkable.

6 A young adult drug addict presents with severe pain in the knee with some redness and swelling. His temperature is not raised. The knee is held in the 'position of comfort' and is very painful to move.

7 A patient who had a hip replacement 5 days ago suffers a minor fall. Forty-eight hours later the hip replacement starts to hurt and they feel generally unwell.

8 A patient from China presents with back pain which is waking him at night and night sweats. Magnetic resonance imaging (MRI) shows a fluid-filled lesion surrounding the L3 vertebra.

9 A motorcyclist who suffered a fracture of the tibia had an intramedullary locked nail inserted to hold the fracture. Shortly after the locking screws and the nail were removed, the patient noticed increasing pain and felt unwell.

→ 3. Bone tumours

A Osteochondroma
B Metastasis
C Giant cell tumour
D Prostate
E Multiple myeloma

Choose and match the correct diagnosis with each of the following scenarios:

1 An elderly patient is found to have fractured through a lytic lesion in the proximal femur following a minor trip. What is the likely cause of the lesion?

2 An elderly patient is found to have a malignant sclerotic lesion in the lumbar spine. What is its likely source?

3 A young adult is found to have a prominent hard lump on the back of her knee attached to the femur, which restricts flexion, but which is now not changing size since she has stopped growing. X-ray shows only a small spike of bone.

4 A patient is found to have many lytic lesions in her skeleton. Biopsy reveals lymphoid-like cells. Her gamma-globulins are raised.

5 A single lytic lesion in a patient's femur is biopsied. The cells are found to be multinucleate osteoclasts.

Answers: Multiple choice questions

Rheumatoid arthritis

1. A, C, E

Rheumatoid arthritis occurs in 3 per cent of women but only 1 per cent of men. Rheumatoid factor is only positive in around 80 per cent of cases, so a negative test does not exclude the diagnosis. The disease is based on a T-cell autoimmune response with release of interleukins, including IL-1 and IL-6, and tumour necrosis factor (TNF). The disease is usually symmetrical and focuses on the small joints of the hands and feet. An inflammatory pannus spreads across, destroying the articular cartilage and eroding the subchondral bone.

2. B, D

The eye problems in rheumatoid arthritis include scleritis and iritis but not retinal detachment. Subcutaneous nodules do occur but these are not Heberden's nodes, which are associated with osteoarthritis. In the heart, myocarditis is well described but rheumatoid arthritis appears to be, if anything, protective of atherosclerosis. Nephritis occurs in the kidneys and can lead to renal failure. Sarcoidosis is not associated with rheumatoid arthritis but amyloid is. There is no evidence that either asthma or early malignant change are more common in rheumatoid arthritis; compression and vascular neuritis are well described.

3. C, E, F, G

There is radial deviation at the wrist with ulnar deviation and subluxation at the metacarpophalangeal joints. It is the extensor tendons which tend to rupture spontaneously, not the flexor tendons. The deformity in the thumb is usually described as a Z-deformity because of its shape. Similarly, in the fingers there can be Boutonnière (hyperflexion of the proximal interphalangeal joint with hyperextension of the distal interphalangeal joint) or swan-neck deformity (hyperextension of the proximal interphalangeal joint with hyperflexion of the distal interphalangeal joint). Carpal tunnel syndrome does occur with hypertrophied synovium around the flexor tendons, but Dupuytren's is not associated with rheumatoid arthritis.

Gout and pseudogout

4. B, C, E, F, G

Gout leads to the deposition of urate crystals. Pseudogout produces pyrophosphate. The crystals can be distinguished microscopically by the fact that pyrophosphate crystals are birefringent, while urate crystals are not. The raised urate levels in the plasma in gout can lead to high levels in the urine and the formation of urate kidney stones. It might be thought that lowering the levels of plasma urate would be the first-line treatment of gout but paradoxically this may actually make the attack worse. The metatarsophalangeal joint is the first to be attacked in around 50 per cent of the presenting cases of gout, so it is by far the commonest joint to be affected. However, in the elderly the commonest cause of acute monoarthritis is pseudogout, which can attack any joint but especially favours large joints such as the hip or knee.

Bone tumours

5. A, B, C, G

Patients presenting with backache with a previous history of malignancy must be treated with a high degree of suspicion that this is metastatic spread. The least that is needed are plain X-rays (the initial investigation of choice in all cases) and routine blood tests. Bone scan is the best way of looking for other metastases, especially remote ones. Metastatic fractures need fixing as quickly as possible to remove pain and to improve mobility in the last precious time left of life. Radiotherapy, surprisingly, does not prevent healing and can be very useful in slowing tumour growth and reducing pain.

When investigating a tumour staging, imaging and blood tests must be completed before biopsy is undertaken so that the correct area is biopsied. The biopsy track must be within the surgical excision zone, and must be excised completely at the time of surgery, so that if there is any tumour seeding it will be removed at definitive surgery.

Local en bloc excision and reconstruction with an endoprosthetic replacement is associated with a slightly higher incidence of local recurrence than primary amputation, but overall the survival is the same in both.

Prostatic metastases are not especially vascular but renal metastases are, and it is these that need to be embolised before surgical approach, as otherwise uncontrollable haemorrhage may result.

Patients with pathological fractures through metastases are often metabolically unwell, with dehydration and hypercalcaemia. Surgery must not be undertaken until their condition has been made as good as possible. Surgery cannot lengthen life but may shorten it.

Answers: Extended matching questions

1. Treatment of rheumatoid arthritis

1D, 2E, 3G, 4F, 5E, 6C, 7B, 8A

A wrist splint can improve hand function in a patient with a painful unstable wrist joint who does not want to consider surgery. In more severe arthritis of the wrist, the distal ulna subluxes posteriorly and becomes very painful. An excision of the distal end of the ulna does not compromise stability but does reduce pain and so improves grip. At the elbow, rheumatoid arthritis can selectively affect the proximal radial head, producing pain on pronation and supination. Once again, excision of the offending bone (this time the proximal radial head) reduces pain and so improves mobility.

Rheumatoid arthritis can create an unstable cervical spine by eroding the facet joints. Fusion of the cervical spine should prevent any further neurological deterioration. The inflammatory pannus can also attack tendons, causing spontaneous rupture. Before this there is obvious tenosynovitis. If this does not respond to medical treatment then synovectomy should be undertaken to prevent rupture of the tendons. If they do rupture then direct repair of these tendons is rarely successful because their healing potential is compromised and so a tendon transfer is more likely to give a good functional result.

If a joint is very stiff and painful as a result of rheumatoid arthritis, it may be best to consider an arthrodesis rather than a joint replacement. The wrist and ankle are especially suitable for this operation as fusion is easy to obtain and function may not be badly compromised. However, the elbow, shoulder, hip and knee have well-proven joint replacements which can give good pain relief while at least preserving some mobility.

2. Diagnosis in arthritis

1E

Ankylosing spondylitis commonly affects middle-aged men who are SLA B27-positive. The condition starts with backache, but rapidly stiffness starts to dominate. The lumbar spine loses its lordosis, becoming stiff and straight, while the hips and knees go into flexion, producing a 'question mark' posture.

2G

There are several reactive arthritides associated with infection of the gastrointestinal or urinary tract by organisms such as *Chlamydia, Shigella* or *Yersinia.* In the latter case, the severity of the joint inflammation is inversely proportional to the severity of the original bowel infection.

3F

Psoriasis and other autoimmune conditions can also cause arthritis, and in the case of psoriasis the spine is commonly affected with massive osteophyte formation reminiscent of DISH (diffuse idiopathic spinal hyperostosis) or Forestier's disease.

4B

Juvenile rheumatoid arthritis usually affects young girls under 5 and affects growth. The knees are commonly severely affected, as is the temporomandibular joint so that they have difficulty opening their mouths. This may make intubation for surgery difficult and dangerous.

5H

Systemic lupus erythematosus can produce joint pains but the steroids used to treat it can also cause avascular necrosis, which in the early stages shows no changes on X-ray.

6I

Drug addicts and patients who are immunocompromised are especially susceptible to septic arthritis. It is most common in the knee. The patient may not be systemically unwell, but the characteristic feature is extreme pain on the slightest movement.

7C

Septic arthritis in an artificial joint usually occurs within a short period after surgery and presents with a low-grade fever and pain in the joint. A minor fall may be a red herring or, some think, may activate the infection. If the diagnosis is suspected, the joint must be opened and biopsies taken for culture. The joint should then be thoroughly washed out and the patient started on high-dose intravenous antibiotics if the joint is to be saved.

8A

Pain which wakes a patient at night and night sweats are caused by either tumour or infection until otherwise proven. The fluid collection on MRI suggests infection and the country of origin and the location in the spine all support the possible diagnosis of tuberculosis.

9D

The introduction of metalwork into bone always carries the risk that the bone may become contaminated with bacteria. In the presence of an implant, low-virulence bacteria may form a biofilm and lie dormant until activated by some major change (such as removal of metalware). The situation may then develop into a full-blown osteomyelitis.

→ 3. Bone tumours

1B

A pathological fracture in an elderly patient through a lytic lesion is likely to be a metastasis. These are far commoner than primary bone tumours.

2D

A malignant lesion in the spine is again likely to be a metastasis. Sclerotic lesions commonly come from the prostate and go to the spine via the venous plexus of Batson.

3A

This lump is not growing so is likely to be benign. It appears to be an outgrowth from the bone, but on X-ray is almost completely invisible. This means that it is mainly a cartilage cap on a bone stalk. This is the characteristic picture of an osteochondroma, which should be removed if it is causing problems.

4E
After metastases, the next most common lesion in the skeleton is plasmacytoma (solitary), which is called multiple myeloma when there are many lesions. These consist of lymphoid tissue.

5C
A solitary lesion full of large multinucleate osteoclasts is a giant cell tumour. It is a benign tumour (it does not metastasise) but is locally quite aggressive and so needs early treatment.

38 Paediatric orthopaedics

Multiple choice questions

Paediatric orthopaedics – general

1. **Which of the following statements are true?**

A The Heuter–Volkmann principle states that compressive forces stimulate growth.
B Wolff's law states that bone is deposited and resorbed according to the loads placed on it.
C Limb bud embryogenesis starts at month 4.
D In-toeing can be caused by persistent femoral neck anteversion.
E All children start with knock-knees which then become bow legs by the time that they are 2 or 3 years old.
F All children under the age of 3 years have flat feet.
G If toe-walking develops after the child has started walking normally, a neurological problem should be suspected.

Developmental dysplasia of the hip

2. **Which of the following statements regarding developmental dysplasia of the hip are true?**

A It is more common in boys than in girls.
B It occurs in up to 20 per cent of breech deliveries.
C It is more common in the first-born.
D It does not run in families.
E It is not associated with spina bifida.
F It is best diagnosed by X-ray.
G It is best treated early by non-operative means.
H The goal of surgery is to get the head concentric within the acetabulum.

Perthes' disease

3. **Which of the following statements regarding Perthes' disease are true?**

A Perthes' disease is a spontaneous avascular necrosis of the hip.
B It is most common in boys around puberty.
C The condition frequently settles spontaneously.
D A similar problem can occur in children with sickle cell disease.
E The prognosis is best in those children in whom the condition develops late.

Slipped upper femoral epiphysis

4. **Which of the following statements regarding slipped upper femoral epiphysis are true?**

A It may present with pain in the knee.
B It can best be diagnosed on an anteroposterior (AP) X-ray.
C It occurs in boys around the age of puberty.
D Perfect reduction must be obtained.
E The other hip is also commonly involved.

Hand abnormalities

5. **Which of the following statements regarding hand abnormalities are true?**

A Surgery to correct hand abnormalities should be deferred until it is clear how much disability the problem is causing.
B Radial club hand tends to occur in isolation of other deformities.
C Radioulnar synostosis requires surgery to restore pronation and supination.
D Congenital radial head dislocation is anterior.

Case study – shoulder pain

6. **A young child presents with pain in her shoulder. There is no history of trauma. She screams if the arm is moved. She is toxic and pyrexial.**

(a) **What is the likely diagnosis?**
A Gout
B Irritable joint
C Septic arthritis
D A fracture
E A dislocation.

(b) **What investigations would you organise?**
A Serum urate
B Full blood count
C Erythrocyte sedimentation rate (ESR) and C-reactive protein (CRP)
D Gamma-globulins
E Blood cultures
F Ultrasound
G X-ray.

(c) **What treatment should be started?**
A Splintage
B Aspiration
C Analgesia
D Anti-inflammatories
E Intravenous antibiotics
F Steroids.

Osteomyelitis

7. **Which of the following statements regarding osteomyelitis are true?**
A It is usually caused by haematogenous spread.
B In neonates, septic arthritis of the hip is effectively synonymous with osteomyelitis.
C Pus forming in medullary bone cannot penetrate cortical bone and so tracks centrally.
D If a sterile aspirate is obtained from what appears to be a septic joint, there may be osteomyelitis nearby.
E Pus collection in bone should not under any circumstances be drained as bone necrosis will result.
F An involucrum is a dead fragment of bone following an attack of osteomyelitis.

Case study – injury in a child

8. **A 2-year-old disabled child is brought to the A&E department with a bucket-handle metaphyseal fracture of the distal femur. There is also callus from a previous tibial fracture. The parents did not see exactly what happened but think he fell from a sofa onto the floor the day before when playing with his older brothers. On examination he is a quiet child who has more than his fair share of bruises on him, of varying ages. What is the diagnosis that must be most carefully investigated?**
A Osteogenesis imperfecta
B Non-accidental injury (NAI)
C Exuberant older brothers
D Fracture through a benign bone cyst
E Pathological fracture through a metastasis from a nephroblastoma.

Extended matching questions

1. Knee problems

A Blount's disease
B Discoid meniscus
C Osgood–Schlatter disease
D Osteochondritis dissecans
E Chondromalacia patellae

Choose and match the correct diagnosis with each of the following scenarios:

1 A young man complains of clunking and locking of the knee. MRI shows that a fragment of the femoral condyle has broken off and is jamming in the joint.

2 A child has a knee which clunks and locks. An MRI shows an abnormal lateral meniscus which is a solid disc rather than a crescent.

3 A child presents with a painful lump over the tibial tubercle.

4 A teenage girl has pain which appears to arise from patellofemoral maltracking.

5 A West Indian child presents with varus bowing of the tibia.

2. Foot problems

A Serial plasters
B Excision
C Soft-tissue releases with correction of the bone alignments of the foot
D Soft-tissue releases
E Regular massage and stretching

Choose and match the correct treatment with each of the following scenarios:

1 A child presents at birth with a clubfoot which can be partially corrected.

2 A child presents at 2 years of age with a stiff clubfoot deformity.

3 A child presents with characteristic rocker-bottom foot of the congenital vertical talus.

4 A child presents with curly toes. They are causing no pain or disability but look unsightly.

5 A school child presents with a stiff and painful foot. CT confirms a tarsal coalition. It is not settling and the first signs of degenerative change in the coalition are starting to appear.

3. Spine and neurological problems in children

A Polio
B Torticollis
C Congenital abnormality of a vertebra
D Spina bifida
E Spondylolisthesis
F Muscular dystrophy
G Cerebral palsy
H Idiopathic scoliosis
I Leg-length inequality
J Scheuermann's disease
K Brachial plexus injury

Choose and match the aetiology or diagnosis with each of the following scenarios:

1 A young child presents with a sharp curve of the spine at T12.

2 A teenager presents with a curve of the spine which produces a rib hump when they tip forward to touch their toes.

3 A child has a curve in the spine which seems to vanish when they sit down.

4 A teenager starts to develop sloping shoulders and a prominent thoracic kyphosis.

5 A patient with backache is found to have the L4 vertebral body displaced forward 30 per cent on the L5.

6 A child is born with the head fixed to one side, due to a contracture of the sternocleidomastoid.

7 After a difficult breech birth, a child is noted to have a flaccid arm.

8 A child is noticed to have a hairy tuft at the base of the spine, and lower motor neuron signs in the lower legs.

9 A child who had a febrile illness now has marked motor weakness and wasting in the lower legs but no sensory loss.

10 A child has flexion contractures of both lower limbs with very high muscle tone. Intelligence is normal.

11 A child presents with progressive muscular weakness in the limbs.

Answers: Multiple choice questions

→ Paediatric orthopaedics – general

1. B, D, F, G

Bones grow in part according to the Heuter–Volkmann principle and Wolff's law. The Heuter–Volkmann principle states that compressive forces inhibit growth while tensile ones stimulate it. Wolff's law states that bone is deposited and resorbed according to the loads placed upon it.

Limb bud embryogenesis starts very early (around week 4) and is complete by week 8 (all within the first trimester). This is the same time as some internal organs, such as the heart, are forming. This means that certain limb bud abnormalities are associated with specific cardiac abnormalities because both are the result of the same insult to the embryo at that critical time.

In-toeing can indeed be caused by persisting femoral neck anteversion, but can also be caused by tibial torsion and metatarsus varus. Most of these conditions correct themselves as the child grows.

Children actually start with bow legs. These then become knock-knees by the time that they are 2 or 3 years old. At the same time, it is true that all normal children start off with flat feet. The arch of the foot only develops with time. Many normal children also start walking on their toes, but if they start walking plantigrade and then go on to their toes as they grow older, this is an ominous neurological sign.

→ Developmental dysplasia of the hip

2. B, C, G, H

Developmental dysplasia of the hip is more common in girls than in boys and occurs in 20 per cent of breech deliveries. It is more common in the first-born and runs in families as well as certain racial groups. It is associated with other congenital abnormalities, especially spina bifida and arthrogryposis. X-ray is of no use in diagnosis early on, because neither the femoral head nor the acetabulum can be visualised at birth as they have not yet ossified. Ultrasound is the examination of choice, as it is possible to see if the femoral head fits snugly in the acetabulum and, if not, then what position allows a reduction to be sustained. If a safe position can be found where the hip can be held properly located, it is much better to hold this position non-operatively using double nappies or a harness. Providing the hip is held concentric in the acetabulum, the two will develop normally and the hip will become stable.

→ Perthes' disease

3. A, C, D

Perthes' disease is believed to be a spontaneous avascular necrosis of the hip. It is commonest in boys but develops long before puberty in children aged around 6 years. Providing that the femoral head revascularises before it collapses, the condition settles spontaneously. Avascular necrosis of the hip can also develop in many other conditions, including sickle cell disease, skeletal dysplasia, following infection, and the use of high-dose steroids. The prognosis is worse the later it develops.

➜ Slipped upper femoral epiphysis

4. A, C, E

Hilton's law states that the nerve supply to a joint is the same as the muscles acting over it. This results in pathology in the hip sometimes presenting as pain in the knee. The slip of the femoral head tends to be mainly backwards and so, although the slip can be seen on the AP (usually in retrospect), a lateral or 'frog's leg view' is the most important for making the diagnosis and must always be requested. The condition is commonest in boys around the age of puberty. If an attempt is made to reduce the slip, there is a major risk of damaging the blood supply to the femoral head and causing the disastrous diagnosis of avascular necrosis. Therefore, in all but the most acute slips, the head is fixed in its slipped position using pins which are designed to prevent the slip going any further. As the other hip is commonly involved, many surgeons will choose to prophylactically pin the other hip before it has a chance to slip.

➜ Hand abnormalities

5. A

Hand abnormalities are a cosmetic and functional problem, but a functional and disfigured hand is much better than a useless but cosmetically normal one. It is therefore important to wait until the child develops hand dominance and shows what they can do with a deformed upper limb before embarking on what may only be cosmetic surgery, which may carry the complication of reducing functionality.

Radial club hand is classically associated with a series of other abnormalities (VACTERL). These involve the vertebrae, anus, cardiovascular system, trachea, renal and limb buds.

Congenital radioulnar synostosis prevents pronation and supination, but unfortunately surgery cannot lead to the recreation of this movement. In Monteggia fractures the dislocation of the radial head is anterior, but in congenital radial head dislocation it is in the opposite direction, posterolateral.

➜ Case study – shoulder pain

6. (a) C; (b) B, C, E, F, G; (c) A, B, C, E

The most likely and most serious diagnosis, which needs to be excluded quickly here, is septic arthritis, as time is of the essence if permanent damage is to be avoided. There is no history of trauma so fracture and dislocation are unlikely. Irritable shoulder does not produce extreme pain, and gout in children does not occur. The blood investigations of choice are full blood count, ESR, CRP and blood cultures. X-rays will not show changes in early septic arthritis but may show other abnormalities, such as underlying osteomyelitis. Ultrasound is the imaging modality of choice as it will show a joint effusion which can then be aspirated under ultrasound control.

Aspiration is both diagnostic and therapeutic. The joint will need splinting for comfort and the patient will need strong analgesia. High-dose intravenous antibiotics should be started at once empirically then changed if necessary once the culture and sensitivities are back. If there is not rapid improvement, the joint should be opened and washed out.

➜ Osteomyelitis

7. A, B, D, F

Osteomyelitis usually arises from haematogenous spread. When the pus starts to accumulate, the pressure rises and the pus appears able to punch its way through cortical bone. This means that the metaphyses of bones which are intra-articular (such as the proximal end of the femur) can produce septic arthritis-like symptoms (with a sterile hip effusion) and/or a full-blown septic arthritis as well. As soon as a collection of pus is suspected, the bone must be opened and the pus drained out. If this is not done, the pus will lift the periosteum killing the bone beneath (a sequestrum) and creating a new outer layer of abnormal bone under the periosteum (the involucrum).

Case study – injury in a child

8. B

Non-accidental injury is most common in children under the age of 3 years and especially if they are disabled. The mechanism of injury here is improbable, there is a delay in presentation, and the injury was not witnessed. These are all characteristic of a history of NAI. The presence of bruises of different ages, especially pinches, is another feature of NAI. Certain fractures, such as the bucket-handle of chip fracture of the metaphysis, are also commonly found in NAI, as is the finding that there are previous healed fractures. There are therefore at least nine features in this case which point towards NAI and this is far more than the threshold needed to activate further investigate by the appropriate authorities.

Answers: Extended matching questions

1. Knee problems

1D

Fragments of the femoral condyle can be lost in a condition called osteochondritis dissecans. These loose fragments can jam in the joint and cause locking.

2B

A second possibility for a clunking, locking knee is the congenital abnormality of the lateral meniscus called discoid meniscus. In these cases the cartilage is not a crescent but has a solid-centre-like a disc. This meniscus is susceptible to tears and then causes locking in the knee.

3C

A painful lump over the tibial tubercle in an adolescent is Osgood–Schlatter disease, an inflammation of the epiphysis under the tibial tubercle. It usually settles spontaneously.

4E

Pain and possible maltracking of the patella is called chondromalacia patellae. It is most painful when going up and down stairs and after sitting still for a long period.

5A

Varus bowing in a West Indian child might be caused by rickets, but is more likely to be Blount's disease, an abnormality of growth of the proximal tibial epiphysis.

2. Foot problems

1A/E, 2D, 3C, 4D, 5B

There are two types of clubfoot. The first is supple and is called physiological. It is probably caused by abnormal position in the uterus. Regular massage and stretching should lead to a rapid improvement. A more rigid form of clubfoot relates to some kind of developmental abnormality of the posteromedial structures of the foot and the calf. The key to treatment is to get the bones of the hindfoot into the correct relationship with each other so that they can grow normally. Careful serial plastering allows this correction to be obtained and sustained (the Ponsetti technique), but if presentation is late or the clubfoot is very rigid, then surgical release of the soft tissues which are tethering the deformity will be needed, followed by plasters designed to hold that position.

A similar treatment regime will be needed for the congenital vertical talus (rocker-bottom foot), as only surgery allows the correct alignment of the bones to be achieved.

Curly toes tend to be a benign condition and, if possible, should be left alone, but if the patient insists on something being done then soft-tissue releases should allow the toes to straighten out. A tarsal coalition will give a pathological flatfoot. The stresses on the abnormal bone bridge will lead to pathological fractures. If this pseudoarthrosis starts to become arthritic, it should be excised.

3. Spine and neurological problems in children

1C, 2H, 3I, 4J, 5E, 6B, 7K, 8D, 9A, 10G, 11F

Failure of the vertebral bodies to develop normally can lead either to a hemivertebra (one side does not develop) or to a fusion on one side of two adjacent vertebrae. Either way, as the child grows, there will be a progressive sharp curve in the spine.

Idiopathic scoliosis is primarily a rotatory deformity of the spine, which develops in the rapidly growing spine and is, in effect, a buckling of the spine. In this condition, the spine rotates more as the child bends forward, creating the characteristic rib hump.

A second growth abnormality of the spine is Scheuermann's disease, which also develops during the adolescent growth spurt. In this case, the spine curves anteriorly (convex posteriorly), producing a stooping gait and droopy shoulders.

A slip between two vertebral bodies (spondylolisthesis) is caused by a failure of the pedicles between the vertebrae. This can be congenital, traumatic or commonly a stress fracture following repeated load, such as weight-lifting.

A twisted neck is called torticollis and in this case it is congenital and is caused by contracture and even a fibrous mass in the sternocleidomastoid muscle. It is associated with other congenital abnormalities such as developmental dysplasia of the hip.

A child with a flaccid arm after birth may have suffered injury to the brachial plexus. This is especially common following a breech delivery.

There are many types of muscular dystrophy affecting different muscle groups, but their characteristic is that they are progressive disorders.

A hairy tuft at the base of the spine is another congenital abnormality which needs checking for at birth. It is a sign of spina bifida. If this is affecting the spinal roots, there will be lower motor neuron signs in the lower legs.

Polio presents as a febrile illness which then goes on to permanently damage the anterior horn cells of the spinal cord, causing muscle weakness but no sensory changes. The motor signs are lower not upper and they are not progressive. By contrast, cerebral palsy produces upper motor neuron signs with spasticity, but once again there should be no sensory impairment.

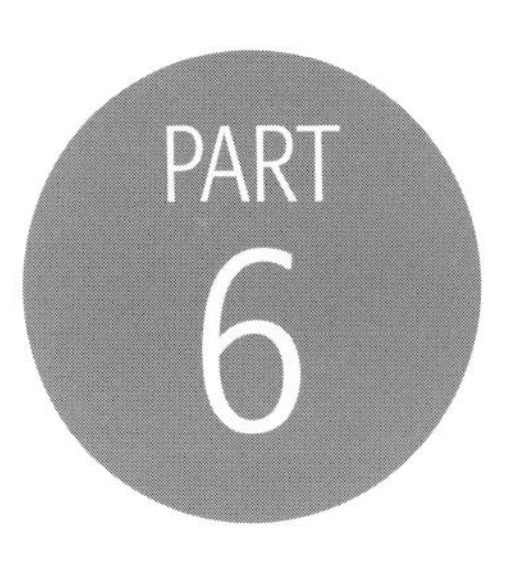

Skin and subcutaneous tissue

39 Skin and subcutaneous tissue 273

39 Skin and subcutaneous tissue

Multiple choice questions

Anatomy

1. **Which of the following statements are true?**
   A The epidermis accounts for the major part of the skin.
   B The majority of epidermal cells are keratinocytes.
   C Melanocytes are cells found in the dermis.
   D Sweat glands are of two types: eccrine and apocrine.
   E Adnexal structures span the epidermis and dermis.

Ulcer edges

2. **Which of the following descriptions of ulcer edges denote malignancy?**
   A Sloping
   B Overhanging
   C Everted
   D Punched out
   E Rolled.

Malignant melanoma

3. **Which of the following are not types of malignant melanoma?**
   A Superficial spreading
   B Salmon patch
   C Nodular
   D Giant congenital pigmented naevus
   E Lentigo maligna
   F Acral lentiginous.

4. **Which of the following statements are false?**
   A The vast majority of malignant melanoma form in pre-existing naevi.
   B Change in colour, shape, size and surface in a naevus should be looked upon with suspicion.
   C Incision biopsy should be done in all suspicious lesions.
   D Superficial spreading melanoma is the most common type.
   E Exposure to ultraviolet rays is a major cause of malignant melanoma.

Necrotising fasciitis

5. **Which of the following statements are false with regard to necrotising fasciitis?**
   A This is a surgical emergency.
   B It is a polymicrobial synergistic infection.
   C To confirm the diagnosis a plain X-ray is done to look for air.
   D 80 per cent of cases have a history of trauma or previous infection.
   E A period of observation is advisable to see if the condition spreads.
   F It can rapidly progress to septic shock.
   G Urgent measures necessary are resuscitation, antibiotics and surgical debridement.
   H The mortality rate is 30–50 per cent

Extended matching questions

1. Definitions

A Ulcer
B Sinus
C Fistula

Choose and match the correct term with each of the following descriptions:

1 An abnormal communication between two epithelial-lined surfaces. The communication or tract may be lined by granulation tissue but in chronic cases it may be epithelialised.

2 A blind-ending tract that connects a cavity lined with granulation tissue (usually an abscess) with an epithelial surface.

3 A discontinuity of an epithelial surface.

2. Infections

A Impetigo
B Erysipelas
C Cellulitis/lymphangitis
D Necrotising fasciitis
E Purpura fulminans

Choose and match the correct condition with each of the following descriptions:

1 A polymicrobial synergistic infection most often caused by group A beta-haemolytic *Streptococcus*.

2 In this lesion there is intravascular thrombosis producing haemorrhagic skin infarction.

3 This is a highly infectious skin lesion, usually affecting children, caused by *Staphylococcus* and/or *Streptococcus*.

4 This is a generalised bacterial infection of the skin and subcutaneous tissue, usually preceded by trauma or ulceration.

5 This produces a well-demarcated infection by streptococci, usually on the face.

3. Benign skin tumours

A Basal cell papilloma
B Papillary wart
C Junctional naevus
D Compound naevus
E Keratoacanthoma

Choose and match the correct condition with each of the following descriptions:

1 A maculopapular pigmented lesion that is most prominent at puberty. It is a junctional proliferation of naevus cells with nests and columns in the dermis.

2 A deeply pigmented macular or papular lesion commonly seen in childhood. It is caused by a dermo-epidermal proliferation of naevus cells and progresses in the older person to form a compound or intradermal naevus. It has no malignant potential.

3 A benign skin tumour caused by the human papillomavirus (HPV) which also causes plantar warts and condylomata acuminata.

4 A soft, warty lesion which is often pigmented and arises from the basal layer of the epidermal cells containing melanocytes. This is one of the commonest benign skin lesions in the elderly.

5 A lesion (Fig. 39.1), usually found on the head, neck and face, shaped like a cup with the centre filled with a keratin plug. The lesion has a short history, measured in weeks. The aetiology is unclear but may be caused by infection of a hair follicle by a papillomavirus. Although it

regresses spontaneously, it is better to excise it for a superior cosmetic outcome and also to differentiate it from squamous cell carcinoma.

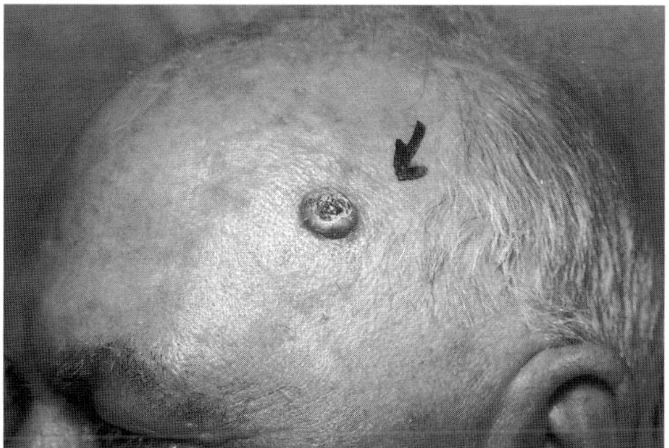

Figure 39.1 Keratoacanthoma.

4. Premalignant and malignant skin lesions

A Bowen's disease
B Extramammary Paget's disease
C Basal cell carcinoma (BCC)
D Squamous cell carcinoma (SCC)
E Malignant melanoma (MM)

Choose and match the correct condition with each of the following descriptions:

1 This is a slow-growing, locally invasive tumour (hence also called a rodent ulcer, as it behaves like a rodent burrowing into neighbouring tissues) of a few years' duration. The edges are typically raised and rolled and occur more often on the face, head and neck.

2 This occurs in the genital or perianal regions or in skin rich in apocrine glands, such as the axilla. It is a form of intraepidermal adenocarcinoma.

3 This is an ulcerated skin lesion of a few months' duration, with a raised, everted edge and an indurated inflamed surrounding area. A minority may have enlarged regional lymphadenopathy from metastasis.

4 There is a pigmented skin lesion on the scalp that has recently changed in colour and has become itchy and started to bleed. There are a few small black spots irregularly scattered around the lesion.

5 There is a slowly enlarging erythematous scaly patch on the dorsum of the right hand of an elderly male.

Answers: Multiple choice questions

Anatomy

1. B, D, E

The epidermis accounts for 5 per cent of the total skin, while the dermis accounts for 95 per cent. The epidermis is composed of keratinised, stratified, squamous epithelium. From superficial to deep it has five layers: stratum corneum, stratum lucidum, stratum granulosum, stratum spinosum and stratum basale. The dermis consists of a superficial papillary layer and a deeper reticular layer.

The majority of epidermal cells are keratinocytes. The basal epidermis also contains melanocytes. Keratinocytes are classified according to their depth and degree of differentiation.

Melanocytes originate from the neural crest and are found in the basal epidermis. Each melanocyte synthesises the pigment melanin, which protects the cell nuclei from ultraviolet radiation. The keratinocytes in the strata granulosum and spinosum contain the melanin. Differences in skin colour are determined by variations in the amount and distribution of melanin within the keratinocytes.

The sweat glands, eccrine and apocrine, open into pores in the hair follicles. Eccrine glands are present throughout the entire body surface, except for the lips. They secrete sweat in response to sympathetic activity such as emotion and are responsible for thermoregulation. In hyperhidrosis, where there is excessive sweating (commonly seen in the palms, axilla and lower limbs), the condition can be cured by performing a sympathectomy. Apocrine glands are found in the axillary and groin areas and become active at puberty. Persistent infection of these glands causes hydradenitis suppurativa.

Adnexal structures, such as hair follicles, sebaceous and sweat glands, span epidermis and dermis. In injuries where epidermis is lost, re-epithelialisation occurs from these structures.

➜ Ulcer edges

2. C, E

➜ Malignant melanoma

3. B, D

4. A, C

➜ Necrotising fasciitis

5. E

Answers: Extended matching questions

➜ 1. Definitions

1C

A fistula is an abnormal communication lined by granulation tissue between two epithelial lined surfaces. These may be congenital, as in tracheo-oesophageal or rectourethral fistulae, or acquired, as in enterocolic, colovesical, enteroenteric fistulae.

2B

A sinus is a blind tract connecting a cavity with an epithelial surface. The cavity is usually an abscess. It may be classified as congenital, as in a remnant of a thyroglossal tract that becomes a cyst which gets infected and bursts which, although called a 'fistula', is strictly a sinus. Acquired causes are a retained foreign body, specific chronic infection, inflammation and malignancy.

3A

An ulcer is a discontinuity of an epithelial surface characterised by gradual destruction with a base that may be necrotic, granulating or malignant. These can be classified as specific, non-specific and malignant.

2. Infections

1D

Necrotising fasciitis used to be called synergistic gangrene. It results from polymicrobial infection, most commonly group A beta-haemolytic *Streptococcus* along with *E. coli*, *Pseudomonas*, *Proteus*, *Bacteroides* or *Clostridium*. The majority occur following trauma or infection, particularly in a smoker or a diabetic. The typical signs are oedema beyond the skin erythema, woody hard induration of the subcutaneous tissue, inability to distinguish between fascial planes and muscle groups, soft-tissue crepitus and severe pain. This must be treated very promptly with resuscitation, antibiotics and surgical debridement; otherwise the patient may go into septic shock.

2E

Purpura fulminans is a rare condition, usually occurring in children, where intravascular thrombosis produces haemorrhagic skin infarction. It can rapidly progress to septic shock. There are three types: acute infectious purpura fulminans caused by either acute bacterial or viral infection and which may result in extensive tissue loss requiring limb amputation; neonatal purpura fulminans; and idiopathic purpura fulminans.

3A

Impetigo is a very infectious superficial skin lesion, usually affecting children. The infection produces blisters that rupture and join up and is covered by honey-coloured crust. Treatment is washing of the area and application of topical or broad-spectrum oral antibiotics.

4C

Cellulitis/lymphangitis is a generalised bacterial infection of the skin and subcutaneous tissue associated with trauma or ulceration. The patient has fever with a red, swollen, tender area with overlying reddish streaks of lymphangitis; *Streptococcus* is the commonest causative organism. Treatment is the prompt administration of the appropriate intravenous antibiotics with rest and elevation to the affected part.

5B

Erysipelas is a well-localised streptococcal infection of the superficial lymphatics, usually associated with trauma to the skin of the face. The area is red and oedematous and the patient has fever with leucocytosis. The appropriate broad-spectrum antibiotic is the treatment of choice.

3. Benign skin tumours

1D, 2C, 3B, 4A, 5E

4. Premalignant and malignant skin lesions

1C

The duration of this slow-growing lesion (rodent ulcer) is usually in years and caused by exposure to ultraviolet light. It most often occurs on the head, neck and face (see Fig. 39.2). It has a raised, rolled edge which may look like a pearl. Although there are several clinical types, by far the commonest is the nodular and nodulocystic type, which is localised. The generalised types are superficial spreading, multifocal or infiltrative, sometimes called geographical type. Surgical excision and primary closure, if possible, or skin grafting or use of rotational flaps by a plastic surgeon comprise the optimum treatment. Although the condition is radiosensitive, this form of treatment is rarely used because the location of the tumour precludes the use of radiotherapy to prevent damage to neighbouring vital structures, such as the lens and cartilages of the ear or nose.

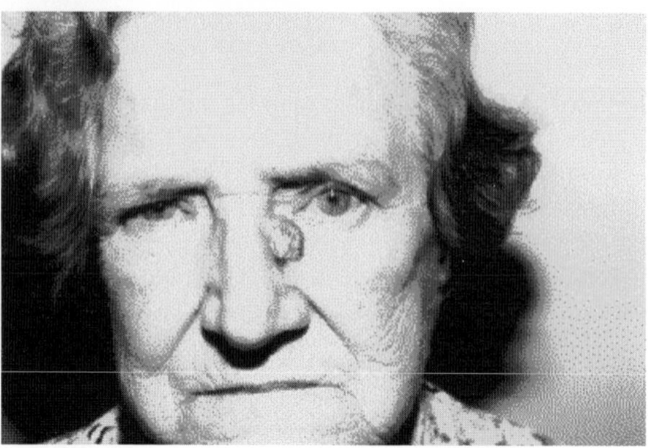

Figure 39.2 Basal cell carcinoma.

2B

This is an intraepidermal adenocarcinoma occurring in the genital or perianal regions or axilla (extramammary Paget's disease: Sir James Paget 1814–1899, surgeon, St Bartholomew's Hospital, London). About a quarter of them are associated with an underlying invasive neoplasm. Surgical excision is the treatment.

3D

Squamous cell carcinoma (SCC), the second most common form of skin cancer, arises from the keratinising cells of the epidermis or its appendages and usually affects the elderly (see Fig. 39.3). The usual causes are prolonged exposure to sun, chronic inflammation, scars of burns and immunosuppression. The duration is usually in months. The lesion is an ulcer with a raised everted edge with the surrounding area red and indurated. Regional lymphadenopathy is more often due to infection as only 2 per cent metastasise.

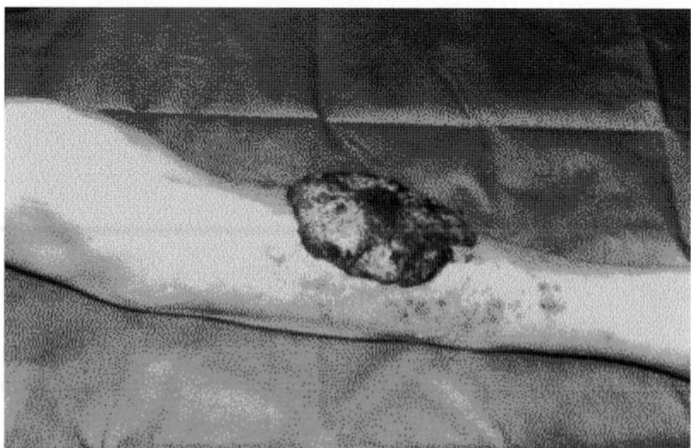

Figure 39.3 Squamous cell carcinoma.

The histology of the excised lesion should include the pathological pattern, the cellular morphology, the Broders' grade (Albert Compton Broders, 1885–1964, American pathologist), the depth of invasion, the presence of any perineural or vascular invasion and the vertical and circumferential excision margin clearance. Depending upon the size and the location, the surgical management should be a multidisciplinary team effort between the plastic surgeon, the radiation oncologist and the pathologist.

4E

This is a MM with satellite nodules (see Fig. 39.4). It is a malignant tumour arising from the melanocytes. Therefore it can arise from any organ where melanocytes are present, such as the choroid of the eye, leptomeninges and the bowel mucosa. Although it accounts for less than 5 per cent of skin malignancy, it is responsible for over 75 per cent of deaths caused by skin malignancy. MM accounts for 3 per cent of all malignancies worldwide and is the commonest cancer in 20–39 year-olds.

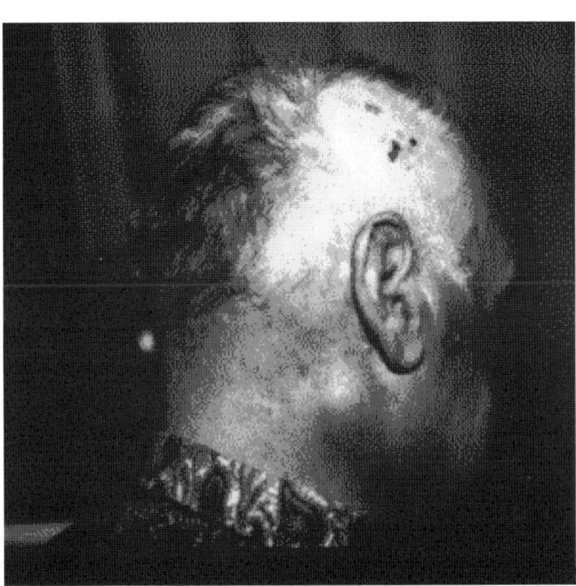

Figure 39.4 Malignant melanoma of scalp showing satellite lesions with cervical lymphnodal metastasis.

Exposure to ultraviolet rays is the major cause whilst the risk factors are enhanced in xeroderma pigmentosum, family history, previous melanoma, large number of naevi, dysplastic naevi, red hair, giant congenital pigmented naevus and immunocompromised patients. The various types are: superficial spreading (70 per cent), nodular (15 per cent), lentigo maligna melanoma (5–10 per cent) and acral lentiginous melanoma (2–8 per cent). The presenting features in a naevus suggesting MM are change in shape, size, colour, surface, itchiness and serosanguinous discharge. MM also occurs underneath the nail bed; these are usually a superficial spreading type and confirmation is by biopsy of the nail matrix. Amelanotic melanoma usually occurs in the gastrointestinal tract.

In a suspected MM regional lymph node metastasis should be sought, besides evidence of distant spread. Confirmation is done by excision biopsy with a 2 mm margin of skin and subdermal fat. Histology is reported according to the Breslow thickness (Alexander Breslow, 1928–1980, American pathologist). This is a guide to further definitive treatment and indicates prognosis. Radical regional lymph node dissection is done when there is metastasis.

Clinically, impalpable lymph nodes may have microscopic metastasis, particularly in those where the Breslow thickness is more than 1 mm. Therefore, in such patients, sentinel lymph node biopsy (SLNB) should be offered and in node-positive patients block dissection is carried out. Of those with SLNB-positive disease, 70–80 per cent will have no other involved regional nodes. In those with clinically involved nodes, 70–85 per cent will have occult distant metastases, such as in the lung or liver.

5A

This is a squamous carcinoma in situ first described in 1912 by John Templeton Bowen, professor of dermatology at Harvard University. It is elevated from the skin surface, red and scaly and spreads locally (see Fig. 39.5). A minority of these lesions may progress to SCC. Chronic exposure to sun, HPV 16 and inorganic arsenic compounds have been thought to be possible causes. When the condition occurs on the glans penis, it is called Queyrat's erythroplasia (Parisian dermatologist Auguste Queyrat described the condition in 1911, although Paget described the same disease 50 years earlier). Treatment is by topical application of 5-fluorouracil or surgical excision.

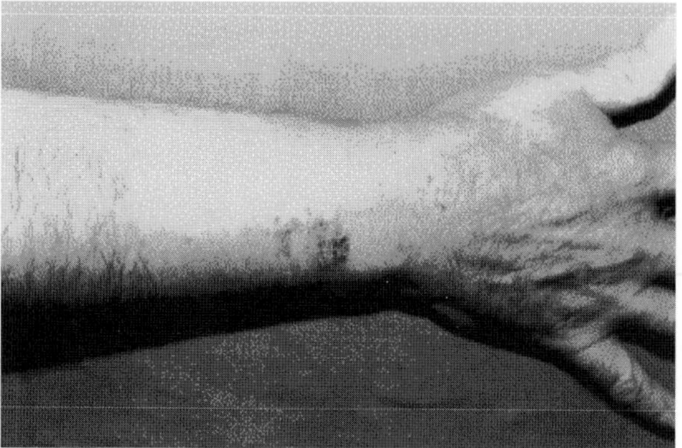

Figure 39.5 Bowen's disease: squamous carcinoma in situ.

PART 7

Head and neck

40 Elective neurosurgery 283

41 The eye and orbit 292

42 Cleft lip and palate: developmental abnormalities of face, mouth and jaws 302

43 The nose and sinuses 309

44 The ear 319

45 Pharynx, larynx and neck 330

46 Oropharyngeal cancer 341

47 Disorders of the salivary glands 351

40 Elective neurosurgery

Multiple choice questions

Intracranial pressure

1. **Which of the following statements about intracranial pressure (ICP) in a normal adult are true?**

A ICP varies from 5 to 15 mmHg at rest.
B ICP decreases with coughing.
C ICP decreases with normal inspiration.
D ICP increases with an increase in arterial $P\text{CO}_2$.
E ICP increases with an increase in $P\text{O}_2$.

Cerebral oedema

2. **Which of the following statements about cerebral oedema are true?**

A It may be either vasogenic or cytotoxic.
B It causes increased ICP.
C It causes brain shift.
D It can be treated with steroids.
E It can be treated with phenytoin.

Brain metabolism

3. **Which of the following statements are true?**

A The brain is dependent on glucose and oxygen for energy.
B The brain has considerable stores of glucose.
C The brain can switch easily to anaerobic metabolism.
D Brain blood flow is 55 mL/100g per min.
E The brain can utilise proteins for energy production.

Papilloedema

4. **Which of the following statements about papilloedema are true?**

A It can be seen in raised ICP.
B It can be associated with retinal haemorrhages.
C It is always present if ICP is greater than 25 mmHg.
D It can cause blindness if left untreated.
E It can be caused by optic nerve compression.

Hydrocephalus

5. **Which of the following statements about hydrocephalus are true?**

A It is the diagnosis when the ventricles are enlarged on CT scan.
B It may present with a 6th nerve palsy.
C It may present with sunsetting eyes and a bulging fontanelle in infants.
D It can cause head enlargement in infants.
E It can cause papilloedema.

Cerebrospinal fluid (CSF) physiology

6. **Which of the following statements are true?**

A The total volume of CSF in adults is 150 mL.
B The total volume of CSF in the normal ventricular system is 35 mL.
C Normal production of CSF is 0.33 mL/min.
D CSF is produced by the choroid plexus alone
E CSF is absorbed in the arachnoid villa and superior sagittal sinus.

Obstructive hydrocephalus

7. **What can cause obstructive hydrocephalus?**

A Meningitis
B Tumours of the fourth ventricle
C Intraventricular haemorrhage

D Encephalitis
E Tumours of the midbrain.

Lumbar puncture

8. Which of the following statements about lumbar puncture are true?

A It is contraindicated in cases of supratentorial mass lesions.
B It can be done to measure ICP.
C It can be done to diagnose meningitis.
D It can be used to treat communicating hydrocephalus.
E It is usually done under general anaesthetic.

Ventriculoperitoneal shunt

9. Which of the following are complications of ventriculoperitoneal (VP) shunt?

A Infection (ventriculitis)
B Blockage of the proximal catheter
C Breakage of the distal catheter
D Intraventricular haemorrhage
E Seizures.

Cerebral abscesses

10. Which of the following statements about cerebral abscesses are true?

A They can be caused by direct spread from an air sinus infection.
B They can be blood-borne (secondary to septicaemia).
C They are a recognised complication of subacute bacterial endocarditis.
D There is an increased risk in patients with cyanotic congenital heart disease.
E Mixed anaerobic and aerobic organisms are common.

Tuberculous meningitis

11. Which of the following statements about tuberculous (TB) meningitis are true?

A CSF classically shows increased lymphocytes, increased protein and slightly low glucose.
B CSF classically shows increased polymorphs, increased protein and markedly reduced glucose.
C It can be detected by polymerase chain reaction.
D It is usually treated with antibiotics.
E It can cause hydrocephalus.

Creutzfeldt–Jakob disease (CJD)

12. Which of the following statements about CJD are true?

A The transmissible agent is an abnormal prion protein.
B Variant CJD has been diagnosed in UK since 1970.
C Instruments used when operating on definite cases must be discarded.
D The infectious agent is present in CSF and brain.
E The infectious agent is present in white blood cells and tonsil tissue.

Brain tumours

13. With which of the following may brain tumours present?

A Seizures
B Focal neurological deficits
C Endocrine dysfunction
D Intracranial bleeds
E Visual loss.

Brain lesions

14. What may be caused by dominant parietal lobe lesions?

A Left to right disorientation
B Foot drop on the opposite side
C Gerstmann's syndrome
D Acalculia and agraphia
E Hand weakness on the same side.

15. What may be caused by dominant temporal lobe lesions?

A Memory dysfunction
B Contralateral superior quadrantanopia
C Ipsilateral hemiparesis
D Dysphasia
E Blindness in the ipsilateral eye.

Pituitary adenomas

16. Which of the following statements about pituitary adenomas are true?

A In their early stages, they may cause a superior quadrantanopia.
B They may present with galactorrhoea.

C They can cause reduced cortisol production.
D They often present with a bitemporal hemianopia.
E They can cause Cushing's disease.

Astrocytomas

17. Which of the following statements are true?
A Astrocytomas are gliomas.
B Astrocytomas can present with seizures.
C The cell of origin is the oligodendrocyte.
D Astrocytomas are radiosensitive tumours.
E Astrocytomas can usually be completely excised.

18. Which of the following statements regarding pilocytic astrocytomas are true?
A They often present in the posterior fossa in children.
B They are WHO grade 2 tumours.
C They have a poor prognosis.
D They are radiosensitive tumours.
E They are not usually found in adults.

Meningiomas

19. Which of the following statements regarding meningiomas are true?
A They are usually benign.
B 80 per cent are supratentorial.
C They can cause cytotoxic brain oedema.
D The 10-year recurrence rate after complete resection is approximately 10 per cent.
E They are often slow-growing.

Cerebral metastases

20. Which of the following statements regarding cerebral metastases are true?
A 40 per cent are from primary lung tumours.
B Cerebral metastases from colon and renal tumours are rare.
C They affect 1 in 4 cancer sufferers.
D 15 per cent have no obvious source lesion – 'unknown primary'.
E Breast cancer is the second most common type.

Aneurysmal subarachnoid haemorrhage

21. Which of the following statements regarding aneurysmal subarachnoid haemorrhage (SAH) are true?
A The incidence is 150 per 100 000 of the population in UK.
B It presents with a sudden severe headache and vomiting.
C Patients usually have a family history of SAH.
D Risk factors are hypertension, cocaine abuse and fibromuscular dysplasia.
E Risk factors are diabetes, obesity and hypercholesterolaemia.

22. What are the typical presenting features of SAH?
A Gradual onset of severe headache
B Neck pain and stiffness
C Third nerve palsy
D Photophobia
E Purpuric rash

23. Which of the following statements regarding diagnosis of SAH are true?
A CT scan is positive in over 90 per cent of cases in the first 24 h.
B False-positives can occur if the lumbar puncture (LP) is traumatic.
C LP can be negative if done less than 12 h after the bleed.
D A bilirubin peak on spectrophotometry is diagnostic.
E Xanthochromia may be detected by the naked eye in many cases if the LP is done within 2 h of the bleed.

Arteriovenous malformations

24. Which of the following statements regarding arteriovenous malformations (AVMs) are true?
A The risk of rebleed is 2–4 per cent per year.
B They can cause epilepsy.
C The risk of rebleeding is greater if aneurysms are present on the feeding vessels.
D They are often associated with hydrocephalus.

E They can be treated with stereotactic radiosurgery

Epilepsy surgery

25. Which of the following statements regarding epilepsy surgery are true?

A Corpus callosotomy can cure drop attacks.
B Good surgical targets are cortical dysplasias and low-grade tumours.
C Mesial temporal sclerosis affects the hippocampus.
D Ictal SPECT (single photon emission computed tomography) can be helpful in identifying a seizure onset zone in the cortex.
E The amygdala is in the frontal lobe.

Parkinson's disease

26. Which of the following statements regarding Parkinson's disease are true?

A It can be treated with L-dopa.
B It can be treated with deep brain stimulation.
C Stimulation targets include the hypothalamus.
D Stimulation targets include the globus pallidus.
E Symptoms include tremor and dystonia.

Trigeminal neuralgia

27. Which of the following statements regarding trigeminal neuralgia are true?

A It is a painful condition affecting the arm.
B It can be caused by vascular compression of the 5th cranial nerve near its root entry zone.
C It can be caused by multiple sclerosis.
D It causes chronic, constant severe facial pain.
E It is often associated with a red eye and runny nose on the affected side.

Carpal tunnel syndrome

28. Which of the following statements regarding carpal tunnel syndrome are true?

A It is caused by entrapment of the median nerve at the wrist.
B Flexion of the wrist bringing on symptoms is known as Tinel's sign.
C Risk factors include hypothyroidism and pregnancy.
D Patients often wake with pain and paraesthesiae in the thumb, index and middle fingers.
E Wrist splints worn at night can be helpful in mild cases.

Answers: Multiple choice questions

Intracranial pressure

1. A, C, D

Intracranial pressure in a normal adult varies between 5 and 15 mmHg at rest. It rises during coughing and straining. Anything that increases intrathoracic pressure will cause ICP to rise. Inspiration is accompanied by a reduction in intrathoracic pressure and therefore ICP falls. An increase in $P\text{CO}_2$ will cause cerebral blood vessels to vasodilate and will increase ICP.

Cerebral oedema

2. A, B, C, D

Cerebral oedema is an increase in brain water and can be cytotoxic or vasogenic. Cytotoxic oedema is caused by an increase in intracellular water. Vasogenic oedema is caused by leakage of water from blood vessels. Tumours such as gliomas and meningiomas cause vasogenic oedema. This increases the mass effect and subsequent brain shift. Cerebral oedema can be treated with steroids such as dexamethasone. Phenytoin is an anticonvulsant and has no effect on cerebral oedema.

Brain metabolism

3. A, D

The brain is dependent on glucose and oxygen for its energy and does not have large stores of either. The brain cannot switch to anaerobic metabolism and brain function will cease if brain blood flow falls below 20 per cent of normal. Normal cerebral blood flow is 55 mL/100 ml per min. After 48 h of starvation, the brain can switch to using ketone bodies as an energy source.

Papilloedema

4. A, B, D

Papilloedema is graded from stage 1 to 4. In its later stages it can be associated with retinal exudates and haemorrhages. Untreated papilloedema will cause visual loss. Papilloedema is not always present in cases of raised ICP. Optic nerve compression can cause optic atrophy but does not cause papilloedema.

Hydrocephalus

5. B, C, D, E

Enlarged ventricles are not always indicative of hydrocephalus. Cerebral atrophy can cause dilatation of the ventricles as an *ex vacuo* effect. The ventricles tend to increase with age due to loss of brain substance.

Hydrocephalus can present with symptoms and signs of raised ICP – headache, vomiting, double vision due to 6th nerve palsy, papilloedema. Ataxia, memory loss and incontinence can be due to hydrocephalus in the elderly. The 6th nerve has a long intracranial course and is prone to stretch with brain shifts or hydrocephalus.

In infants, the presenting features may be increasing head circumference, bulging fontanelle, sunsetting eyes, irritability, vomiting and failure to thrive.

Cerebrospinal fluid (CSF) physiology

6. A, B, C, E

Cerebrospinal fluid is made by the choroid plexus of the lateral, third and fourth ventricles and by diffusion of extracellular fluid from the brain. The production of CSF by the choroid plexus is an energy-dependent process. The rate of production is 0.33 mL/min. An average adult will produce 475 mL/24 h. The ventricles hold 35 mL. The rest of the CSF is in the lumbar theca and subarachnoid space of the brain.

Obstructive hydrocephalus

7. B, C, E

Hydrocephalus can be divided into different types. It can be 'obstructive', i.e. does not communicate with the basal cistern or subarachnoid space, or 'communicating', where the level of obstruction is within the basal cisterns, subarachnoid space or arachnoid villi.

Obstructive hydrocephalus is caused by, for example, tumours blocking the foramen of Monro, cerebral aqueduct or fourth ventricle. Midbrain tumours often obstruct the cerebral aqueduct. Intraventricular haemorrhage can obstruct the aqueduct or the foramen of Monro.

Meningitis often causes adhesions at the base of the brain in the basal cisterns and therefore causes communicating hydrocephalus. Encephalitis is an infection or inflammation of the brain and is not usually a cause of hydrocephalus.

Lumbar puncture

8. A, B, C, D

Lumbar puncture is the insertion of a needle into the lumbar subarachnoid space, below the level of the conus (usually done at L4/5 or L5/S1) to obtain a specimen of CSF, e.g. for culture and microscopy in cases of meningitis. CSF pressure can also be measured. If the patient is lying flat, with the head at the same level as the back, and there is no block to CSF circulation, this pressure will be the same as ICP. The procedure is usually done under local anaesthetic.

Lumbar puncture is contraindicated in the presence of intracranial mass lesions, as removal of CSF from the lumbar subarachnoid space can provoke 'coning' of the brainstem. In cases of communicating hydrocephalus, CSF can be drained from the lumbar theca to treat the hydrocephalus. This is often done in patients with subarachnoid haemorrhage.

→ Ventriculoperitoneal shunt

9. A, B, C, D, E

Complications of VP shunt include the following:

- Infection of the shunt catheter and intraventricular CSF. This is known as ventriculitis. The walls of the ventricles become very inflamed. The shunt has to be removed. The infection is treated with IV and intrathecal antibiotics.
- The proximal catheter which lies in the ventricle is the commonest site of shunt blockage. It is often blocked by choroid plexus.
- The catheters can break, especially in children. A common place for this is in the neck.
- There is a 1 per cent risk of causing intraventricular haemorrhage during shunt insertion.
- Any neurosurgical procedure where the cortex is breached can cause seizures.
- The shunt valve can stop working or become blocked with debris or red blood cells.
- Shunts can over-drain and cause low-pressure headaches or subdural haemorrhages.

→ Cerebral abscesses

10. A, B, C, D, E

Cerebral abscesses can be caused by direct spread from an infected sinus (frontal or mastoid) or by blood-borne spread. Any condition which causes a septicaemia can cause brain abscess, e.g. subacute bacterial endocarditis. Severe tooth decay or gum disease can also be a source of organisms in the bloodstream. Patients with left-to-right shunts in the heart are at increased risk, as blood will bypass the lungs which mop up a lot of organisms. Mixed aerobic and anaerobic organisms are common.

→ Tuberculous meningitis

11. A, C, D, E

Tuberculous meningitis can be difficult to diagnose. CSF classically shows increased lymphocytes, increased protein and a slightly low glucose. TB bacilli may not be seen. Detection by polymerase chain reaction of bacterial DNA is becoming more common. It can cause hydrocephalus due to adhesions in the basal cisterns. It is treated with antibiotics.

→ Creutzfeldt–Jakob disease

12. A, C, D, E

Creutzfeldt–Jakob disease is transmitted by an abnormal prion protein which is present in brain, CSF, white blood cells and tonsil tissue. Variant CJD has been diagnosed in the UK since 1986. It appears to have spread from cows infected with bovine spongiform encephalitis which then entered the food chain. It was not recognised as an entity in 1970.

Instruments used during surgery in known CJD cases that came into contact with CSF, tonsil, blood or brain have to be discarded.

→ Brain tumours

13. A, B, C, D, E

Brain tumours can present in many ways. They are often associated with seizures or focal neurological deficits. Pituitary and hypothalamic tumours can cause endocrine dysfunction. Some tumours have a propensity to bleed and may present as a life-threatening intracerebral bleed. Visual loss can be caused by the tumour itself or present secondary to raised pressure and papilloedema.

→ Brain lesions

14. A, C, D

The parietal lobe is essentially a sensory lobe. Dominant parietal lobe lesions cause left–right disorientation, finger agnosia, acalculia and agraphia. Gerstmann's syndrome is when these occur together.

The foot part of the motor cortex is in the posterior frontal cortex on the upper medial side next to the falx. The hand part of the motor cortex is lower down in the posterior frontal lobe.

15. A, B, D

The temporal lobe structures are very involved in memory, speech and hearing. The temporal lobe is closely applied to the posterior frontal lobe at the Sylvian fissure, which carries the middle cerebral artery. Part of the optic radiation passes around the temporal lobe and can be affected by temporal lobe lesions. A contralateral superior quadrantanopia is seen in these cases.

Temporal lobe lesions would not cause blindness in the ipsilateral eye or an ipsilateral hemiparesis – the motor cortex is in the posterior frontal lobe but supplies the contralateral limbs.

→ Pituitary adenomas

16. A, B, C, D, E

Pituitary adenomas can be secreting or non-secreting. A tumour secreting adrenocorticotrophic hormone will cause Cushing's disease. A tumour secreting prolactin will cause galactorrhoea. Non-secreting tumours tend to be larger at presentation and often present with visual failure. Pressure on the normal pituitary gland will cause loss of normal secretion and hypopituitarism. Patients often have a low cortisol.

A pituitary tumour will grow out of the pituitary fossa and compress the optic nerve or chiasm from below. In the early stages this will cause a superior temporal quadrantanopia. In the later stages a bitemporal hemianopia is usual.

→ Astrocytomas

17. A, B, D

Astrocytomas are gliomas. The cell of origin is the astrocyte. Other types of glioma include oligodendroglioma (cell of origin is the oligodendrocyte) and ependymoma. These tumours are diffuse infiltrative tumours and it is difficult to completely excise them. They can present with seizures. Gliomas are graded 1–4. The most malignant type (grade 4) is glioblastoma multiforme. Many astrocytomas are radiosensitive.

18. A, D

Pilocytic astrocytomas are WHO grade 1 astrocytomas with a very good prognosis (90 per cent 10-year survival). They often occur in the posterior fossa in children. They are radiosensitive tumours but complete excision is often possible in the posterior fossa and is the treatment of choice. Pilocytic astrocytomas can also be found in adults.

Meningiomas

19. A, B, D, E

Meningiomas are usually benign tumours; 80 per cent are found supratentorially. They can cause vasogenic brain oedema and seizures as well as focal neurological deficits. They arise from the meninges of the brain. They are often slow-growing but a small proportion show atypical features on microscopy. These may grow more rapidly and have an increased risk of recurrence.

If a meningioma is completely excised, the recurrence rate is approximately 10 per cent unless a wide margin of associated dura can also be excised.

Cerebral metastases

20. A, B, C, D, E

The commonest primary tumour that gives rise to cerebral metastases is bronchogenic carcinoma, closely followed by breast cancer. Brain metastases from renal and colon cancers are much rarer. The commonest type of brain tumour is a secondary tumour. In 15 per cent of cases the primary lesion is undiagnosed.

Aneurysmal subarachnoid haemorrhage

21. B, D

The incidence of aneurysmal SAH is 15/100 000 population in the UK. There are other causes of SAH, e.g. trauma, bleed from an arteriovenous malformation. SAH usually presents with a severe, sudden, headache associated with nausea and vomiting, neck stiffness and photophobia. Neck pain may also be present. Some patients lose consciousness. The severity of the bleed is scored using the WFNS scoring system. Grade 1 is a good grade and grade 5 is the worst. Prognosis depends on the initial grade, among other things.

Most patients with SAH do not have a family history of SAH. Risk factors are hypertension, cocaine abuse and fibromuscular dysplasia, which leads to weakness of blood vessel walls and predisposes to aneurysm formation.

22. B, C, D

The presenting features are typically severe, sudden, headache associated with nausea and vomiting, neck stiffness and photophobia. Neck pain may also be present. Some patients lose consciousness. The features need to be distinguished from meningitis (headache comes on more slowly, with rash and fever often present). A posterior communicating aneurysm may present with a painful third nerve palsy with the pupil being affected before eye movements. This is due to rapid expansion of the aneurysm, causing it to press on the third cranial nerve. It is a neurosurgical emergency as the aneurysm may rupture at any time.

23. A, B, C, D

With third-generation CT scanners, SAH can be diagnosed on CT scan alone with >90 per cent accuracy within the first 24 h after the bleed. If the history is good and the CT scan is negative, LP must be performed. LP should not be performed too early as xanthochromia takes time to develop. A traumatic tap can cause confusion. Spectrophotometry of CSF is very helpful. A bilirubin peak is diagnostic of SAH. Xanthochromia will not be detectable to the naked eye 2 h after the bleed. It is usual to perform LP 12 h after the onset of headache.

Arteriovenous malformations

24. A, B, C, E

The risk of rebleed is 2–4 per cent per year. This is greater if aneurysms are seen on the feeding vessels. AVMs often cause epilepsy but are not usually associated with hydrocephalus. They can be treated by surgery, endovascular techniques or stereotactic radiotherapy. It often takes a combination of these to fully treat a large AVM.

Epilepsy surgery

25. A, B, C, D

Corpus callosotomy can often cure drop attacks. Focal abnormalities such as cortical dysplasias and low-grade tumours can be good surgical targets. Mesial temporal gliosis affects the hippocampus. This can be seen to be abnormal on MRI scan. Ictal SPECT is being increasingly used to identify seizure foci. The amygdala is a medial temporal structure.

Parkinson's disease

26. A, B, D, E

Parkinson's disease presents with tremor (pill-rolling) and dystonia. The usual treatment for Parkinson's disease is L-dopa. Some patients can be treated with deep brain stimulation. Targets for stimulation include the subthalamic nucleus and globus pallidus. The hypothalamus is not involved in Parkinson' disease.

Trigeminal neuralgia

27. B, C

Trigeminal neuralgia is a painful condition affecting one-half of the face. It can affect one or more divisions of the trigeminal nerve. The pain is severe and episodic. The pain can be precipitated by eating or brushing teeth or by light touch. It can be caused by multiple sclerosis but in many cases a vascular loop can be seen in contact with the 5th nerve, close to its root entry zone.

A red eye and runny nose is not typical of trigeminal neuralgia.

Carpal tunnel syndrome

28. A, C, D, E

Carpal tunnel syndrome is caused by compression of the median nerve at the wrist. Causes include age (due to 'wear and tear' changes in the carpal bones and thickening of the tendon sheaths and transverse carpal ligament), hypothyroidism and pregnancy. Patients typically wake at night with pain and paraesthesia in the thumb, index and middle fingers. Symptoms can be provoked by driving and reading a newspaper in many cases. Flexion of the wrist may well bring on the symptoms. This is known as Phalen's test. Tinel's test is performed by tapping the nerve over the carpal tunnel and eliciting paraesthesia.

In milder cases, wrist splints worn at night can be helpful. The diagnosis can be confirmed with nerve conduction tests. Sometimes surgery is required to decompress the carpal tunnel.

41 The eye and orbit

Multiple choice questions

➜ Tears

1. **How do tears produced in the lacrimal gland enter the conjunctival sac?**

A Through the nasolacrimal duct
B Through the lacrimal duct
C Through the 10–15 lacrimal gland ducts
D Through the meibomian orifices
E Through the ducts of Moll.

➜ Spread of infection

2. **What is a potential route of spread of infection from the eyelid skin to the intracranial cavity?**

A Orbital lymphatics
B Ophthalmic veins
C Subperiosteal potential spaces
D Facial artery
E Perineura of branches of the trigeminal nerve.

➜ Meibomian cysts

3. **What does a meibomian cyst consist of?**

A A meibomian eyelash follicle infection
B A sebaceous ('meibomian') cyst of the eyelid margin skin
C A meibomian sweat gland inclusion cyst
D Chronic granulomatous inflammation of a meibomian gland
E An epidermoid cyst of embryonic meibomian structures.

4. **How are persistent meibomian cysts treated?**

A Incision and curettage from the conjunctival surface
B Incision and curettage from the eyelid margin surface
C Incision and insertion of a small pack
D Long-term oral antibiotic therapy
E Excision biopsy.

➜ Basal cell carcinoma

5. **How should a recent-onset suspected basal cell carcinoma of the eyelid skin be treated?**

A Photograph and clinical follow-up
B Liquid nitrogen cryotherapy
C Curettage
D Excision biopsy
E Radiotherapy.

➜ Infection of the tear sac

6. **What is the typical cause of acute infection of the tear sac (acute dacryocystitis)?**

A Spread of infection from the ethmoid sinus
B Nasolacrimal duct obstruction
C Spread of infection from the maxillary sinus
D Spread of infection from the nasal mucosa
E Viral infection of the lacrimal gland.

➜ Dysthyroid exophthalmos

7. **In acute dysthyroid exophthalmos, when should urgent orbital decompression surgery be considered?**

A Diplopia is present.
B Raised intraocular pressure is present.
C Fat prolapse into the eyelids is present.
D Eyelid oedema is present.
E Compressive optic neuropathy is present.

➜ Retinoblastoma

8. **How does retinoblastoma, a malignant tumour of the retina, commonly present in young children?**

A Reduced vision
B Pain

C A swollen eye
D A white pupil reflex
E Regional lymphadenopathy.

➜ Ocular tumour

9. What is the most common ocular tumour in adults?

A Lung carcinoma metastases to the retina
B Choroidal malignant melanoma
C Choroidal sarcoma
D Retinal glioma
E Choroidal epithelioma.

➜ Herpes simplex infection of the cornea

10. How is herpes simplex infection of the cornea typically diagnosed?

A Viral culture of cases of conjunctivitis.
B The presence of typical herpetic vesicles on the eyelid skin.
C The presence of a branching pattern of epithelial fluorescein staining.
D The presence of a herpetic vesicle of the corneal epithelium on fluorescein staining.
E The presence of an inflamed 'phlycten' lump at the junction of the cornea and sclera.

➜ Fracture of the orbit

11. How is a 'blow-out' fracture of the orbit typically seen on radiography?

A Fracture of the ethmoid lamina papyraceum
B Blood in the ethmoid sinus
C Blood in the maxillary antrum
D Air in the orbit
E Soft-tissue prolapse in the maxillary antrum.

➜ Hyphaema

12. What does the finding of hyphaema following blunt trauma indicate?

A That the anterior chamber should be washed out promptly, in order to prevent corneal staining.
B That thrombolytic treatment should be given immediately in order to prevent the development of glaucoma.
C That strict bedrest, with bandaging of the affected eye, should be instituted immediately in order to prevent secondary haemorrhage.
D That associated intracranial haemorrhage is likely, and a cranial CT scan should be ordered immediately.
E That the eye should be carefully examined for associated injuries, especially of the retina.

➜ Irregular pupil

13. A front-seat passenger in a road traffic accident presents with facial lacerations and an irregular pupil in one eye. What is the most likely cause of the irregular pupil?

A A perforating injury of the globe, with some iris prolapse
B Blunt trauma to the pupil sphincter
C A partial third cranial nerve injury
D Traumatic Horner's syndrome
E Distortion of the anterior lens capsule due to traumatic cataract development.

➜ Intraocular foreign body

14. When an intraocular foreign body due to a hammer and chisel injury is suspected, which of the following imaging techniques should not be ordered?

A Plain radiograph of the eye and orbit
B Ultrasound examination of the eye
C Magnetic resonance imaging (MRI) scan of the eye and orbit
D Computed tomography (CT) scan of the eye and orbit
E Optical tomography of the eye.

➜ Tissue burns with ischaemic necrosis

15. Which of the following are most likely to cause severe tissue burns with ischaemic necrosis?

A Acid chemicals
B Alkaline chemicals
C Ultraviolet radiation
D Thermal energy
E Ionising radiation.

Herpes simplex corneal infection

16. Which of the following topical treatments are contraindicated for herpes simplex corneal infection?

A Aciclovir ointment
B Atropine eye drops
C Steroid eye drops
D Chloramphenicol eye drops
E Non-steroidal anti-inflammatory eye drops.

Painful, red eye

17. Which of the following may cause a painful, red eye accompanied by vomiting?

A Conjunctivitis
B Iritis
C Acute glaucoma
D Episcleritis
E Keratitis.

Investigation of loss of vision

18. Which of the following suspected diagnoses requires immediate measurement of erythrocyte sedimentation rate (ESR) and C-reactive protein (CRP) level?

A Retinal detachment
B Central retinal vein occlusion
C Posterior vitreous detachment
D Cranial arteritis
E Macular degeneration.

Surgical techniques

19. What does LASIK refer to?

A Laser in situ keratomileusis
B Laser-assisted interstitial keratectomy
C Long-acting stromal inhibition keratotomy
D Laser epithelial keratomileusis
E Lateral segment interstitial keratotomy.

20. Following cataract surgery, how might thickened posterior lens capsule tissue be cut?

A Ruby laser capsulotomy
B Photodisruptive YAG (yttrium aluminium garnet) laser capsulotomy
C Photoablative argon laser capsulotomy
D Photodisruptive eximer laser capsulotomy
E Diode laser capsulotomy.

21. What is removed in the operation of eyeball evisceration?

A The intact eyeball, along with short portions of the extraocular muscles
B The complete contents of the orbit, within the orbital periosteum
C The vitreous body of the eye
D The crystalline lens and the vitreous body of the eye
E The cornea and the contents of the eye within the sclera.

22. What is used in incision and curettage of a meibomian cyst?

A A skin incision tangential to the lid margin
B A skin incision radial to the lid margin
C A tarsal conjunctiva incision tangential to the lid margin
D A tarsal conjunctiva incision radial to the lid margin
E An eyelid crease skin incision.

Extended matching questions

1. Initial investigations

A Arrange plain skull X-rays.
B Measure blood pressure, random blood glucose and full blood count.
C No investigations. Contact the duty ophthalmologist.
D Arrange urgent CT scan of the orbits.
E Send blood for ESR and CRP.
F Arrange urgent abdominal ultrasound.
G Send blood for connective tissue diseases screen.

H Discuss urgent MR angiogram with the duty neuroradiologist.
I Request urgent measurement of ophthalmic artery perfusion using Doppler ultrasound.
J Measure blood pressure, random blood glucose and request carotid duplex ultrasound.

Choose the correct action to be taken by the A&E doctor with each of the following scenarios:

1 An 83-year-old woman presents with sudden loss of vision on the right eye, and gives a 3-week history of scalp tenderness. On ophthalmoscopy the right optic disc is pale and oedematous. You suspect cranial arteritis. What initial investigation(s) would you arrange?

2 A 63-year-old male presents with an acute-onset, complete right third cranial nerve palsy and headache. You are concerned about a possible intracranial aneurysm. What initial investigation(s) would you arrange?

3 A 67-year-old female presents with a painful left eye and vomiting. The symptoms have been present for 18 h. The eye is red, the cornea is hazy, the pupil is large and does not react, and the eye feels hard to palpation. What initial investigation(s) would you arrange?

4 A 70-year-old female presents with acute loss of vision in the right eye. On ophthalmoscopy there are numerous retinal haemorrhages in the eye, and a central retinal vein occlusion is suspected. What initial investigation(s) would you arrange?

5 A 70-year-old male presents with acute loss of vision in the left eye. On ophthalmoscopy the retina is pale, with a cherry red spot at the fovea. You suspect a central retinal artery occlusion. What initial investigation(s) would you arrange?

→ 2. Eyelid lumps

A Squamous cell carcinoma
B Lacrimal sac mucocele
C Molluscum contagiosum
D Lacrimal gland tumour
E Sebaceous cyst
F Dermoid cyst
G Preseptal cellulitis
H Meibomian cyst
I Cyst of Moll
J Basal cell carcinoma

Choose the correct diagnosis for each of the scenarios given below:

1 A 2-year-old child presents with acute swelling and redness of the eyelids of the left eye. The underlying eye and orbit appear normal.

2 A 16-year-old male presents with a slightly red, firm lump deep to the skin of the left lower eyelid. It has been present for several months and remains unchanged in size. It is not painful.

3 A 72-year-old female presents with a tense, fluctuant swelling just medial to the medial canthus of the left eye.

4 A 9-year-old girl presents with a small, firm lump at the margin of the left upper eyelid. The left eye has been intermittently red and irritable for 6 weeks.

5 A 70-year-old male presents with a slowly enlarging pearl-coloured, firm, smooth lump on the skin of the right lower eyelid. The lump has a small, central crater that tends to bleed at times.

3. Causes of red eye

A Acute angle closure glaucoma
B Allergic conjunctivitis
C Subconjunctival haemorrhage
D Uveitis
E Scleritis
F Bacterial conjunctivitis
G Adenovirus conjunctivitis
H Bacterial keratitis
I Scleritis
J Herpes simplex keratitis.

Choose the correct diagnosis for each of the scenarios given below:

1 A 23-year-old male presents with pain and photophobia of the right eye. On examination the vision is slightly reduced, there is pink coloration around the edge of the cornea, and the pupil is small and irregular.

2 A 33-year-old female presents with an irritable right eye. The vision is slightly blurred and the eye is slightly red. When fluorescein dye is instilled, there is an area of branching-shaped staining of the corneal epithelium.

3 A 63-year-old female presents with a bright red discoloration of the temporal part of the sclera of the right eye. Her vision is normal and she has no discomfort.

4 A 12-year-old girl presents with red, sticky eyes. On awakening in the morning, the eyelids are crusted and stuck together. Her vision remains normal.

5 A 55-year-old female presents with moderately severe pain in the right eye. On examination the temporal and superior sclera is a deep red colour, with some overlying oedema.

4. Management of ocular trauma

A Instil antibiotic ointment and place an eye pad over the eye.
B Commence prophylactic intravenous antibiotics and perform a temporary tarsorrhaphy.
C Instil local anaesthetic and perform irrigation of the cornea and of the conjunctival sac with saline
D Arrange plain X-ray or CT scan of the eyes.
E Arrange ultrasound examination of the orbits.
F Arrange a CT scan of the facial and orbital bones, to include coronal views.
G Arrange an MRI scan of the eyes and orbits.
H Arrange examination under anaesthetic and surgical repair as required.
I Take a corneal scrape for bacterial culture.
J Irrigate the cornea and conjunctiva with weak acetic acid, until the pH is neutral.

Choose the correct management actions for each of the scenarios given below:

1 A 23-year-old male was punched in the right eye. There is some bruising of the eyelids, but the eye is intact. However, he complains of double vision and has restricted eye movement on attempted upward gaze.

2 A 48-year-old male was grinding metal and presents with a metal foreign body adherent to the cornea. You instil local anaesthetic, and remove the foreign body with a needle.

3 A 36-year-old male was hammering a metal block with a chisel. He was not wearing eye protection. His right eye suddenly became painful, with blurred vision. There is a small conjunctival laceration just lateral to the cornea, with associated subconjunctival haemorrhage.

4 A 33-year-old male was washing out a glass container that contained alkaline liquid. Some of the liquid splashed into his right eye and the eye is now very painful.

5 A 55-year-old man was punched in the right eye during a fight. The vision is reduced and there is a large volume of subconjunctival haemorrhage. The pupil is distorted, the anterior chamber is shallow and you think there may be some prolapsed iris tissue.

Answers: Multiple choice questions

→ Tears

1. C

The lacrimal gland lies under the upper, outer orbital rim and opens into the upper conjunctival fornix through 10–15 ducts. Trauma, surgery or inflammatory scarring in this area can result in a dry eye.

→ Spread of infection

2. B

The orbit contains branches of the ophthalmic veins, which anastomose anteriorly with the face and posteriorly with the cranial cavity. These channels can provide a route for the spread of sepsis.

→ Meibomian cysts

3. D

The meibomian glands are situated within the tarsal plates, and open at the eyelid margin. Retention cysts of the meibomian glands result in the accumulation of granulomatous reaction around meibomian lipid secretions. A meibomian cyst is a chronic granulomatous inflammation of a meibomian gland.

4. A

Meibomian cysts often resolve spontaneously over a period of months. However, persistent meibomian cysts may be treated by inclusion and curettage from the conjunctival surface. Atypical or recurrent cysts should be biopsied.

→ Basal cell carcinoma

5. D

Recent-onset basal cell carcinoma may be treated by excision biopsy, with histological confirmation that the excision has been complete. More extensive lesions may require treatment with Mohs' micrographic surgical excision.

→ Infection of the tear sac

6. B

Obstruction of the nasolacrimal duct may lead to formation of a mucocele within the tear sac. If this becomes infected, acute dacryocystitis occurs. Following initial antibiotic treatment, a dacryocystorhinostomy bypass operation should be performed.

→ Dysthyroid exophthalmos

7. E

Orbital decompression surgery may be needed when compression of the optic nerve results in reduced vision. Systemic glucocorticoid therapy may be used to provide temporary control, pending surgery.

Retinoblastoma

8. D

These tumours are often calcified, and frequently present with the appearance of a white pupil reflex. They may also present with a squint, and all children with a squint should have a careful fundus examination performed.

Ocular tumour

9. B

Malignant melanoma of the uvea (iris, ciliary body, choroid) is the most common tumour in adults. It most often arises in the choroid, and the prognosis is less good for choroid lesions than for the iris. Treatment by brachytherapy or proton beam irradiation may be performed in order to preserve the eye, but enucleation is needed in some cases. The most common site of metastasis is the liver.

Herpes simplex infection of the cornea

10. C

Fluorescein staining of the corneal epithelium, viewed in blue light, demonstrates any epithelial disturbance. Herpes simplex infection causes a typical branching ('dendritic') pattern of staining.

Fracture of the orbit

11. E

The floor of the orbit is the weakest point when the orbital pressure is acutely elevated by blunt trauma. This results in a 'blow-out' fracture, with downward prolapse or the inferior orbital tissues. Reduced upward eye movement results.

Hyphaema

12. E

Hyphaema refers to blood in the anterior chamber following blunt trauma. Hyphaema can be followed by secondary haemorrhage, with related raised intraocular pressure. However, associated injuries to other structures of the eye, especially the retina, may be present.

Irregular pupil

13. A

Perforating eye injuries are less common when seatbelts are worn. Perforating injuries of the cornea and adjacent sclera result in areas of iris prolapse. The pupil becomes distorted, due to displacement of the iris. The eye should not be extensively examined, but should be protected with a shield, pending examination under anaesthetic and primary surgical repair.

Intraocular foreign body

14. C

Intraocular foreign bodies are often composed of ferrous metal in this situation. A magnetic field will result in movement of the foreign body within the eye, with resulting iatrogenic trauma.

Tissue burns with ischaemic necrosis

15. B

Alkaline chemicals penetrate tissues quickly, and can cause extensive ischaemia and necrosis. Immediate irrigation is required, and should be continued until a neutral pH is obtained.

Herpes simplex corneal infection

16. C

Herpes simplex corneal infections show a characteristic branching ('dendritic') pattern when stained with fluorescein dye. They should be treated with topical antiviral preparations such as aciclovir ointment. Steroid eye drops cause marked worsening of the infection, which may result in severe corneal scarring.

Painful, red eye

17. C

Acute elevation of intraocular pressure results in an oedematous cornea and a hard eye on palpation. The severe, visceral pain that accompanies acute glaucoma may cause vomiting, and the condition may be mistaken for an acute abdominal diagnosis.

Investigation of loss of vision

18. D

The ESR and CRP are often very elevated in cranial arteritis. Prompt diagnosis, leading to prompt therapy with glucocorticoids, can prevent blindness due to bilateral arteritic anterior ischaemic optic neuropathy.

Surgical techniques

19. A

A superficial corneal flap is cut, and a layer of corneal stroma is ablated with an eximer laser. The flap is then repositioned.

20. B

Short pulses of YAG laser energy produce photodisruption, with no thermal effect. Tissues such as the posterior lens capsule, the iris and vitreous bands may be divided.

21. E

Evisceration refers to removal of all tissues within the sclera. The cornea is excised, and all intraocular tissues are removed with a curette. All fragments of the uveal tract (iris, ciliary body and choroid) are removed.

22. D

The incision is made on the inner surface of the eyelid, in order to avoid a visible scar. The incision is radial to the lid margin, in line with the affected meibomian gland, in order to avoid cicatricial shortening of the tarsal plate.

Answers: Extended matching questions

1. Initial investigations

1E

A high index of suspicion should be maintained for cranial arteritis. The ESR and CRP are usually elevated. Prompt treatment with glucocorticoids may prevent bilateral blindness.

2H

The combination of acute third cranial nerve palsy and pain is suggestive of an intracranial aneurysm. Prompt treatment may prevent catastrophic subarachnoid haemorrhage.

3C

Acute angle closure glaucoma causes severe pain, which may result in vomiting and be mistaken for an acute abdominal pathology.

4B

Underlying causes for central retinal vein occlusions include hypertension, diabetes and hyperviscosity syndromes (and glaucoma). These should be treated, if detected, and the patient should be referred for a 'soon' ophthalmology outpatient appointment.

5J

In addition to asking if the patient smokes, causes of arteriosclerosis should be sought. Therapy is based on reduction of cardiovascular risk factors, aspirin and assessment for possible carotid endarterectomy surgery.

2. Eyelid lumps

1G

Cellulitis of the eyelids is often due to underlying sinus disease. Aggressive antibiotic treatment is needed.

2H

Meibomian cysts are retention cysts of the meibomian glands, and contain sebaceous material. They slowly resolve spontaneously, but may be incised on the inner aspect of the eyelid, and curetted if this is desired.

3B

A mucocele of the lacrimal sac occurs when proximal and distal outflow from the sac are occluded. Recurrent infection may occur, and the definitive treatment consists of dacryocystorhinostomy surgery.

4C

Viruses shed from molluscum contagiosum lesions cause a recurring viral conjunctivitis. The lesion may be curetted, excised or treated with cryotherapy.

5J

Basal cell carcinomas are a common form of eyelid skin neoplasia. They are locally invasive, and must be fully excised with a generous margin.

3. Causes of red eye

1D

Anterior uveitis, in which the iris is inflamed, results in spasm of the pupil sphincter muscle and adhesions between the iris and the lens. Deposits of inflammatory cells may be seen on the inner surface of the cornea. Treatment is with pupil-dilating eye drops and steroid eye drops.

2J

Herpes simplex infection of the corneal epithelium typically causes a branching-patterned disturbance of the corneal epithelium. Treatment is with aciclovir ointment. Steroid treatment must be avoided, as this will cause severe worsening of the condition and permanent scarring.

3C

Subconjunctival haemorrhages look dramatic but are of no functional significance. They may occur following straining, coughing, sneezing or minor trauma. They are said to be associated with hypertension. However, typically no underlying cause is evident.

4F
Bacterial conjunctivitis is a common, self-limiting condition. Typically there is a purulent exudation. Antibiotic eye drops slightly shorten the duration of the infection, but are unnecessary, as the condition is self-limiting.

5E
Scleritis is a form of connective tissue inflammation, frequently associated with rheumatoid arthritis. The inflammation may be controlled with non-steroidal anti-inflammatory drugs, but in more severe cases, glucocorticoids are needed.

4. Management of ocular trauma

1F
The clinical features are typical of 'blow-out' fracture of the floor of the orbit, with entrapment of soft tissues attached to the inferior rectus muscle. The fracture, and soft tissues prolapsed into the maxillary antrum, will be demonstrated with coronal CT scan views of the orbital floor.

2A
After removal of a corneal foreign body, there is risk of infection and the eye is painful. Antibiotic ointment and an eye pad are generally used in this circumstance. This treatment is also appropriate for a corneal abrasion.

3D
There is a high likelihood of the presence of a metallic intraocular foreign body in this circumstance. Even very small radio-opaque foreign bodies may be demonstrated with a plain X-ray or CT scan. Ultrasound examination may be done very gently, but there is a risk of causing further injury by pressing on the eye. MRI scanning is absolutely contraindicated, as a magnetic field will cause movement of an intraocular ferrous foreign body, with further injury.

4C
A large volume of saline should be used to irrigate the eye, until all traces of alkaline chemical have been removed. Alkaline substances are much more damaging than other chemicals, as they denature proteins and penetrate deeply into the tissues.

5H
It is very likely that the eye has been ruptured. Attempts to examine the eye in further detail may result in further injury. A more complete examination should be performed under anaesthetic. The injury should be explored, and a primary repair performed.

Cleft lip and palate: developmental abnormalities of face, mouth and jaws

Multiple choice questions

➜ Cleft palate – general

1. **Which of the following statements about cleft palate are true?**
   - A The incidence of cleft lip and palate is 1 in 6000 live births.
   - B The incidence of cleft palate is 1 in 1000 live births.
   - C The typical distribution of cleft lip alone is 35 per cent.
   - D The typical distribution of isolated cleft palate is 40 per cent.
   - E Cleft palate alone is more common in males.

➜ Orofacial congenital abnormalities

2. **Which of the following statements regarding congenital abnormalities are true?**
   - A The most common congenital abnormalities of the orofacial structures are cleft lips, alveolus and palate.
   - B They are also an associated feature in over 300 recognised syndromes.
   - C There is an increased incidence in the black population.
   - D Genetics and the environment both play a part in causation.
   - E Family history with a first-degree relative affected increases the risk to 1 in 100 live births.

➜ Causes and syndromes

3. **Which of the following statements regarding causal factors of cleft lip and palate are true?**
   - A Environmental factors are less important for cleft palates than for cleft lip/palate.
   - B Environmental maternal epilepsy is one factor not associated with clefts.
   - C Down's syndrome may be associated with clefts.
   - D Apert's and Treacher–Collins syndromes are not associated with clefts.
   - E An isolated cleft palate is more commonly associated with a syndrome than cleft lip alone.

➜ Pierre Robin syndrome

4. **Which of the following statements are true?**
   - A Pierre Robin syndrome is the commonest syndrome associated with clefts.
   - B Pierre Robin syndrome includes glossoptosis.
   - C Retrognathia is not a feature of the Pierre Robin syndrome.
   - D Pierre Robin syndrome is named after the first patient in whom the condition was described in 1729.
   - E Pierre Robin syndrome is associated with early respiratory and feeding difficulties.

➜ Muscle and structural considerations

5. **Which of the following statements are true?**
   - A In cleft lip there is disruption of the 2 groups of muscles of the upper lip and nasolabial region.
   - B In bilateral cleft lip, the disruption is associated with a prolabium.
   - C Prolabial tissue contains muscle tissue.

D The secondary palate is defined as the structures anterior to the incisive foramen.
E Cleft palate results in failure of fusion of the 2 palatine shelves.

➜ Further anatomical consideration

6. Which of the following statements are true?

A In a complete cleft palate, the nasal septum and vomer are completely separated from the palatine processes.
B In a cleft of the soft palate, the muscle fibres are orientated wrongly but insert into the posterior edge of the hard palate.
C In a submucous soft-palate cleft, the mucosa is not intact.
D The LAHSHAL system of classification describes the features of a cleft.
E Using the LAHSHAL classification, the incomplete right unilateral cleft lip and incomplete cleft of soft palate extending onto the hard palate are represented by lahSh.

➜ Use of scans in clefts and respiratory and nutritional considerations

7. Which of the following statements are true?

A Antenatal scans are useful in the early diagnosis of cleft palates.
B As a result of scan results, the parents-to-be should get appropriate support and counselling.
C Diagnosis by scan of a cleft can be made before 15 weeks of gestation.
D Most babies born with a cleft lip and palate feed well and thrive.
E Major respiratory problems occur exclusively in Pierre Robin syndrome.

➜ Pierre Robin syndrome problems and muscle structure in clefts

8. Which of the following statements are true?

A Labioglossopexy is not a procedure used in Pierre Robin syndrome problems.
B Hypoxia is more likely to occur in the awake Pierre Robin baby than during sleep.
C In cleft surgery the emphasis is repair of the muscles.
D There are 4 muscles of the soft palate.
E Tensor palati is a soft palate muscle.

➜ Repair of cleft lip and palate

9. Which of the following statements are true?

A Restoration of normal anatomy does not encourage normal facial growth in cleft surgery.
B Cleft lip repair is usually performed between 3 and 6 months of age.
C Cleft palate repair is frequently performed between 19 and 24 months.
D A two-stage repair of cleft palate means more tissue damage occurs.
E The Delaire method of repair of a cleft lip is the only satisfactory method for cleft lip closure.

➜ Team approach in clefts and care of the ear

10. Which of the following statements are true?

A Management of clefts requires a multidisciplinary team approach.
B Long-term review is not required.
C In cleft palate, Eustachian tube dysfunction is not the cause of otitis media.
D Early (6–12 months) prophylactic myringotomy and grommet insertion temporarily eliminate middle ear effusion.
E Regular audiology tests should always be done during childhood.

➜ Speech problems

11. Which of the following statements regarding speech problems in cleft patients are true?

A Speech problems are common in cleft palate patients.
B Assessment should be performed at 18 months.

C Speech problems are not associated with airflow.
D Velopharyngeal incompetence is associated with hyponasal speech.
E Speech problems are managed by speech and language therapy, surgery and speech training devices.

Dental care

12. Which of the following statements regarding dental care in cleft patients are true?

A Tooth management is not usually an issue in cleft cases.
B Orthodontic care should only be done in cases where dentition is diseased or poorly maintained.
C. An abnormal number or eruption problems of teeth rarely occur in cleft patients.
D Orthodontic treatment is commonly carried out at 8–10 years and 14–18 years.
E Expansion of the maxillary arches is done at 14–18 years.

Revisional surgery

13. Which of the following statements are true?

A Revisional lip surgery in previously repaired cleft lips should usually be delayed for 2 years unless the original muscle repair has been judged inadequate.
B Nasal deformity confirms incomplete reconstruction of skin deformity.
C The Cupid's bow is an important cosmetic area of the soft palate.
D Alveolar bone grafts should be performed long before orthodontics are considered.
E Alveolar bone grafts are useful in closing residual fistula of the anterior palate.

Bone grafts

14. Which of the following statements are true?

A Alveolar bone grafts are able to receive an osseointegrated dental implant.
B Alveolar bone grafts cannot be used with simultaneous secondary lip revision.
C Alveolar bone grafts are obtained from the humerus and femur.
D It is useful to ensure a tooth erupts into the alveolar bone graft.
E Failure of D results in bone absorption in the long term.

Surgical repair

15. Which of the following statements are true?

A Orthognathic surgery is designed to correct poor mid-face growth.
B Elective setback of the maxilla is the method of choice to correct the mid-face problem.
C Mandibular advancement may also help.
D Orthognathic surgery does not commence until the age of 6 years.
E Major osteotomies are required in Apert's and Crouzon's syndromes when a craniofacial team working in designated centres must be involved.

Role of nasal surgery and audit

16. Which of the following statements are true?

A Open rhinoplasty is not a procedure to be done after orthognathic surgery.
B Open rhinoplasty is indicated when there is dislocation of cartilaginous septum into the cleft nostril.
C Open rhinoplasty is also indicated when there is collapse of the lower lateral cartilage on the cleft side.
D Tip projection of the nose cannot be improved by a postauricular onlay graft.
E Meticulous record-keeping, including speech recordings and audits, are essential in the overall care of cleft patients.

Tooth structure in cleft lip patients

17. Which of the following statements regarding tooth structure are true?

A Partial anodontia is not found in cleft lip patients.

B Removal of supernumerary teeth encourages eruption of secondary dentition.
C Genetic disorders can cause changes in structure and attrition of teeth.
D Measles does not cause defects in the structure of teeth
E Tetracycline can cause defects in the structure of teeth.

Tooth eruption

18. Which of the following statements regarding tooth eruption are true?

A Eruption of teeth may be impaired by a dentigerous cyst.
B Eruption of teeth is not a problem in cleidocranial dysostosis.
C Management of partial anodontia is not possible.
D Management of unerupted teeth involves removal of any obstruction, including overcrowding caused by supernumerary teeth.
E The most common site for supernumerary teeth is in the mandible.

Mandible and maxilla problems

19. Which of the following statements are true?

A Dental occlusion problems can arise when there is disproportion in growth between the maxilla and the mandible.
B Class 11 occlusion deformity is associated with over development of the mandible.
C Condylar hyperplasia is an idiopathic condition occurring between 35 and 45 years of age.
D Condylar hyperplasia causes asymmetrical growth of the jaw in both the vertical and horizontal planes.
E Facial disproportionate growth is not a feature of Treacher–Collins syndrome.

Deformities of the jaw – investigation and treatment plans

20. Which of the following statements are true?

A A bone scan is a useful investigation in condylar hyperplasia.
B Orthognathic surgery is the term given to surgical correction of deformities of the jaw.
C A combination between orthodontic and maxillofacial surgeons is important in orthognathic surgery.
D Treatment planning usually begins with orthodontic treatment at the age of 17–18 years.
E Cephalometric studies are of little value in the above planning.

Answers: Multiple choice questions

Cleft palate – general

1. B, D

The incidence of cleft lip and palate is 1 in 600 live births and that of isolated cleft palate is 1 in 1000 live births. Cleft lip alone comprises 15 per cent of all clefts while cleft palate alone comprises 40 per cent. The latter is more common in females.

Orofacial congenital abnormalities

2. A, B, D

The commonest orofacial congenital abnormalities are cleft lips, alveoli and cleft palates. There are at least 300 recognised syndromes that have associated cleft problems. The black population does not have an increased cleft incidence, but it is increased in ethnic Chinese and is highest among the Native American tribes of Montana, USA. Both genetic and environmental factors play a part in causation. A family history of a cleft in a first-degree relative increases the risk to 1 in 25 live births.

Causes and syndromes

3. C, E

The environment is of greater importance in cleft palate than in cleft lip and palate. Environmental factors implicated in clefts include maternal epilepsy and drugs, including steroids, diazepam and phenytoin. Down's, Apert's, and Treacher–Collins syndromes can be associated with clefts, especially an isolated cleft palate.

Pierre Robin syndrome

4. A, B, E

Pierre Robin was a professor of dentistry, who described the syndrome in 1929. Glossoptosis and retrognathia in this syndrome contribute to early respiratory and feeding problems. It is the commonest syndrome associated with clefts.

Muscle and structural considerations

5. A, B, E

Cleft lip is caused by disruption of the nasolabial and bilabial muscles with this more profound and symmetrical in bilateral clefts. The prolabium has no muscle tissue and is associated with bilateral cleft lips. The secondary palate is found posterior to the incisor foramen and a cleft palate is the result of failure in fusion of 2 palatine shelves.

Further anatomical consideration

6. A, B, D

In complete cleft palate, the nasal septum and the vomer are separated from the palatine processes. The attachment of the muscle fibres is into the posterior edge of the hard palate in a cleft of the soft palate. In submucous clefts of the soft palate, the mucosa is intact and a groove occurs as a result of muscle abnormality. Classification of clefts can be simplified using the LAHSHAL system – lahSh is an incomplete right unilateral cleft lip and alveolus with a complete cleft soft palate extending partly onto the hard palate.

Use of scans in clefts and respiratory and nutritional considerations

7. B, D, E

Antenatal scans are of use in diagnosing cleft lips but they are of no value in the diagnosis of cleft palates. Appropriate counselling should be given to prospective parents when the diagnosis has been made. Ultrasonic scans and diagnosis of cleft lips can be made after 18 weeks' gestation but not before. Feeding and thriving in cleft lip and palate babies are usually normal. Major respiratory problems occur in the Pierre Robin syndrome.

Pierre Robin syndrome problems and muscle structure in clefts

8. C, E

A technique that may be useful in preventing respiratory complications in Pierre Robin cases is labioglossopexy. In that syndrome, hypoxia occurs while asleep, not awake. Repair of muscle is the crucial thing in cleft repairs. There are 5 muscles that control activity in the soft palate, one of which is the tensor palati muscle.

Repair of cleft lip and palate

9. B

It is important in cleft surgery to encourage normal facial growth by restoring normal anatomy. Cleft lip repair is done at the age of 3–6 months, while cleft palates are repaired at 6 months.

When there are combined cleft lip and palates, usually there are 2 operations, the 2nd being the repair of the hard palate with or without lip revision at 15–18 months. A 2-stage repair of palatal clefts is sensible as well as being less destructive than a single-stage one. There are several techniques available for cleft repairs and the Millard methods have become popular in recent years.

Team approach in clefts and care of the ear

10. A, D, E

A multidisciplinary team approach is essential in the management of clefts as is long term review including audit of results. Otitis media is associated with cleft palate and Eustachian tube problems. Elective myringotomy and insertion of grommets at 6–12 months can eliminate middle ear effusion. Audiology tests should be always be done throughout childhood to check on potential hearing problems.

Speech problems

11. A, B, E

Speech problems are commonly found in cleft patients and are associated with airflow problems. They are assessed at the age of 18 months. Velopharyngeal incompetence is associated with hypernasal speech. The management of speech problems involves surgery, therapists, and speech training devices.

Dental care

12. D

Problems with teeth are common in cleft patients – orthodontic care is used to prevent disease and abnormal dentition, including eruption problems or abnormal numbers of teeth. It is done at 8–10 and 14–18 years of age. Expansion of the maxilla is done earlier than 14–18 years; this is when surgery to correct a malpositioned or retrusive maxilla by osteotomy is performed.

Revisional surgery

13. A, E

Any revision of previously repaired cleft lips is considered after 2 years. Nasal cleft deformities are the result of incomplete reconstruction of the nasolabial muscle ring. The Cupid's bow is an important cosmetic feature of the upper lip repair – and the normal lip. Alveolar bone grafts are done as a rule, though not always, after a period of orthodontics and can be useful in closing a fistula of the anterior palate.

Bone grafts

14. A, D, E

Alveolar bone graft can receive an osseointegrated dental implant and can be performed at the same time as secondary lip revision. Bone for grafting is obtained from the iliac crest or tibia. It is useful to get any teeth to erupt into the graft and failure for this to happen will result in bone absorption in the long term.

Surgical repair

15. A, E

Orthognathic surgery is used to correct poor mid-face growth problems. The mandible is set back while the maxilla is set forward when mid-face retrusion exists. This type of surgery is not performed at the age of 5 years but is best done before the canine tooth erupts – between 8 and 11 years. Major osteotomies in Apert's or Crouzon's syndromes are operated on by specialised craniofacial surgeons in designated centres.

Role of nasal surgery and audit

16. C, E

Open rhinoplasty is usually performed after orthognathic surgery has corrected facial structure and deformities. It is done when there is dislocation of the central septum into the non-cleft nostril and/or there is collapse of the lower lateral cartilage on the cleft side. Tip projection is done by using cartilage onlay graft material, which can be obtained from the ear – by either a postauricular or a preauricular approach. Meticulous record-keeping and audit and analysis over many years are essential in the overall management of cleft patients.

Tooth structure in cleft lip patients

17. B, C, E

Partial anodontia can be found in clefts, and removal of supernumerary teeth will encourage the eruption of secondary dentition. Genetic disorders can cause changes in the structure and attrition of teeth. Diseases, such as measles, and drugs, such as tetracycline, can also cause disorders of teeth.

Tooth eruption

18. A, D

Dentigerous cysts can cause non-eruption of teeth and this is also a feature of cleidocranial dysostosis. The management of partial anodontia is possible and management of unerupted teeth by removal of any obstruction including supernumerary teeth is very helpful. The most common site of supernumerary teeth is in the maxilla and not the mandible.

Mandible and maxilla problems

19. A, D

Dental occlusion disparity causes growth problems for the mandible and maxilla. In class 11 dental occlusion, the mandibular teeth are placed posterior to the maxillary teeth. Condylar hyperplasia occurs in the 15–30 year age group and causes abnormal growth of the jaw in both vertical and horizontal planes. Treacher–Collins syndrome is associated with facial growth disparity.

Deformities of the jaw – investigation and treatment plans

20. A, B, C

A bone scan is a useful method of examination in cases of condylar hyperplasia. The correction of jaw deformities is orthognatics surgery and the combination of orthodontics and maxillofacial surgery is important in orthognathic surgery. Orthodontic care should be done earlier than the age of 17–18 years. Cephalometric investigations are helpful and important in abnormalities of facial growth.

43 The nose and sinuses

Multiple choice questions

In the following, choose the single best answer.

➜ Anatomy of the nose and paranasal sinuses

1. **Which of the following sinuses do not open on to the lateral wall of the nose?**
   A Maxillary sinus
   B Ethmoid sinus
   C Frontal sinus
   D Sphenoid sinus
   E Septal sinus.

2. **Via which route does the greater palatine artery supply the nasal septum?**
   A Foramen rotundum
   B Vidian canal
   C Incisive canal
   D Sphenopalatine foramen
   E Cribriform plate.

3. **Intracranial drainage of venous blood from the nose and sinuses passes to the cavernous sinus via which route?**
   A Ophthalmic vein
   B Pharyngeal plexus
   C Pterygoid plexus
   D Facial vein
   E Supratrochlear vein.

➜ Imaging of the paranasal sinuses

4. **Which view(s) are necessary on computed tomography (CT) for detailed assessment of the sinuses?**
   A Coronal
   B Axial
   C Coronal and axial
   D Coronal and sagittal
   E Coronal, axial and sagittal.

➜ Trauma to the nose and paranasal sinuses

5. **Injury to which blood vessel is associated with severe post-traumatic epistaxis?**
   A External carotid artery
   B Facial artery
   C Sphenopalatine artery
   D Anterior ethmoid artery
   E Nasal artery.

6. **How can clear nasal discharge be confirmed as cerebrospinal fluid (CSF) rather than nasal mucus?**
   A High-resolution CT scanning
   B Glucose stick testing
   C T2-weighted MRI scanning
   D Endoscopic examination
   E Increased production with dependent head position.

7. **How should suspected nasal bone fracture be managed?**
   A Facial X-rays
   B Immediate manipulation
   C Review in clinic at 4–5 days
   D Arrangements for rhinoplasty
   E Examination under anaesthetic with or without manipulation.

8. **Which of the following is not a complication of nasal septal haematoma?**
   A Meningitis
   B Septal abscess
   C Cosmetic deformity
   D Cavernous sinus thrombosis
   E Ischaemia of the soft palate.

The nasal septum

9. **Which of the following procedures involve correction of a deviated nasal septum with preservation of cartilage?**
   A Submucous resection
   B Septoplasty
   C Turbinectomy
   D Submucous diathermy
   E Septodermoplasty.

10. **Which of the following is not included in the aetiology of nasal septal perforation?**
   A Allergy
   B Infection
   C Vasculitis
   D Malignancy
   E Toxic irritation.

11. **Which of the following are not complications of nasal septal perforation?**
   A Epistaxis
   B Whistling
   C Nasal obstruction
   D Nasal polyps
   E Cosmetic deformity.

Epistaxis

12. **Which of the following regarding Wegner's granulomatosis are true?**
   A It affects the nose alone
   B It is best diagnosed by CT scanning
   C It can affect the nose, lungs and kidneys
   D It is treated surgically
   E It tends to spare nasal septal cartilage.

13. **Which of the following is not a cause of epistaxis?**
   A Trauma
   B Foreign bodies
   C Infections
   D Granulomatous disorders
   E Old age.

14. **What gender/age group does juvenile angiofibroma tend to affect?**
   A Boys aged 10–14
   B Girls aged 10–14
   C Boys aged 14–18
   D Girls aged 14–18
   E Children aged 10–14.

15. **Which of the following statements about juvenile angiofibroma are true?**
   A It requires biopsy for diagnosis.
   B It should initially be treated medically.
   C It is associated with vascular malformations of the meninges.
   D It is diagnosed with imaging.
   E It may be cured by embolisation.

16. **What may be involved in the management of life-threatening epistaxis?**
   A Ligation of the facial artery
   B Ligation of the lingual artery
   C Ligation of the external carotid artery above the origin of the lingual artery
   D Ligation of the external carotid artery below the origin of the lingual artery
   E Ligation of the internal carotid artery.

17. **What should be included in the management of hereditary haemorrhagic telangiectasia (HHT)-related epistaxis?**
   A Nasal packing
   B Nasal cautery
   C Oestrogen creams
   D Ligation of the anterior ethmoidal artery
   E Platelet transfusion.

Nasal polyps

18. **Where do the majority of nasal polyps arise from?**
   A Maxillary sinuses
   B Ethmoid sinuses
   C Frontal sinuses
   D Sphenoid sinuses
   E Nasal septum.

19. **Which of the following is associated with nasal polyps?**
   A Penicillin allergy
   B Chronic bronchitis
   C Aspirin allergy
   D Gastric polyps
   E Medullary thyroid cancer.

20. **Which of the following are not commonly associated with nasal polyps?**
   A Epistaxis
   B Nasal obstruction

C Ansomia
D Rhinorrhoea
E Sinus infection.

21. Which of the following should be suspected in unilateral nasal polyps?
A Cystic fibrosis
B Malignancy
C Allergy
D Fungal infection
E Cocaine abuse.

22. Which of the following statements regarding surgery for nasal polyps are true?
A It is recommended in all patients fit for surgery.
B It is recommended as a long-term cure.
C It is recommended after failure of steroid treatments.
D It is recommended prior to CT scanning of the sinuses.
E It is performed through an external incision to allow excision with clear margins.

Sinusitis

23. What is the most likely organism in maxillary sinusitis?
A *Staphylococcus aureus*
B *Pseudomonas aeruginosa*
C *Streptococcus pneumoniae*
D *Chlamydia trachomatis*
E *Staphylococcus epidermidis.*

24. Where is a trochar usually inserted in antral lavage?
A Through the canine fossa
B Through the inferior meatus
C Through the middle meatus
D Percutaneously
E Through the natural maxillary sinus ostium.

25. In acute sinusitis, pus may be seen draining from which of the following?
A Inferior meatus
B Middle meatus
C Superior meatus
D Supreme meatus
E Nasolacrimal duct.

26. Which of the following is not a complication of acute frontoethmoidal sinusitis?
A Periorbital sinusitis
B Meningitis
C Extradural abscess
D Intracerebral abscess
E Gingivitis.

Tumours of the nose and sinuses

27. Which of the following statements about nasal tumours is true?
A The uncommon nature of symptoms from nasal tumours facilitates early diagnosis.
B Early cosmetic deformity allows for early diagnosis in nasal tumours.
C Missed diagnosis is common in nasal tumours given the non-specific symptoms.
D Nasal tumours tend to present with bilateral symptoms.
E Nasal tumours rarely grow sufficiently to cause nasal obstruction.

28. Which of the following statements regarding transitional cell papillomas are true?
A They only affect the nasal cavity.
B They have no association with malignancy.
C They are treated surgically as for simple polyps.
D They are sometimes diagnosed following routine nasal polypectomy.
E They do not erode bone.

29. Which of the following statements regarding adenocarcinoma of the nasal cavity are true?
A It is associated with exposure to hard wood dust
B It tends to arise from the nasal septum.
C It can be diagnosed on CT scanning.
D It is associated with watery rhinorrhoea.
E It tends to present in the early stages of disease.

30. **Which of the following statements is false?**
   - A Malignant tumours of the sinuses require a multidisciplinary approach.
   - B Malignant tumours of the sinuses require detailed cross-sectional imaging.
   - C Malignant tumours of the sinuses are treated with surgery alone.
   - D Malignant tumours of the sinuses should not be biopsied due to the risk of bleeding.
   - E Malignant tumours of the sinuses may present with locally invasive disease.

Extended matching questions

→ 1. Imaging of the nose and paranasal sinuses

- A Culture and sensitivity of nasal mucus
- B Facial X-rays
- C Non-contrast-enhanced CT scan of sinuses
- D Contrast-enhanced CT scan of sinuses
- E Mucosal biopsy and blood test for ESR and ANCA
- F Antral lavage
- G Biopsy under endoscopic control in clinic
- H Plain sinus X-rays
- I Sweat testing for cystic fibrosis
- J Outpatient review in 4–7 days.

Choose the most appropriate action for each of the clinical scenarios below:

1. An 18-year-old male attends the emergency department following alleged assault. Following clinical assessment, an isolated nasal fracture is suspected.
2. A 35-year-old female with simple nasal polyps has failed maximal medical therapy and wishes to consider surgical management.
3. A 16-year-old male presents with unilateral nasal obstruction and intermittent unilateral epistaxis.
4. A 25-year-old male presents with a 10-day history of unilateral facial pain, rhinorrhoea and systemic upset with opacification of the maxillary sinus on X-ray, unresponsive to antibiotics.
5. A 46-year-old female presents with bloodstained nasal discharge, nasal obstruction, haematuria and shortness of breath. Examination reveals a septal perforation and granulations on the nasal mucosa.

→ 2. Anatomy of the nose and paranasal sinuses

- A Anterior ethmoidal artery
- B Posterior ethmoidal artery
- C Sphenopalatine artery
- D Inferior meatus
- E Middle meatus
- F Superior meatus
- G Nasolacrimal duct
- H Maxillary sinus
- I Ethmoid sinus
- J Sphenoid sinus.

Choose the correct response for each question below:

1 Which vessel is most likely to cause significant post-traumatic epistaxis?

2 Where does the maxillary sinus ostium lie?

3 From which sinus does periorbital cellulitis usually spread?

4 What structure lies in the inferior meatus

5 Where do the openings of the posterior ethmoid sinuses lie?

Answers: Multiple choice questions

Anatomy of the nose and paranasal sinuses

1. D
2. C
3. A

Imaging of the paranasal sinuses

4. E

Both coronal and axial views are required to assess the sinuses prior to surgery. The coronal views are the most important and may require digital reconstruction. They allow accurate assessment of the cribriform plate, the insertion of the uncinate and the medial orbital wall (lamina papyracea). Axial views allow assessment of the posterior ethmoid cells and their relationship to the optic nerve. Sagittal views allow assessment of the frontal recess and should be inspected prior to surgery in this area.

Trauma to the nose and paranasal sinuses

5. D

The anterior ethmoid artery can be injured in trauma and splinted open by bony fragments of the lacrimal, ethmoid and frontal bones. Soft-tissue swelling may splint the vessel closed until the oedema subsides, leading to a delayed torrential haemorrhage. An external approach to this artery allows for control, through an incision placed at the midpoint between the medial canthus and the midline of the nose.

6. B

Clear rhinorrhoea following head trauma should raise the suspicion of CSF leak, which can be tested for using glucose sticks. A more accurate measure is beta-2-transferrin, which is present only in CSF and the aqueous humour. This requires specialised analysis and cannot be performed at the bedside.

Depending on the nature of the trauma, CSF leaks may be managed spontaneously in the first instance. Those that fail to cease spontaneously can be investigated using high-resolution CT, T2-weighted MRI or intrathecal fluorescein. Following identification of the site of the leak, the method of closure is dependent on site, size and surgical expertise. Transnasal approaches avoid an external scar and prevent retraction of the brain, but may not be suitable in all cases.

7. C

Although nasal fractures can be assessed and managed immediately, within the first hour, soft-tissue swelling prevents accurate assessment of the bony skeleton. It is very unusual for the clinician to see patients in time to treat these injuries at the first visit. Following a full assessment for associated injuries, and particularly for septal haematoma, which requires urgent treatment, arrangements should be made for review after 4–7 days when swelling has subsided. X-ray assessment was popular in the past, but clinical assessment is sufficient to diagnose the injury and false-negatives are common due to visible bony suture lines, so they are uncommonly performed today.

If a nasal injury is seen within a week and a fracture associated with a change in nasal shape is identified, simple manual manipulation under local or general anaesthetic arranged in the first 2–3 weeks allows for fracture reduction without the need to resort to rhinoplasty. Eighty per cent of patients will be satisfied with the results, and those who are not can be considered at that point for formal rhinoplasty.

8. E

Septal haematoma is generally a complication of nasal trauma, including surgery. Bleeding results from fracture of the nasal septum and blood collects between the mucoperichondrial flaps which surround the septum on both sides. The septum derives its blood supply from these flaps, and without these nutrients, the cartilage undergoes necrosis, leading to septal perforation. This loss of support can lead to collapse of the nasal skeleton with both cosmetic and functional effects.

The haematoma often becomes infected to form a septal abscess, which will result in increasing pain and pyrexia. Sepsis from this area drains to the cavernous sinus and can result in intracerebral sepsis, which in turn may be life-threatening. It is for this reason that the clinician must have a high index of suspicion of septal haematoma following injury. Treatment of septal haematoma involves aspiration under local anaesthetic, or incision and drainage under general anaesthetic, with nasal packing as required.

→ The nasal septum

9. B

Septoplasty involves straightening of the bony and cartilaginous nasal septum whilst aiming to preserve cartilage. Submucous resection was a procedure which predated septoplasty and involved resection of the deviated cartilage. Turbinectomy involves resection of the inferior turbinate, performed for enlarged turbinates, and submucous diathermy involves monopolar diathermy to the submucosal tissue of the inferior turbinate to encourage scarring and a reduction in turbinate volume. Septodermoplasty is a procedure rarely performed for persistent epistaxis in HHT patients. The mucosa of the nasal septum is excised and replaced with split-thickness skin grafts.

10. A

As with all conditions, the surgical sieve can be applied to septal perforation. Allergy, however, is not a recognised cause of perforation. Common causes include trauma, from surgery, nose picking and cocaine abuse. TB and syphilis infection should be considered as well as granulomatous conditions such as Wegener's granulomatosis and malignancy.

Investigation of septal perforations will be guided by history, but may include chest X-ray, bloods for antineutrophil cytoplasmic antibodies (ANCA) and syphilis serology, as well as biopsy of the perforation for histology.

11. D

Septal perforations are commonly asymptomatic; however, a feeling of nasal obstruction and crusting is common. As crusts break off, the exposed raw mucosa often bleeds repeatedly. Small anterior perforations can cause a whistling as air passes by. Large perforations can reduce the support of the nasal dorsum, leading to a saddle nose deformity with collapse of the middle third of the nose. This can lead to cosmetic and functional problems.

Treatment for septal perforation will be tailored to the complaints and many patients require no treatment at all. Crusting and bleeding can be treated with barrier creams such as soft liquid paraffin. Larger perforations can be fitted with a silastic obturator which occludes the perforation and can improve crusting and the feeling of obstruction. Patients who cannot tolerate such treatment can be considered for surgical closure of the perforation. Many procedures have been described, which is an indication that none has proven to be uniformly successful.

Epistaxis

12. C

Wegener's granulomatosis results in a vasculitis which can affect any organ in the body, but commonly involves the nose, lungs and kidneys. Diagnosis requires histology, which can be achieved by renal biopsy or biopsy of active nasal granulomata. Nasal manifestations include bloodstained nasal discharge and nasal obstruction. Granuloma may lead to septal perforation and further complications. Treatment is medical and often coordinated by the physician rather than the ENT surgeon. Surgical correction of a nasal septal perforation should not be considered unless the disease has been in long-term remission.

13. E

Specific causes of epistaxis are often impossible to identify. Although trauma, infection, foreign bodies and granulomatous conditions can cause bleeding, it is more common that the cause is idiopathic. Factors such as hypertension and anticoagulation are associated with epistaxis and result in heavier bleeding. Such patients often have a lower physiological reserve to cope with the haemodynamic stress that results.

Treatment of epistaxis should include identification and treatment of any underlying causes. Bleeding points can be treated with local cautery or directed nasal packing. Those who do not respond to such treatment can be considered for postnasal packs, which compromise the airway. These patients may be best managed in a high-dependency setting. Surgical treatment includes sphenopalatine and anterior ethmoidal ligation and, if unsuccessful, internal maxillary artery ligation; if life-threatening, consider ligation of the external carotid above the level of the lingual artery.

14. C

Juvenile nasal angiofibroma tends to affect adolescent boys and presents with nasal obstruction and intermittent epistaxis. Staging relies on examination and imaging. Biopsy is not routinely indicated as it can be associated with significant haemorrhage. If required, biopsy should be performed in a theatre setting with the appropriate equipment for arrest of haemorrhage and resuscitation.

Management involves surgical excision following detailed imaging to delineate the vascular supply to the tumour. Preoperative embolisation of these tumours has been used to minimise perioperative blood loss, not as a curative treatment.

15. D

16. C

The lingual artery is an end artery, and ligation below this level can jeopardise the blood supply to the ipsilateral tongue. Identification of branches of the external carotid also ensures that the vessel ligated is not the internal carotid, which has no branches in the neck.

17. C

Epistaxis related to HHT is a difficult condition to treat. Cautery to the bleeding vessel may be effective in the short term, but the long-term nature of the condition results in multiple attempts at cautery and septal perforation. Nasal packs may be used to control bleeding in the short term but removal of packs can lead to traumatic haemorrhage. Oestrogen creams result in metaplasia of the pseudostratified columnar epithelium to a stratified squamous type, which can provide more protection for the fragile vessels. Laser treatment to bleeding points can be successful, although it needs to be repeated as the telangiectasia returns with time. Septodermoplasty involves replacing the nasal mucosa with split-skin grafts, although the condition can also affect the skin graft with time. Young's procedure involves surgically closing the nostril. This reduces trauma to the septum from turbulent airflow and is reserved for resistant cases.

➜ Nasal polyps

18. B

Most simple nasal polyps arise from the ethmoid sinuses. As they grow they fill the middle meatus and may involve the mucosa of all sinuses.

19. C

Sampter's triad describes an association between aspirin allergy, asthma and nasal polyps.

20. A

Although patients with nasal polyps can develop epistaxis, it is not a common complaint. Obstruction, rhinorrhoea and sinus infection are common problems, as is loss of sense of smell (anosmia). Treatment with nasal steroids is particularly useful for managing nasal obstruction. Anosmia is often upsetting for patients and is difficult to treat. A course of oral steroids may be successful in reducing polyp bulk and allowing access to the olfactory cleft. Rhinorrhoea is treated with topical steroid sprays, antihistamines and anticholinergics.

21. B

Simple nasal polyps tend to be bilateral. Unilateral polyps are an indication for endoscopic examination of the nose which may reveal bilateral disease that is hidden on anterior rhinoscopy. Truly unilateral polyposis is suggestive of malignancy, especially if associated with bleeding, pain or cranial nerve dysfunction. Identification of unilateral polyposis requires imaging with CT and biopsy.

22. C

Treatment of nasal polyps is medical in the first instance. Polyps cannot be cured, but the symptoms they cause can often be controlled with topical nasal steroids and short courses of oral steroids. Patients who fail a course of maximal medical therapy should be considered for surgical treatment.

Current surgical standards require preoperative CT scanning in an attempt to minimise the risks of surgery, which include damage to the orbital structures and skull base with CSF leak. An endoscopic approach to simple nasal polyps is common, although some practitioners use a headlight to illuminate the nasal cavity. The goal of surgical treatment is to reduce the bulk of the disease, improve patients' symptoms and avoid complications. Following surgery, patients will be asked to continue on nasal steroid sprays in an attempt to reduce or delay symptom recurrence. Standard polypectomy does not involve external incisions. More radical forms of surgery are required for malignant disease of the nose and sinuses.

➜ Sinusitis

23. C

24. B

Antral lavage is used in acute sinusitis to wash pus from the maxillary sinus. A trochar is inserted under the inferior turbinate and passed through the thin bone in the inferior meatus in the direction of the ipsilateral tragus. The trochar can then be used to aspirate air to confirm its position. Saline is used to wash out the sinus and provide pus for culture. This procedure was used regularly in the past for the treatment of chronic sinusitis but has been superseded by modern techniques of functional sinus surgery, which aim to spare mucosa and preserve the natural function of the paranasal sinuses. By opening the drainage pathways of the sinuses through the middle meatus, function of the mucociliary transport mechanism is aided. This promotes the natural function of the sinus mucosa and allows access for topical medication to the sinuses.

25. B
All sinuses other than the posterior ethmoids and the sphenoid sinus drain into the middle meatus.

26. E
Acute sinusitis can spread directly by infected thrombophlebitis or through dehiscences in the walls of the sinus to the orbit or cranial cavity. Haematogenous spread from infected sinuses is also possible. The presence of one complication should alert the clinician to the possibility of synchronous complications. Patients with periorbital cellulitis who require imaging should have contrast-enhanced imaging of the sinuses, orbit and cranial cavity to exclude intracranial complications.

Orbital cellulitis presents with chemosis and erythema of the preseptal tissues. As the infection progresses, proptosis and limitation of gaze may develop, suggesting abscess formation. As the pressure in the orbit increases, ischaemia of the optic nerve, with irreversible damage and blindness, can occur. For this reason early identification and treatment with antibiotics and drainage of any abscess should be a priority. The development of intracranial sepsis in the form of extradural abscess, subdural abscess, intracerebral abscess, meningitis or venous sinus thrombosis should be identified and managed with cooperation from a neurosurgical team.

Tumours of the nose and sinuses

27. C
Nasal tumours tend to present with nasal obstruction and epistaxis. These symptoms are common in the general population and very rarely associated with malignant disease. For this reason, nasal tumours are often missed and present late. As the tumour grows in the sinus and extends out of the bony confines, it involves the surrounding structures, including the cranial nerves (e.g. the infraorbital nerve), orbit and cribriform plate. Symptoms tend be unilateral in the first instance but can be bilateral in advanced disease.

Staging of sinonasal malignancy is crucial in multidisciplinary management. CT and MRI give the best results allowing estimation of bony destruction, as well as cranial nerve, orbital and dural involvement. Management of sinonasal malignancy tends to be surgical with postoperative radiotherapy. Some units have published good results using a debulking surgical approach and repeated topical chemotherapeutic applications.

28. D
Transitional cell papilloma involves the mucosa of the nose and sinuses. It tends to grow from the lateral wall of the nose to involve the middle meatus and osteomeatal complex, and grows out through the pterygomaxillary fissure into the infratemporal fossa. The disease is benign but tends to recur locally following excision. There is a quoted association with malignancy of between 5 and 10 per cent, although it is uncertain whether the benign lesion becomes malignant or a second lesion develops separately.

Staging with CT +/– MRI is required to plan treatment, which can be performed either endonasally or via an open approach to afford wider exposure and more complete excision. Long-term follow-up with endoscopic examination of the postoperative cavity is required with biopsies of any suspicious tissue.

29. A
Adenocarcinoma has an association with the hardwood dust involved in furniture manufacture. Nasal obstruction and epistaxis are presenting features. It tends to arise from the nasal sinuses and

is diagnosed on biopsy. As with other sinus disease, cross-sectional imaging is important in staging the disease, and the treatment tends to be surgical.

30. C

Answers: Extended matching questions

→ 1. Imaging of the nose and paranasal sinuses

1J

Although X-rays of the nasal bones have been used in assessment of nasal fractures, they are not required and add little to assessment of nasal trauma. Review in around 1 week allows for assessment once post-injury oedema has settled and leaves time for manipulation within 2–3 weeks prior to fracture healing.

2C

CT scans without contrast allow assessment of the bony anatomy of the sinuses and are used as a 'road map' for surgery. Sinus surgery should not be performed without preoperative CT scan.

3D

Examination reveals a mass lesion in the ipsilateral nasal cavity. Contrast-enhanced imaging of juvenile angiofibroma allows for assessment of the tumour, its bony confines and its vascular supply. Imaging can be combined with preoperative embolisation to reduce perioperative blood loss.

4F

The history is one of unilateral maxillary sinusitis. Endoscopic examination with decongestion of the middle meatus may be sufficient to allow drainage of sinus content through the natural ostium. If this is unsuccessful, X-ray of the sinuses will show opacification and pus may be obtained from antral lavage.

5E

The suspected diagnosis here is of Wegener's granulomatosis. The condition may be confirmed by biopsy of an active granulation; ESR and ANCA may also be useful to diagnose the condition. These patients should be managed in conjunction with a physician due to the multisystem nature of the disease. Management is unlikely to involve surgery.

→ 2. Anatomy of the nose and paranasal sinuses

1A, 2E, 3I, 4G, 5F

44 The ear

Multiple choice questions

In the following, choose the single best answer.

Surgical anatomy of the ear

1. **Which of the following statements is true?**
   A The external ear canal is approximately 2 cm in length.
   B The outer third of the ear canal is cartilaginous, the inner two-thirds bony.
   C The epithelium of the outer ear canal migrates outwards from the tympanic membrane.
   D The pinna consists of fibrocartilage.

2. **What does the tympanic membrane consist of?**
   A Two layers: epithelial and mucosal.
   B An upper portion called the pars tensa and a lower portion called the pars flaccid.
   C A single layer of stratified squamous epithelium.
   D Three layers: epithelial, fibrous and mucosal.
   E Two layers: mucosal and hyaline cartilage.

3. **Where does the facial nerve exit the temporal bone?**
   A Stylomastoid foramen
   B Internal acoustic meatus
   C Petrotympanic fissure
   D Facioparotid foramen
   E Foramen ovale.

4. **Which of the following statements regarding the cochlea are true?**
   A It contains endolymph, which communicates with cerebrospinal fluid (CSF).
   B It contains perilymph, which communicates with CSF.
   C It contains both endolymph and perilymph, which communicate with CSF.
   D It contains both endolymph and perilymph, which are not in communication with CSF.
   E It contains endolymph and perilymph, which have a high potassium concentration.

5. **Which of the following statements regarding the vestibular semicircular canals are true?**
   A They contain otoconial membranes.
   B They receive innervation from the greater auricular nerve.
   C They are embedded in the skull positioned in a single plane.
   D They are supplied by the cochlear nerve.
   E They react to angular acceleration.

6. **What nerve does not supply sensation to the external ear?**
   A Cranial nerve V
   B Cranial nerve VII
   C Cranial nerve VIII
   D Cranial nerve IX
   E Cranial nerve X

Radiological investigation of the ear

7. **Which of the following statements are true?**
   A Computed tomography (CT) is the investigation of choice for identification of lesions of cranial nerve VIII.
   B Magnetic resonance imaging (MRI) is the investigation of choice for identification of lesions of cranial nerve VIII.
   C MRI is the investigation of choice for imaging cholesteatoma.

D The resolution of CT scanning is insufficient to show bony abnormality in the middle ear.
E Bony abnormalities should be excluded by preoperative MRI scanning.

Conditions of the external ear

8. Where does the external ear develop from?
A The first branchial arch
B The second branchial arch
C The third branchial arch
D The first and second branchial arches
E The second and third branchial arches.

9. Which of the following statements regarding an auricular haematoma are true?
A It will resolve spontaneously.
B It is caused by a collection of blood between the skin and perichondrium.
C It should be treated with aspiration.
D It should be treated with incision and drainage.
E It will result in only short-lasting cosmetic deformity.

10. Which of the following statements regarding otitis externa are true?
A It can be distinguished from otitis media by pain on movement of the pinna.
B It is best treated initially with oral antibiotics.
C It is commonly caused by streptococcal infection.
D It should not be treated with microscopic aural toilet, to avoid damage to the skin.
E It should not be treated with steroids, due to the risk of overwhelming sepsis.

11. Which of the following statements regarding necrotising otitis externa are true?
A It tends to run an indolent course.
B It tends to be bilateral.
C It spares cranial nerve VII.
D It is caused by streptococcal infection.
E It should be suspected in elderly diabetics.

12. Which of the following statements about malignant lesions of the external ear are true?
A They are most commonly melanoma.
B They are most commonly carcinoma.
C They metastasise first to the submandibular region.
D They are best treated with chemotherapy.
E They are unlikely to have spread from surrounding structures.

Conditions of the middle ear

13. Which of the following statements regarding trauma of the middle ear are true?
A Traumatic perforation of the tympanic membrane usually heals spontaneously.
B Blood in the ear canal should be suctioned clear to allow inspection of the canal.
C Dislocation of the ossicular chain usually affects the smallest ossicle, the stapes.
D CT scanning of the middle ear cannot identify abnormalities which can be corrected surgically.
E Damage to the ossicular chain cannot currently be repaired surgically.

14. Which of the following statements regarding acute suppurative otitis media are true?
A It is most common in adults.
B It is most painful immediately following rupture of the tympanic membrane.
C It is commonly caused by streptococcus pneumonia.
D It is not associated with mastoiditis.
E It is associated with a sterile middle ear effusion.

15. Which of the following statements regarding otitis media with effusion are true?
A It is uncommon in children.
B It results in perforation of the tympanic membrane.
C It causes systemic upset in the child.
D It is due to Eustachian tube dysfunction.
E It presents with otalgia.

16. **Which of the following regarding treatment of otitis media with effusion in children are true?**
   A Urgent treatment of effusion once diagnosed improves outcome.
   B Medical treatment of otitis media with effusion has been proven effective.
   C Grommet insertion requires later grommet removal in most children.
   D Following grommet insertion, children should not swim for around 1 year.
   E A watch-and-wait policy results in improvement in 50 per cent over 6 weeks.

17. **Which of the following statements regarding middle ear effusion in adults are true?**
   A It is a common finding.
   B It tends to persist.
   C If persistent, it should be treated medically.
   D It may be the presenting feature of nasopharyngeal carcinoma.
   E It responds to adenoidectomy.

18. **What are the typical presenting symptoms associated with chronic otitis media?**
   A Otorrhoea and hearing loss
   B Pain and discharge
   C Dizziness and hearing loss
   D Tinnitus and dizziness
   E Pain and tinnitus.

19. **What is cholesteatoma?**
   A A benign condition which is self-limiting
   B A benign condition which can be locally destructive
   C A malignant ear condition without metastasis
   D A malignant condition with metastasis
   E An infection more common in the immunocompromised patient.

20. **Which of the following is not a recognised complication of chronic otitis media?**
   A Meningitis
   B Intracerebral abscess
   C Periorbital cellulitis
   D Extradural abscess
   E Subdural abscess.

21. **Which of the following statements regarding otosclerosis are true?**
   A An abnormal ear drum suggests the diagnosis.
   B Men are more commonly affected.
   C The malleus is the ossicle most commonly affected.
   D Surgical treatment is unlikely to be effective.
   E The disease is often bilateral.

22. **Which of the following statements about middle ear tumours are true?**
   A The most common middle ear tumour is squamous cell carcinoma.
   B The most common middle ear tumour is a glomus tumour.
   C Vascular middle ear tumours tend to present with a constant tinnitus.
   D Squamous cell carcinoma of the middle ear tends to spare the facial nerve.
   E Because of the bony anatomy, palsies of the cranial nerves in the jugular foramen do not occur in association with middle ear tumours.

→ Conditions of the inner ear

23. **Which of the following statements regarding congenital anomalies of the inner ear are true?**
   A Children cannot be formally assessed with hearing tests, so treatment should be based on clinical suspicion.
   B Children with profound hearing loss should not be offered hearing aids due to the social stigma of these devices.
   C In correctly selected cases, cochlear implantation offers significant benefits.
   D Most cases of profound sensorineural hearing loss are due to maldevelopment of the cochlear nerve.
   E A child with a congenital hearing loss will also have an abnormal middle ear.

24. **Which of the following statements about presbycusis are true?**
   A A condition which tends to affect adolescents
   B A condition which tends to affect the elderly
   C A condition which results in a low-frequency hearing loss

D A condition caused by loss of cochlear hair cells at the apex of the cochlea
E A condition which is unlikely to be helped by hearing aids.

25. Following temporal bone fracture, which of the following are true?
A It is important to asses and document facial nerve function.
B Hearing loss is very uncommon.
C Sensorineural hearing loss will tend to recover given time.
D Plain X-rays allow preoperative assessment of temporal bone anatomy.
E Examination of the ear canal will add nothing to the examination.

26. Which of the following statements is true regarding ototoxic drugs?
A Aminoglycoside-containing ear drops must be avoided in perforated tympanic membranes.
B Ototoxic drugs selectively impair cochlear function over vestibular function.
C Ototoxicity will manifest during treatment.
D Renal function may be an important factor in ototoxicity.
E Loop diuretics should be used when the risk of ototoxicity is high.

27. Which of the following statements regarding benign paroxysmal positional vertigo are true?
A It causes vertigo lasting hours.
B It is associated with intermittent tinnitus.
C It can only be diagnosed in the absence of recent head injury.
D It causes vertigo in the absence of nystagmus.
E It may be helped with a repositioning manoeuvre.

28. Which of the following statements regarding the vertigo associated with Ménière's disease are true?
A It lasts for days to weeks.
B It lasts for minutes to hours.
C It lasts for seconds to minutes.
D It is an isolated symptom.
E It is caused by recurrent infection.

29. In patients presenting with facial palsy, which of the following should be done?
A Examination should include the ear, the parotid and the cranial nerves.
B Antibiotics should be prescribed.
C Bell's palsy should be diagnosed if the ear is discharging.
D Patients should be warned that recovery is unlikely.
E During treatment, patients should be advised to keep the affected eye open to prevent deterioration in vision.

➜ Neoplasms

30. Which of the following regarding the management of acoustic neuroma are true?
A Hearing will be lost during treatment for this condition.
B Predictable tumour growth allows for appropriately timed treatment.
C Treatment options are complex and involve factors including tumour size and hearing levels.
D CT scanning is the investigation of choice.
E Following diagnosis, treatment is mandatory.

Extended matching questions

➜ 1. Otological sepsis

A Prescribe nasal decongestant sprays
B Prescribe nasal steroid sprays
C Prescribe analgesia with systemic antibiotics if symptoms do not settle within 48 h
D Topical antibiotic and steroid drops
E Topical antibiotic drops with a prolonged course of intravenous (IV) antibiotics
F Surgical repair of the ear drum

G Surgery to exteriorise the disease
H Urgent contrast-enhanced CT scan of temporal bones and brain
I Plain X-ray of the affected temporal bone
J MRI of internal acoustic meatus

Choose the most appropriate action for each of the clinical scenarios given below:

1 A 4-year-old who is pulling at their ear presents with pyrexia, systemic upset and a bulging red ear drum.

2 A 36-year-old patient with eczema presents with a unilateral itchy, painful ear and associated discharge following a recent holiday.

3 A 76-year-old diabetic presents with severe otalgia, otorrhoea and facial nerve palsy.

4 A 52-year-old presents with a chronic perforation of the tympanic membrane and a first episode of otorrhoea.

5 A fit 68-year-old presents with atticoantral chronic otitis media (cholesteatoma) and persistent foul-smelling discharge.

6 A 28-year-old with a history of recent viral illness followed by otalgia presents to casualty with a pyrexia and a Glasgow Coma Scale of 9.

→ 2. Applied anatomy of the ear

A First and second branchial arches
B Second and third branchial arches
C Cranial nerve VII
D Cranial nerve IIX
E Cranial nerve X
F Stylomastoid foramen
G Internal acoustic meatus
H Incus
I Stapes
J Jugular foramen

Choose the most appropriate response for the questions below:

1 Where does the facial nerve enter the temporal bone?

2 Which area is most commonly affected by otosclerosis?

3 The external ear develops from which embryological structures?

4 Which structure explains the presence of vesicles in the ear canal in Ramsay Hunt syndrome?

5 Otalgia may be a presenting feature of laryngeal cancer due to pain referred through which structure?

Answers: Multiple choice questions

→ Surgical anatomy of the ear

1. C

The external ear canal is approximately 3 cm in length, the outer two-thirds are cartilage, extending from the elastic cartilage of the pinna to the bony medial third. Epithelium migrates from the tympanic membrane outwards along the ear canal, making the ear self-cleaning.

2. D

The tympanic membrane consists of an inner mucosal, middle fibrous and an outer stratified squamous epithelial layer. The inferior section of the membrane, below the lateral process of the malleus, is called the pars tensa, and the section superior to the lateral process is called the pars flaccid.

3. A

The facial nerve enters the temporal bone at the internal acoustic meatus, winding its way through labyrinthine, tympanic and mastoid segments in the bony fallopian canal. It exits the skull at the stylomastoid foramen, which is identified during parotid surgery.

4. B

The cochlea is a spiral consisting of two and three-quarter turns. Within this bony space, perilymph and endolymph are separated by Reissner's membrane. The perilymph is in communication with the CSF, whilst the endolymph has a high potassium concentration. Hair cells on the basilar membrane within the cochlea vibrate and transduce mechanical energy into electrical energy.

5. E

The three semicircular canals lie within the temporal bone at right angles to one another. They react to angular acceleration, whilst the utricle and saccule react to linear acceleration and gravity. As in the cochlea, shearing forces produce hair cell movement which is transduced into electrical activity carried in the vestibular nerve.

6. C

Sensory supply to the ear comes from cranial nerves V, VII, IX and X, as well as from branches of C2,3. This variation of sensory supply explains the varied causes of referred otalgia, classically laryngeal cancer. It also explains the presence of vesicles in the ear canal in association with herpes zoster infection of CN7 – Ramsay Hunt syndrome.

→ Radiological investigation of the ear

7. B

Computed tomography shows bony lesions and MRI shows soft tissue lesions most accurately. MRI is used to identify lesions of the acoustic nerves such as schwannomas. CT is useful to identify the bony anatomy of the middle ear preoperatively, although not all surgeons use it as routine. The definition of high-resolution CT scanning allows identification of most bony abnormalities, which can be confirmed during surgery.

→ Conditions of the external ear

8. D

9. D

Auricular haematomas tend to follow blunt trauma to the pinna. The shearing of the perichondrium from the cartilage results in bleeding into the space which develops. As cartilage derives its blood supply from this perichondrium, cartilage necrosis can occur, resulting in a lasting deformity. Although aspiration of a haematoma will result in temporary resolution, recurrence is the rule and incision and drainage with antibiotic cover and postoperative pressure dressing forms the treatment of choice.

10. A

Otitis externa is a generalized inflammatory condition of the external ear canal. Pathogens including pseudomonas can be involved. Pain on movement of the pinna is typical, which is not seen in otitis media. Topical antibiotics and steroids are the initial treatment of choice, followed by debris removal with microscopic assistance if this fails. Systemic treatment is rarely required.

11. E

This condition, which results in osteomyelitis of the skull base, presents with unilateral severe otitis externa. Patients are often immunocompromised, and elderly diabetics with otitis externa should be suspected of the condition. As the condition spreads it can involve cranial nerves VII, IX and X. Treatment is systemic and prolonged with 6 week courses of antibiotics common.

12. B

Most malignancies of the external ear are basal cell or squamous cell carcinomas. They tend to present as slow-growing, crusting lesions. The ear canal, which is surrounded on all sides, may be invaded by tumours from the parotid gland or postnasal space. Most resectable tumours should be treated primarily with surgery.

→ Conditions of the middle ear

13. A

Traumatic perforations tend to heal spontaneously, although perforations secondary to welding and blast injuries do worse. In ossicular trauma the incus is usually involved, and ossicular damage can be reconstructed by reshaping the damaged ossicle or by using a prosthetic implant. CT scanning can show the position of the ossicles prior to surgery, although it is not mandatory.

14. C

Suppurative otitis media is most common in children, and results in a purulent fluid building up behind an intact tympanic membrane. The rise in pressure results in pain, which subsides on perforation of the ear drum. *Streptococcus pneumoniae* and *Haemophilus influenzae* are the most common organisms involved. Treatment will depend on the state of the child, as the role of antibiotics is controversial. Almost all episodes will resolve without antibiotics, and current practice guidelines suggest the provision of an antibiotic prescription to the parents with instructions to use only if symptoms do not settle within 48 h. The mastoid air cells communicate freely with the middle ear and so mastoiditis is associated with otitis media.

15. D

The majority of children will have an episode of otitis media with effusion. It is thought to be due to poor Eustachian tube function, leading to a negative middle ear pressure and collection of a transudate fluid in the middle ear space. If a perforation is present, the fluid cannot collect. The child tends to present with fluctuating hearing loss and possible delayed speech with behavioural problems. Pain is rare in this condition.

16. E

Most middle ear effusions will resolve naturally. Children at risk of missing out on educational opportunities are those who have a bilateral persistent effusion. These children can be identified by serial examinations and audiological assessment. Medical treatments are of limited value. Grommet insertion and adenoidectomy are surgical options. Grommets grow out in around 6–18 months and there is no need to avoid swimming during this time.

17. D

Middle ear effusion is rare in adults and when present tends to resolve quickly. Persistent effusion should be viewed as suspicious as neoplastic obstruction of the Eustachian may be the cause. These patients should have an examination +/− biopsy of the nasopharynx as a joint procedure if considering grommet insertion. The adenoid is small in adults, and the post nasal space large, which makes adenoid obstruction of the Eustachian tube uncommon in this age group.

18. A

Chronic otitis media typically presents with intermittent discharge and a mild conductive hearing loss. Pain is unusual, and dizziness or vertigo is associated with advanced disease affecting the vestibular labyrinth. Tinnitus can be associated with hearing loss but is not a typical feature of chronic otitis media.

19. B

Cholesteatoma results from a collection of squamous epithelium in a retraction pocket of the tympanic membrane. The pocket prevents normal epithelial migration, which results in accumulation of cells and gradual enlargement of the retraction pocket. As the disease progresses, a low-grade osteomyelitis develops, and chronic foul discharge can be both seen and smelt. The disease can erode through local structures, including the ossicles, cochlea, vestibule and the bony partitions between the ear and the middle and posterior cranial fossae. This puts the patient at risk of hearing and balance dysfunction as well as intracranial sepsis.

20. C

Chronic otitis media can lead to intracerebral, extradural and subdural abscess. Other intracranial complications of otitis media include meningitis and sigmoid sinus thrombosis. Periorbital cellulitis is a complication of sinusitis not otitis media.

21. E

In otosclerosis, abnormal bone deposition in the temporal bone occurs, most commonly affecting the stapes in the oval window. This reduces the mobility of the stapes in the oval window and leads to a conductive hearing loss. Women are more commonly affected, and the disease is often bilateral. Treatment options include reassurance, hearing aid and surgery, which is successful in over 90 per cent of cases. Rare complications include sensorineural hearing loss and balance disturbance.

22. B

The most common middle ear tumour is a glomus tumour, from the non-chromaffin paraganglionic tissue. They are highly vascular and tend to present with a pulsatile tinnitus and hearing loss. The ear drum may have a classic cherry-red appearance and cranial nerve palsies (VII, IX, X, XI and XII) are not uncommon. Squamous cell carcinoma tends to present with a deep-seated pain and bloody discharge. Facial paralysis often occurs.

→ Conditions of the inner ear

23. C

Congenital inner ear disorders can exist with or without middle ear abnormalities. Most cases of profound sensorineural hearing loss are due to loss of cochlear hair cells. Any parent who has concerns about their child's hearing should be taken seriously. Paediatric audiology is a skilled field and includes both subjective and objective testing. Objective testing is now routine in neonates in the UK, which has improved the detection of children who are hearing-impaired. The auditory system develops with the child and it is important that children with a hearing loss are provided with hearing aids during this period of neural plasticity to optimise their development. Patients with a profound hearing loss may be candidates for cochlear implantation, which can offer significant benefits. Children who would otherwise be permanently deaf can attend mainstream schools and perform at a similar level to their normal hearing peers.

24. B

Presbycusis is characterised by the loss of hearing in the high frequencies. It tends to affect the elderly and is the result of hair cell loss starting at the basal turn of the cochlea. It is generally bilateral and can be associated with tinnitus. Hearing aids are used in the treatment of the disability caused by this condition.

25. A

The temporal bone is the hardest bone in the body, but it can be fractured in severe head trauma. Classically fractures are described in relation to the ear canal as longitudinal or transverse.

Structures within the temporal bone which may be damaged include the facial nerve and the cochlea. Transverse fractures have a higher rate of damage to these structures than do longitudinal fractures. Examination of the ear canal may reveal a fracture in the roof of the canal, confirming the diagnosis. Hearing loss is common, either from conductive loss related to blood in the canal, haemotympanum or ossicular disruption, or from sensorineural loss, which is permanent if the cochlea has been disrupted. Assessment of the facial nerve is essential. If immediate total paralysis is present, the nerve is likely to have been damaged and surgical intervention should be considered. If the nerve is functional, either partially or completely, its integrity can be assumed and any later loss of function is secondary to oedema, so will not be improved with surgery. Some patients will be unconscious at the time of assessment, and facial nerve function will not be recorded. If these patients wake with a complete palsy, decision-making is more complicated. Any intervention should be preceded by high-resolution CT scanning of the temporal bone anatomy.

26. D
Many drugs are potentially ototoxic, with some affecting the cochlea and some the vestibular system. Aminoglycosides and cisplatin are commonly encountered in clinical practice and cause an irreversible hearing loss. Aspirin produces a reversible hearing loss. Patients with poor renal function are at particular risk, and loop diuretics potentiate the ototoxic effects of aminoglycosides. Ototoxicity may be a delayed phenomenon, and some patients may be unable to report problems if they are critically ill during the time of treatment. There has been controversy over the use of aminoglycoside drops in the presence of a perforation, however there is little evidence that, during an active infection, short courses cause significant damage. A recent consensus statement from UK experts supported their use, although many would be cautious, especially in an only hearing ear.

27. E
Benign paroxysmal positional vertigo (BPPV) is probably caused by fragments of the otoconial membrane floating into the semicircular canals. This interferes with their function and produces vertigo and nystagmus which lasts for seconds and is provoked by head movement. It may follow head injury but may also be spontaneous. The condition tends to be self-limiting, lasting around 3 months, but particle repositioning manoeuvres such as the Epley manoeuvre can be used to hasten the resolution of symptoms.

28. B
Ménière's disease describes an intermittent vertigo which lasts for minutes to hours and is associated with tinnitus, hearing loss and a feeling of aural fullness. The cause is unclear although it may be related to pressure changes within the inner ear. Investigation will include MRI to exclude mass lesions at the cerebellopontine angle, which may mimic the condition. Treatment includes diuretics which may help lower the inner ear pressure, injection of gentamicin to the middle ear to perform a pharmaceutical larbyrinthectomy or more destructive surgical interventions to destroy the labyrinth or the nerves that supply it.

29. A
Viral infection of the facial nerve is a common cause of unilateral palsy. The most common of these is Bell's palsy, which results in swelling of the nerve within its bony canal and subsequent dysfunction. Around 85–95 per cent of patients make a good recovery with evidence suggesting that steroid treatment improves outcome. Bell's palsy can only be diagnosed if no other cause for the paralysis can be found. It should be remembered that the facial nerve exits the brainstem, runs through the temporal bone and out into the parotid gland before reaching the facial muscles. All areas should be examined, including the cranial nerve. The presence of active ear infection should prompt urgent referral for intravenous antibiotics. The presence of a parotid mass or other cranial nerve palsies should prompt further investigation.

Neoplasms

30. C

Acoustic neuroma is the most common tumour of the cerebellopontine angle. It is normally a schwannoma of the vestibular nerve. Growth of these tumours is slow and unpredictable. Treatment options are complex and will include observation with interval scanning, surgery or radiotherapy. MRI is the investigation of choice. Patients should be made aware of the risks of surgery to their hearing and facial nerve in particular. Different surgical approaches to this area have been described, each of which has advantages and disadvantages. Radiotherapy with the gamma knife can be used to arrest the growth of the tumour, although the patient will require lifelong interval scans. Some patients will decide not to have treatment, while others will not be fit to undergo such a major procedure.

Answers: Extended matching questions

1. Otological sepsis

1C

Acute otitis media is the likely diagnosis. Current treatment guidelines suggest the provision of antibiotics and reassurance. A prescription for antibiotics may be provided with advice that the symptoms normally resolve spontaneously. If they are not improving within 48 h, the parents are advised to use the prescription. There is no evidence that nasal decongestants or nasal steroids are helpful in acute otitis media.

2D

The diagnosis is otitis externa, often precipitated by swimming whilst on holiday. The initial treatment should include topical antibiotics and steroid drops. If this does not lead to symptom resolution, aural toilet may be required.

3E

The diagnosis is of necrotising otitis externa. This condition is more common in the immunocompromised and leads to osteomyelitis of the skull base. As the disease progresses to involve the bone, the cranial nerves which traverse the skull base can be affected. Treatment involves parenteral and topical antibiotics targeted against Pseudomonas, until culture results are available. Aural toilet is also important. Treatment will be long term and patients may require 6 weeks of IV antibiotics.

4D

This patient has chronic otitis media with perforation and should be treated with an antibiotic and steroid drop. Short courses of aminoglycoside-containing drops can be used safely in such patients. The decision as to whether to operate to close the perforation in the long term will depend on the severity of symptoms.

5G

In cholesteatoma, keratin debris collects in a retraction pocket of the tympanic membrane. This debris becomes infected and gives rise to a foul-smelling discharge. If allowed to continue, the disease will increase in size and may damage the ossicles, the cochlea and the vestibule and can lead to intracranial sepsis. Appropriate treatment is surgical and involves exteriorisation of the disease.

6H

This patient may have developed an intracranial complication of acute otitis media. These include meningitis, subdural abscess, extradural abscess, intracerebral abscess and venous sinus thrombosis. An urgent contrast-enhanced CT scan will allow assessment of intracranial disease.

2. Applied anatomy of the ear

1G

The seventh cranial nerve enters the temporal bone at the internal acoustic meatus and exits at the stylomastoid foramen. During its course within the temporal bone, it can be divided into labyrinthine, tympanic and mastoid parts.

2I

Otosclerosis results in bone deposition within the temporal bone. The site most commonly affected is the footplate of the stapes, where it articulates with the oval window. The excess bone interferes with the rocking movement of the stapes, resulting in a conductive hearing loss.

3A

4C

Ramsay Hunt syndrome is a varicella zoster infection of the facial nerve which leads to facial palsy. The infection also affects fibres from the facial nerve which supply the ear canal. When vesicles form and break down, a painful otitis externa develops which often requires topical treatment and aural toilet.

5E

Otalgia is an ominous sign in head and neck cancer, as it suggests cranial nerve involvement. In laryngeal cancer, involvement of the vagus nerve (cranial nerve X) may lead to otalgia. Glossopharyngeal nerve (cranial nerve IX) involvement in oropharyngeal tumours may also present with ipsilateral otalgia.

45 Pharynx, larynx and neck

Multiple choice questions

In the following, choose the single best answer.

Clinical anatomy and physiology

1. **The pharynx extends from the level of the skull base to which vertebra?**
   - A Fourth cervical vertebra
   - B Fifth cervical vertebra
   - C Sixth cervical vertebra
   - D Seventh cervical vertebra
   - E First thoracic vertebra.

2. **Infection of the parapharyngeal space places the patient at risk of:**
   - A Otitis media
   - B Acute tonsillitis
   - C Dental infection
   - D Mediastinitis
   - E Epiglottitis.

3. **The superior and recurrent laryngeal nerves are branches of which cranial nerve?**
   - A Eighth cranial nerve
   - B Ninth cranial nerve
   - C Tenth cranial nerve
   - D Eleventh cranial nerve
   - E Twelfth cranial nerve.

4. **Which of the following is not a function of the larynx?**
   - A Preparation of fold bolus for swallowing
   - B Protection of the lower respiratory tract
   - C Phonation
   - D Control of pressure during respiration
   - E Fixation of the chest.

5. **What does the level system for describing the neck refer to?**
   - A A system for describing skin lesions involving the neck
   - B A system for describing lymph nodes of the neck
   - C A system for describing the salivary glands
   - D A system for describing movement of the larynx during swallowing
   - E A system for describing venous drainage of the neck.

Diseases of the pharynx

6. **Which of the following is an indication for adenoidectomy?**
   - A Hyponasal speech
   - B Velopharyngeal insufficiency
   - C Recurrent epistaxis
   - D Cleft palate
   - E Obstructive sleep apnoea.

7. **In which patients presenting with unilateral nasal obstruction and recurrent epistaxis should angiofibroma be suspected?**
   - A Elderly male smokers
   - B Adolescent patients of Chinese origin
   - C Middle-aged patients with atopy and asthma
   - D Adolescent males
   - E Immunocompromised patients.

8. **Which virus is associated with nasopharyngeal carcinoma?**
   - A Epstein–Barr virus
   - B Varicella zoster
   - C Human papillomavirus (HPV) 6 and 11
   - D Herpes simplex
   - E Rhinovirus.

9. **Treatment of a peritonsillar abscess requires:**
   - A Tonsillectomy
   - B Transoral incision and drainage

C Transcervical incision and drainage
D Endoscopic de-roofing
E Ultrasound/CT-guided aspiration.

10. How should retropharyngeal abscess be treated?
A Under local anaesthetic in the sitting position
B Under local anaesthetic with the patient supine
C Under general anaesthetic with the patient head down
D With antibiotics alone
E As an outpatient.

11. A pharyngeal pouch develops in an area of weakness – where?
A At the point the superior laryngeal nerve penetrates the thyrohyoid membrane
B At the potential space between the superior constrictor and skull base
C At the weakness where the pharyngeal constrictors meet the midline raphe
D Created following tonsillectomy
E Between the lower border of the inferior constrictor and cricopharyngeus muscles.

12. Squamous cell carcinoma (SCC) of the oropharynx is associated with:
A Cigarette smoking
B Epstein–Barr virus
C Consumption of salted fish
D Exposure to hardwood dust from the furniture industry
E Poorly fitting dentures.

13. Which of the following statements regarding SCC of the hypopharynx are true?
A It carries a relatively good prognosis due to early presentation.
B It can be adequately assessed in the outpatient clinic.
C It rarely spreads to cervical lymph nodes.
D It is associated with submucosal spread.
E It may present with otalgia referred through cranial nerve XI.

→ Diseases of the larynx

14. In paediatric suspected acute epiglottitis, which of the following is contraindicated?
A Antibiotics
B Examination of the mouth with headlight and spatula
C Examination under general anaesthetic
D Emergency intubation
E Tracheostomy.

15. Which of the following are not indications for tracheostomy?
A Acute upper airway obstruction
B Potential upper airway obstruction
C Tension pneumothorax
D Protection of the lower airway
E Prolonged artificial ventilation.

16. Which of the following are advantages of a tracheostomy?
A A decrease in alveolar ventilation
B An increase in the work of breathing
C Increased rate of moisture exchange from the upper airway
D Reduced mucus production
E Reduction of anatomical dead space.

17. Which of the following are not features of a modern tracheostomy tube?
A A low-pressure cuff
B An inner tube
C An outer flange
D A port for nasogastric feeding
E A speaking valve attachment.

18. Which of the following is true of cricothyroidotomy?
A The procedure requires a high level of surgical expertise.
B It may be associated with subglottic stenosis.
C It is a long-term solution to airway obstruction
D It involves excision of the anterior cricoid cartilage
E It should routinely be converted to a tracheostomy.

19. **What is the preferred treatment for vocal fold nodules?**
A Speech therapy
B Surgical excision
C Radiotherapy
D Steroid injection
E Inhaled corticosteroid.

20. **Which statement is true of unilateral vocal cord palsy?**
A It is most commonly right-sided.
B It should be investigated by CT larynx.
C It may be associated with a normal voice.
D It requires tracheostomy.
E It leaves the vocal cord fully adducted.

21. **Early laryngeal cancer presents with:**
A Otalgia
B Lymph node metastasis
C Hoarseness
D Dysphagia
E Weight loss.

22. **Which of the following statements regarding laryngectomy is true?**
A The procedure involves separation of the airway from the GI tract.
B The procedure can treat malignancy without affecting the voice.
C The surgical tracheostomy may be closed once postoperative swelling subsides.
D It prevents patients from speaking.
E It is the recommended treatment for early laryngeal cancer.

The neck

23. **Which of the following applies to branchial cysts?**
A They usually present in the neonatal period.
B They present in the midline of the neck.
C Infection of the cyst leads to an increase in size, facilitating surgical excision.
D They are found at the junction of the upper and middle third of the sternomastoid muscle.
E They contain clear fluid.

24. **Which of the following is true of a cystic hygroma?**
A They present during puberty.
B They are brilliantly translucent.
C They are firm on palpation.
D Cosmetic concern is the only indication for treatment.
E They undergo a predictable growth pattern.

25. **A thyroglossal duct cyst is a remnant of which structure?**
A The thyrocervical trunk
B The cervical sinus
C The track of the thymus through the neck in to the mediastinum
D The fourth branchial pouch
E The track of the thyroid from the tongue base to the neck.

Trauma to the neck

26. **Following blunt laryngeal trauma, which of these statements is true?**
A The anatomy of the larynx allows for significant swelling prior to loss of function.
B Endotracheal intubation should be performed prior to the formation of oedema and maintained until swelling subsides.
C Fractured cartilages should be left untouched to optimise laryngeal function.
D Low tracheostomy should be considered.
E If a laryngeal stent is placed, an open procedure is required for removal.

27. **Ludwig's angina describes which condition?**
A Submandibular swelling with inflammatory oedema of the floor of mouth
B Spreading cellulitis of the lower neck with dark discoloration in patches related to necrosis
C Gingivostomatitis
D Retrosternal chest pain related to swallowing
E Cellulitis secondary to zoster lesions in the cervical dermatomes.

28. A collar-stud abscess refers to which disease process?

A Bacterial cervical lymphadenitis
B Infection of a necrotic malignant cervical lymph node
C Tuberculous cervical lymphadenitis
D Tracking of a peritonsillar abscess into the parapharyngeal space
E A postoperative wound infection which drains through the collar incision of thyroidectomy.

Primary tumours of the neck

29. Which of the following statements about carotid body tumours is true?

A 90 per cent of patients have a family history.
B They are more common in populations living at high altitude.
C They are hormonally active.
D The mass can be moved up and down but not side to side.
E Preoperative fine-needle aspiration (FNA) confirms the diagnosis.

30. A procedure which removes all lymph nodes on one side of the neck but preserves the accessory nerve, jugular vein and sternomastoid muscle is called:

A A radical neck dissection
B A classical neck dissection
C A selective neck dissection
D A subtotal neck dissection
E A modified radical neck dissection.

Extended matching questions

1. Investigation of the pharynx, larynx and neck

A FNA
B Open excision
C Ultrasound
D CT scan of the neck and chest
E MRI scan
F Positron emission tomography (PET) scan
G Barium swallow
H Examination under anaesthetic
I Referral for radiotherapy
J Laryngectomy

Choose the most appropriate action for each of the scenarios listed below:

1 A 72-year-old presents with recurrent aspiration pneumonia and reflux of undigested food which occurs hours after meals.

2 A 60-year-old male smoker presents with a 3 cm palpable cervical lymph node and no other abnormality on examination.

3 A 46-year-old presents with a pulsatile mass in the left neck which moves side to side but not up and down.

4 A 58-year-old smoker presents with hoarseness and an ulcerated area on the left vocal cord.

5 A 66-year-old smoker presents with a new-onset left vocal cord palsy.

2. Investigation and management of the acute airway case

A Ultrasound-guided aspiration

B Per-oral incision and drainage

C Early tracheostomy

D Intubation until swelling subsides

E Cricothyroidotomy

F Insertion of an oral airway

G Transfer to theatre with experienced anaesthetist and surgeon

H Endoscopic excision of lesions

I A short course of steroids

J Soft tissue neck X-ray

Choose the most appropriate management for each of the scenarios listed below:

1 A stertorous 16-year-old with tonsillitis and a positive test for glandular fever fails to improve with antibiotics, fluids and analgesia.

2 A 3-year-old presents with a short history of fever, drooling and stridor.

3 A 21-year-old with sore throat, fever and trismus has deviation of the tonsil and uvula to the contralateral side.

4 A 28-year-old who came off his motorbike and struck his neck on a lamp post presents with increasing stridor.

5 A 4-year-old who presents with hoarseness and stridor has papillomatous lesions affecting the larynx.

Answers: Multiple choice questions

Clinical anatomy and physiology

1. C

The pharynx is a muscular tube which extends from skull base to the level of the sixth cervical vertebra, which corresponds to the lower level of the cricoids cartilage. At this point the pharynx is continuous with the cervical oesophagus.

2. D

The deep spaces of the neck lie between fascial planes which allow for the spread of infection in predictable patterns. Pus can track through these potential spaces to the para-oesophageal region and the superior mediastinum. The most common sources of suppuration in the parapharyngeal lymph nodes are dental and tonsil infections.

3. C

The sensory and motor innervation of the larynx is derived from branches of the vagus nerve. The superior laryngeal nerve supplies sensation to the larynx above the true vocal folds, and motor supply to the cricothyroid muscle. The recurrent laryngeal nerve supplies sensation to the larynx below the vocal folds and all other intrinsic laryngeal muscles. Damage to the recurrent laryngeal nerve during thyroidectomy will produce a cord paralysis and resulting hoarseness. Damage to branches of the superior laryngeal nerve, which runs close to the superior pole of the thyroid, will cause a change in voice, which may only be detectable whilst singing.

4. A

The primary function of the larynx is to protect the lower respiratory tract. It acts as a sphincter which closes during swallowing at the laryngeal inlet, the false cords and the glottis. It also helps in the cessation of respiration during the swallow and is involved in the cough reflex. The human larynx is well developed for phonation, but also helps control pressure during the respiratory cycle, with vocal cord abduction during inspiration. Closure against raised subglottic pressure splints the chest and aids in lifting, climbing and defaecation.

5. B

The level system describes the lymph nodes of the neck. Squamous cell carcinoma of the upper aerodigestive tract metastasises to predictable areas of the neck. Historic treatment of metastatic SCC of the head and neck involved radical neck dissection, a procedure which comprised removal of all lymphatics of the neck with sacrifice of the sternocleidomastoid muscle, the internal jugular vein and the accessory nerve. As our understanding of patterns of metastasis have evolved, procedures have been developed which spare these structures, particularly the accessory nerve. These modified radical neck dissections reduce the morbidity of the procedure (shoulder pain related to division of cranial nerve XI) without reducing disease control.

➜ Diseases of the pharynx

6. E

Adenoidectomy for obstructive sleep apnoea in children with postnasal obstruction is often combined with tonsillectomy. The risks of adenoidectomy include velopharyngeal insufficiency, which results in reflux of liquids into the nose whilst swallowing. Patients with cleft palate, either clinically obvious or a submucous cleft, are at higher risk.

7. D

Juvenile nasal angiofibroma tends to present in adolescent males. The tumour often involves the nasopharynx, and, as it enlarges, causes local damage, including to the optic nerve, which can result in blindness. Nasopharyngeal SCC is more common in Chinese populations. Nasal polyps tend to be bilateral.

8. A

Nasopharyngeal carcinoma is associated with Epstein–Barr virus, as well as there being a genetic susceptibility and an association with traditional diets containing salted fish. Serological investigation for Epstein–Barr virus-associated antigenic markers can be used in disease detection and as tumour markers to detect recurrence. IgA to antiviral capsid antigen has found use as a screening tool in southern China when applied to high-risk groups.

9. B

Peritonsillar abscess or quinsy describes an infective process which results in a collection of pus in the peritonsillar space. The tonsil and uvula are pushed medially and there is often significant trismus due to inflammation around the pterygoid muscles. Supportive treatment with fluids, analgesia and antibiotics are often required, but definitive treatment is with transoral incision and drainage under local anaesthetic. In children, a general anaesthetic is required and tonsillectomy is often performed at the same time.

10. C

Retropharyngeal abscess most commonly affects children under the age of 1 year. It is associated with infection of the tonsil, oropharynx or nasopharynx. Patients will show the signs of infection and may have severe airway compromise. The abscess may be seen on examination. Treatment involves admission, with parenteral antibiotics and fluids, however incision and drainage are indicated. Discussion with a senior anaesthetist is advised and orotracheal intubation should be performed in the head-down position so that accidental perforation of the abscess during intubation does not result in aspiration of pus. The abscess cavity can usually be accessed through the oral cavity, although transcervical approaches can be used.

11. E
A pharyngeal pouch develops at Killian's dehiscence, which lies between the inferior fibres of the inferior constrictor muscle and the cricopharyngeus muscle. The cause of this condition is not clear but may relate to incoordination of relaxation of the upper oesophageal sphincter or abnormalities of the pharyngeal contraction wave.

12. A
Cigarette smoking is the most significant risk factor for SCC of the head and neck, including SCC of the oropharynx. Alcohol consumption is a less significant risk factor, although in combination with cigarette smoke, the effects have been shown to be synergistic.

13. D
Hypopharyngeal cancer is classified according to the site of probable origin. It often presents late, with vague symptoms including dysphagia, hoarseness and otalgia (referred through cranial nerve IX and X). Assessment involved flexible endoscopy in the clinic, laryngoscopy under general anaesthetic and radiological investigations – CT/MRI as well as videofluoroscopy and chest X-ray to detect as second primary. Lesions can spread submucosally, which makes determining surgical margins challenging. The hypopharynx receives a rich, bilateral lymphatic supply, making cervical metastasis common, although not always palpable.

→ Diseases of the larynx

14. B
Children with epiglottitis will be febrile and often drooling due to the pain related to swallowing. They present with stridor and require urgent treatment. They should be nursed in a quiet environment and with a parent present to encourage them to remain calm. Any measures which may upset the child, including examination with a spatula and intravenous (IV) cannulation, should be avoided as this may precipitate a respiratory arrest. An expert anaesthetist and ENT surgeon should be summoned and the child transferred to the operating theatre for examination under general anaesthetic. Intubation should be attempted, but if unsuccessful, a tracheostomy may be required. Once a safe airway has been secured, the child will be managed in an intensive care unit with IV antibiotics until the swelling subsides.

15. C
Tracheostomy involves producing an entrance to the trachea through the skin of the neck. It can be done in cases of airway obstruction above the level of the tracheostomy in cases of epiglottitis. In such cases, the indication is usually urgent or life-saving. The time to perform a tracheostomy is when you first think it might be necessary! Following head injury or coma, patients are at risk of aspiration and a tracheostomy can be used to place a cuffed tube and protect the lower airway. This also allows access for pulmonary toilet. Patients who are intubated and ventilated for a prolonged period may be suitable for tracheostomy, which allows a reduction in sedative medications and is more comfortable for the patient.

16. E
The anatomical dead space is reduced by around 50 per cent following tracheostomy. The work of breathing decreases and alveolar ventilation increases. Drying of the tracheal epithelium occurs due to loss of the heat and moisture exchange functions of the upper airway, and there is an increase in mucus production which can lead to obstruction of the tube. Splinting of the larynx can lead to aspiration during swallowing.

17. D
Modern tracheostomy tubes are made of plastic or silver. They are available in a range of inner and outer diameters, and with a single tube, or with an inner tube and outer tube. The advantage of a removable inner tube is that removing it to clean the tube does not leave the tracheostomy empty. This makes cleaning the tube easier for the nursing staff and patient. Tubes can be cuffed or uncuffed, and have an outer flange to connect tapes which pass around the neck to secure the tube's position. Speaking valves prevent exhaled air from leaving the tube, diverting it up through the larynx thus allowing phonation. Tracheostomy tubes can interfere with feeding, however feeding tubes must not be placed in the trachea.

18. B
Cricothyroidotomy is performed through a vertical skin incision and involves division of the cricothyroid membrane for 1 cm immediately above the cricoid cartilage. It can be performed quickly and little surgical expertise is required. It can be used for emergency access to the airway. Its use is controversial and it may be associated with long-term voice change and subglottic stenosis. The point of entry to the trachea lies immediately below the glottis, and scarring at this point is likely to result in pathological changes to the delicate vocal fold.

19. A
Vocal nodules result from vocal abuse. They are fibrous thickenings of the vocal fold at the junction of the anterior and middle thirds. This is the point of maximum convexity during phonation. Speech therapy is the preferred treatment, as surgical excision, injection or radiotherapy would result in further scarring of the vocal fold. The underlying lamina propria of the vocal fold is critical to its function, and treatments aim to leave this untouched. If nodules do not settle with speech therapy, microsurgical techniques can be used to remove them, but patients must be aware that their voice may not return to its original state.

20. C
Vocal cord palsy can be unilateral or bilateral. Particularly with a left vocal cord palsy, bronchial malignancy must be suspected given the recurrent laryngeal nerve's route through the chest. Investigation should be with CT of the neck and chest to image the nerve's path to the larynx. Although a unilateral palsy will lead to initial voice change, symptoms may resolve as the contralateral cord compensates. For this reason, post-thyroidectomy follow-up should include visualisation of the larynx to document cord function. Although a unilateral cord palsy will not require a tracheostomy, bilateral palsies, which can follow thyroidectomy, are more likely to require intervention. The cords tend to lie in a paramedian position and compromise the airway in the immediate postoperative period.

21. C
Cancer of the larynx most commonly affects the vocal cord and presents with hoarseness. For this reason patients with persistent hoarseness should be referred to an ENT surgeon for visualisation of the larynx. Otalgia is a sign of advanced disease as pain radiates through the vagus nerve. The glottis itself has no lymphatic supply, so until the disease enlarges to involve the subglottis or supraglottis, lymph node metastasis is rare. Early laryngeal cancer does not impair swallowing, but as the disease progresses it can lead to significant changes in pharyngeal function.

22. A
Laryngectomy involves removal of the larynx, with the trachea brought out on the skin of the neck permanently, and the remaining pharynx closed to separate the airway and the GI tract. The vocal folds are removed which clearly changes the voice, although there are multiple strategies which allow patients to speak following surgery. The electrolarynx can be used to produce sound which is turned into speech by the patient's remaining vocal tract, swallowed air can be regurgitated

as speech or modern valves can be used to divert pulmonary air up through the neopharynx facilitating speech also.

The neck

23. D

Branchial cysts are thought to represent a remnant of the second branchial cleft, although opinions vary. They present in young adults, with a neck mass at the junction of the upper and middle thirds of the sternomastoid muscle. They contain thick turbid fluid containing cholesterol crystals. If they become infected, surgical excision is made more challenging and the procedure should be postponed until the infection resolves.

24. B

Cystic hygroma, a malformation of lymphatics, presents in early infancy. It can sometimes be diagnosed in the prenatal period on ultrasound scanning – and when massive can even interfere with labour. The neck is a common site and these soft compressible masses are brilliantly translucent. Cystic hygromas of the neck behave unpredictably and can interfere with the airway, which is an indication for treatment. Definitive treatment involves excision or sclerotherapy; however, extensive, multicystic disease presents a challenge irrespective of the treatment modality.

25. E

The thyroid descends from the foramen caecum at the junction of the posterior and middle thirds of the tongue to its position in front of the trachea. If a remnant of this thyroglossal tract fails to involute, a thyroglossal duct cyst is formed. The path of the thyroid hooks around the hyoid bone, so surgical treatment requires excision of the middle of the body of the hyoid to prevent recurrence. Excision of these cysts involves a midline neck dissection to include all branches of the cyst, removal of the hyoid, as described, and excision of a cuff of tongue base tissue.

Trauma to the neck

26. D

Following blunt trauma to the larynx, haematoma and swelling can lead to a rapid loss of the airway. Long-term intubation following such an injury will result in a foreign body reaction to the tube which can cause massive permanent fibrosis. Low tracheostomy should be considered with open repair of significant mucosal lacerations and suture repair of displaced cartilage fractures. Laryngeal stents may be left in place for around 5 days and removed endoscopically.

27. A

Ludwig's angina is an infective condition affecting the submandibular space. Oedema of the floor of the mouth elevates the tongue, which compromises the airway. The infection is often polymicrobial and requires broad-spectrum antibiotics. If swelling continues despite treatment, surgical decompression of the submandibular triangles may be required with division of the mylohyoid to decompress the floor of mouth. Tracheostomy should be considered. This condition should not be confused with Vincent's angina, an infective gingivostomatitis.

28. C

Tuberculous adenitis tends to affect the upper deep cervical lymph nodes. A collection can develop in these nodes and, without treatment, pus can erode the deep fascial planes to penetrate up towards the superficial fascia. Here it spreads out within this space and is referred to as a collar-stud abscess. Eventually the abscess will burst and form a discharging sinus. Patients will not show the classic signs of a bacterial abscess (hence the term cold abscess) and ideally incision and drainage should be avoided, as it will also result in a discharging sinus. Appropriate antibiotics and management of renal or pulmonary disease, if coexistent, should be commenced. Occasionally abscesses will fail to resolve, at which point complete surgical excision is the treatment of choice.

Primary tumours of the neck

29. B

Carotid body tumours or chemodectomas are more common at altitude as the chronic hypoxia leads to carotid body hyperplasia. Only 10 per cent have a family history, and although these tumours are associated with phaeochromocytomas, they are not hormonally active themselves. The classic pulsatile mass at the level of the carotid bifurcation can be moved side to side but not up and down. Investigation is with angiogram/MRI, not FNA, which is contraindicated. If the mass presents in the parapharyngeal space, intraoral biopsy is also contraindicated as a haematoma can lead to fatal airway compromise. These tumours are slow-growing and benign so the need for surgical removal should be carefully considered.

30. E

The classical, radical neck dissection involved removal of all nodes, the sternomastoid, jugular and accessory. Selective neck dissections remove only lymphatics, but not all levels. Modified neck dissections can be classed 1–3 depending on the number of structures preserved from the nerve, vein and muscle. Subtotal is not a term applied to neck dissection.

Answers: Extended matching questions

1. Investigation of the pharynx, larynx and neck

1G

The diagnosis is pharyngeal pouch, which can be seen on barium swallow. Symptoms include dysphagia, aspiration, gurgling noises on swallowing and the reflux of pouch contents. Management options include endoscopic or open procedures.

2A

This is suspicious of SCC. The first investigation is FNA. Open biopsy of the node risks seeding malignancy and can compromise prognosis. Having made a diagnosis, the next steps would be scanning with MRI/CT and examination under anaesthetic. There is a growing role for PET scanning in the investigation of patients with metastatic SCC from an unknown origin.

3E

Carotid body tumours should not be biopsied. MRI scans or angiograms will demonstrate the disease and its relationship with the carotid vessels.

4H

Persistent hoarseness and vocal cord changes in a smoker are suspicious of malignancy. Examination under anaesthetic with biopsies allows for a histological diagnosis and accurate staging of malignancy.

5D

The recurrent laryngeal nerve on the left has a long route through the chest and can be damaged at any point along its route. Bronchial carcinoma should be ruled out, but malignancies elsewhere, including the oesophagus and thyroid, should also be considered.

2. Investigation and management of the acute airway case

1I

Stertor is the sound made by upper airway obstruction at a level above the larynx. Epstein–Barr virus can cause tonsillitis, often presenting with a grey/white film over the tonsils. The tonsils can be enlarged sufficiently to threaten the airway. These patients should be monitored carefully, and ideally nursed in a high-dependency area. If they fail to respond to antibiotics, a short course of steroids should be given. Patients whose airway continues to deteriorate should be considered for urgent tonsillectomy.

2G

This child should be considered to have epiglottitis. These patients should be managed in a calm environment, with nothing done to upset them, particularly no attempts to examine the throat which can precipitate respiratory arrest. The patient should be transferred to theatre and examined under anaesthetic with an experienced anaesthetist and a surgeon capable of performing paediatric tracheostomy if required.

3B

This patient has a peritonsillar abscess which can be treated with incision and drainage through the mouth. The mucosa is prepared with a local anaesthetic spray and a scalpel blade is used to incise the abscess wall. These patients will also be managed with antibiotics, fluids and analgesia until their oral intake is sufficient.

4C

Blunt laryngeal trauma can result in loss of the airway, and prompt intervention may be required. Endotracheal intubation should be avoided as the foreign body reaction to the tube can result in permanent laryngeal damage. An early tracheostomy is appropriate, with inspection of the larynx and repair of mucosal and cartilage injuries in an attempt to minimise long-term loss of function.

5H

Recurrent respiratory papillomatosis is a condition caused by HPV 6 and 11. It results in papillomata at sites of epithelial transition such as the vocal folds. Following a biopsy for histological confirmation, the lesions should be excised endoscopically using cold steel or laser. The underlying tissues must not be damaged as this condition often improves after puberty and the aim is to maintain the normal function of the larynx as far as possible.

46 Oropharyngeal cancer

Multiple choice questions

In the following, choose the single best answer.

→ Anatomy and pathology

1. **The posterior border of the oral cavity is:**
   - A The base of the vallecula
   - B The posterior tonsillar pillar
   - C The level of the circumvallate papillae of the tongue
   - D The posterior pharyngeal wall
   - E The lingual surface of the epiglottis.

2. **Which of the following structures is not part of the oropharynx?**
   - A The hard palate
   - B The tonsillar fossa
   - C The superior surface of the hyoid bone
   - D The base of tongue
   - E The posterior pharyngeal wall.

3. **What is the most common malignancy encountered in the oropharynx?**
   - A Adenocarcinoma
   - B Squamous cell carcinoma (SCC)
   - C Adenoid cystic carcinoma
   - D Non-Hodgkin's lymphoma
   - E Salivary gland tumours.

4. **Which of the following conditions is not associated with malignant transformation?**
   - A Erythroplakia
   - B Chronic hyperplastic candidiasis
   - C Sideropenic dysphagia (Paterson–Kelly syndrome)
   - D Angular stomatitis
   - E Oral lichen planus.

5. **The term 'field change' in relation to oral cancer refers to what?**
   - A The wide field radiotherapy techniques which must be applied to the oral mucosa in head and neck cancer patients.
   - B The demarcated mucosal changes seen in patients with oral cancer which resembles the appearance of agricultural fields.
   - C The effect upon the surrounding oral mucosa conferred by long-standing dental caries.
   - D The widespread damage of epithelium leading to mucosal changes and a high incidence of separate tumours.
   - E The requirement to rotate the radiotherapy field during a course of treatment to maximise tissue-sparing effects.

6. **What does the term 'skip metastasis' refer to?**
   - A The tendency of oral cancers to metastasise to the liver without cervical nodal metastasis.
   - B The tendency of oral cancers to metastasise to bone without cervical nodal metastasis.
   - C The tendency of oral cancers to metastasise to lower-echelon cervical lymph nodes without involving the higher echelons.
   - D The tendency of oral cancers to metastasise to the higher-echelon cervical lymph nodes then on to the lower level nodes.
   - E The tendency of oral cancers to metastasise the contralateral cervical nodes.

→ Clinical features, investigation and staging of oropharyngeal cancer

7. **Which of the following statements is true with regard to cancers of the lip?**
   A They tend to present early.
   B They tend to affect the upper lip.
   C Lymph node metastasis tends to involve level V first.
   D Lymph node metastasis occurs early.
   E Disease tends to spread in a vertical direction.

8. **Which of the following is not a feature of oral cancer?**
   A Mouth ulceration >4 weeks
   B Painless neck mass
   C Unexplained tooth mobility
   D Trismus
   E Unilateral tonsillar enlargement.

9. **Which of the following is true of oropharyngeal cancers?**
   A Ease of office examination means examination under anaesthetic is rarely required.
   B The folded mucosal nature of the tonsil and tongue base can render early disease occult.
   C The painless nature of oropharyngeal cancer allows for examination and biopsy without anaesthetic.
   D Early presentation of most cases allows for conservative treatment.
   E As SCC is the most common malignancy, biopsy for histology is seldom required.

10. **Which of the following is true with regard to the investigation of oral/oropharyngeal cancer?**
   A Artefact from dental amalgam limits the usefulness of MRI.
   B The sensitivity of MRI for detecting nodal metastasis greatly exceeds that of CT.
   C MRI allows for better visualisation of soft-tissue infiltration than CT.
   D As MRI is more widely available than CT, it tends to be used for convenience.
   E In patients unable to tolerate CT scanning due to claustrophobia, MRI is the appropriate choice.

11. **Which of the following statements regarding fine-needle aspiration cytology (FNAC) in oropharyngeal cancer is true?**
   A It causes seeding of disease to the skin.
   B It provides reliable results independent of the operator.
   C It is used for diagnosis of primary disease.
   D It is used in assessment of enlarged cervical lymph nodes.
   E It requires adequate fixation for interpretation.

→ Treatment of oropharyngeal cancer

12. **Which of the following factors should not be considered in tailoring treatment for a patient with head and neck cancer?**
   A Chronological age
   B The site of disease
   C The stage of disease
   D The histology
   E Social factors.

13. **Management of premalignant conditions should not include:**
   A Smoking cessation
   B Photographic recording
   C Biopsy from more than one site
   D Surgical excision
   E Radiotherapy.

14. **Which of the following is true of treatments for cancer of the lip?**
   A Small tumours can be managed with shave excision.
   B Surgery and radiotherapy have similar cure rates.
   C Defects of between one and two-thirds of the lower lip require reconstruction with distant flaps.
   D In total lip reconstruction, the neck should not be entered, so as to preserve blood supply to the tissues.

E In closure of lip lesions, the apposition of the mucosal surface is the most important layer.

15. **What effect does the presence of cervical metastasis have on prognosis in head and neck cancer?**
A 10 per cent decrease in survival
B 30 per cent decrease in survival
C 50 per cent decrease in survival
D No effect on survival
E Improved overall survival.

16. **What effect does the degree of differentiation of SCC in head and neck cancer have on overall management?**
A The higher the degree of differentiation, the lower the stage of disease.
B The higher the degree of differentiation, the higher the stage of disease.
C The higher the degree of differentiation, the higher the dose of radiotherapy used.
D The higher the degree of differentiation, the lower the dose of radiotherapy used.
E The degree of differentiation does not directly effect management.

17. **In the management of field change, which of the following statements is true?**
A Radiotherapy allows for widespread superficial treatment without severe side-effects.
B Platinum-based chemotherapy is a recognised treatment.
C Lesions in the mouth should be treated surgically in a combined procedure with neck dissection.
D Multiple surgical excisions are preferred to radiotherapy.
E Treatment is contraindicated.

➜ Reconstructive techniques

18. **Which of the following statements about the principles of oropharyngeal reconstruction is false?**
A Unopposed action of one hypoglossal nerve leads to a compromised swallow.
B Small defects of the lateral tongue may be closed primarily.
C Small defects of the lateral tongue may be left to heal by secondary intention.
D Radial forearm free flaps can be used to provide a thin flap with good results.
E Following total glossectomy, a thick reconstruction flap is beneficial.

19. **Which of the following statements about reconstruction of anterior floor of mouth defects is true?**
A Due to the excellent blood supply of this area, defects rarely require formal reconstruction.
B It is unacceptable to advance the ventral tongue forward to the labial mucosa.
C Microvascular free flap reconstruction is the only option available.
D Defects which require excision of the anterior mandible should be treated by delayed bony reconstruction.
E Treatment of the neck is unlikely to be required.

20. **Which of the following techniques is not part of a stepwise approach to tissue reconstruction?**
A Closure by primary intention
B Closure by secondary intention
C Closure by tertiary intention
D Local flap reconstruction
E Free flap reconstruction.

21. **Which arterial pedicle is harvested to supply a rectus abdominus free flap?**
A The inguinal artery
B The deep inferior epigastric artery
C The circumflex femoral artery
D The deep circumflex iliac artery
E The internal mammary artery.

22. **The composite forearm free flap is based upon which arterial pedicle?**
A The radial artery
B The ulnar artery
C The lateral decubitus artery
D The brachial artery
E The profunda brachii artery.

Management of neck disease

23. Which of the following statements about management of oropharyngeal cancer is true?

A Transoral access makes most primary lesions in this area amenable to surgical treatment.
B Cervical metastases are rare.
C Chemoradiotherapy is contraindicated for tumours in this region.
D In patients with large volume neck disease surgical excision alone is the preferred treatment
E Treatment of the neck alone with surgery, followed by chemoradiotherapy to treat the primary and neck, may be appropriate.

24. Which of the following statements is true?

A The addition of chemotherapy to radiotherapy causes no increase in morbidity versus radiotherapy alone.
B The addition of chemotherapy to radiotherapy for lesions of the tongue base has not been shown to improve survival.
C Using chemoradiotherapy ensures preservation of organ function.
D Frail patients may not tolerate the addition of chemotherapy to radiotherapy.
E Chemoradiotherapy is effective for large volume disease.

25. Which of the following statements is true in the clinically node-negative neck?

A The absence of palpable cervical lymph nodes confirms that the disease has not metastasised.
B The absence of both palpable and radiologically obvious lymph node metastases confirms that the disease has not metastasised.
C Treatment with radiotherapy is equally effective as surgery.
D Radical neck dissection should be performed if there is a risk of occult metastasis.
E The histological findings following planned neck dissection will not influence further treatment.

26. Which of the following statements is true in the clinically node-positive neck?

A N1 disease describes one palpable node whatever the size.
B N2 disease can be unilateral or bilateral.
C N3 disease must include bilateral disease.
D N4 disease involves critical structures.
E All of the above.

Complications and outcomes of treatment

27. Which of the following is not a complication of oropharyngeal resection?

A Xerostomia
B Thoracic duct injury
C Soft-tissue oedema
D Rupture of carotid artery
E Accessory nerve palsy.

28. Which of the following is not a complication of radiotherapy for head and neck cancer?

A Atherosclerosis of the carotid artery
B Trismus
C Visual impairment
D Osteoradionecrosis of the mandible
E Renal toxicity.

29. Which of the following statements is true for patients who complete treatment for oropharyngeal cancer?

A Although physical impairment may be severe, psychological disturbances are uncommon.
B Recurrence following major surgery is likely to be managed best with palliative care.
C Most recurrences occur at around 5 years post-treatment.
D Follow-up is best coordinated by the primary care physician.
E Morbidity following treatment is short-lived.

30. **What is the most significant factor in determining prognosis in oropharyngeal cancer?**
- A Tumour size
- B Patient age
- C Presence of metastasis
- D Concomitant medical conditions
- E Smoking status of the patient.

Extended matching questions

→ 1. Anatomy
- A Vermillion border
- B Buccal surface of the lip
- C Ventral surface of the tongue
- D Junction of anterior 2/3 and posterior 1/3 of the tongue
- E Junction of the hard and soft palate
- F Lingual surface of the epiglottis
- G Posterior pharyngeal wall
- H Upper surface of the hyoid bone
- I Anterior tonsillar pillar
- J Posterior tonsillar pillar

Match the most appropriate anatomical term with the descriptions given below:

1. The anterior border of the oral cavity
2. The posterosuperior border of the oral cavity
3. The inferior border of the oropharynx
4. The posterior border of the oropharynx
5. Line of the circumvallate papillae

→ 2. Treatment and outcomes in oropharyngeal cancer
- A Physiological age of the patient
- B Social class of the patient
- C Smoking status of patient
- D Size of primary lesion
- E Presence of extensive field change
- F Degree of histological differentiation
- G Presence of extracapsular spread
- H Presence of cervical nodal metastasis
- I Bulky neck disease
- J Palsy of accessory nerve

Choose the most appropriate response for the questions below:

1. Which factor will necessitate postoperative radiotherapy in the clinically node-negative neck?
2. Which factor may prevent the addition of chemotherapy to treatment?
3. Which factor has the biggest impact on prognosis?
4. Which factor should encourage surgery over radiotherapy?
5. Which factor will require planned surgery and postoperative radiotherapy?

Answers: Multiple choice questions

Anatomy and pathology

1. C

The oral cavity runs from the skin-vermillion border on the lips to the level of the soft palate superiorly and the circumvallate papillae on the tongue. This line lies at the junction between the anterior two-thirds and the posterior third of the tongue.

2. A

The oropharynx lies posterior to the oral cavity, so the hard palate is outside its boundaries. The oropharynx includes the tonsillar fossae laterally and the base of tongue down to its attachment to the superior border of the hyoid in the vallecula. Posteriorly, the posterior pharyngeal wall from the level of the hard palate to the level of the hyoid is included.

3. B

Squamous cell carcinoma is the most common malignancy in head and neck mucosa. There is a strong association with tobacco consumption and a synergistic effect with alcohol. Different methods of tobacco consumption account for geographic differences in disease distribution. The practice of chewing tobacco on the Indian subcontinent has led to high rates of oral cavity and oropharyngeal cancer.

4. D

Most oral carcinomas do not develop in an area of clinically obvious premalignant disease. Erythroplakia describes a lesion that is a bright red plaque. Chronic hyperplastic candidiasis can result in malignant transformation, and in these patients an immunological defect may coexist. Oral lichen planus has a weak association with malignant transformation.

5. D

Field change refers to the widespread damage to mucosa caused by chronic exposure to tobacco and alcohol. This so-called 'cancerisation' effect results in a high rate of separate tumours within the mucosal field. Fifteen per cent of patients will develop a second primary, most commonly a metachronous lesion. The rate of synchronous tumours is 4 per cent.

6. C

Head and neck cancers tend to metastasise in a predictable manner, however SCC of the oral tongue can present with skip metastasis and disease in the lower-echelon lymph node groups (levels III and IV) without involving the upper echelons (I and II). Oropharyngeal nodes commonly metastasise to levels II, III and IV as well as the contralateral neck. Distant metastases are uncommon.

Clinical features, investigation and staging of oropharyngeal cancer

7. A

Cancer of the lip is unusual in comparison with other oral cancers as it tends to present early. The lower lip is affected more commonly than the upper lip. Disease on the upper lip tends to be more aggressive. Metastasis occurs late and tends to be to nodes in levels I and II. The disease tends to spread laterally over the mucosal surface.

8. E

Late presentation of head and neck cancer results in poor outcome. The presence of a cervical metastasis halves a patient's prognosis. Delays may be due to the elderly and frail nature of these patients and the fact that denture-wearers may be used to discomfort and ulceration within the mouth. Trismus develops from involvement of the pterygoid muscles. The palatine tonsils lie in the tonsillar fossa, which is within the oropharynx not the oral cavity.

9. B

Early mucosal disease involving the tonsil, tongue base and nasopharynx may be impossible to see on clinical examination. Disease can hide in the mucosal folds within these regions and fool the examiner. For this reason complete examination must include palpation. This is often uncomfortable and even exquisitely tender for the patient and requires general anaesthetic in almost all patients. Oropharyngeal cancer often presents late, sometimes as a cervical metastasis without evidence of the primary disease on inspection. Definitive histology should be sought in all cases.

10. C

Magnetic resonance imaging gives excellent soft-tissue definition, which allows superior assessment of tissue invasion for diseases of the oropharynx and oral cavity. CT is more widely available and less claustrophobic but it provides less soft-tissue definition and can be affected by dental artefact. Currently the sensitivity and specificity of MRI and CT for detecting cervical metastases are comparable.

11. D

Fine-needle aspiration cytology has become a routine investigation of cervical disease in the head and neck. It is not used for the primary, where open biopsy through the mouth is preferred. Results are operator-dependent, and if the cytologist is available immediately, no fixative is required. Seeding is not a complication of FNA. Recent work suggests that ultrasound guidance can significantly improve yield.

Treatment of oropharyngeal cancer

12. A

Many factors must be considered before designing a treatment plan. Modern anaesthetic techniques allow major surgery to be performed on patients with significant comorbidities. Head and neck cancer patients will be heavy smokers and may be alcoholics and hence physiological age is more important than chronological age. The treatment options include surgery, radiotherapy and chemotherapy.

13. E

Removing the aetiological factors associated with malignancy is the basis of managing premalignant conditions. Smoking is the most common aetiological factor. Photographic records are valuable and more accurate than clinical diagrams. By taking biopsies from more than one site, a more accurate picture can be built up of disease progression. Lesions can be excised or vaporised with laser but not treated with radiotherapy, which should be reserved for true malignancy.

14. B

Both surgery and radiotherapy offer cure rates of around 90 per cent for cancer of the lip. Small lesions can be managed surgically with V-wedge excisions closed primarily. Excision of one to two-thirds of the lower lip can be closed with local flaps. In total reconstruction of the lip, distant flaps are used which require access to the neck to anastomose vessels to the branches of the external carotid. Neck dissection is likely to be required for such patients who are at high risk of cervical metastasis. In closing the lip, the vermillion border is vital to prevent a poor cosmetic result.

15. C

Cervical metastasis in head and neck cancer carries a 50 per cent reduction in survival rates. Treatment of the neck should be considered both when there is clinically palpable metastatic disease and when the chance of micrometastases (which are impalpable) is greater than 20 per cent. At this level the morbidity of treatment is lower than the impact of potential disease. In practice this means that the cervical nodes should be treated in all cases other than early glottis and lip lesions.

16. E

Differentiation is often commented upon by pathologists, and forms part of the minimum dataset of many cancer groups. The current staging systems used in the UK and USA do not consider the histological differentiation and have little impact on treatment at present. It is likely that, as our understanding of the impact of perivascular and perineural invasion as well as histological differentiation increases, such indicators may be incorporated into staging systems.

17. D

Cases of field change or multiple precancerous lesions should be treated with surgical excision. Radiotherapy would require treatment of a wide field, which would result in severe morbidity and make interpretation of future biopsies from that site less reliable. Chemotherapy is not a recognised treatment for non-malignant disease. In cases of premalignancy, neck dissection would not be warranted, as the disease would not have spread by definition. If, having reviewed the formal histology, a malignancy is discovered, the staging process should be undertaken and the neck treated, if indicated.

→ Reconstructive techniques

18. A

Oropharyngeal resection has an impact on swallowing. Sacrificing both hypoglossal nerves will lead to a loss of function of the tongue and subsequent morbidity. If possible at least one nerve should be preserved to help swallow rehabilitation. Lateral tongue lesions may be closed primarily or left to heal by secondary intention. Free flaps should be chosen depending on the defect created. If there is much tissue loss, a bulky flap such as a rectus abdominus should be chosen to replace the tissue. Radial forearm free flaps can be left thin and pliable so they mould to the contours of the defect.

19. B

Most floor-of-mouth tumours require formal reconstruction. Advancing the ventral tongue to the labial mucosa leads to significant speech and swallowing morbidity, which is considered unacceptable. Options include local and free flap reconstruction. If the anterior mandible is resected, immediate reconstruction is required to prevent severe functional and cosmetic defects. There is a rich, often bilateral, lymphatic supply to this area and treatment of the neck is likely to be required.

20. C

Reconstruction of a defect in the oral cavity or oropharynx should be approached logically. Some lesions may be left to heal by secondary intention, some may be closed primarily. Local flaps were extensively used prior to the advent of procedures to harvest reliable free flaps. The choice of technique will depend on the tissue removed, the tissues remaining, the functional aims and the fitness of the patient.

21. B

22. A

→ Management of neck disease

23. E

The oropharynx is a difficult site to access surgically. Small lesions can necessitate extensive access procedures and resections. Cervical metastases are common. Chemoradiotherapy is a recognised treatment for disease in this area, as it is for other head and neck cancers. It may be used in an organ preservation strategy, designed to prevent the need for glossectomy or laryngectomy. This approach can be used with surgical treatment of the neck in selected cases. The chance of local recurrence is high in patients with large volume neck disease (N2/N3), and postoperative radiotherapy should be used.

24. D

The role of chemotherapy is becoming clearer, with survival benefits being demonstrated for chemoradiotherapy over radical surgery for lesions of the tongue base. The addition of chemotherapy to radiotherapy significantly increases both morbidity and mortality, which is why frail patients may not tolerate the regime. Although chemoradiotherapy avoids surgical treatment, there are post-treatment changes, including fibrosis and reduced vascular supply. These changes can lead to loss of function. Treatment of large-volume disease still requires surgery, if feasible, as chemoradiotherapy is less effective in these cases.

25. C

A neck can be described as negative on palpation, or following radiological assessment, often by CT. Both of these modalities have a sensitivity and specificity (around 70 per cent for palpation and 80–90 per cent for CT). Because of this, micrometastases will always be missed. It is for this reason that treatment of the neck should be considered. Current guidelines suggest that if the chance of a metastasis is 20 per cent or greater, treatment should be advised. In the clinically negative neck, radiotherapy and surgery are equally effective. There is no evidence that radical neck dissection confers a survival advantage over modified radical neck dissection. If the histology shows malignancy with extracapsular or perineural invasion, postoperative radiotherapy should be considered.

26. B

- N0 – no regional nodal metastasis
- N1 – single lymph node metastasis <3 cm
- N2 – single ipsilateral node 3–6 cm/ipsilateral multiple nodes <6 cm/bilateral or contralateral nodes <6 cm
- N3 – any node >6 cm.

Complications and outcomes of treatment

27. A

Xerostomia is dryness of the mouth associated with radiotherapy to the head and neck that involved the salivary glands. Soft-tissue oedema occurs following surgery and is particularly bad following bilateral neck dissection. If both internal jugular veins must be sacrificed, swelling is severe with a significant rise in intracranial pressure.

28. E

Renal toxicity is a complication of chemotherapy which may be added to radiotherapy. All structures within a radiotherapy field are affected by it. Fibrosis of the muscles of mastication results in trismus, damage to the lens or optic nerve can affect vision, and atherosclerosis can develop in the carotid artery. Osteoradionecrosis is a difficult problem which is best avoided by removal of infected teeth in the field, and providing a well-vascularised cover to the mandible as part of treatment.

29. B

Treatment for head and neck cancer can be both physically disfiguring and functionally disabling. The loss of the ability to swallow and speak normally has a tremendous effect on patients' lifestyle. Coupled with cosmetic deformity, these changes can result in severe psychological disturbance. Pre- and post-treatment counselling may minimise the effects, but many of these changes will be long-term or permanent. Support is generally best provided by the team who coordinated treatment, as primary care physicians are unlikely to have great experience of these rare conditions. Most recurrences present within the first 12 months (70 per cent) and 90 per cent within the first 2 years. Patients who present with recurrence following a major resection are unlikely to be suitable for curative treatment and will often be best managed in a palliative care setting. At 5 years many patients can be discharged from oncological surveillance, but may require ongoing support from other members of the team.

30. C

The presence of nodal metastasis is the most significant prognostic factor, although all others will have an impact on the patient, their response to treatment and their subsequent outcome.

Answers: Extended matching questions

1. Anatomy

1A, 2E, 3H, 4G, 5D

2. Treatment and outcomes in oropharyngeal cancer

1G

If histology demonstrates extracapsular spread following a staging neck dissection for the clinically node-negative neck, postoperative radiotherapy is used to reduce the chance of local recurrence.

2A

Chemotherapy adds significantly to the morbidity and mortality of treatment and so it may be contraindicated in frail patients.

3H

The presence of cervical metastases halves the prognosis.

4E

Patients with field change or multiple tumours should be treated with surgery if possible, as radiotherapy involves irradiating a large area with consequent severe morbidity. The radiotherapy changes can also interfere with interpretation of future biopsies if required.

5I

Bulky neck disease responds poorly to single modality treatment and neck dissection with post operative radiotherapy should be considered.

47 Disorders of the salivary glands

Multiple choice questions

In the following, choose the single best answer.

Anatomy, physiology and pathology of the salivary glands

1. **The minor salivary glands contribute what percentage of the total salivary volume?**
   A 10 per cent
   B 20 per cent
   C 30 per cent
   D 40 per cent
   E 50 per cent.

2. **What percentage of minor salivary gland tumours are malignant?**
   A 50 per cent
   B 60 per cent
   C 70 per cent
   D 80 per cent
   E 90 per cent.

3. **Which statement most accurately describes the anatomy of the sublingual glands?**
   A They drain through the sublingual duct which opens into the floor of mouth.
   B They drain either directly on to the floor of mouth or into the submandibular duct.
   C They consist of two lobes separated by the mylohyoid muscle.
   D They are embedded in the intrinsic muscles of the ventral surface of the tongue.
   E They lie in the space between the mandible and the two bellies of digastric.

4. **The term plunging ranula refers to which clinical entity?**
   A A malignant congenital salivary mass arising from the submandibular gland
   B A benign salivary mass involving the parotid and submandibular glands
   C A mucous retention cyst originating from the sublingual glands, limited by the mylohyoid muscle
   D A mucous retention cyst originating from the submandibular and sublingual glands which perforates the mylohyoid muscle to enter the neck
   E A midline neck mass which moves on tongue protrusion.

The submandibular glands

5. **Which of the following structures is not an anatomical relation to the submandibular salivary gland?**
   A The anterior facial vein
   B The facial artery
   C The inferior alveolar nerve
   D The lingual nerve
   E The hypoglossal nerve.

6. **Which structure marks the posterior boundary of the submandibular duct which can safely be accessed via an intraoral approach?**
   A The third molar tooth
   B The body of the submandibular duct
   C The lingual nerve
   D The posterior edge of the mylohyoid
   E The marginal mandibular nerve

7. **Which statement best describes placement of the incision used for submandibular gland excision?**
   A Directly over the palpable position of the gland with the neck extended
   B Between the superior limit of the gland and the mandible
   C At the lower limit of the gland
   D 4 cm below the mandible

E Parallel to the sternomastoid muscle at the level of the gland.

8. **Which structure attaches the deep lobe of the submandibular gland to the lingual nerve?**
A The hypoglossal nerve
B The submandibular ganglion
C The deep cervical fascia
D The tendon of digastric
E The mylohyoid.

9. **Which of the following is not a complication of submandibular gland excision?**
A Frey's syndrome
B Anaesthesia of the ipsilateral tongue
C Weakness of the corner of the mouth
D Anaesthesia of submental skin
E Paralysis of the ipsilateral tongue.

10. **What percentage of submandibular tumours are malignant?**
A 20 per cent
B 30 per cent
C 40 per cent
D 50 per cent
E 60 per cent.

11. **Which of the following is not a feature of salivary malignancy?**
A Facial nerve weakness
B Rapid enlargement
C Induration of the overlying skin
D Cervical node enlargement
E Rubbery consistency.

12. **Which is the most appropriate form of biopsy for a major salivary gland tumour?**
A Open surgical biopsy to allow histology
B Salivary washings
C Frozen section during formal excision
D Fine-needle aspiration cytology (FNAC)
E Biopsy is contraindicated.

➜ The parotid gland

13. **Which of the following structures does not lie in the parotid gland?**
A The facial nerve
B Terminal branches of the external carotid
C The glossopharyngeal nerve
D The retromandibular vein
E Lymph nodes.

14. **Which of the following complications is associated with mumps infection?**
A Secretory otitis media
B Pancreatitis
C Balanitis
D Uveitis
E Inflammatory arthritis.

15. **Which of the following conditions is associated with ascending bacterial sialadenitis?**
A Dental abscess
B Oral thrush
C Dehydration
D Otitis media
E Hyperglycaemia.

16. **Which of the following bacteria is the most common cause of bacterial sialadenitis?**
A Staphylococcus aureus
B Staphylococcus epidermidis
C Streptococcus pyogenes
D Pseudomonas aeruginosa
E Atypical mycobacteria.

17. **In a 4-year-old with recurrent bilateral parotid swelling made worse on eating, what is the most likely diagnosis?**
A Sialolithiasis
B Salivary duct stricture
C Sjögren's syndrome
D Recurrent parotitis of childhood
E HIV-associated parotitis.

18. **Chronic parotitis in children is pathognomonic of what disease?**
A HIV
B Sialolithiasis
C Bacterial parotitis
D Tuberculous parotitis
E Wegener's granulomatosis.

19. **What percentage of salivary stones occur in the parotid gland?**
A 10 per cent
B 20 per cent
C 30 per cent
D 40 per cent
E 50 per cent.

20. **What is the most common site for a parotid tumour?**
A At the anterior border of the masseter
B Inferior to the angle of the mandible
C As a parapharyngeal mass
D Anterior to the ear
E Behind the angle of the mandible.

21. **How should a benign tumour involving the tail of parotid be managed?**
A Enucleation
B Open biopsy prior to formal excision
C Radiotherapy
D Total parotidectomy
E Superficial parotidectomy.

Parotid surgery

22. **Which nerve must be transacted as part of a superficial parotidectomy?**
A The facial nerve
B The hypoglossal nerve
C The greater auricular nerve
D The accessory nerve
E The auriculotemporal nerve.

23. **Which of the following landmarks is used to locate the facial nerve trunk?**
A The insertion of sternomastoid
B The greater horn of the hyoid
C The superior-most portion of the cartilaginous ear canal
D The insertion of digastric
E The insertion of masseter.

24. **Which of the following is not a branch of the facial nerve?**
A Temporal
B Oribtal
C Zygomatic
D Buccal
E Cervical.

25. **Which of the following branches of the facial nerve can be divided without the need for immediate cable graft repair?**
A Temporal
B Oribtal
C Zygomatic
D Buccal
E Cervical.

26. **What is Frey's syndrome following parotidectomy?**
A Gustatory sweating
B Dry mouth due to reduction in salivary flow
C Development of a sialocele over the parotid bed
D Cosmetic deformity due to loss of parotid bulk
E Hyperplasia of the contralateral parotid gland.

Degenerative conditions

27. **Which of the following statements is true of secondary Sjögren's syndrome?**
A It is more common in males.
B It is more common in the elderly.
C It is associated with connective tissue disorders.
D The submandibular glands are more commonly affected.
E The chance of malignant transformation is greater than in primary Sjögren's.

28. **With which malignancy is Sjögren's syndrome associated?**
A Acinic cell carcinoma
B Adenoid cystic carcinoma
C Carcinoma ex pleomorphic adenoma
D Salivary sarcoma
E Lymphoma.

29. **Which of the following is not associated with xerostomia?**
A Depression
B Dehydration
C Sjögren's syndrome
D Radiotherapy to the head and neck
E Cholinergic medications.

30. **Management strategies for drooling include:**
A Botulinium toxin injection into submandibular and parotid glands
B Radiotherapy to the salivary glands
C Submandibular duct repositioning
D Bilateral submandibular gland excision
E Excision of submandibular glands and repositioning of parotid ducts.

Extended matching questions

1. Investigation and management of a parotid mass

A Open biopsy
B FNA
C Frozen section biopsy
D Pleomorphic salivary adenoma
E Warthin's tumour
F Adenoid cystic carcinoma
G Lymphoma
H Greater auricular nerve
I Facial nerve
J Hypoglossal nerve
K Marginal mandibular nerve
L Superficial parotidectomy
M Enucleation of the parotid mass
N Radiotherapy

Study Fig. 47.1 and choose the most appropriate response for the questions below:

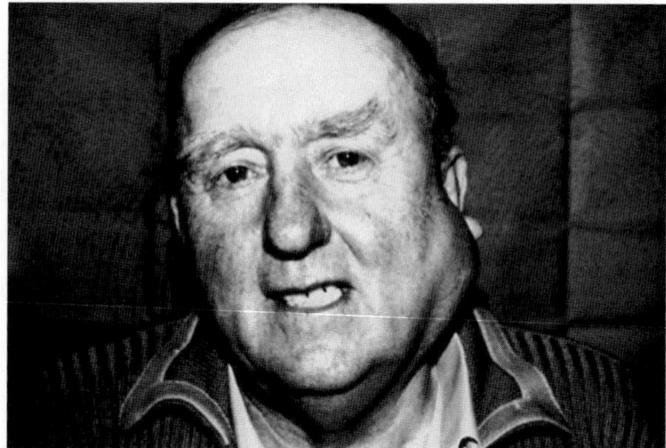

Figure 47.1 Pleomorphic adenoma of the left parotid.

1 What is the most likely diagnosis?

2 What form of biopsy would be most appropriate?

3 Which nerve is it particularly important to test prior to surgery?

4 Which form of treatment would you recommend to this patient?

5 Which structure will be sacrificed during the procedure?

2. Investigation and management of submandibular gland disease

A Sialogram
B Floor of mouth X-ray
C Orthopantogram

D Intermittent pain and swelling
E Weight loss and otalgia
F Dental infection
G Submandibular gland excision
H Transoral stone excision
I Hypoglossal nerve
J Lingual nerve
K Submandibular nerve
L Marsupialisation
M Primary closure
N Stenting of the duct

Study Fig. 47.2 and choose the most appropriate response from the choices below:

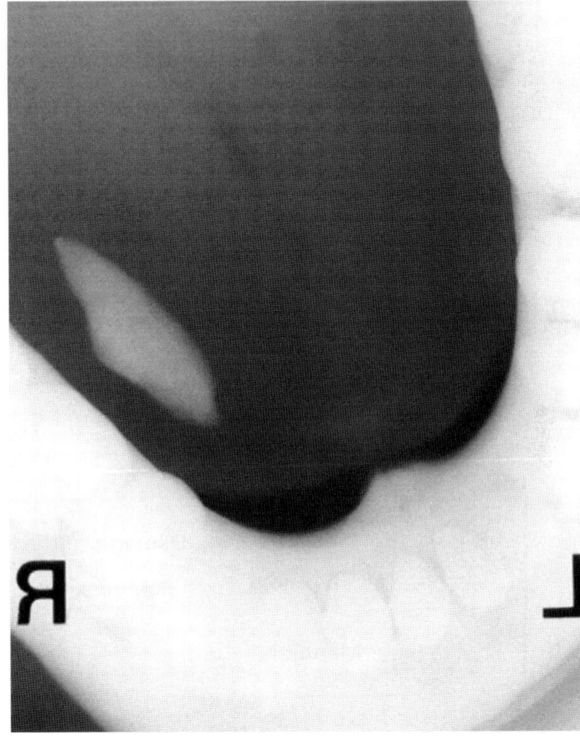

Figure 47.2 Floor of mouth X-ray.

1 What type of X-ray is shown here?

2 What symptoms is the patient likely to present with?

3 What treatment would you suggest?

4 What nerve is at risk?

5 How is ductal stenosis prevented?

Answers: Multiple choice questions

Anatomy, physiology and pathology of the salivary glands

1. A

There are around 450 minor salivary glands distributed through the oral cavity, oropharynx, larynx, trachea and paranasal sinuses. In total they contribute around 10 per cent of the total salivary flow.

2. E

In contrast to the major salivary glands, tumours of the minor salivary glands are highly likely to be malignant. They are often discoloured with a pink, blue or black appearance. If lesions involve the hard palate, treatment involves excision with partial or total maxillectomy.

3. B

4. D

This rare form of mucous retention cyst arises from submandibular and sublingual glands. It expands to perforate the mylohyoid muscle and extend down into the neck. The mass can be seen in the neck and the floor of the mouth. The diagnosis can be confirmed with MRI and treatment consists of excision with the ipsilateral salivary glands.

The submandibular glands

5. C

The submandibular gland consists of two lobes which communicate around the posterior border of mylohyoid. The gland is drained by the submandibular duct, which drains against gravity up to the sublingual papilla in the floor of mouth. The facial vessels are closely related to the gland. On the glands' deep surface, the lingual and hypoglossal nerves are in close proximity. The marginal mandibular nerve is also at risk during surgery on the gland, due to its position in relation to the skin incision. The inferior alveolar nerve enters the mandible and is protected during surgery on the submandibular gland (see Fig. 47.3).

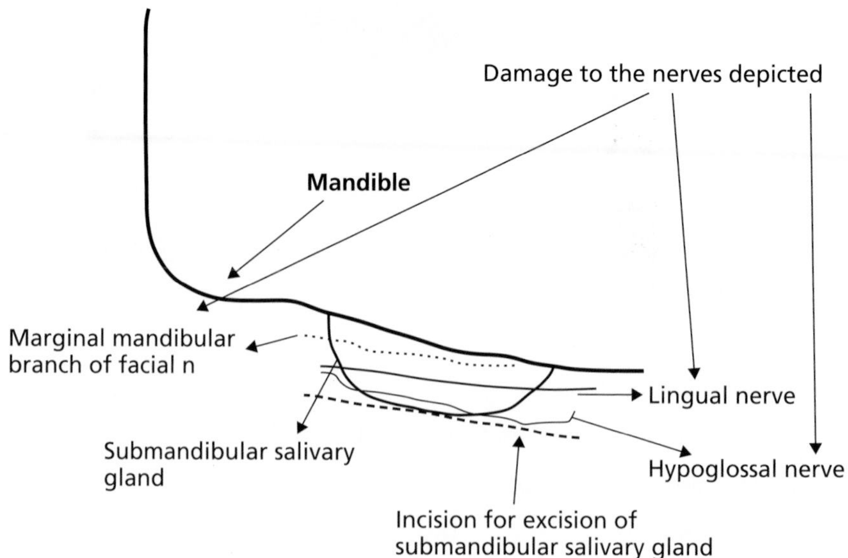

Figure 47.3 Anatomy of the submandibular gland.

6. C
Stones in the submandibular duct may be excised via an intraoral approach if they lie anterior to the lingual nerve, marked by the level of the second molar. The nerve is at risk if the duct is explored behind this level, where calculus disease should be managed with submandibulectomy and excision via a transcervical approach.

7. D
The incision for submandibular gland excision should be placed in a skin crease 4 cm (two fingers' breadths) below the mandible. This avoids damage to the marginal mandibular nerve. It should be no more than 6 cm in length. The incision should be carried through platysma and on through the superficial layer of the deep cervical fascia which protects the marginal mandibular nerve, which lies in a subplatysmal plane.

8. B
The lingual nerve must be identified during excision of the submandibular gland. It lies in the deep surface of the gland and is tethered to it by the submandibular ganglion. This structure relays parasympathetic supply to the gland. The lingual nerve can be seen dipping down towards the deep surface of the gland. There is often a blood vessel associated with the ganglion, and both structures should be clamped and tied. The nerve retracts up into the floor of the mouth, carrying the vessel with it, which can lead to troublesome bleeding.

9. A
Frey's syndrome (gustatory sweating) is due to innervation of sweat glands by cut parasympathetic nerve fibres following parotidectomy. Damage to the lingual nerve causes anaesthesia of the tongue as well as taste disturbance. The marginal mandibular nerve supplies the corner of the mouth. The nerve to mylohyoid supplies sensation to the submental skin, which can be damaged during the dissection. Hypoglossal nerve injury leads to paralysis of the tongue.

10. D
Fifty per cent of submandibular tumours are benign, in contrast with 80 per cent of parotid tumours. The exact diagnosis is often unclear following preoperative work-up.

11. E
The neck mass typically described as rubbery is a lymph node in lymphoma.

12. D
Open biopsy of neck masses is contraindicated unless there is no other option. The procedure leads to seeding of tumour cells, which negatively impacts on prognosis. FNA with a size 18G needle is safe and provides material for cytology. The use of FNA is controversial with some surgeons, indicating that the results rarely alter management. Results are variable and should be audited within departments that use the technique. FNA can be used to identify malignant disease prior to surgery, which can help in obtaining informed consent and planning procedures. Frozen sections are difficult to interpret and are not routinely used.

→ The parotid gland

13. C
The parotid gland is encased in the deep cervical fascia, which splits around it. It lies lateral to the parapharyngeal space, and so the glossopharyngeal nerve lies medial to it.

14. B
The classic conditions associated with mumps (paramyxovirus) infection are orchitis, oophritis, pancreatitis, sensorineural deafness and meningoencephalitis. These conditions are rare and more common in adults than in children.

15. C

Ascending bacterial sialadenitis classically affects the dehydrated elderly patient. The condition results from salivary stasis and presents with pain, swelling and erythema over the parotid gland. The pain is exacerbated by eating or drinking. Pus may be milked from the parotid duct.

16. A

Staphylococcus aureus and *Streptococcus viridians* are the most common organisms in bacterial sialadenitis. Treatment should be with fluids, analgesia and antibiotics. If the gland becomes fluctuant, aspiration is preferable to incision and draining. If incision and drainage are required, the incision should be short and low to avoid the facial nerve, dissection should be blunt and a drain should be placed for up to 72 h.

17. D

Recurrent parotitis of childhood is a condition of unknown aetiology. It tends to affect children aged 3–6 years but can affect older children who are more likely to respond to conservative measures, which include short courses of antibiotics. If symptoms persist, a longer course of prophylactic antibiotics should be considered, with surgery in cases which fail to respond.

18. A

HIV can also present with parotid cysts. The presentation is very similar to Sjögren's syndrome, although with a negative autoantibody screen. The glands tend to be painless and surgery should only be considered for cosmesis if glands are enlarged due to cystic lesions demonstrated on MRI.

19. B

The majority of stones occur in the submandibular duct. This is said to occur as the gland drains against gravity, so promoting salivary stasis and stone formation. The mucinous form of saliva produced by the submandibular gland is also said to promote sialolithiasis.

20. E

Parotid tumours can present throughout the gland; however, they are often behind the angle of the mandible, inferior to the lobule of the ear. Deep lobe tumours can present in the parapharyngeal space with medialisation of the tonsil. These should not be biopsied through a transoral approach due to the airway risk and the differential diagnosis, which includes vascular tumours.

21. E

There is no place for enucleation in modern practice. The aim of parotid surgery should be to perform excision with a cuff of normal tissue. The terms superficial and total parotidectomy refer to the position of the resected specimen in relation to the facial nerve. Although enucleation is an attractive proposition, the high levels of recurrence mean revision surgery is often required, which puts the nerve at high risk due to the scarred nature of the parotid bed.

→ Parotid surgery

22. C

As the gland is mobilised and a plane is developed between its posterior border and the anterior border of the sternomastoid muscle, the greater auricular must be sacrificed. All patients should be warned of the anaesthesia of the ear lobule which results. This is more of a problem in male patients, as it can make shaving in this area more challenging.

23. D

The main landmarks used are the insertion of the digastric muscle and the inferior portion of the cartilaginous ear canal. Control of bleeding at the time of identification is vital, as any blood in the enclosed space developed hampers the surgical view.

24. B (see Fig. 47.4)

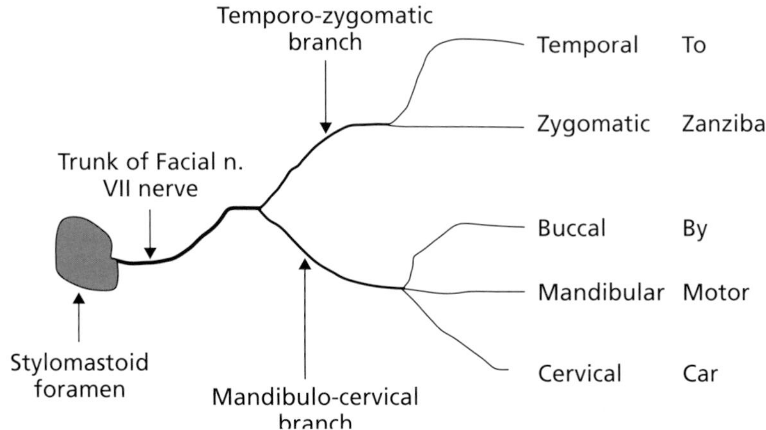

Figure 47.4 Branches of the facial (seventh cranial) nerve. The aide-memoire is To Zanzibar By Motor Car.

25. D
The integrity of the facial nerve should be preserved at all costs; however, if it is clearly involved in disease and the function is compromised, it may require elective division. Under these circumstances, or if a section of nerve is damaged accidentally, repair must be undertaken. The buccal branch is an exception, as it has a less vital role and the presence of multiple cross branches in this region results in some postoperative function.

26. A
The procedure involves division of the postganglionic parasympathetic fibres which would innervate the glandular tissue of the parotid. As these fibres regenerate, they grow towards the sweat glands in the skin flap. This leads to gustatory sweating. It is very common following parotidectomy, but it is uncommon for patients to complain about it.

Degenerative conditions

27. C
Sjögren's syndrome presents with dry mouth (xerostomia) and dry eyes (keratoconjunctivitis sicca). In the primary disease there is no association with connective tissue disorders. The salivary glands rarely get swollen or infected, however the parotid is more commonly affected than the submandibular glands. The chance of malignant transformation is higher in the primary form of the disease.

28. E
There is an association with lymphoma (B-cell type) which is heralded by immunological changes within the blood.

29. E
Anticholinergics, in particular antidepressants, are associated with xerostomia. Management of the condition depends on the underlying cause. Following radiotherapy to the head and neck it can be particularly troublesome. Treatment involves increased fluid intake, carrying a bottle of water and using forms of artificial saliva.

30. B
Most droolers are children with cerebral palsy. Conservative measures should be employed with speech therapy and thought given to posture. If these are unsuccessful, botox can be considered. It tends to give a short-term response. Surgery can be used to reposition the submandibular ducts to the tonsillar fossa, or to excise the gland completely. The parotid ducts can also be repositioned. Care must be taken to ensure safety of swallow prior to repositioning procedures, as there is a danger of turning a drooler into an aspirator. The submandibular glands produce the most saliva in the resting state, so most attention is paid to these.

Answers: Extended matching questions

1. Investigation and management of a parotid mass

1D
The most common diagnosis in a parotid mass in this age group is pleomorphic salivary adenoma. Warthin's tumour is another benign mass which is less common and can be bilateral.

2B
Fine-needle aspiration is the biopsy of choice. Not all surgeons perform a biopsy prior to surgery, as they argue it does not alter management; however, it may allow identification of a malignant tumour which can aid in surgical planning and consent.

3I
The facial nerve is at risk during surgery and it is important to document its function prior to the procedure.

4L
The treatment will be superficial parotidectomy. Most lesions lie superficial to the facial nerve. Further confirmation could be obtained by preoperative MRI. The position of the nerve is estimated to be at the level of the retromandibular vein which can be seen on the scan. Enucleation leads to unacceptably high levels of recurrence.

5H

2. Investigation and management of submandibular gland disease

1B
This is a floor of mouth X-ray. Submandibular stones are often radio-opaque (>80 per cent), unlike parotid stones.

2D
Although the patient may present with overt infection, or having palpated the stone themselves, the most common symptoms will be intermittent unilateral pain and swelling. This will be exacerbated by eating.

3H
This stone is well anterior to the second molar which is the surface marking for the lingual nerve. For that reason transoral excision is recommended. Under local anaesthetic a suture is passed under the duct, posterior to the stone to prevent dislodging the stone back into the body of the gland. An incision is then made over the stone which can be delivered into the floor of mouth.

4J

5L
Primary closure of the duct is likely to be followed by stricture formation. Marsupialisation prevents stricture occurrence.

PART 8 Breast and endocrine

48 Thyroid and the parathyroid gland 363

49 Adrenal glands and other endocrine disorders 375

50 The breast 385

48 Thyroid and the parathyroid gland

Multiple choice questions

➜ Non-thyroidal illness

1. Which of the following are true with regard to sick euthyroid syndrome?

A It can present as high T3 and T4.
B It is often seen in the ITU setting.
C Thyroid-stimulating hormone (TSH) may be high.
D TSH is usually suppressed.
E Thyroid replacement is favoured.

➜ Hyperthyroidism

2. How does hyperthyroidism usually present?

A Graves' disease
B Toxic nodule
C Thyroid malignancy
D De Quervain's thyroiditis
E Toxic multinodular goitre.

➜ Thyrotoxicosis

3. What are the manifestations of thyrotoxicosis?

A Irritability
B Hair loss
C Muscle weakness and wasting
D Hyperkinesias
E Heart failure.

➜ Clinical features of hyperthyroidism

4. Which of the following are associated with Graves' disease?

A Pretibial myxoedema
B Exposure keratitis
C Optic neuropathy
D Chemosis
E Lymphoid hyperplasia.

➜ Medical therapy for hyperthyroidism

5. Which of the following are true regarding medical therapy for thyrotoxicosis?

A Propranolol and nadolol reduce free T3 (fT3) and free T4 (fT4) levels.
B Antithyroid drugs most often cure thyrotoxicosis due to a toxic nodule.
C Carbimazole can be safely given in pregnancy and lactation.
D Agranulocytosis is an uncommon problem with antithyroid drugs.
E Patients with ophthalmopathy respond best to medical management.

➜ Surgery for thyrotoxicosis

6. Surgery is the preferred option of treatment in which of the following cases of thyrotoxicosis?

A A diffuse toxic nodule
B Severe manifestations of Graves' ophthalmopathy
C Pregnant mothers not adequately controlled with medications
D Relapse of Graves'
E Presence of local compressive symptoms.

➜ Radioiodine treatment

7. Which of the following are indications for radioiodine treatment?

A Relapsed Graves' disease
B Thyrotoxicosis in young children
C Multinodular goitre
D Severe ophthalmopathy
E Pregnancy and lactation.

Neonatal hypothyroidism

8. Which of the following are true in neonatal hypothyroidism?

A Endemic cretinism is due to iodine deficiency.
B Macroglossia is a clinical feature.
C Biochemical screening for hypothyroidism is carried out on all neonates in the UK.
D Radioactive iodine treatment is safe after the first trimester of pregnancy.
E Women on antithyroid drugs may give birth to a hypothyroid baby.

Myxoedema

9. Myxoedema can present as:

A Complete heart block
B Ventricular tachycardia
C Mania
D Shortness of breath
E Sepsis.

Biochemical features of hypothyroidism

10. Biochemically hypothyroidism can be associated with:

A Hyponatraemia
B Hyperlipidaemia
C Thyroid peroxidase (TPO) autoantibodies
D Raised TSH
E Low fT3 and fT4.

Classification of hypothyroidism

11. Hypothyroidism could be a presenting feature in which of the following conditions?

A Sarcoidosis
B Pituitary lesions
C Benzodiazepine treatment
D Thyroiditis
E Iodine deficiency.

Thyroid cancer

12. Which of the following statements regarding thyroid neoplasms are true?

A Papillary carcinoma is the most common.
B Men and women are equally affected.
C Thyroid cancer is commonest after the age of 70 years.
D Medullary carcinoma originates from the C-cells.
E Anaplastic carcinoma is the least common.

Thyroglobulin

13. Which of the following statements regarding thyroglobulin are true?

A It is part of normal thyroid function tests.
B It is secreted only by cancerous cells.
C Autoantibodies may interfere with its levels.
D It is a sensitive marker of recurrence of thyroid cancer.
E Radioiodine treatment affects its concentration.

Papillary and follicular cancers

14. Which of the following statements are true?

A Lymph node metastasis is commoner in follicular cancer than in papillary cancer.
B Papillary cancer is associated with increased incidence of nodal metastasis.
C Distant metastasis is commoner in the follicular variety.
D Hurthle cell carcinoma is a type of follicular cancer.
E Papillary carcinoma is usually non-encapsulated and slow-growing.

Differentiated thyroid cancers

15. Which of the following statements are true when a preoperative diagnosis of a differentiated thyroid cancer is made?

A Whole-body MRI or CT imaging is essential.
B Lobectomy is recommended for tumours less than 2 cm.
C Selective nodal dissection may be performed.
D Routine central compartment node clearance is not essential for small tumours.

E Rising thyroglobulin levels are an indication for completion thyroidectomy.

Medullary carcinoma of the thyroid

16. **Which of the following statements regarding medullary thyroid cancers are true?**
   A It can present as multiple endocrine neoplasia.
   B It is not TSH-dependent
   C It is associated with a poor prognosis
   D Diarrhoea is a common feature
   E High levels of calcitonin and carcinoembryonic antigen (CEA) are typical

Primary hyperparathyroidism

17. **Which of the following statements are true?**
   A Primary hyperparathyroidism is usually sporadic.
   B Hypercalcaemia triggers the release of parathyroid hormone (PTH).
   C Familial hyperparathyroidism commonly presents as an adenoma.
   D Familial hyperparathyroidism is mostly sporadic.
   E Hyperparathyroidism can be associated with a pituitary adenoma.

Calcium

18. **Which of the following suggest a biochemical diagnosis of primary hyperparathyroidism?**
   A Raised ionised calcium and suppressed PTH levels
   B Raised total calcium and elevated PTH levels
   C Low serum phosphate levels
   D Low urine calcium level
   E Raised ionised calcium and elevated PTH levels.

Hypercalcaemia

19. **Which of the following are associated with hypercalcaemia?**
   A Thyrotoxicosis
   B Chronic renal failure (CRF)
   C Familial hypocalciuric hypocalcaemia (FHH)
   D Sarcoidosis
   E Milk alkali syndrome.

Parathyroidectomy

20. **Which of the following are operative indications for primary hyperparathyroidism?**
   A Renal stones
   B Low bone density
   C Renal impairment
   D Serum calcium of 2.75
   E Young age.

Primary hyperparathyroidism

21. **Regarding operation for primary hyperparathyroidism, which of the following statements are correct?**
   A Permanent hypoparathyroidism is likely.
   B PTH can be measured intraoperatively.
   C Recurrent laryngeal nerve damage can occur in about 5–7 per cent of cases.
   D Endoscopic technique is the most favoured operative mode.
   E Gamma probes can be used for exploratory purposes.

Multiple endocrine neoplasia

22. **A 60-year-old retired nurse presents with weight loss, fainting episodes and tiredness. A blood glucose performed was 2.5 mmol/L. An insulinoma is suspected. What are the appropriate tests?**
   A A short synacthen test
   B Insulin levels
   C C-peptide levels
   D A 24 h fast
   E All of the above.

Imaging and the parathyroid

23. **Which of the following statements regarding imaging of the parathyroid gland are true?**
   A High-frequency ultrasound can identify nearly 75 per cent of enlarged glands.

B Technetium-99m-labelled sestamibi isotope (MIBI) scan identifies around 90 per cent of enlarged glands.
C Single photon emission computed tomography (SPECT) scan can influence surgical approach.
D CT and MRI must be undertaken prior to first-time neck exploration.
E Adenomas weighing less than 500 mg show reduced concordance with imaging.

→ Operative strategies for the parathyroid

24. Which of the following statements are true regarding operative strategies for the parathyroid?

A In a conventional approach, a transverse collar incision is made.
B In a targeted approach, a 2–3 cm incision is made over the site of the adenoma.
C In patients with four-gland disease, transcervical thymectomy is not recommended.
D In multiple endocrine neoplasia type 1 (MEN-1), total parathyroidectomy reduces the risk of recurrence.
E Preoperative imaging can identify nearly 10 per cent of patients with mediastinal adenoma.

→ Hypoparathyroidism

25. Which of the following statements are correct?

A Serum calcium must be checked within 24 h of total thyroidectomy.
B Serum calcium levels below 1.90 mmol/L can pose a medical emergency.
C Chvostek's sign is suggestive of hypercalcaemia.
D DiGeorge syndrome is a medical cause of hypoparathyroidism.
E Cardiac arrhythmias can occur during an episode of hypocalcaemia.

→ Management of hypercalcaemia

26. Which of the following statements are true regarding medical management of primary hyperparathyroidism?

A Use of diuretics could reduce serum calcium levels by increasing their excretion via the kidneys.
B Cinacalcet is a bisphosphonate used to reduce calcium levels.
C Palmidronate is a bisphosphonate used to reduce calcium levels.
D Intravenous saline is the first line of management in hypercalcaemia.
E Serum calcium over 3.5 mmol/L is a medical emergency.

Extended matching questions

→ 1. Causes of hypercalcaemia and hypocalcaemia

A Dehydration
B Primary hyperparathyroidism
C FHH
D Hypoparathyroidism
E Vitamin D deficiency

Choose and match the correct diagnosis with each of the scenarios given below:

1 A 70-year-old man presents with constipation and confusion. His serum calcium is 3.7 mmol/L and his phosphate is 0.5 mmol/L.

2 A 40-year-old banker attends a well-man clinic. His serum calcium is 2.9 mmol/L and his phosphate is 0.8 mmol/L. His PTH levels are 9 pmol/L. The urine calcium creatinine ratio is very low.

3 An elderly man is recovering from a hernia repair. His bloods are as follows: urea 10.7 mmol/L, creatinine 84 μmol/L, calcium 3.20 mmol/L.

4 A young woman underwent a thyroidectomy for a large multinodular goitre. Eight hours after the operation, she developed tingling and numbness around her mouth.

5 An elderly woman who is mostly house-bound was admitted following a hip fracture. Her serum calcium is 1.8 mmol/L, phosphate is 0.7 mmol/L and serum alkaline phosphatase is 640 IU/L.

→ 2. Hyperthyroidism

A Graves' disease
B Human chorionic gonadotrophin (HCG) effect
C Thyrotoxicosis
D Sick euthyroid disease
E Toxic nodule

Reference values for thyroid function tests (TFTs) are as follows:

TSH 0.5 – 4 mIU/ L
fT3 3.5 – 6.5 pmol/ L
fT4 10 – 23 pmol/ L

Choose and match the correct diagnosis with each of the scenarios given below:

1 An elderly woman presents with sweating and confusion. Her biochemistry is as follows: TSH < 0.1 mIU/ L; fT3, 15.8 pmol/ L; fT4, 1.0 pmol/ L.

2 A 10-week pregnant woman has severe vomiting. Her TFTs are as follows: TSH, 0.02mIU/ L; T3, 5.2 pmol/ L; T4, 11 pmol/ L.

3 A middle-aged man is in ITU following emergency laparotomy for a bleeding ulcer. His TFTs are as follows: TSH < 0.01 mIU/ L; T3, 2.0 pmol/ L; T4, 0.5pml/ L.

4 A 22-year-old woman with a smooth goitre presents with sweating and weight loss. Her TFTs are as follows: TSH, 0.01mIU/ L; T3, 8.0 pmol/ L; T4, 41 pmol/ L.

→ 3. Hypothyroidism

A Autoimmune thyroiditis
B TSH-secreting adenomas (TSHoma)
C Amiodarone-induced thyroid disease
D Myxoedema
E Heterophil antibodies interference

Choose and match the correct diagnosis with each of the scenarios given below:

1 An elderly woman presets to A&E with third-degree heart block. She is overweight, has dry skin and slow reflexes.

2 A 44-year-old man underwent chemical cardioversion for atrial fibrillation (AF). His baseline TFTs were normal. He is now hypothyroid.

3 A GP is having difficulty trying to treat a 62-year-old woman for hypothyroidism. Despite thyroxine dosage of 200 μg, her thyroid functions are suggestive of hypothyroidism.

4 A young woman with rheumatoid arthritis has discordant TFTs, with TSH, fT3 and fT4 all elevated.

5 A 40-year-old woman presents with hypothyroidism and elevated TPO antibodies.

→ 4. Goitre

A Toxic nodule
B Multinodular goitre

C Follicular carcinoma of the thyroid
D Graves' disease.

Choose and match the correct diagnosis with each of the scenarios given below:

1 A middle-aged woman presents with a long-standing goitre. Her right lobe is more enlarged than the left. She is clinically euthyroid.

2 A young woman presents with a firm enlarged goitre with bruit. She complains of grittiness in the eye.

3 A 60-year-old presents with a firm thyroid nodule. Isotope scan shows increased uptake by the nodule.

4 A 55-year-old presents with thyroid nodule and left-sided total ophthalmoplegia and absent corneal reflexes.

→ 5. Thyroid cancers

A Papillary thyroid cancer
B Anaplastic carcinoma
C Lymphoma
D Medullary carcinoma

Choose and match the correct diagnosis with each of the scenarios given below:

1 An 82-year-old woman presents with a thyroid nodule, weight loss, backache and hypercalcaemia.

2 An elderly woman with previous history of Hashimoto's thyroiditis presents with an irregular, hard nodule in her right thyroid lobe.

3 A 12-year-old boy presents with a nodule and regional lymph node enlargement.

4 A 28-year-old has a parathyroid adenoma and elevated levels of calcitonin.

Answers: Multiple choice questions

→ Non-thyroidal illness

1. B, D

Non-thyroidal illness is synonymous to sick euthyroid syndrome. It appears in the context of severe illness, such as severe infections, renal failure, liver failure and malignancies. It is characterised by low T3 and T4 and an inappropriately suppressed TSH. The evidence so far is not clear if replacement benefits such cases.

→ Hyperthyroidism

2. A, B, D, E

Graves' disease is a common autoimmune condition that usually occurs in young women and is associated with eye signs. Abnormal TSH receptor antibodies produce a disproportionate and prolonged effect. It can be associated with other autoimmune conditions such as Addison's disease, type 1 diabetes, pernicious anaemia and coeliac disease. Toxic nodular goitre is often seen in middle age or in the elderly and is rarely associated with eye signs. A solitary toxic nodule is often autonomous and its hypertrophy/hyperplasia is not associated with TSH receptor antibodies. Thyroid cancer very rarely presents as hyperthyroidism. Thyroid inflammation, especially postpartum, can cause hyperthyroidism.

Thyrotoxicosis

3. A, B, C, D, E

Thyrotoxicosis is characterised by the clinical, physiological and biochemical changes that result when tissues are exposed to excess thyroid hormone. It can present with symptoms of hyperactivity, insomnia and heat intolerance, weight loss with increased appetite, palpitations and fatigue. The signs often are fine tremor, warm moist skin, proptosis palmar erythema, onycholysis, hair loss, high output heart failure and, rarely, periodic paralysis which is associated with hypokalaemia.

Clinical features of hyperthyroidism

4. A, B, C, D, E

The exophthalmos in thyroid eye disease is due to retrobulbar infiltration of tissues with fluid and round cells. Oedema of the eyelids and conjunctival injection may be worsened by compression of ophthalmic veins. Urgent action (orbital decompression) is needed in the case of corneal ulceration, congestive ophthalmopathy or optic neuropathy. Treatment with steroids and orbital radiotherapy is sometimes needed. Thyroid dermopathy is caused by deposition of hyaluronidase in the dermis and cutis.

Medical therapy for hyperthyroidism

5. D

Carbimazole (first drug of choice) and propylthiouracil (given during pregnancy and lactation) are the common antithyroid drugs that are used; 30–40 per cent of patients remain euthyroid 10 years after discontinuation of therapy. However, rarely relapses are corrected with medication. Large goitres, younger patients and very elevated fT3 and fT4 rarely benefit from medical management. A toxic nodule is autonomous in nature and will relapse if medications are stopped. Agranulocytosis occurs in only 0.1–0.5 per cent of patients on antithyroid drugs. Beta-blockers reduce the adrenergic effects of thyroxine in peripheral tissues

Surgery for thyrotoxicosis

6. A, B, C, D, E

Cure can be offered by surgery, reducing the mass of overactive tissue. However, there is a risk of permanent hypothyroidism in total thyroidectomy and recurrence of toxicity in subtotal resections. Recurrence can also occur in 5 per cent of cases if less than a total thyroidectomy has been performed. Parathyroid insufficiency occurs in <5 per cent of cases undergoing surgery. The following are also indications for surgery: presence of suspicious thyroid nodule by FNAC; pregnant women inadequately controlled on medications; and large thyroid glands with relatively low radioiodine uptake.

Radioiodine treatment

7. A, C

Radioiodine treatment recommends the administration of enough radioiodine to achieve normal thyroid status. Hypothyroidism occurs in 15–20 per cent at 2 years. It is contraindicated in young children, pregnant and lactating mothers. It is the definitive choice of treatment in cases of relapsed Graves' disease and in multinodular goitre and adenomas.

Neonatal hypothyroidism

8. A, B, C, E

Cretinism is a consequence of inadequate thyroid hormone production during the foetal and early neonatal periods. Endemic cretinism is due to dietary deficiency, whereas sporadic cases are due to either inborn error of thyroid metabolism or complete or partial agenesis of the gland. Immediate diagnosis and treatment are essential to prevent long-term physical and mental developmental delay. In hyperthyroid pregnant women, drugs such as propylthiouracil are preferred as they limit ability to induce hypothyroidism in the foetus.

Myxoedema

9. A, B, C, D, E

Myxoedema is associated with accentuated signs and symptoms of hypothyroidism. There is often a malar flush, yellow tinge to the skin and altered mental state. It can present as bradycardia and hypothermia with its associated tachy- and bradyarrhythmias. Heart failure and infections are associated with increased mortality.

Biochemical features of hypothyroidism

10. A, B, C, D, E

Biochemically hypothyroidism is characterized by low free t3 and free t4 hormones. As a compensatory attempt, the pituitary secretes TSH, which is elevated. It can present as hyponatraemia and raised total cholesterol and LDL cholesterol.

Classification of hypothyroidism

11. A, B, D, E

Hypothyroidism can be classified as: goitrous (iodine deficiency, Hashimoto's thyroiditis or drugs such as lithium, amiodarone, iodides and aminosalicylic acid); non-goitrous (atrophic thyroiditis, post-radiation); pituitary-related (panhypopituitarism); neoplastic; infiltrative (sarcoidosis); or infective (rare).

Thyroid cancer

12. A, D

Depending on the cells of origin, thyroid cancers can be classified as originating from:

- papillary cells
  - differentiated such as papillary and follicular carcinoma
  - undifferentiated anaplastic carcinomas
- lymphocytes – lymphoma
- C-cells – medullary carcinoma.

The relative incidence of primary malignant tumour of the thyroid cancer is as follows: papillary cancer, 60 per cent; follicular carcinoma, 20 per cent; anaplastic cancer, 10 per cent; medullary and malignant lymphoma, 5 per cent each. The annual incidence of thyroid cancer is 3.7 cases per 100 000 population and the female:male sex ratio is 3:1. It is commonest in adults aged 40–50 years.

Thyroglobulin

13. C, D

Thyroglobulin is secreted by normal thyroid tissue and is a sensitive marker of recurrence of thyroid cancer. Following surgery and radioiodine treatment, levels must be undetectable at <2 ng/L. Its measurement can be made difficult by the presence of antithyroglobulin antibodies.

Papillary and follicular cancers

14. B, C, D, E

Compared with most cancers, the prognosis in differentiated thyroid cancers is excellent. Papillary cancers are encapsulated, slow-growing and spread to adjacent structures (nodes). They are confined to the neck in >95 per cent of cases. Follicular cancer arises from the epithelium. It is capsular and is more likely to spread via the haematogenous route rather than local invasion. Hurtle cell carcinoma is an aggressive type of follicular cancer with a poor prognosis.

Differentiated thyroid cancers

15. B, C, D, E

There are several controversies regarding treatment for differentiated cancers. However, following a FNAC that shows differentiated thyroid cancer, imaging of the neck with MRI or CT is suggested. Total thyroidectomy is recommended for tumours greater than 2 cm and those with nodal involvement or metastasis. Lobectomy is recommended for the remainder. Functional selective node dissection of involved node levels is performed, if required.

Medullary carcinoma of the thyroid

16. A, B, D, E

Medullary carcinoma refers to tumours of the parafollicular cells. It is characterised by high levels of serum calcitonin and CEA. Diarrhoea is present in 30 per cent of cases and may be due to 5-hydroxytryptamine produced by tumour cells. Like many endocrine neoplasms, the progression of disease may be slow. It can occur with phaechromocytoma and hyperparathyroidism in a syndrome called multiple endocrine neoplasia type 2A (MEN 2A).

Primary hyperparathyroidism

17. A, E

The prevalence of primary hyperparathyroidism increases with advancing age. Most cases are sporadic. Nearly 85 per cent of these patients have an adenoma; 13 per cent have hyperplasia of the glands; and a very small proportion have multiple adenomas or cancer. Familial hyperparathyroidism is genetically determined and associated with MEN-1 (primary hyperparathyroidism, pituitary adenoma and pancreatic tumours such as insulinoma, gastrinoma and VIPoma) and MEN 2 (primary hyperparathyroidism, medullary carcinoma of thyroid and phaeochromocytoma). The familial variety can also exist as isolated hyperparathyroidism and exists as hyperplasia.

Calcium

18. B, C, E

Hypercalcaemia normally suppresses the release of PTH by the parathyroid gland. Calcium circulates in the plasma mostly bound to albumin; however, it is the ionised or free calcium that is biologically active. Measurement of ionised calcium is tedious and albumin-adjusted (corrected) calcium is just as good. Hyperparathyroidism is associated with raised serum calcium, low serum phosphate and hypercalciuria.

Hypercalcaemia

19. A, B, C, D, E

Chronic renal failure is associated with vitamin D deficiency and hypocalcaemia initially; these result in stimulation of the parathyroid gland and release of PTH, causing secondary hyperparathyroidism. However, long-standing stimulation of the parathyroid results in autonomous secretion of PTH by the gland, causing tertiary hyperparathyroidism. Granulomatous conditions such as tuberculosis and sarcoidosis cause hypercalcaemia.

Parathyroidectomy

20. A, B, C, E

Surgery is the only curative option for this condition. Medical therapy such as calcium receptor agonists and bisphosphonate therapy are helpful along with eradication of drugs that induce hypercalcaemia (diuretics, lithium). Surgery is indicated in the presence of hypercalcaemia with serum calcium over 2.9 mmol/L (especially in the presence of symptoms), presence of falling bone density or the presence of osteoporosis and renal stone disease or renal impairment.

Primary hyperparathyroidism

21. A, B, E

Preoperative discussion for a parathyroidectomy must include the possibility of recurrent laryngeal nerve injury (1 per cent), postoperative haemorrhage (1 per cent), recurrent and permanent hypoparathyroidism. PTH has a very short half-life and will disappear within a few minutes of excision of the gland. High levels, despite excision, suggest residual gland. PTH levels are measured in an operative setting to guide the surgeon if the gland has been completely removed. A conventional thyroidectomy incision is most frequently used. A gamma probe can be used to guide exploration following preoperative injection of MIBI.

Multiple endocrine neoplasia

22. B, C, D

An insulinoma is a tumour which originates from the pancreas; it is biochemically confirmed by demonstrating hyperinsulinaemia despite hypoglycaemia with elevated levels of proinsulin and C-peptide. It is often very difficult to diagnose, as imaging with MRI may not always pick up these small lesions (<4 mm). A supervised 24 h fast may be necessary. Insulinoma can be a part of MEN associated with hyperparathyroidism and pituitary adenoma (type 1) and medullary carcinoma (type 2). Assessment of bone profile, PTH levels and genetic testing are other tests required.

Imaging and the parathyroid

23. A, C, E

High-frequency ultrasound is non-invasive and can identify 75 per cent of enlarged glands. However, despite good resolution it has poor penetrance and cannot visualise the mediastinum. Technetium-99m-labelled sestamibi isotope scans can identify 75 per cent of glands and the area scanned must include the mediastinum to detect ectopic glands. SPECT scan gives a three-dimensional approach and can influence surgical approach.

Operative strategies for the parathyroid

24. A, B, D

Confident preoperative localisation permits a 2–3 cm incision located over the site of the adenoma. This is placed to permit extension to a formal bilateral exploration incision if the imaging is suboptimal. In a conventional approach, the patient is positioned in reverse Trendelenburg and a transverse incision is made, the subplatysmal plane is developed superiorly and, inferiorly, the deep cervical fascia is incised. In four-gland disease, a transcervical thymectomy is considered to reduce the risk of recurrence or recurrent primary hyperparathyroidism. Preoperative imaging identifies around 1 per cent of patients with a mediastinal adenoma.

Hypoparathyroidism

25. A, B, D, E

Signs and symptoms of hypocalcaemia are related to the duration and level of hypocalcaemia. It could range from mild circumoral and digital numbness to tetany with carpopedal spasm, neuromuscular excitability, cardiac arrhythmias and seizures. Serum calcium below 1.90 must be treated as an emergency and 10 mL or 10 per cent calcium gluconate must be given IVI slowly; 10 per cent magnesium infusion is also considered. In milder cases, 1 g of oral calcium can be given 3 or 4 times daily.

Management of hypercalcaemia

26. C, D, E

Medical management of primary hyperparathyroidism involves a low calcium diet and withdrawal of drugs that aggravate hypercalcaemia, such as diuretics and lithium. Cinacalcet is a calcium receptor agonist and reduces calcium levels. Intravenous saline to correct dehydration and a bisphosphonate such as palmidronate is essential.

Answers: Extended matching questions

1. Causes of hypercalcaemia and hypocalcaemia

1B

Primary hyperparathyroidism is associated with raised serum calcium and low phosphate levels. The PTH levels are not suppressed despite the hypercalcaemia.

2C

Familial hypocalciuric hypocalcaemia is another differential for primary hyperparathyroidism. It causes the same biochemical features as primary hyperparathyroidism apart from low urinary calcium excretion. Most patients are asymptomatic and the problem is in the calcium-sensing receptors in the parathyroid gland.

3A

Dehydration is a very common cause for mild hypercalcaemia.

4D

Serum calcium levels can come down when the parathyroid glands are inadvertently removed. Levels must always be checked within 24 h of any thyroid surgery.

5E

Vitamin D deficiency is common in house-bound and institutionalised individuals. It causes hypocalcaemia and hypophosphataemia in severe cases. Alkaline phosphatase is elevated in osteomalacia. However, recent fracture could also raise the ALP levels.

2. Hyperthyroidism

1C

T3 toxicosis can present with all features of thyroid excess. Due to rapid conversion of T4 to T3, T4 levels are often low.

2B

Pregnancy can be associated with hyperthyroidism. Beta-HCG increases exponentially in early pregnancy. This itself causes suppression of TSH. The thyroid-binding globulin levels are altered as well.

3D

Thyroid functions are not helpful in the immediate period after an acute illness or stress. Sick euthyroid disease causes suppression of both TSH and free thyroid hormones.

4A

Graves' disease is an autoimmune condition characterised by a smooth goitre, a strong family history and a female preponderance.

3. Hypothyroidism

1D

Myxoedema can present with heart block, hypothermia and sometimes coma.

2C
Amiodarone is a popular antiarrhythmic. It contains a very high iodine load, however, and can cause both over-activation and under-stimulation of the thyroid gland.

3B
TSHoma is a rare tumour from the anterior pituitary secreting TSH. Thyroid hormone resistance is another cause of elevated TSH levels despite adequate thyroxine replacement.

4E
Autoantibodies, especially found in rheumatoid arthritis, can interfere in the fT4 levels and cause discordant TFTs. They can be corrected by performing tests on another analyser or the use on heterophil-blocking antibodies.

5A
Thyroid peroxidase antibodies (TPO) are associated with autoimmune hypothyroidism.

4. Goitre

1B
Simple multinodular goitre is due to relative iodine deficiency. It is long-standing. FNAC should be undertaken if there is a doubt about the diagnosis.

2D
Graves' disease is an autoimmune disease due to the presence of TSH receptor antibodies. Exophthalmos, diffuse goitre with a bruit with clinical and biochemical hyperthyroidism, is characteristic.

3A
Solitary toxic nodule could represent a single active nodule in a multimodal goitre, a thyroid adenoma (scan shows normal or decreased uptake) or a toxic adenoma (increased uptake with hyperthyroid features).

4C
Follicular carcinoma of the thyroid is the second commonest after papillary carcinoma. It arises later in life and is prone to blood-borne metastasis. Secondaries to the cavernous sinus result in the relevant eye signs.

5. Thyroid cancers

1B
Anaplastic carcinoma tends to occur in the elderly and is malignant and poorly differentiated.

2C
Lymphoma can arise in a gland affected by Hashimotoís thyroiditis.

3A
Papillary thyroid cancers occur in childhood and middle age. They are well differentiated and show metastasis to the regional lymph nodes.

4D
Medullary carcinoma of the thyroid can form part of the MEN syndrome. It occurs in young adults and carries a good prognosis. These carcinomas secrete calcitonin from the parafollicular cells.

49 Adrenal glands and other endocrine disorders

Multiple choice questions

➜ Anatomy of the adrenal gland

1. **Which of the following statements are correct?**

A The right adrenal is located on top of the upper pole of the right kidney.
B The left adrenal is covered by the pancreatic tail.
C The right adrenal vein drains into the renal vein.
D It is difficult to cannulate the left adrenal vein.
E The inner layer of the adrenals is called the zona reticularis.

➜ Hormones and the adrenals

2. **Which of the following statements regarding the adrenal gland are true?**

A The zona glomerulosa secretes aldosterone.
B The zona reticularis consists of chromaffin cells.
C Cortisol is produced in the adrenal medulla.
D Aldosterone is a mineralocorticoid.
E Catecholamines are only formed in para-adrenal glands.

➜ Adrenal hormones

3. **Which of the following tests are indicated in the hormonal evaluation of an adrenal mass?**

A Catecholamine estimation in blood
B Measurement of aldosterone in blood
C Urinary electrolyte analysis
D 24 h urinary cortisol
E 24 h urinary catecholamines.

➜ Adrenal masses

4. **Which of the following statements is false?**

A All adrenal masses need to be biopsied
B The likelihood of a mass being malignant increases with increasing size.
C Nearly 80 per cent of adrenal masses are non-functioning.
D Conn's disease accounts for 1 per cent of adrenal adenoma.
E The non-functional adenoma should not undergo surgical resection.

➜ Primary hyperaldosteronism

5. **Which of the following are true in primary hyperaldosteronism?**

A Hypokalaemia is always present.
B Plasma renin activity is increased.
C Plasma aldosterone is increased.
D Drugs such as beta-blockers have to be discontinued before the test.
E If a biochemical diagnosis is reached, no imaging is required.

➜ Adrenal vein catheterisation

6. **Which of the following statements regarding adrenal vein catheterisation (AVC) are true?**

A Samples for catecholamines are sampled from the inferior vena cava (IVC).
B Samples for aldosterone are sampled from the IVC.
C Samples for aldosterone are sampled from the adrenal veins.
D AVC must only be considered if surgery is planned.
E It is technically difficult to cannulate the left adrenal vein.

Cushing's syndrome

7. How is Cushing's syndrome clinically characterised?

A Central obesity
B Osteoporosis
C Hirsutism
D Hypokalaemia
E Hyperkalaemia.

8. Which tests are indicated in the diagnosis of Cushing's syndrome?

A 24 h urinary cortisol
B 9am cortisol
C Midnight cortisol
D Serum adrenocorticotrophic hormone (ACTH)
E Dexamethasone suppression test.

Surgery in Cushing's disease

9. Which of the following statements are true?

A Patients with Cushing's are at increased risk of hospital-acquired infections.
B Patients do not require prophylactic anticoagulation.
C Following surgical removal of unilateral adrenal adenomata, cortisol supplementation is not necessary.
D Nelson's syndrome is a cause of Cushing's disease.
E Cushing's-associated medical conditions need not be treated medically preoperatively.

Congenital adrenal hyperplasia

10. Which of the following regarding congenital adrenal hyperplasia (CAH) are true?

A Virilisation is characteristic.
B Girls are affected more than boys.
C Some children are affected in puberty.
D 17-hydroxylase is the commonest enzyme deficiency.
E Cortisol excess is a common feature.

Short synacthen test

11. A short synacthen test was performed in a 26-year-old male admitted to the ITU with multi-organ failure. The results are as follows: 0 min, 300 mmol/L; 30 min, 450 mmol/L; 60 min, 390 mmol/L. What is this suggestive of?

A Adrenal failure
B Pituitary failure
C Sepsis
D Cushing's syndrome
E None of the above.

Multiple endocrine neoplasia

12. Which of the following statements are true regarding multiple endocrine tumours (MEN)?

A They are always benign in nature.
B They are mostly inherited.
C The mode of inheritance is autosomal dominant.
D MEN-1 could be caused by mutations in the menin gene.
E MEN 2 is caused by mutations in the RET proto-oncogene.

Pancreaticoduodenal endocrine tumours

13. Which of the following statements are true?

A Insulinomas are the commonest form of pancreaticoduodenal endocrine tumours (PETs).
B Diarrhoea is a common presentation in gastrinomas.
C Peptic ulcers in gastrinomas are solitary.
D VIPomas present with diarrhoea.
E PETs occur in 50–60 per cent of MEN-1 patients.

MEN-1

14. Which of the following statements regarding operative management are correct?

A All MEN-1 parathyroid adenomas must be operated on.
B MEN-1 gastrinomas must be operated on.
C MEN-1 insulinoma must be operated on.
D Distal pancreatectomy is the procedure of choice in most gastrinomas.
E Non-functioning PETs need not be operated on.

Neuroendocrine tumours

15. Which of the following are true regarding neuroendocrine tumours (NETs)?

A They are found as single cells in the mucosa of bronchi.
B Peptide hormones such as serotonin and gastrin are stored in its granules.
C Chromogranin A is a tumour marker.
D Catecholamines are the major metabolites of serotonin.
E Nearly 40 per cent of NETs are located in the appendix.

16. Which of the following statements regarding NETs of the bronchi are true?

A The bronchi and lung constitute 1 per cent of all NETs.
B The diagnosis is mostly made due to symptoms of cough and airway obstruction.
C A highly undifferentiated NET must be treated as lung cancer.
D 5-HIAA is often very elevated in these cases.
E Patients do not suffer from carcinoid syndrome despite metastasis.

Extended matching questions

1. Hypoadrenalism

A Meningococcal septicaemia
B Nelson's syndrome
C Addison's disease
D Congenital adrenal hyperplasia
E Adrenal haemorrhage

Choose and match the correct diagnosis with each of the scenarios given below:

1 A 17-year-old girl with type 1 diabetes presents with weakness and generalised pigmentation.

2 An 80-year-old male has marked pigmentation of skin and scar tissues. He has abdominal scars of bilateral adrenalectomy.

3 An elderly man on warfarin therapy presents with hypotension and an international normalised ratio (INR) of 4.2.

4 A 4-day-old neonate develops seizures. Blood tests show Na of 124 mmol/L and K of 6.1 mmol/L.

5 A university student is brought to A&E resuscitation area moribund. She has a purpuric non-blanchable rash on her legs.

2. Hypercortisolism

A Cushing's disease
B Cushing's syndrome
C Multiple endocrine neoplasia
D Non-endocrine tumour
E Conn's syndrome

Choose and match the correct diagnosis with each of the scenarios given below:

1 A 40-year-old chronic smoker presents with weight loss, ankle oedema and hypokalaemic alkalosis.

2 A long-standing asthmatic with frequent exacerbations has gradually developed hirsutism, truncal obesity and bruising.

3 A 48-year-old man presents with visual disturbance, headache and hypertension.

4 Paramedics are called to the home of a young woman who suffered from a seizure. Her blood glucose was found to be 2.3 mmol/L. Her family mention that she has collapsed on a few occasions in the recent past.

5 A 36-year-old man is being investigated for resistant hypertension.

3. Sex hormones

A Hypogonadotrophic hypogonadism
B Teratoma
C 21-hydroxylase deficiency
D Arrhenoblastoma
E Polycystic ovarian syndrome

Choose and match the correct diagnosis with each of the scenarios given below:

1 A 21-year-old woman who is obese (body mass index, BMI, 37 kg/m^2) develops hirsutism and oligomenorrhoea. Her serum testosterone is mildly elevated.

2 A 42-year-old woman presents with a short history of hirsutism, clitoromegaly and deep hoarse voice. Her serum testosterone levels are markedly elevated.

3 A 3-day-old female child shows features of ambiguous genitalia.

4 A young man was testing his partner's pregnancy kit and his urine tested repeatedly positive for the pregnancy test.

5 A 50-year-old presents with poor libido and loss of body hair.

4. Carcinoid tumours

A Pulmonary stenosis
B Pancreatic carcinoid
C Carcinoid syndrome
D Cushing's syndrome
E Carcinoid tumour

Choose and match the correct diagnosis with each of the descriptions given below:

1 Tumours that arise from the enterochromaffin cells

2 Liver metastasis of tumours that arise from the enterochromaffin cells

3 Associated fibrotic lesions

4 Ectopic hormone secretion causing weight gain, hypertension and diabetes

5 These tumours can present with hypoglycaemia.

5. Hypertension and hypokalaemia

A Urine K^+, laxative and diuretic screen
B 24 h urinary cortisol
C Plasma renin activity
D MRI scan
E Reassurance

Choose and match the correct management with each of the scenarios given below:

1 A young man presents with recent-onset severe hypertension, diabetes, weight gain and muscle weakness.

2 A 52-year-old man presents with hypertension, abdominal pain and tachycardia. His dexamethasone suppression test suggests cortisol excess.

3 A middle-aged, overweight, sedentary City of London worker is found to have borderline hypertension. He has been commenced on a diuretic. His serum K is 3.2 mmol/ L. Other electrolytes are normal.

4 A 32-year-old woman presents with resistant hypertension.

5 A 23-year-old fitness enthusiast gives a history of tiredness, weight loss and hypokalaemia.

Answers: Multiple choice questions

Anatomy of the adrenal gland

1. B, C, D

The right adrenal gland lies between the right lobe of the kidney and the diaphragm, close to the inferior vena cava (IVC). The left adrenal lies on the upper pole of the left kidney and is covered by the pancreatic tail and the spleen. A large adrenal vein drains into the IVC on the right side, and the left adrenal vein drains into the renal vein on the left. Hence it is difficult to sample from the left adrenal vein due to it anatomic position during adrenal venous sampling. This procedure is performed to differentiate biochemically between primary hyperaldosteronism and bilateral hyperplasia.

Hormones and the adrenals

2. A, B, D

Embryologically and histologically, the adrenal cortex is made up of the cortex and medulla. The cortex itself has three zones: the zona glomerulosa, which secretes aldosterone, a mineralocorticoid; the zona fasciculata, which secretes cortisol, a glucocorticoid; and zona reticularis, which secretes the sex steroids. The medulla consists of large chromaffin cells that store catecholamine granules.

Adrenal hormones

3. B, C, D, E

The purpose of hormonal evaluation is to demonstrate hormonal excess. A 24 h urinary cortisol and 24h urinary catecholamines are the first-line investigations. A dexamethasone suppression test and loss of circadian rhythm (thus a morning and midnight cortisol) are diagnostic of hypercortisolism. Serum electrolytes, plasma renin activity, aldosterone, serum sex steroids such as testosterone and dehydroepiandrosterone (DHEA) are essential. Urine K^+ is an easy and informative test in the work-up towards primary hyperaldosteronism where there is excessive loss of K^+ in urine despite hypokalaemia.

Adrenal masses

4. A, E

An adrenal mass must not be biopsied until a phaeochromocytoma has been excluded biochemically; otherwise it can result in fatal activation of target organs such as the cardiovascular system. Most often the indications for an adrenal biopsy are to confirm metastasis, which accounts for 2 per cent of adrenal tumours. The probability of an adrenal mass being a carcinoma increases with the size of the mass. Non-functioning adenomas greater than 4 cm must be considered for surgical resection.

Primary hyperaldosteronism

5. B, C, D

A unilateral adenoma (Conn's syndrome) is the commonest cause of primary hyperaldosteronism (PHA). Hypokalaemia is not always present. In normokalaemic PHA, 70 per cent have hyperplasia of the adrenal cortex. Demonstration of lack of suppression of renin activity despite high aldosterone levels points towards this diagnosis. Several drugs affect the renin–angiotensin–aldosterone pathway. Beta-blockers, however, significantly suppress renin activity. Alternative agents to control hypertension such as alpha-blockers have to be considered. Despite biochemical diagnosis, imaging has to be performed to distinguish unilateral from bilateral disease.

Adrenal vein catheterisation

6. B, C, E

Adrenal vein catheterisation is considered before a decision regarding surgical or non-surgical management is considered. An apparent unilateral mass could be non-functioning in the presence of bilateral hyperplasia. During this procedure, samples for cortisol and aldosterone are obtained from the IVC and the right and left adrenal veins. The aldosterone:cortisol ratio is determined in each of these samples. A significant increase in the ratio on one side indicates unilateral disease. The left adrenal vein drains first into the renal vein, which subsequently drains into the IVC; the right adrenal vein drains directly into the IVC and is easier to cannulate.

Cushing's syndrome

7. A, B, C, D

Clinically Cushing's syndrome is characterised by features of cortical excess, such as obesity, hypertension, diabetes, skin changes and hirsutism. Patients often present with muscle weakness and hypokalaemia.

8. A, B, C, D, E

The key to diagnose hormonal excess is demonstration of lack of suppression and/or loss of circadian rhythm (see Fig. 49.1). Serum ACTH levels will discriminate ACTH-dependent causes from ACTH-independent causes. If ACTH levels are elevated, the pituitary is imaged with MRI. If MRI is negative, an inferior petrosal sinus may be sampled. The chest and abdomen are imaged to look for tumours that may secrete ectopic ACTH. If the ACTH is suppressed, the adrenals must be imaged as it is likely to be the source of hormonal excess.

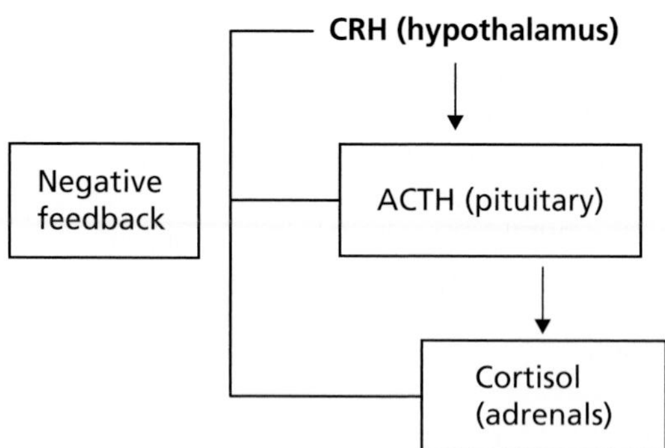

Figure 49.1 Hypothalamic-Pituitary-Adrenal axis.

Surgery in Cushing's disease

9. A

Patients with steroid excess can be immunocompromised and are at increased risk of infection. They are also at increased risk of thromboembolic disease. Associated diabetes and hypertension must be well controlled prior to surgery to improve outcome. In case of unilateral adenomata, there is suppression of the contralateral gland which takes several months to recover. Steroid cover is required in the immediate postoperative and for several months after as well. Nearly 10 per cent of patients who undergo bilateral adrenalectomy develop an aggressive pituitary tumour, producing Nelson's syndrome, characterised by hyperpigmentation and marked elevation in ACTH.

→ Congenital adrenal hyperplasia

10. A, C

Congenital adrenal hyperplasia is an autosomal recessive condition. Males and females are equally affected with an incidence of 1 in 5000 live births. 21-hydroxylase is the deficient enzyme in 95 per cent of cases. The condition is marked by reduced cortisol and excessive ACTH secretion, which can lead to increased production of androgenic precursors. It can present as ambiguous genitalia in a female infant. Male infants are diagnosed later with virilising features. Milder enzyme deficiencies present later in life or during periods of stress such as puberty.

→ Short synacthen test

11. A

A synacthen test is performed to assess adrenal reserve. A basal cortisol level is performed and samples taken again 30 and 60 min after ACTH administration. In case of adrenal failure there is an insufficient increase in cortisol after synacthen (synthetic ACTH) administration. If the rise in cortisol is < 500 nmol/L and less than twice the basal value, adrenal insufficiency is suspected. A synacthen test does not test pituitary function.

→ Multiple endocrine neoplasia

12. B, C, D, E

MEN are inherited syndromes presenting as benign and malignant tumours in various endocrine glands. MEN-1 involve the anterior pituitary (presenting as prolactinoma, non-functioning pituitary adenomas), hyperplasia of the parathyroid and pancreaticoduodenal tumours. It is caused by germ-line mutations in the menin gene located on chromosome 11, while MEN 2 is subdivided into 2a (medullary carcinoma of thyroid, primary hyperparathyroidism and phaeochromocytoma) and 2b (medullary thyroid carcinoma, phaechromocytoma and characteristic facial and mucoid neuromas accompanied by a marfanoid habitus).

→ Pancreaticoduodenal endocrine tumours

13. B, D, E

Pancreaticoduodenal endocrine tumours occur in 50–60 per cent of MEN-1 patients. They are often multiple and recur after surgery. Gastrinoma is the most common of the PETs, followed by insulinoma. Gastrinomas often present as multiple peptic ulcers that are refractory to treatment. Malabsorption and diarrhoea are common presentations due to acid-related inactivation of enzymes and mucosal damage of the upper small bowel. VIPomas present with produce watery diarrhoea which is secretory in nature.

→ MEN-1

14. B, C

The indications for surgery in MEN-1 primary hyperparathyroidism follow the same criteria as in sporadic disease, i.e. degree of hypercalcaemia, renal stone presence etc. MEN-1 gastrinomas and insulinomas have to be operated on to prevent distant metastasis. Most gastrinomas are located in the duodenum or pancreatic head (gastrinoma triangle); pylorus-preserving partial pancreaticoduodenostomy is recommended. If located on the body or tail of the pancreas, distal pancreatectomy is considered.

Neuroendocrine tumours

15. B, C, E

Neuroendocrine tumours arise from the diffuse neuroendocrine cells that can be found in the mucosa of the bronchi, stomach, gut, biliary tree, urogenital system and the pancreas. The cells secrete different neuroendocrine markers such as synaptophysin, chromogranin and neuron-specific enolase. NET of the jejunum and ileum excrete 5-hydroxyindoleacetic acid (5-HIAA), a serotonin metabolite. Forty per cent of NETs are located in the appendix, nearly 25 per cent in the small bowel and 15 per cent in the rectum.

16. C, E

Ten per cent of the NET occurs in the lung. The diagnosis is easier in centrally located lung tumours (which present with cough and obstruction) than in peripherally located tumours, which remain indolent for a long time. Diagnosis is often made by radiography. Foregut tumours do not secrete serotonin and 5-HIAA is not elevated. This is why they don't have typical features of flushing, wheezing etc. despite the presence of liver metastasis.

Answers: Extended matching questions

1. Hypoadrenalism

1C

Addison's disease is autoimmune adrenal failure. It is associated with other autoimmune conditions such as type 1 diabetes, pernicious anaemia, premature ovarian failure and autoimmune thyroiditis.

2B

Nelson's disease occurs due to excessive ACTH stimulation (lack of negative feedback), following bilateral adrenalectomy. ACTH has a direct action on melanocytes due to its similarity to melanocyte-stimulating hormone (MSH).

3E

Adrenal haemorrhage can occur in cases when the INR is prolonged.

4D

Congenital adrenal hyperplasia is seen in 1:2500 live births. It presents as salt-wasting in severe cases. Exacerbations resemble an adrenal crisis with hypotension, hyponatraemia and hyperkalaemia. It occurs due to deficiency of enzymes (21-hydroxylase) required in the biosynthesis of cortisol.

5A

Meningococcal sepsis can result in adrenal infarction and haemorrhage and is called Waterhouse–Friderichen syndrome.

2. Hypercortisolism

1D

Oat cell carcinoma of the bronchus produces ACTH. The degree of hypokalaemia is particularly severe in cases of ectopic ACTH production.

2B

Cushing's syndrome is associated with excess cortisol. It typically causes a moon face, truncal obesity, hirsutism, easy bruising and proximal muscle weakness. Diabetes and hypertension are frequent associations.

3A

Cushing's disease is ACTH-dependent. It is caused by pituitary or hypothalamic lesions.

4C

An islet cell tumour secreting insulin (insulinoma) is associated with MEN. Demonstration of elevated insulin levels (despite hypoglycaemia) and C-peptide levels is diagnostic.

5E

Primary hyperaldosteronism is a cause in approximately 1 per cent of all hypertensives.

3. Sex hormones

1E

Polycystic ovarian syndrome presents with oligomenorrhoea, weight gain and hirsutism. Biochemically the testosterone, prolactin and LH could be mildly elevated. Ultrasound demonstrates the cystic changes in the ovaries.

2D

Malignant tumours of the adrenals and the ovaries can result in marked elevation of testosterone and masculinisation. Arrhenoblastoma is an ovarian tumour which also produces other androgens such as androstenedione.

3C

21-Hydroxylase deficiency causes hypocortisolism. The cortisol precursors are shunted down the sex steroid pathway, resulting in virilising effects in the neonate.

4B

Germ cell tumours such as teratoma produce HCG and alpha-fetoprotein (AFP).

5A

Hypogonadotrophic hypogonadism is associated with low pituitary (follicle-stimulating hormone, luteinising hormone (LH)) and low testicular hormones (testosterone).

4. Carcinoid tumours

1E

Carcinoid tumours arise from the enterochromaffin cells and are most commonly found in the appendix, ileum, rectum, lungs, gonads and duodenum.

2C

Carcinoid tumours from the ileum, stomach and duodenum can metastasise to the liver and impede hepatic clearance of metabolites such as serotonin and bradykinins. This can result in cutaneous flushing and diarrhoea.

3A

Chronic increase in metabolites such as 5-hydroxytryptamine results in endocardial fibrosis and heart failure. There are predominant right-sided heart lesions such as pulmonary stenosis and tricuspid regurgitation.

4D

Ectopic humoral syndromes occur in ACTH-producing bronchial carcinoids.

5B

Hypoglycaemia occurs in insulin-producing pancreatic carcinoid.

5. Hypertension and hypokalaemia

1B

The symptoms are suggestive of cortisol excess. In the first instance a 24 h urinary cortisol must be performed. If increased cortisol is excreted in the urine, an overnight dexamethasone test can be performed to confirm the excess (failure to suppress cortisol despite exogenous administration of steroid). A high-dose dexamethasone test confirms the source of the loss.

2D
Following biochemical diagnosis of hypercortisolism, imaging must be considered.

3E
This is not an unusual finding in essential hypertension. Diuretics such as thiazides are often used in the treatment and can cause mild hypokalaemia.

4C
Resistant hypertension (requiring over four medications achieving control) must be investigated, with evaluation of the renin–angiotensin–aldosterone axis.

5A
Diuretics and laxative abuse can present as hypokalaemia resistant to supplementation. Bartter syndrome is a differential diagnosis in this case.

50 The breast

Multiple choice questions

Investigations in breast cancer

1. Which of the following statements are true?

A Five per cent of breast cancers are missed by population-based mammographic screening.
B Ultrasound can also be used as a screening tool.
C Magnetic resonance imaging (MRI) can be a useful imaging tool.
D Fine-needle aspiration cytology (FNAC) and core biopsy are equally useful diagnostically.

Benign breast disease

2. Which of the following statements are false?

A Benign breast disease is the most common cause of breast problems.
B Lipoma is a common condition of the breast.
C Traumatic fat necrosis can be mistaken for a carcinoma.
D 30 per cent of breast cysts recur after aspiration.
E Non-cyclical mastalgia is more common in postmenopausal women.

Breast cancer

3. Which of the following conditions have an increased risk of breast carcinoma?

A Breast cyst
B Duct ectasia
C Florid hyperplasia
D Atypical ductal or lobular hyperplasia
E Fibroadenoma.

4. In a patient with nipple discharge which of the following statements are true?

A Clear, serous discharge may be physiological.
B Bloodstained discharge occurs in carcinoma, duct ectasia and duct papilloma.
C Mammography is an important investigation.
D Microdochectomy is the treatment once cancer has been excluded.
E Paget's disease causes discharge from the surface.

5. In breast carcinoma, which one of the following statements is false?

A Ductal carcinoma is the most common variant.
B Lobular carcinoma occurs in 15 per cent.
C There may be a combination of lobular and ductal features.
D Colloid, medullary and tubular carcinomas carry a poor prognosis.
E Paget's disease is a superficial manifestation of an underlying breast carcinoma.

6. In the treatment of breast cancer, which of the following statements are false?

A There is a higher rate of local recurrence after conservative surgery and radiotherapy.
B After mastectomy, radiotherapy to the chest wall is not indicated.
C Sentinel lymph node biopsy should be done in clinically node-negative disease.
D Besides treating the patient, the role of axillary surgery is to stage the patient accurately.

E Lymph node-positive women and higher-risk node-negative women should have adjuvant chemotherapy.

F There is no role for preoperative chemotherapy.

Extended matching questions

➜ Benign breast disease

A Fat necrosis
B Breast abscess
C Tuberculosis
D Mondor's disease
E Duct ectasia
F Aberrations of normal development and involution (ANDI)
G Breast cyst
H Galactocele
I Fibroadenoma
J Phyllodes tumour

Choose and match the correct diagnosis with each of the scenarios given below:

1 A 42-year-old woman presents with a large irregular lump, about 12 cm in diameter, in her right breast, of 4 months' duration. The lump is very mobile and is stretching the skin and about to ulcerate.

2 A 25-year-old woman presents with a discrete lump in the left breast. She found it accidentally 3 weeks ago. She can move the lump about within the breast tissue.

3 A 40-year-old Asian woman, recently arrived in the UK, complains of a lump in her right breast of several months' duration. There is no pain. In her ipsilateral axilla she also has a discharging abscess, which tends to clear up and recur again.

4 A 45-year-old woman complains of pain in her left breast of 2 weeks' duration. On examination she has a tender string-like band with overlying prominent veins.

5 A 28-year-old lactating woman noticed a tender lump deep to her areola. The lump is cystic.

6 A 40-year-old woman complains of a lump in her right breast that she noticed accidentally 3 weeks ago. This has not changed since her period a week ago. It is mobile and tender.

7 A 50-year-old woman noticed a lump in her left breast 4 weeks ago. She has a firm, slightly tender lump which is not mobile. On questioning about trauma, she recalls having been hit on her breast by her grandchild at about the same time.

8 A 30-year-old woman complains of a tender, painful right breast with fever. She gave birth to her third child 2 weeks ago. On examination she feels hot with a red, tender, indurated and diffuse lump underlying the areola.

9 A 44-year-old woman complains of greenish nipple discharge on and off for 4 months. On examination she has an irregular, firm lump deep to the areola which looks indrawn.

10 A 38-year-old woman complains of painful breasts of some 6 months' duration. She noticed a lump in her right breast 6 weeks ago and feels that the size of the lump waxes and wanes with her periods, which are regular.

Answers: Multiple choice questions

Investigations in breast cancer

1. A, C

A normal mammogram does not exclude the presence of a carcinoma as 5 per cent of breast cancers are missed on population screening. In mammography, soft-tissue radiographs are taken by placing the breast in direct contact with ultrasensitive film and exposing it to low-voltage, high-amperage X-rays. The radiation dose is about 0.1 cGy. This investigation is more sensitive in the older age group as the breast becomes less dense. Digital mammography and tomo-mammography are being used as more advanced techniques.

Ultrasound is not useful as a screening tool and is highly operator-dependent. It is particularly useful in young women with dense breasts to distinguish between a cyst and a solid lesion. This technique is also being used to look for and biopsy impalpable axillary lymph nodes. MRI is an extremely useful imaging modality to distinguish scar tissue from recurrence in a patient who has had breast conservation carried out. It is the best imaging technique for breasts which have had implants inserted.

Fine-needle aspiration cytology is the least invasive technique of obtaining a cytological diagnosis; the accuracy increases with the experience of the operator and cytologist. However, false-negatives do occur. A core biopsy gives far more information: it gives a definitive preoperative diagnosis, differentiates between ductal carcinoma in situ and invasive cancer, and allows the receptor status to be determined to help in neoadjuvant chemotherapy.

Benign breast disease

2. B, E

Breast cancer

3. C, D

4. A, B, D, E

5. D

6. B, F

After mastectomy, radiotherapy to the chest wall is indicated in patients in whom the risks of local recurrence are high, such as those with large tumours, patients with large numbers of positive nodes and extensive lymphovascular invasion.

Primary neoadjuvant chemotherapy is used for large operable tumours, the aim being to shrink the tumour to enable breast-conserving surgery to be carried out. This approach is successful in up to 80 per cent of cases.

Answers: Extended matching questions

1. Benign breast disease

1J

This lady has a Phylloides tumour, so called because it is leaf-like (Phylloides in Greek = leaf-like) in appearance. The size can vary. It has an irregular bosselated surface with the overlying skin stretched. The tumour is also called cystosarcoma phyllodes although it is neither cystic nor a sacrcoma. Sir Benjamin Brodie (1783–1862, Surgeon, St George's Hospital, London) described it in 1840 as sero-cystic disease of breast. After triple assessment, it is treated by enucleation, wide local excision or simple mastectomy depending upon the size.

2I

This 25-year-old lady has a fibroadenoma – an incidental, mobile lump. After reassurance with triple assessment, it needs to be removed only in case of inconclusive cytology or if the patient wishes removal.

3C
Tuberculosis (TB) of the breast is usually associated with pulmonary TB or TB cervical adenitis. It is almost unknown in the indigenous British population but still common in developing countries. The discharging sinus in her axilla is from TB lymphadenitis. The diagnosis is confirmed by triple assessment. Treatment is antituberculous chemotherapy, while mastectomy is reserved for persistent residual infection.

4D
This patient suffers from thrombophlebitis of the superficial veins of the chest. The condition, called Mondor's disease (Henri Mondor, 1885–1962, a Parisian surgeon) is associated with a cord-like subcutaneous band made clinically obvious by stretching the skin on raising the arm. All diagnostic efforts must be made to exclude an underlying occult carcinoma causing lymphatic permeation.

5H
This lady has a galactocele – a rare condition; sub-areolar cystic lump which she dates from the start of her lactation. Confirmation is by aspiration of milk.

6G
This woman typically suffers from a breast cyst. It is essential to exclude malignancy by triple assessment. Aspiration of the cyst following which it completely disappears will give both physical and psychological relief.

7A
Traumatic fat necrosis usually occurs in middle-aged women after blunt trauma. A painless lump appears which may feel like a carcinoma. There may even be skin-tethering and nipple retraction. Just because there is a history of trauma, the diagnosis may not be fat necrosis, because the trauma might have drawn the patient's attention to the presence of the lump which is a carcinoma. The full triple assessment should be carried out to be sure of the diagnosis.

8B
A breast abscess is most often associated with lactation and usually caused by Staphylococcus aureus. A segment of the breast is inflamed, red, very painful, tender and indurated. In the early stage, cellulitis is present. An appropriate antibiotic is used after aspiration of pus. Under antibiotic cover, repeated aspirations with ultrasound guidance, good support to the breast and analgesia comprise the treatment of choice. Rarely, if the skin is thinned and the abscess is about to burst, a radial incision and drainage are carried out. If antibiotic is used without drainage of the pus, an 'antibioma' – a sterile, brawny, oedematous swelling – may form which can take weeks to resolve.

9E
This patient has the typical features of duct ectasia – nipple discharge (not bloodstained), deformed nipple with retraction, and a subareolar indurated mass which may mimic carcinoma. The condition is caused by dilatation and inflammation of the ducts, leading to periductal mastitis. A carcinoma must be excluded by triple assessment. Treatment is by surgical removal of all terminal ducts.

10F
The Cardiff Breast Clinic described a condition called aberrations of normal development and involution (ANDI). The symptoms are generalised lumpiness of breasts, less often confined to one quadrant; changes being cyclical with the periods; and sometimes a discrete lump, which may be a cyst or a fibroadenoma. Mastalgia may be quite disabling and the pain should be distinguished from that referred from the chest wall. The underlying pathological features are cyst formation, fibrosis, hyperplasia and papillomatosis. Triple assessment is done to exclude carcinoma. Examination at a different time of the menstrual cycle followed by reassurance supplemented by conservative measures is the overall management.

PART 9

Cardiothoracic

51 Cardiac surgery 391

52 The thorax 397

51 Cardiac surgery

Multiple choice questions

➜ Cardiopulmonary bypass

1. Which of the following statements is false?

A Cardiopulmonary bypass has brought about remarkable progress in cardiac surgery.
B The cardiopulmonary bypass circuit consists of a venous reservoir, oxygenator, heat exchanger, filter and roller pump.
C Cardiopulmonary bypass is not used outside cardiac surgery.
D Patients require full-dose heparin with the use of cardiopulmonary bypass.
E Cardiopulmonary bypass can cause serious systemic complications.

➜ Ischaemic heart disease

2. Which of these is not a risk factor for ischaemic heart disease?

A Smoking
B Obesity
C Advancing age
D Reduced physical activity
E Female gender.

➜ Coronary artery bypass surgery

3. Which of the following statements are true?

A Coronary artery bypass surgery affords symptomatic and prognostic benefit for subsets of patients with ischaemic heart disease.
B Myocardial infarction is an indication for emergency coronary artery bypass surgery.
C Selective coronary angiography is the 'gold standard' investigation and demonstrates coronary stenosis and coronary characteristics helpful in planning surgery.
D An estimate of the operative mortality can be calculated using risk scoring systems.
E The left internal mammary (or thoracic) artery has a better 10-year patency rate than long saphenous vein grafts.

➜ Valvular heart disease

4. Which of the following statements are false?

A The indication for surgery in mitral valve disease (regurgitation and stenosis) is severe symptoms, as assessed by the New York Heart Association (NYHA) functional classification.
B Acute and chronic mitral regurgitation have similar pathophysiology and clinical presentation.
C Mitral stenosis causes left atrial enlargement, pulmonary hypertension, atrial fibrillation and haemoptysis.
D Mitral valve repair is superior to mitral valve replacement but more technically demanding.
E All of the above.

5. Which of the following statements is false?

A Aortic stenosis is associated with a risk of sudden death related to the severity of stenosis.
B Rheumatic heart disease can cause both aortic stenosis and aortic regurgitation.
C Distinguishing between aortic stenosis and chronic aortic regurgitation is usually difficult on clinical grounds alone.
D Aortic valve repair is not a common practice like mitral valve repair.
E None of the above.

Prosthetic heart valves

6. Which of these statements are true?

A Biological valves are obtained from animals (xenograft or heterograft), dead humans (allograft or homograft) and the patient (autograft).

B Mechanical valves are more durable than biological valves.

C Lifelong anticoagulation is required for all prosthetic valves.

D Age is the only determinant of the choice of prosthetic valve.

E Biological valves are not at risk of prosthetic valve endocarditis.

Congenital heart disease

7. Which of the following statements is false?

A Cyanotic heart diseases are often more complex compared with acyanotic diseases, and result from a right-to-left shunt or a pulmonary circulation that runs in parallel to systemic circulation, or abnormal connection of blood vessels to the heart.

B Acyanotic heart diseases are more common that cyanotic heart diseases, and usually cause heart failure in infancy.

C The coexistence of ventricular septal defect, overriding aorta, pulmonary stenosis and right ventricular hypertrophy is referred to as Fallot's tetralogy.

D Four types of atrial septal defects are perimembranous, muscular, atrioventricular and subarterial.

E In septal defects (atrial and ventricular) a left-to-right shunt causes an increase in pulmonary blood flow and pulmonary vascular resistance. Progressive changes occur if the defects are not closed, leading to Eisenmenger's syndrome.

8. Which of these are not acyanotic heart diseases?

A Patent ductus arteriosus

B Total anomalous pulmonary venous drainage

C Transposition of the great vessels

D Patent foramen ovale

E Coarctation of the aorta.

The thoracic aorta and pericardial disease

9. Which one of these statements is false?

A Common causes of thoracic aortic aneurysm are atherosclerosis and connective tissue disorders.

B Indication for surgery in thoracic aneurysm depends on the part of the thoracic aorta involved.

C Paraplegia, renal failure and ventricular dysfunction are some complications of descending aneurysm repair.

D Stanford types A and B aortic dissection require emergency repair.

E Pericardial effusion causes an increase in intrapericardial pressure and compression of the atria when this pressure exceeds the atrial pressure. This decreases venous return, cardiac output and blood pressure (cardiac tamponade).

Extended matching questions

1. Cardiac disease

A Echocardiography

B Computed tomography (CT) scan of the chest

C Ischaemic heart disease

D Mitral regurgitation

Choose and match the most appropriate diagnosis or investigation for the clinical scenarios below:

1 A 72-year-old female with chronic stable angina presents with new-onset dyspnoea on mild exertion, bilateral basal crepitations and a new loud apical pansystolic murmur. Chest radiograph shows cardiomegaly and pulmonary congestion, and electrocardiography confirms recent myocardial infarction. What is the likely diagnosis?

2 Clinical examination of a 35-year-old man who has Marfan's syndrome with aneurysmal dilatation of the ascending aorta reveals wide pulse pressure, water-hammer pulse and a mid-diastolic murmur. What procedure is appropriate at this stage in the management of this patient?

3 A 66-year-old male is informed during consent for a procedure for a cardiac disease that, in addition to a procedure-related mortality of about 2 per cent, there is a risk of neurological dysfunction of less than 2 per cent, cardiac arrhythmia up to 30 per cent and significant bleeding up to 5 per cent. What condition is this procedure for?

4 On routine chest radiography, a 78-year-old male is suspected of having an aneurysm of the descending thoracic aorta. What is the appropriate investigation?

Answers: Multiple choice questions

Cardiopulmonary bypass

1. C

Cardiopulmonary bypass provides cardiac and respiratory support when the function of the heart and lungs needs to be temporarily interrupted. Whereas cardiac surgery remains its principal domain, it can be used in the management of patients outside cardiac surgery. For example, it facilitates the resection of renal and hepatic tumours invading the inferior vena cava, highly vascular tumours and extensive arteriovenous malformations.

Ischaemic heart disease

2. E

Male gender is a risk factor for ischaemic heart disease. However, studies have shown that female gender is associated with a worse outcome of coronary artery bypass surgery.

Coronary artery bypass surgery

3. A, C, D, E

Survival benefit of surgery over angioplasty and stenting has been demonstrated in patients with:

- >50 per cent stenosis of the left main stem
- >70 per cent stenosis of the proximal left anterior descending artery
- >70 per cent stenosis of all three major coronary arteries (right coronary, left anterior descending and circumflex)
- coronary artery stenosis with poor left ventricular function.

Selective coronary angiography demonstrates coronary anatomy and enables the visualisation of coronary artery size, evaluation of the site, extent and complexity of stenosis, and assessment of the distal coronary to help plan surgery. It also allows an estimation of left ventricular function. Rare lesions that can affect outcome of surgery, such as coronary artery aneurysm and fistula, are also revealed. Selective coronary angiography provides comprehensive information, not possible with other imaging techniques, that is useful in developing a strategy for surgery.

Risk scoring systems like the European System for Cardiac Operative Risk Evaluation (EuroSCORE), which allocate scores to risk factors in a patient, is routinely used to estimate the risk of operative mortality. This predicted operative mortality forms part of a patient's informed consent.

Venous and arterial conduits are used for coronary artery bypass surgery. The long saphenous vein is the most common vein conduit used and the left internal mammary artery is the most common arterial conduit, and the graft of choice for the left anterior descending artery. Venous grafts are susceptible to atherosclerosis, resulting in a 10-year patency rate of 50–60 per cent for the long saphenous vein. By comparison, arterial grafts are better protected against atherosclerosis. The left internal mammary artery has a 10-year patency rate of 90 per cent.

Valvular heart disease

4. A, B

Surgery is performed in mitral valve disease to relieve symptoms and to improve survival (prognostic). Severe symptoms, therefore, are not the only indication for surgery. For mitral regurgitation, progressive left ventricular dilatation and/or dysfunction and severe onset of regurgitation are the other indications. For mitral stenosis, the other indications are the severity of stenosis (moderate and severe stenosis with valve area of $\leq$1.5 cm^2) and systemic embolisation.

The onset of mitral regurgitation has implications for changes in cardiac morphology and function, and consequently the strategy for surgical correction. In mitral regurgitation, retrograde ejection leads to an increase in left ventricular volume load. The amount of retrograde ejection increases slowly in chronic mitral regurgitation, allowing adaptive changes like progressive left ventricular dilatation and hypertrophy, and left atrial dilatation, to develop without substantial pressure increase. As a result the pulmonary circulation is protected from developing a sudden increase in pressure. Acute mitral regurgitation does not allow time for these compensatory changes. High-volume retrograde flow into a small left atrium causes a sudden surge in left atrial pressure and a back pressure increase affecting the pulmonary venous circulation, leading to pulmonary congestion and oedema. Chronic mitral regurgitation, however, ultimately causes congestive cardiac failure when the compensatory mechanisms are overwhelmed.

Acute mitral regurgitation presents with sudden onset and rapidly progressive dyspnoea with clinical and radiological evidence of pulmonary oedema. Chronic mitral regurgitation is usually asymptomatic until pulmonary congestion and left ventricular failure develop. Then symptoms like fatigue, dyspnoea on exertion, orthopnoea and atrial fibrillation (due to left atrial enlargement) occur, and left ventricular enlargement becomes apparent radiologically. A loud apical pansystolic murmur is audible in both acute and chronic mitral regurgitation.

5. C

Aortic stenosis and chronic aortic regurgitation are usually asymptomatic until cardiac decompensation occurs. Compensatory mechanisms include ventricular hypertrophy (increase in wall thickness) to overcome the left ventricular outflow obstruction of aortic stenosis, and left ventricular dilatation to accommodate the increased left ventricular volume load due to aortic regurgitation. With cardiac decompensation, and acute aortic regurgitation, patients develop exertional dyspnoea and angina. Syncope is also common with aortic stenosis.

Marked differences exist with clinical findings. A harsh systolic ejection murmur, heard loudest in the aortic area and radiating to the carotids, is typical of aortic stenosis.

The distinctive features of aortic regurgitation are due largely to a wide pulse pressure and include:

- collapsing pulse (water-hammer pulse)
- visible capillary pulsation in the nail bed (Quincke's sign)
- pulsatile head bobbing (de Musset's sign)
- visible pulsation of neck arteries (Corrigan's sign)
- 'pistol shot' sound on auscultation of the femoral artery (Traube's sign)
- uvular pulsation (Müller's sign).

In aortic regurgitation also, the apex beat is often visible and displaced laterally. The characteristic murmur of aortic regurgitation is high-pitched, mid-diastolic and best heard at the left sternal border. The electrocardiographic and radiological appearances are not usually distinctive.

Prosthetic heart valves

6. A, B

Biological valves are made or obtained from animal or human tissue. While valves obtained from humans (homograft and autograft) are harvested and implanted without major alteration of the configuration, valves made from animal tissue (heterograft) are constructed to resemble human valves and are mounted on a frame (stented) or frameless (stentless). Among biological valves, heterografts are most commonly used; specifically, stented heterografts are the most frequently implanted. Biological valves are non-thrombogenic so do not require lifelong anticoagulation.

Biological valves, unlike mechanical valves, are subject to degenerative changes which lead to structural failure, and hence their durability is limited. Younger patients are probably more vulnerable. The need to replace a prosthetic valve also arises if there is a paravalvular leak causing haemodynamic instability or haemolytic anaemia, thrombosis of the valve, thromboembolism related to the valve and infection of the valve (prosthetic valve endocarditis). Homografts and autografts (entirely human tissues) are less susceptible to thrombosis/thromboembolism and infection. Mechanical valves and the other biological valves have low risks of paravalvular leak, infection and thrombosis/thromboembolism.

Congenital heart disease

7. D

Three main types of atrial septal defect (defect in the septum between the right and left atria) described are: ostium secundum, ostium primum and sinus venosus.

The defects listed in D (perimembranous, muscular, atrioventricular and subarterial) are the four types of ventricular septal defects. In both atrial and ventricular septal defects, a left-to-right shunt occurs and in the long term can cause Eisenmenger's syndrome from high-volume pulmonary blood flow, high pulmonary pressure and reversal of shunt.

8. B, C

In total anomalous pulmonary venous drainage, pulmonary venous return is into the systemic venous circulation usually through a communication with the inferior vena cava, superior vena cava, coronary sinus or right atrium, instead of the left atrium. The typical presentation is cyanosis after the first week of life. If there is a coexistent atrial septal defect, cyanosis is minimal even with high pulmonary flow.

The aorta arises from the right ventricle and the pulmonary artery from the left ventricle in transposition of the great vessels. This arrangement allows the pulmonary and systemic circulation to run in parallel rather than in series. As oxygenated blood is confined to the pulmonary circulation and deoxygenated blood to the systemic circulation, this condition is not compatible with life. Associated defects like foramen ovale and ventricular septal defect provide channels for mixing of blood. Transposition of the great vessels is the most common congenital heart disease, causing cyanosis in the newborn period, and, in general, the second most common cyanotic congenital heart disease after tetralogy of Fallot.

The thoracic aorta and pericardial disease

9. D

Aortic dissection originating (defect or intimal flap) in the ascending aorta is type A, and one that originates in the descending aorta (beyond the origin of the left subclavian artery) is type B, according to the Stanford classification. Type A requires emergency surgical intervention but type B is best managed conservatively initially. The indications for surgery in type B aortic dissection include:

- worsening chest pain indicating imminent rupture
- progressive expansion of lesion on serial chest imaging (radiograph or CT scan)
- malperfusion syndrome resulting in organ dysfunction, such as renal failure, or limb and neurological complications.

Answers: Extended matching questions

→ 1. Cardiac disease

1D

Even with stable symptoms due to adequate medical therapy, ischaemic heart disease can still cause morphological complications and remains a common cause of mitral regurgitation (ischaemic mitral regurgitation) as a result of its local or global effects. Regional myocardial ischaemia and myocardial infarction cause papillary muscle dysfunction or rupture. Global myocardial ischaemia causes left ventricular dysfunction and dilatation, which pulls the mitral leaflets apart so that functional mitral regurgitation occurs in the presence of grossly normal mitral valve leaflets.

2A

Marfan's syndrome is associated with cystic medial necrosis of the vessel wall, causing weakness and dilatation of the vessel. The aortic root and ascending aorta are commonly affected. Aortic regurgitation due to aortic root dilatation is common. The presence of clinical features of aortic regurgitation in the setting of ascending aortic aneurysm warrants further investigation. Echocardiography assesses the severity of regurgitation, the diameter of the aortic root, aortic valve morphology and left ventricular dimensions and function. The information provided by echocardiography is vital in deciding the optimal type of surgical repair.

3C

Surgical revascularisation for ischaemic heart disease is achieved by coronary artery bypass grafting, one of the most investigated surgical procedures with well and consistently documented complications. An estimate of the operative mortality can be calculated using risk stratification systems like the EuroSCORE. Surgery for mitral valve disease is associated with higher operative mortality, approximately 5–6 per cent.

4B

The diagnosis of thoracic aneurysm can be confirmed by CT of the chest. The site, size and presence of thrombi can be assessed. As descending thoracic aneurysm is often managed conservatively, CT is useful for serial assessment of the aneurysm to determine when surgery is indicated, due to acute enlargement or progressive increase in size to over 6 cm.

52 The thorax

Multiple choice questions

➜ Anatomy and physiology

1. **Which of the following statements is false?**

A The lungs are derivatives of the primitive foregut.

B The left lung has more lobes and segments than the right lung.

C Bronchial arteries arise directly from the thoracic aorta to provide systemic blood supply to the trachea and bronchi.

D Anatomical differences between the right and left main bronchi favour the inhalation of foreign bodies into the right.

E Pulmonary function tests assess the functional capacity, the severity of pulmonary disease and help to predict response to treatment.

➜ Pleural space disease

2. **Which of the following statements are true?**

A Tension pneumothorax can cause haemodynamic compromise.

B Pleural effusions due to cardiac failure, renal failure, hepatic disease, inflammatory disease and malignancy have different protein content.

C Infection of the pleural space (empyema) results from iatrogenic and non-iatrogenic causes.

D Video-assisted thoracoscopic surgery (VATS) plays a major role in the management of pleural space diseases.

E Chest drains are no longer critical to the management of chest disease.

➜ Primary lung cancer

3. **Which one of these statements is false?**

A Lifetime cigarette smoking, quantified as 'pack-years', is a major risk factor for bronchial carcinoma.

B Compared with non-small-cell cancer, small-cell lung cancer, formerly known as oat cell cancer, is less common, metastasises early and is less amenable to surgery.

C Finger clubbing and hypertrophic pulmonary osteoarthropathy, sometimes described as clinical features of lung cancer, are usually incidental findings and not due to primary lung cancer.

D The appropriate treatment strategy is dependent on tumour type, tumour stage, and the general fitness and lung function of the patient.

E Late survival has a direct relationship with the tumour stage at the time of treatment.

➜ Investigating bronchial carcinoma

4. **Which one of these statements is true?**

A Chest radiograph yields very useful information about primary lung cancer.

B Computed tomography (CT) is only useful for guiding fine-needle aspiration.

C Positron emission tomography (PET) has high specificity for bronchial carcinoma.

D Sputum cytology has a high sensitivity.

E Invasive procedures such as mediastinoscopy, mediastinotomy and thoracoscopy are not staging procedures.

➜ Non-malignant conditions

5. **Which of the following statements is false?**

A Bronchopulmonary carcinoid tumours usually arise from neuroendocrine cells in major bronchi, are very vascular and slow-growing, and, although benign, sometimes metastasise.

B Surgery has a limited role in the treatment of bronchiectasis and tuberculosis.
C Blunt and penetrating chest trauma can cause death from hypovolaemia, hypoxaemia and tamponade.
D Diaphragmatic hernia through the foramen of Morgagni is usually posterior, while herniation through the foramen of Bochdalek lies more anteriorly.
E Pectus carinatum and pectus excavatum are chest wall deformities that require surgery mainly for cosmetic reasons.

Extended matching questions

1. Management of thoracic disease

A Thoracotomy
B Chest drain insertion
C Bronchoscopy
D CT scan of the chest
E None of the above

Choose and match the appropriate answer for the following questions:

1 A middle-aged male patient presents with spontaneous recurrent haemoptysis, and clinical examination reveals no abnormal findings. Her chest radiograph is normal. What is the procedure of choice?

2 After reading the information booklet about his proposed procedure, an anxious 45-year-old female patient being consented for a procedure is worried about the post-procedural complications of pain and possible rib fractures. What procedure is this patient planned to have?

3 Following a right pneumonectomy, the postoperative recovery of a 52-year-old male patient is complicated by bronchopleural fistula, which presents with pyrexia, expectoration of large amounts of purulent sputum and a high fluid level on chest radiograph. In addition to positioning the patient to lie on the operated side, what procedure is urgently required?

4 A mediastinal mass is found incidentally on the chest radiograph of a 65-year-old female non-smoker who is otherwise healthy, with no significant past medical history. Which option would you recommend to this patient at this time?

5 Which procedure is required to assess the fitness for lung resection of a 73-year-old male with left upper lobe lung cancer and emphysema?

Answers: Multiple choice questions

Anatomy and physiology

1. B

The left lung is divided into an upper lobe and a lower lobe by the oblique fissure. There are five segments in the upper lobe and five in the lower lobe. Each segment is an anatomically defined unit with named bronchi, pulmonary artery branch and pulmonary vein tributary.

The right lung, on the other hand, has three lobes. An oblique fissure separates the upper and lower lobes. The upper lobe is further separated from a middle lobe by a horizontal fissure. The right lung also has 10 segments distributed as follows: three in the upper, two in the middle and five in the lower lobe.

Pleural space disease

2. A, B, C, D

In tension pneumothorax, positive pressure builds up in the hemithorax as air accumulates through a breach in the visceral pleura, which acts like a valve allowing a unidirectional flow of air out of the lung. The high intrapleural pressure results in compression of the ipsilateral lung, flattening of the hemidiaphragm, mediastinal distortion and shift, and impairment of venous return to the heart and hence a reduction of cardiac output.

Pleural effusion results from interference with either the mechanisms of pleural fluid production by capillaries of parietal pleura or absorption by the capillaries of the visceral pleura. Depending on the protein concentration, pleural effusions are classified as transudates (less than 30 g/L) or exudates (30 g/L or more).

In cardiac failure, the pulmonary capillary pressure is elevated, leading to increased production of pleural effusion with low protein content.

Renal and hepatic failure are associated with low plasma protein and intravascular oncotic pressure. The pleural effusion that results from reduced pleural fluid absorption is low in protein content. Inflammatory diseases increase pleural capillary permeability to cause the accumulation of fluid and protein. Malignancy obstructs the lymphatic system and causes a protein-rich pleural effusion.

The pleural cavity is sterile but the bronchial tree is not. A breech of the sterile barrier between the pleura and the bronchial system on one hand (endogenous), and between the pleura and the external environment (exogenous) on the other, increases the risk of empyema (infection within the pleural space). Iatrogenic introduction of bacteria into the pleural space can occur during aspiration of effusions, insertion of chest drains, thoracoscopy and thoracotomy. Traumatic haemothorax provides a favourable culture medium for infection. Endogenous spread can occur from pneumonia, bronchiectasis, tuberculosis, fungal infections and lung abscess.

Video-assisted thoracoscopic surgery is a less invasive method for investigating and treating thoracic pathologies, including pleural diseases such as pneumothorax, pleural effusion and empyema. It plays a major role in the management of thoracic diseases.

Intercostal chest drains are fundamental to the management of chest disease. The insertion of chest drains can be life-saving, and they are used as either sole therapeutic interventions or adjunctive to other thoracic procedures.

Primary lung cancer

3. C

Finger clubbing and hypertrophic pulmonary osteoarthropathy are clinical findings seen in some patients with primary lung cancer. The direct association with lung cancer is demonstrated by regression of these muscular and skeletal abnormalities when the cancer is resected.

Investigating bronchial carcinoma

4. A

Most lung cancer lesions or their secondary effects are detected on chest radiograph. Pleural effusion, distal lung collapse or consolidation due to bronchial obstruction, and raised hemidiaphragm due to invasion of phrenic nerve are some secondary effects of lung cancer seen on chest radiograph.

Computed tomography is central to further characterisation of primary lung cancer with regard to site, tumour size (T stage), proximity to chest wall and mediastinal structures, and mediastinal lymph node status (N stage). It also facilitates percutaneous biopsy.

Positron emission tomography shows high uptake of fluorodeoxyglucose (FDG) by lesions with high metabolism, so in addition to cancer, infections and other inflammatory lesions show avid update of FDG.

Sputum cytology has a high false-negative rate because it relies on the probability of obtaining a sample with exfoliated tumour cells which can be low for peripheral lung cancers.

Mediastinoscopy, mediastinotomy and thoracoscopy are frequently used to assess the extent of tumour spread (staging) and sometimes for establishing histological diagnosis.

➜ Non-malignant conditions

5. D

Non-traumatic herniation of abdominal viscera through the diaphragm commonly occurs at two congenital sites, namely the foramen of Morgagni, which is an anterior defect between sternal and costal attachments of the diaphragm, and the foramen of Bochdalek, which lies posteriorly in the dome of the diaphragm.

Answers: Extended matching questions

➜ 1. Management of thoracic disease

1C

Haemoptysis is commonly caused by bronchopulmonary trauma, infection or neoplastic (benign and malignant) lesions of pulmonary system. The underlying pathologies are usually in direct or indirect communication with the bronchial tree. Bronchoscopy affords the ability to visualise the lesion, the potential to obtain biopsies or treat, or the insight to plan further treatment. The flexible bronchoscope can be advanced into segmental bronchi and is useful for obtaining sputum and tissue biopsies. As the calibre is small and suction is limited, flexible bronchoscopes may not have optimal diagnostic and therapeutic yield soon after an episode of haemoptysis because blood clots obscure visualisation. Rigid bronchoscopy overcomes these setbacks but requires general anaesthesia.

2A

Thoracotomy involves muscle cutting, rib spreading and parietal pleura breeching. Sometimes rib fractures occur and the intercostal nerves are bruised during rib spreading. In the early postoperative period, therefore, thoracotomy pain can be severe and difficult to control. The functional consequence of post-thoracotomy pain leads to other complications such as impairment of mobilisation, normal breathing and gas exchange. The strategies commonly used to manage early post-thoracotomy pain include oral analgesia, and either intravenous opiates used as patient-controlled analgesia (PCA) or local anaesthesia delivered via catheters into the paravertebral or extrapleural space.

3B

Morphological changes such as mediastinal shift, elevation of the hemidiaphragm and crowding of the ribs occur after pneumonectomy to contract the pneumonectomy space, which fills with tissue fluid. Dehiscence of the bronchial stump occurs in bronchopleural fistula to establish communication between colonised bronchial tree and the sterile pneumonectomy space. Invariably, the pneumonectomy space and fluid get infected in bronchopleural fistula. Signs of systemic infection (pyrexia) with clinical (expectorating purulent sputum) and radiological (high fluid level) evidence of infected collection in the chest warrant immediate chest drain insertion to control the source of sepsis. Further management of bronchopleural fistula is undertaken in specialised centres.

4D

A mediastinal mass on chest radiograph deserves further investigation with CT of the chest to define the site, size, nature and attachments of the mass and surrounding structures, and, where possible, to obtain a guided percutaneous biopsy for histological diagnosis. On the basis of the location in the mediastinum, the possible cause of the mass can be suspected. Common mediastinal masses in the different parts of the mediastinum are:

- superior mediastinum – lymphoma, thyroid and parathyroid
- anterior mediastinum – thymoma, lymphoma and germ cell tumour
- middle mediastinum – cystic lesions, lymphoma and mesenchymal tumours
- posterior mediastinum – neurogenic tumours, cystic lesions and mesenchymal tumours.

5E

In order to determine the fitness of patients for lung resection, and the extent of resection they can tolerate, pulmonary function test is necessary. Peak expiratory flow rate, forced expiratory volume in 1 sec (FEV_1), forced vital capacity (FVC) and arterial blood gases provide useful information. In general, a patient is fit for lobectomy if the FEV_1 is >1.5 L and pneumonectomy if >2.0 L.

PART 10 Vascular

53 Arterial disorders 405

54 Venous disorders 411

55 Lymphatic disorders 416

53 Arterial disorders

Multiple choice questions

➜ Claudication

1. **Which of the following statements are true?**
   A Intermittent claudication may be present at rest.
   B Intermittent claudication is commonly relieved by getting out of bed.
   C Intermittent claudication is most commonly felt in the calf.
   D Intermittent claudication distance is usually inconsistent on a day-to-day basis for a given patient.
   E Intermittent claudication is thought to be due to nerve compression in the leg muscle compartments.

➜ Critical ischaemia

2. **Which of the following statements are true?**
   A Rest pain is commonly found in the calf in critical limb ischaemia.
   B Rest pain is often relieved by getting out of bed and taking a few steps.
   C Hypoaesthesia is a feature of pregangrene.
   D Absence of foot pulses implies critical ischaemia.
   E Paralysis of the leg may suggest an acutely ischaemic leg.

➜ Aorto-iliac disease

3. **Which of the following are true in aorto-iliac disease?**
   A Impotence is common.
   B It may be the cause of thigh and calf claudication.
   C It is very unlikely in the presence of femoral pulse.
   D Surgical intervention has the poorest results in aorto-iliac disease when compared with infra-inguinal disease.
   E Bruits are commonly found in the lower abdomen.

➜ Investigations

4. **Which of the following statements are true?**
   A Doppler ultrasound works on the basis of a frequency shift when sound waves hit moving red blood cells.
   B ABPI means 'ankle brachial pulsatility index'.
   C An ABPI of greater than 0.9 is probably normal.
   D Duplex scans are a combination of waveform analysis and B-mode ultrasound.
   E Carotid surgery is often performed on the basis of duplex scans without further imaging.

5. **Which of the following statements regarding angiography are true?**
   A It is only done once it is considered that intervention may be appropriate.
   B Compared with conventional angiography, the digital subtraction angiograms require an increased contrast load for reliable images.
   C Magnetic resonance angiography (MRA) is largely replacing conventional angiography for routine imaging.
   D Neurological dysfunction is a potential complication of arteriography.
   E Routine aortography cannot be performed via the femoral artery.

➜ Drugs

6. **Which of the following drugs have been shown to improve claudication?**
   A Beta-blockers
   B Aspirin
   C Oxpentifylline

D Simvastatin
E Prostacyclin.

Abdominal aortic aneurysms

7. **Which of the following statements are true?**
A Abdominal aortic aneurysms (AAAs) are usually symptomatic.
B Older chronological age is not a bar to surgery.
C Ultrasound has a high degree of sensitivity and specificity for AAAs.
D The size of the aneurysm is best assessed by angiography.
E Most AAAs will eventually rupture, resulting in the patient's death.

8. **Which of the following statements regarding complications of AAA surgery are true?**
A Colonic ischaemia may occur in up to 10 per cent of postoperative patients.
B Renal failure is uncommon following elective AAA repair.
C Most elective deaths are from respiratory failure.
D Endovascular aneurysm repair has a perioperative mortality equivalent to open repair.
E Graft infection is seen in less than 1 per cent of elective cases.

9. **Ruptured abdominal aortic aneurysms**
A Most patients die following ruptured AAA.
B Most ruptures occur anteriorly into the peritoneal cavity.
C Patients with a rupture should be immediately and aggressively resuscitated prior to surgery.
D CT scan is always needed preoperatively to confirm the diagnosis.
E Ruptures are rarely seen in aneurysms of less than 5 cm.

Acute arterial occlusion

10. **Acute arterial occlusion may be caused by:**
A Compartmental swelling
B Damage to the intima only following external trauma
C Intra-abdominal swelling
D Intramural haemorrhage
E Arterial spasm.

Gangrene

11. **Which of the following is not a cause of gangrene?**
A Buerger's disease
B Infection
C Intra-arterial drug injection
D Frostbite
E Deep vein thrombosis insufficiency.

Amputation

12. **Which of the following are indications for major amputation?**
A Clostridium infection of the lower leg.
B Severe trauma
C Neurofibroma
D Knee flexion contracture
E Severe rest pain without gangrene.

13. **Which of the following regarding amputations are true?**
A Toe amputations usually heal well in diabetics.
B Transmetatarsal amputation can relieve rest pain.
C Above-knee amputation is generally a better choice than below-knee in large-vessel occlusive disease.
D A Gritti–Stokes amputation is performed at the ankle level.
E Below-knee amputations are not 'end-weight-bearing' amputations.

Raynaud's phenomenon

14. **Which of the following statements are true?**
A Primary Raynaud's phenomenon often results in digital gangrene.
B Primary Raynaud's is most commonly seen in young girls.
C Primary Raynaud's may be associated with vibrating tools.
D Systemic lupus erythematosus (SLE) is a common underlying cause of secondary Raynaud's.
E Sympathectomy is an effective treatment of Raynaud's phenomenon.

Extended matching questions

1. Emboli

A Air embolism
B Fat embolism
C Mycotic embolism
D Foreign body embolism
E Cholesterol embolism
F Popliteal arterial embolism
G Acute aortic thrombosis

Choose and match the correct diagnosis with each of the scenarios given below:

1 A 22-year-old male involved in a motorcycle accident presents to A&E with a fractured femur and, following fixation, is noted to have become disorientated with several areas of petechial haemorrhage.

2 A 75-year-old female presents with a sudden episode of acute pain in the right leg. On examination she has an irregular tachycardia of 120 beats/min and a white, paraesthetic right lower leg. She has no palpable pulses below the groin but her left leg pulses are present and normal.

3 A 59-year-old male presents to A&E with paralysis and paraesthesia of his lower limbs. On examination there are no femoral pulses and he has mottling of the skin of the lower abdomen.

4 A 65-year-old woman presents to her GP with several recent episodes of temporary left eye blindness which resolved on each occasion after about 5 min. Retinoscopy shows several areas of poor filling in the retinal arteries.

5 A 40-year-old IV drug abuser presents with fevers, breathlessness and pain in his right buttock. His temperature is 38°C and examination reveals marked mottling over the right gluteal area and thigh. He has a grade V aortic murmur.

Answers: Multiple choice questions

Claudication

1. C

Intermittent claudication is pain that is only present following exercise. It is rest pain that is relieved by getting out of bed. The commonest site for intermittent claudication is the calf, and the claudication distance is remarkably consistent on a day-to-day basis. Intermittent claudication is due to relative ischaemia of the muscles during exercise with stimulation of pain pathways via cytokines etc.

Critical ischaemia

2. B, C, E

Rest pain is pain found in the toes or forefoot of the foot because of severe ischaemia. It can be relieved by dependency, which is often achieved by getting out of bed and walking around. Hypoaesthesia is often present in threatened limbs, but where paralysis is present this is likely to be due to an acutely ischaemic leg or an acute-en-chronic ischaemia. The absence of foot pulses is commonly present in patients with vascular disease and does not in itself imply critical ischaemia.

Aorto-iliac disease

3. A, B, E

Impotence is commonly found in patients with aorto-iliac disease, although it is not always due to arterial insufficiency. Both thigh and calf claudication can be caused by aorto-iliac disease and the presence of a femoral pulse does not eliminate the possibility of iliac arterial pathology. The results following aorto-iliac reconstruction are very much better than found in smaller vessel disease, such as in the femoropopliteal segment, and bruits are commonly found when listened for in the lower abdomen as a consequence of aorto-iliac occlusive disease.

Investigations

4. A, C, D, E

The Doppler principle depends on frequency shift of reflected ultrasound waves hitting red cells. ABPI means ankle brachial pressure index, and generally an ABPI > 0.9 would be regarded as normal. Duplex scans are now the gold standard assessment of carotid arterial flow and are a combination of waveform analysis and B-mode ultrasound.

5. A, C, D

Angiography should not be performed unless intervention is seriously being considered. Digital subtraction arteriograms require a reduced contrast load compared with conventional arteriography, although it should be noted that intravenous digital subtraction angiograms do indeed require a very significant contrast load. MR angiography is increasingly taking over as the initial imaging modality of choice, although conventional angiography is still generally needed for subsequent intervention, such as angioplasty. Neurological complications, though rare, are a recognised complication of arteriography. The vast majority of arteriograms are now done using the Seldinger technique via the femoral artery and can routinely image the aorta.

Drugs

6. C

Beta-blockers actually reduce muscle blood flow and can worsen claudication. Aspirin and Simvastatin are routinely prescribed for cardiovascular risk factors but do not affect claudication distance. Prostacyclin is occasionally used for critical limb ischaemia but has no effect on claudication distance. Oxpentifylline has been shown to have a marginal benefit on walking distance but is not often prescribed nowadays.

Abdominal aortic aneurysms

7. B, C

The majority of AAAs are usually asymptomatic. They are more common with increasing age, which in itself is not a bar to surgery. Ultrasound is the standard investigation for aortic aneurysm and has a very high degree of sensitivity and specificity, as well as reproducibility. Angiography is a very poor method of assessing size as much of the aneurysm contains clot. Most patients will actually die from other causes with their aneurysm intact as the majority of aneurysms are relatively small when first found and the growth rate is only approximately 0.2 cm/year.

8. A, B, E

Transient colonic ischaemia is surprisingly common following elective aneurysm repair. Fortunately it rarely presents with a major problem. Renal failure is extremely uncommon following elective repair although it is quite common following ruptured repair. Most elective deaths are secondary to myocardial ischaemia and the death rate from endovascular repair is probably only one-third of that using an open technique. Graft infection is very rarely seen in AAA repair, particularly where the graft is confined to the abdominal cavity and does not extend to the femoral arteries.

9. A, E

The majority of patients will die from ruptured aneurysm before they ever reach hospital. Of those who do reach hospital, 30–50 per cent may still die. Most ruptures occur posteriorly, giving some time for intervention to be performed. Intraperitoneal rupture is often fairly rapidly fatal. Patients with ruptures should not be aggressively resuscitated, but rather a programme of controlled hypotension should be initiated. Although useful, CT scan should never be done in patients who are significantly hypotensive, and these patients should be taken straight to theatre. The incidence of ruptures in patients with aneurysms of less than 5 cm is less than 1 per cent over the first year.

Acute arterial occlusion

10. A, B, D

Compartment syndrome is a well-recognised cause of arterial occlusion and is commonly seen following major trauma and crush injuries. Following blunt trauma, it is possible to get intimal tears without significant injury to the rest of the arteries. Although arterial spasm can give rise to temporary cessation of blood flow, it does not in itself result in arterial occlusion. Likewise intra-abdominal swelling can never be tense enough to occlude the major arteries in the abdomen. Intramural haemorrhage within the plaque is, however, a relatively common complication of atheroma and is frequently seen in, for example, the carotid bifurcation.

Gangrene

11. E

Deep vein thrombosis insufficiency on its own will not cause gangrene. Venous gangrene may occasionally occur but this is due to very extensive deep vein thrombosis thrombosis.

Amputation

12. A, B, D, E

Neurofibromas are benign tumours of the nerves and, in themselves, would not be an indication for amputation. Clostridium infection (gas gangrene) is an emergency often requiring guillotine amputation. Likewise, severe trauma may, on occasions, require major amputation. Some patients with knee flexion contractures are better off with major amputation, particularly where there is coexistent vascular disease. Revascularisation in the presence of a knee contracture is pointless. Some patients with severe rest pain and non-reconstructable disease will only obtain relief following major amputation.

13. A, E

In contrast to large-vessel disease, toe amputations often heal very well in diabetics provided that they are not primarily closed at the time of surgery. In the presence of rest pain, a below-knee amputation is usually required to relieve the symptoms. Below-knee amputations provide a much better quality of life and opportunity for prosthetic fitting than above-knee amputations and should be the preferred choice. A Gritti–Stokes amputation is at the knee joint level and below–knee amputations transfer the weight via a suction socket taking pressure on the anterior tibial tuberosity and patella tendon primarily.

Raynaud's phenomenon

14. B, C, D

Primary Raynaud's occurs in young girls and never results in ulceration or digital gangrene. It may be associated with vibration tools, the more extreme example of this being hand-arm vibration syndrome. SLE and other connective tissue disorders commonly have secondary Raynaud's phenomenon. Although used historically, a sympathectomy has little role to play in the treatment of Raynaud's phenomenon.

Answers: Extended matching questions

→ 1. Emboli

1B
This is a classical presentation of fat emboli following fracture and long bone fixation. Given the cerebral symptoms, high dose oxygen +/− ventilation may be essential here.

2F
This is a classical example of arterial embolism to the popliteal artery in a patient who has almost certainly got atrial fibrillation. Emergency femoral or popliteal embolectomy is absolutely indicated, followed by anticoagulation.

3G
Acute aortic thrombosis is a very serious, life-threatening condition with a poor prognosis. Classically, mottling is seen up to the umbilicus in these patients.

4E
Amaurosis fugax secondary to either small clots or cholesterol emboli is quite a common presentation. The cholesterol emboli can often be seen on retinoscopy.

5C
Increasingly, intravenous drug addicts present with arterial complications. In this case, it is likely that the patient has developed aortic valve vegetations and infection and mycotic embolisation to the buttocks and thigh.

54 Venous disorders

Multiple choice questions

➜ Venous leg ulcers

1. **Which of the following statements regarding venous leg ulcers are true?**

A Less than 10 per cent of patients will get a recurrence within 5 years after healing.
B Superficial venous surgery reduces the risk of subsequent ulceration.
C Venous ulcers are best managed by 'two layer' bandaging.
D Greater than 60 per cent of all leg ulcers are venous in origin.
E A class 2 stocking provides about 50 mmHg pressure at the ankle.

➜ Venous thrombosis

2. **Which of the following statements regarding venous thrombosis are true?**

A Between 5 and 10 per cent of the population may have a thrombophilia.
B Virchow's triad describes extra luminal, intramural and intraluminal obstructive causes.
C A family history of venous thrombosis is a risk factor for a patient.
D Risk can be abolished by effective prophylaxis.
E Homan's sign is pathognomonic in this condition.

3. **Which of the following regarding diagnosis of deep vein thrombosis (DVT) are true?**

A Clinical findings are a reliable way of establishing the diagnosis.
B A raised D-dimer level is high specific for venous thrombosis.
C Duplex scanning is the investigation of choice for DVT.
D Radioiodine-labelled fibrinogen is commonly used in the diagnosis of DVT.
E Computed tomography (CT) pulmonary angiography is the definitive test for pulmonary embolism.

4. **Which of the following regarding treatment of DVT are true?**

A Warfarin helps remove clot from the veins.
B Low-molecular-weight heparin is now the standard initial treatment for DVT.
C INR stands for 'intrinsic notional ratio'.
D Warfarin is generally continued for 3–6 months following DVT.
E Most patients with an iliofemoral DVT will need a caval filter.

➜ Varicose veins

5. **Which of the following regarding varicose veins are true?**

A Varicose veins may cause venous claudication.
B Varicose veins may be associated with the *fOXC2* gene.
C The prevalence of varicose veins is twice as common in women than in men.
D Right leg varicose veins are more common than left leg varicose veins.
E Handheld Doppler provides an accurate assessment of saphenopopliteal competence.

6. **Which of the following are indications for surgery in varicose veins?**

A Recurrent haemorrhage
B Skin changes such as lipodermatosclerosis or ulceration
C Itching
D Cosmesis
E Deep vein thrombosis.

7. Which of the following statements regarding complications of surgical treatment of varicose veins are true?

1 Drop foot may occur.
2 DVT occurs in about 5 per cent of cases.
3 Causalgia is an infrequent complication.
4 Saphenous nerve injury may lead to paraesthesia of the forefoot.
5 Numbness of the heel may be caused by tibial nerve neuropraxia.

Extended matching questions

→ 1. Ulcers

A Diabetes
B Deep vein thrombosis insufficiency
C Marjolin's ulcer
D Systemic lupus erythematosus (SLE)
E Diabetes
F Neuropathy
G Arterial disease

Choose and match the correct diagnosis with each of the scenarios below:

1 A 55-year-old woman presents with brown discoloration and induration around the ankle and a 3-cm-diameter ulcer lying just above the medial malleolus.

2 A 60-year-old man presents with a history of pins and needles in his left foot following multiple back operations and an ulcer over the plantar aspect of his second metatarsal head.

3 A 70-year-old lifelong male smoker presents with a painful ulcer over the head of his first metatarsal where he is noted to have a mild hallux valgus.

4 A 65-year-old man presents with a chronic ulcer of seven years lying over the medial aspect of his calf and which has recently become painful and enlarged.

5 A patient presents with small punched-out, painful ulcers over the dorsum of her foot.

→ 2. Varicose veins

A Endovascular laser treatment (EVLT)
B Valve surgery
C Foam sclerotherapy
D Saphenofemoral ligation, stripping and stab avulsions
E Class 2 support stockings
F Anticoagulation
G Thromboembolic deterrent (TED) stockings and prophylactic Fragmin
H Palma procedure
I Thrombolysis

Choose and match the most appropriate management with each of the scenarios below:

1 A 75-year-old man presents with a history of DVT 5 years ago and a recently healed venous ulcer. Duplex scan demonstrates isolated popliteal venous reflux.

2 An 80-year-old woman presents with a recently fractured neck of femur and a swollen painless warm leg; all peripheral pulses are palpable.

3 A 42-year-old woman presents with primary varicose veins and severe symptoms with a needle phobia. Duplex scan shows an isolated saphenofemoral junction incompetence and long saphenous vein reflux.

4 A 48-year-old man has a body mass index (BMI) of 37 and is a heavy smoker. He has primary symptomatic varicose veins with skin changes and duplex scan demonstrates an isolated saphenopopliteal junction incompetence and short saphenous reflux.

5 A 40-year-old man has a BMI of 30 and a previous idiopathic iliofemoral DVT. Duplex scan shows complete external iliac vein occlusion. He has significant venous claudication and leg swelling which interferes with his working life.

Answers: Multiple choice questions

➜ Venous leg ulcers

1. B, D

After successful management there is a 20–30 per cent incidence of re-ulceration within the first 5 years after healing. Superficial venous surgery does reduce, but not eliminate, the risk of subsequent ulceration. Three- or four-layer bandaging is regarded as the gold standard, although class 2 support stockings can offer an equivalent compression regime. Class 2 stockings may provide up to 30 mmHg pressure at the ankle.

➜ Venous thrombosis

2. A, C

Activated protein C deficiency, associated with factor V Leiden, occurs in about 7 per cent of the population. In addition, there are deficiencies of AT3 and protein S as well as lupus and antiphospholipid antibodies, all of which can predispose to thrombosis. Virchow described changes in the vessel wall (endothelial damage), stasis as a result of diminished blood flow and increased coagulability of blood as the three elements predisposing to thrombosis. A family history of venous thrombosis is important, and although risk can be reduced by effective prophylaxis, it cannot be eliminated. Homan's sign, which is resistance of the calf muscles to dorsiflexion, is generally unhelpful as it is commonly found in other conditions as well.

3. C, E

Many patients have no symptoms and few signs of DVT on presentation. At least half of patients with a suspected clinical DVT have another cause of their symptoms. D-dimers are not specific for venous thrombosis, being an acute-phase protein. As such, they will be raised following events such as surgery, and care must be taken in the interpretation of levels. Duplex scanning is nowadays the gold standard investigation for DVT. It has almost completely replaced radioiodine-labelled fibrinogen and ascending venography. CT pulmonary angiogram is the investigation of choice in a patient suspected of having a pulmonary embolism.

4. B, D

Warfarin on its own does not remove clot from veins (thrombolysis). If this is being considered then tissue plasminogen activator or streptokinase is needed. Low-molecular-weight heparin is nowadays regarded as a standard initial treatment for DVT. It has largely replaced unfractionated heparin in this area. INR stands for international normalised ratio and is a measure of warfarin activity. Generally speaking, warfarin is continued for 3–6 months in DVT. The indications for a caval filter are a contraindication to anticoagulation or occurrence of pulmonary emboli despite adequate anticoagulation. An iliofemoral DVT alone is not sufficient justification.

➜ Varicose veins

5. B

Venous claudication is uncommon and caused by deep vein thrombosis obstruction. Varicose veins are not a cause, although they are very common, affecting some 5 per cent or more of the adult population. In patients with a definite family history, there may be an abnormality in the *fOXC2* gene; and although women present more commonly with varicose veins, the distribution is roughly equal between men and women. Left leg varicose veins are actually more common than in the right leg, though it is not clear why this is the case. Handheld Doppler, while very useful in the groin, is inaccurate over the saphenopopliteal region and duplex scanning is required to demonstrate saphenopopliteal incompetence.

6. A, B
Bleeding and skin changes are regarded as genuine indications for surgery. Deep vein thrombosis is often a contraindication to surgery and cosmesis is not an appropriate indication. Itching is very common in patients and, on its own, is rarely an indication for surgery.

7. A, C, E
A drop foot is an infrequent complication of saphenopopliteal exploration and is a consequence of bruising or damage to the common peroneal (lateral popliteal) nerve. Bruising or damage to the tibial nerve in this procedure can give rise to heel numbness while saphenous nerve injury generally causes numbness of the medial aspect of the calf and ankle. Occasionally these nerve injuries can give rise to severe causalgia, which can be extremely debilitating for patients.

Answers: Extended matching questions

→ 1. Ulcers

1D
Classical venous ulcers occur on the medial aspect of the calf, rarely extending into the foot or the upper calf. Venous ulcers generally have surrounding lipodermatosclerosis where there is thickening pigmentation and induration of the skin. This pigmentation is secondary to haemosiderin deposition. Deep vein thrombosis insufficiency is often present on duplex scan but some ulcers can be secondary to superficial venous disease.

2F
Peripheral neuropathy may commonly present with ulceration over bony prominences. In patients with dysfunctional foot architecture, such as loss of the transverse arch, these ulcers can commonly occur over the second or third metatarsal head. Protection of the ulcer by orthotic fitting and arch support is often highly successful.

3G
In a patient with ulcers over a bony prominence where there is no neuropathy and a clear history of smoking, arterial disease should be suspected and pulses palpated. In addition, ankle brachial pressure indices should be obtained to confirm or rule out arterial disease.

4C
Long-standing ulceration may give rise to a Marjolin's type of ulcer (squamous or basal cell carcinoma). Biopsies (traditionally four quadrants) are indicated in such ulcers.

5D
Small punched-out ulcers are often suspicious of vasculitis, such as is found in SLE. In such patients, an antibody screen should be obtained, particularly where diabetes and major arterial disease have been ruled out.

→ 2. Varicose veins

1E
In an older patient with a history of DVT and deep vein thrombosis reflux, the main stay of management is compression support stockings. This improves symptomatology and reduces the risk of future ulceration.

2G

This woman with a recent fractured neck of femur is at high risk of DVT and should be treated with thromboembolic stockings and prophylactic Fragmin.

3D

This patient would be best served with conventional saphenofemoral ligation, stripping and stab avulsions because of her needle phobia and symptomatic varicose veins.

4A

This man could either have EVLT or conventional saphenopopliteal ligation. EVLT might be the better option in view of his BMI.

5H

This man has symptomatic deep vein thrombosis obstruction and if he is to have any treatment then the Palma cross-femoral bypass using the opposite long saphenous vein would the optimum choice. Unfortunately this operation has modest results.

55 Lymphatic disorders

Multiple choice questions

→ Lymphatics

1. Which of the following statements are true?

A Lymphatics contain endothelium.
B Lymphatics may be surrounded by smooth muscle.
C Lymphatics contain valves.
D Flow is from superficial to deep in the limbs.
E Lymphatics communicate with arterials in the capillary bed.

→ Lymphangitis

2. Which of the following statements are true?

A Lymphangitis is usually caused by *Pseudomonas*.
B Lymphangitis is indicated by red streaking in the limb.
C Lymphangitis may predispose to further attacks.
D Lymphangitis is less common in patients with lymphoedema.
E Lymphangitis may often result in bacteraemia.

→ Lymphoedema

3. Which of the following statements regarding lymphoedema are true?

A Primary lymphoedema occurs in more than 5 per cent or the population.
B Early treatment is usually successful.
C Early treatment includes surgical drainage.
D Fluid is relatively low in protein in lymphoedema.
E Lymphoedema often involves the muscle compartments.

4. Causes of lymphoedema include:

A Metastatic carcinoma in lymph nodes
B Arterial insufficiency
C Deep vein thrombosis (DVT)
D Radiotherapy
E Sedentary occupation.

5. Which of the following is not a risk factor for lymphoedema?

A Limb surgery (e.g. varicose vein operation)
B Obesity
C Family history
D A Baker's cyst
E Air travel.

6. Which of the following statements regarding filariasis are true?

A Filariasis is the commonest cause of secondary lymphoedema.
B It may lead to elephantiasis.
C It may be eradicated by antibiotics.
D Once treated, the lymphoedema resolves.
E The mosquito is heavily implicated in this disorder.

7. Which of the following are true regarding the treatment of lymphoedema?

A Surgery will be required in about 10 per cent of patients.
B The mainstay of management is bedrest.
C Compression stockings should provide a pressure of 40–60 mmHg at the ankle.
D Early treatment of infected episodes with penicillin is important.
E Exercise is contraindicated because of increased swelling.

Extended matching questions

1. Lower limb swelling

A Congestive cardiac failure
B Lymphoedema
C DVT
D Cellulitis
E Calf muscle tear
F Compartment syndrome
G Critical ischaemia

Choose and match the correct diagnosis with each of the following scenarios:

1 A 70-year-old man has had severe pain at night in his right leg for the past 5 weeks and is unable to sleep. He relieves the pain by sleeping in a sitting position and presents with leg swelling.

2 A 45-year-old woman with a pansystolic murmur and bilateral painless limb leg swelling presents to her GP with breathlessness.

3 A 25-year-old fit male presents with pain and swelling of the leg following a football match.

4 A 60-year-old man has marked leg swelling 1 day after undergoing a femoral distal bypass for critical ischaemia. Pulses are present but the calf is tense and tender.

5 A 30-year-old woman presents with a 1-year history of progressive painless swelling in her left leg. There is no history of DVT or injury.

6 A 50-year-old man presents with a history of an ingrown toenail which has been exquisitely tender over the past 48 h. The lower leg is hot and swollen.

7 An 80-year-old woman presents with a painful swollen right leg 6 days after admission for a left hemispheric stroke which has left her bed-bound

2. Investigations in lymphatic disorders

A Lymphangiography
B Lymphoscintigraphy
C Computed tomography (CT)
D Magnetic resonance imaging (MRI)
E Ultrasound
F Biopsy of nodes

Choose and match the investigation that corresponds best with each of the following statements:

1 This is best for distinguishing between venous and lymphatic causes of a swollen limb.

2 This is best for diagnosing malignancy in lymph nodes.

3 This is best to exclude a pelvic or intra-abdominal mass causing leg swelling.

4 This provides the best reflection of lymphatic function.

5 This is no longer used as a first-line test for lymphoedema.

6 This can provide useful information on venous abnormalities.

Answers: Multiple choice questions

➜ Lymphatics

1. A, B, C

Lymphatics are indeed lined by endothelial cells and the larger lymph channels are surrounded by smooth muscle, which is an important element in the movement of lymph of the limbs. These lymph channels contain valves that augment this process. Unlike veins, flow is actually from the deep to the superficial system, although lymph channels run alongside veins commonly. Unlike veins, lymph channels are blind-ending sacks and do not communicate with the capillary bed directly.

➜ Lymphangitis

2. B, C, E

Lymphangitis is commonly caused by streptococcal infection or, less commonly, *Staphylococcus*. It classically presents with superficial red streaks along the lines of the lymphatic channels and is much more likely to recur in patients with underlying lymphoedema. Once a patient has one attack, further attacks are more likely, owing to damage of the lymph channels and lymph nodes. Untreated lymphangitis may often result in bacteraemia and even septicaemia.

➜ Lymphoedema

3. B

Primary lymphoedema occurs in less than 1 per cent of the population. If identified early and treated appropriately, patients generally do very well. Surgical treatment (which does not include drainage) is rarely performed and is reserved for the most extreme of cases. Lymphoedema fluid is classically high in protein content and although 40 per cent of lymph is formed within skeletal muscle, the oedema rarely involves the muscle compartments.

4. A, C, D

Arterial insufficiency is not a cause of lymphoedema *per se*. Likewise, sedentary occupation is not known to be associated with lymphoedema. Radiotherapy, DVT and metastatic carcinoma are all well-documented causes of lymphoedema.

5. D

Baker's cyst is the correct answer. All the others have been associated directly with lymphoedema, including, interestingly, air travel.

6. A, B, E

Filariasis affects about 100 million people worldwide and is caused by a nematode, *Wuchereria bancrofti*. This is spread by the common mosquito. It may indeed lead to elephantiasis and the treatment is not antibiotics but diethylcarbamazine. Unfortunately this does not reverse the lymphatic changes and the patient will still require treatment for their lymphoedema.

7. C, D

Surgery is very rarely required in the treatment of lymphoedema. Whilst bedrest has a role in severe exacerbations, the mainstay of management is compression stockings, which should provide a pressure of between 40 and 60 mmHg at the ankle. In patients who experience an episode of infection or cellulitis, early treatment with penicillin is mandatory. Flucloxacillin may need to be added to this in cases which are thought to be due to *Staphylococcus*. Gentle exercise is positively encouraged in cases of lymphoedema, as it aids the return of lymph up the remaining lymph channels.

Answers: Extended matching questions

1. Lower limb swelling

1G
Patients with critical ischaemia and rest pain often sleep either sitting up or with one leg dangling over the edge of the bed. This effectively results in a gravitation oedema of the limb which can be confusing to the uninformed.

2A
Bilateral leg swelling and breathlessness in the absence of pain would suggest a cardiac cause in this case, possibly due to mitral or tricuspid incompetence.

3E
Simple trauma is a common explanation for acute leg swelling in otherwise fit young individuals. The treatment is ice compression and elevation.

4F
Ischaemia perfusion resulting in a compartment syndrome can be a very serious cause of acute leg swelling in vascular patients and such patients may need urgent fasciotomy.

5B
This is likely to be lymphoedema tarda and, provided it is recognised and treatment instituted early, the outcome is likely to be very good.

6D
This is a classical example of cellulitis secondary to a distal infective cause and requires bedrest, elevation and antibiotics.

7C
Stroke patients are at very high risk of DVT and any patient with a painful swollen leg presenting within a few days of their stroke should be considered to have had a DVT until proven otherwise.

2. Investigations in lymphatic disorders

1D
Magnetic resonance imaging is particularly useful and can show clear images of lymphatic channels. It is possible to show lymphatic hyperplasia with MRI and it is helpful in distinguishing between venous and lymphatic causes of limb swelling.

2F
If malignancy is suspected in a lymph node, this should be confirmed either by fine-needle aspiration or surgical biopsy.

3C
Computed tomography scan is the investigation of choice when looking for pelvic or intra-abdominal malignancy, which might be responsible for limb swelling or lymphoedema.

4B
Lymphoscintigraphy has replaced lymphangiography as the primary diagnostic technique for investigating the lymphatic system. It provides a useful measure of lymphatic function.

5A
Lymphangiography is now rarely performed. It does, however, allow for an anatomical picture of the lymphatic channels and as such is still seen as the gold standard for showing structural abnormalities. It is, however, painful for the patient and technically difficult to perform.

6E
Ultrasonography, specifically duplex, is a very important investigation in assessment of the venous circulation, particularly in the lower limb.

PART 11 Abdominal

56 History and examination of the abdomen 423

57 Hernia, umbilicus and abdominal wall 425

58 The peritoneum, omentum, mesentery and retroperitoneal space 432

59 The oesophagus 437

60 Stomach and duodenum 441

61 The liver 451

62 The spleen 458

63 The gall bladder and bile ducts 461

64 The pancreas 468

65 The small and large intestines 474

66 Intestinal obstruction 488

67 The vermiform appendix 495

68 The rectum 499

69 The anus and anal canal 504

56 History and examination of the abdomen

Multiple choice questions

→ Conditions causing abdominal pain

1. Which of the following medical conditions is not a cause of abdominal pain?

A Diabetic ketoacidosis
B Porphyria
C Angina
D Pneumonia
E Coeliac disease
F Herpes zoster.

→ Parietal peritoneum

2. Which of the following statements are true?

A The parietal peritoneum is innervated by somatic nerves.
B The parietal peritoneum is innervated by autonomic nerves.
C Pain originating in the parietal peritoneum is poorly localised.
D Pain from the parietal peritoneum may radiate.

Extended matching questions

→ 1. Sources of abdominal pain

A Splenic rupture
B Testicular pain
C Ureteric colic
D Appendicitis
E Cholecystitis
F Pancreas

Match the following sources of pain to the site of radiation:

1 Back

2 Umbilicus

3 Lower angle of scapula

4 Loin

5 Groin

6 Left shoulder tip

Answers: Multiple choice questions

→ Conditions causing abdominal pain

1. E

An insulin-dependent diabetic should always raise the suspicion of ketosis causing abdominal pain. An urgent blood sugar and urine examination should give the diagnosis. Violent intestinal colic may occur in porphyria, a congenital abnormality of haemoglobin metabolism. Patients may present with anaemia, photosensitivity, hypersplenism and constipation.

Epigastric pain can mimic angina. A careful history followed by an ECG should give the diagnosis. Pain in the upper quadrant may be the presentation of lower-lobe pneumonia. Pyrexia with signs in the chest are the diagnostic pointers.Coeliac disease causes malnutrition and abdominal pain is not a feature.

Herpes causes pain across the abdomen without guarding or rebound tenderness along a dermatome; pain precedes vesicular skin eruption.

→ Parietal peritoneum

2. A, D

The parietal peritoneum is innervated by the relevant somatic nerves through the spinal nerves in the distribution of the overlying dermatomes. Pain is well localised to the site of inflammation. Pain from parietal peritoneal inflammation may radiate along the line supplied by the somatic nerve, as in acute cholecystitis when the pain radiates to the back.

Answers: Extended matching questions

→ 1. Sources of abdominal pain

1F, 2D, 3E, 4B, 5C, 6A

57 Hernia, umbilicus and abdominal wall

Multiple choice questions

→ Predisposing factors for hernia

1. Which of the following is not a predisposing factor for a hernia?

A Chronic obstructive pulmonary disease
B Obesity
C Urinary stones
D Pregnancy
E Peritoneal dialysis.

→ Causes of hernia

2. Which of the following are more common in multiparous women?

A Indirect inguinal hernia
B Lumbar hernia
C Umbilical
D Direct inguinal hernia
E Femoral hernia.

→ Complications of hernia

3. Which of the following is not a complication of an inguinal hernia?

A Irreducibility
B Inflammation
C Strangulation
D Obstruction
E Bleeding.

→ Strangulated hernia

4. Which of the following is not true in relation to strangulated hernias?

A They present with local and then generalised abdominal pain and vomiting.
B A normal hernia can strangulate at any time.
C This is more common in femoral hernia.
D They can be reliably excluded in irreducible hernias on clinical examination.
E They require urgent surgery.

→ Anatomy of the inguinal canal

5. Regarding the anatomy of the inguinal canal, which of the following are true?

A In infants the internal and external rings are almost superimposed.
B The inferior epigastric vessels lie posterior and lateral to the internal ring.
C The inguinal canal is about 10 cm long and is directed downwards, medially and forwards.
D In males, the normal constituents of the inguinal canal are the spermatic cord, the inguinal nerve and the genital branch of the genitofemoral nerve.
E The internal ring is a U-shaped opening in the external oblique aponeurosis 1.25 cm above the mid-inguinal point.

→ Sliding inguinal hernia

6. Which of the following are true about a sliding inguinal hernia?

A It is far more common in men.
B It should be suspected clinically in small hernias confined to the inguinal canal.
C It is more common in the young patient.
D It is impossible to control with a truss, and hence an operation is indicated.
E It is unnecessary to excise the sac and attempts to dissect the bowel wall can be dangerous.

→ Femoral hernia

7. Which of the following statements regarding a femoral hernia are true?

A It is more common in women.
B The femoral canal occupies the most lateral component of the femoral sheath.

C It can be easily controlled by truss.
D Strangulation is the initial presentation in 40 per cent of patients.
E An operation is only occasionally required.

➜ Umbilical hernia

8. Which of the following statements are true regarding umbilical hernia?

A The umbilical hernia in an infant is through the umbilical cicatrix but is usually paraumbilical in adults.
B Men are affected more frequently than women.
C Irreducibility is common due to omental adhesions.
D Mayo's operation involves mesh repair of the hernia.
E Infantile umbilical hernias need immediate surgery.

➜ Umbilical discharge

9. Which of the following are causes of umbilical discharge?

A Persistent vitellointestinal duct
B Persistent urachus
C Pilonidal sinus
D Omphalitis
E Endometrioma.

➜ Burst abdomen

10. Which of the following are true regarding 'burst abdomens'?

A The incidence is around 10–15 per cent.
B Midline and vertical incisions are more likely to burst than transverse incisions.
C Catgut is associated with a lower risk of burst abdomen.
D A serosanguinous discharge is the forerunner of disruption in half of these cases.
E Most cases are managed conservatively.

Extended matching questions

➜ 1. Diagnosis of various abdominal wall hernias

A Direct inguinal hernia
B Femoral hernia
C Umbilical hernia
D Incisional hernia
E Indirect inguinal hernia
F Paraumbilical hernia
G Epigastric hernia
H Divarication of recti
I Spigelian hernia

Choose and match the correct diagnosis with each of the scenarios given below:

1 A 6-month-old infant is brought by his mother with a history of lump over the belly-button, which increases in size when the baby is crying.

2 A 26-year-old builder presents with a lump over his left groin which has been there for the last 3 years. Examination reveals cough impulse and a reducible hernia over the left groin extending to the scrotum. Internal ring occlusion test is positive.

3 A 60-year-old obese woman is referred with a history of painful lump around her umbilicus. Examination reveals an irreducible lump just above the umbilicus.

4 A 78-year-old woman is referred to your clinic with a 6-week history of suspected enlarged left groin lymph node. Examination reveals a 2 cm hard and irreducible lump over the medial aspect of the left groin. There is no cough impulse.

5 A 40-year-old woman is referred to your clinic with a history of a gradually increasing lump over the lower abdomen. She has had three caesarean sections in the past. Clinical examination reveals a Pfannenstiel scar. There is cough impulse and a reducible lump over the right lateral aspect of this scar extending to the right groin.

6 A 76-year-old man is referred to you with a 2-year history of lumps over both his groins. These are only causing him minimal discomfort. Clinical examination confirms reducible hernias over both his groins. Internal ring occlusion test is negative.

7 A 50-year-old man presents with a lump below the umbilicus and lateral to the rectus. A cough impulse is felt over the area and the lump reduces with difficulty.

8 A 22-year-old fit male presents with an epigastric bulge. This becomes prominent while exercising in the gym. It is otherwise asymptomatic. Clinical examination reveals a midline gutter in the upper abdomen.

9 A 30-year-old female presents with a localised sharp pain in the upper abdomen. Clinical examination reveals a button-like soft swelling equidistant between the xiphisternum and the umbilicus. There is no cough impulse and the lump is not reducible.

→ 2. Complications of hernia

A Strangulation
B Obstruction
C Incarceration
D Perforation
E Irreducibility

Choose and match the correct diagnosis with each of the scenarios given below:

1 A 70-year-old male is referred to your clinic with a long-standing left inguinal hernia. He has not noticed any recent changes in his hernia and his bowels have been normal. On examination you see a giant inguinoscrotal hernia which is not completely reducible.

2 A 40-year-old male is referred with irreducibility and increasing pain over his right inguinal hernia over the past 8 h. On examination the hernia is extremely tender with signs of peritonitis.

3 A 60-year-old female is referred with a history of increasing abdominal pain and distension over the past 2 days. She has been vomiting repeatedly over this period. Clinical examination reveals a right groin lump which is not reducible and abdominal examination reveals a distended but soft abdomen with increased bowel sounds.

4 A 50-year-old male is referred with irreducibility and discomfort over his right inguinal hernia over the past 3 h. His bowels have been normal. An irreducible hernia is confirmed on examination. The abdomen is soft, non-tender and not distended.

5 A 90-year-old woman with a long-standing history of incisional hernia presents to the emergency with faeculant discharge from the hernia site. Examination reveals excoriated and ulcerated skin over the incarcerated long-standing hernia.

→ 3. Treatment of abdominal wall hernias

A Wait and watch
B Transabdominal preperitoneal (TAPP) repair
C Open mesh repair
D Open/laparoscopic mesh repair
E Non-surgical

F Total extraperitoneal (TEP)/TAPP repair
G Mayo repair
H Open suture repair

Choose and match the most appropriate operation with each of the conditions given below:

1 Primary unilateral inguinal hernia

2 Primary bilateral inguinal hernia

3 Recurrent inguinal hernia – post-open repair

4 Infantile umbilical hernia

5 Recurrent inguinal hernia – post-laparoscopic repair

6 Divarication of recti

7 Incisional hernia

8 Epigastric hernia

9 Paraumbilical hernia

Answers: Multiple choice questions

→ Predisposing factors for hernia

1. C

Any cause of increased abdominal pressure will predispose to an abdominal hernia. Prostatism with obstructive urinary symptoms can predispose to hernia but uncomplicated urinary stones do not. Other causes of straining include chronic constipation and work-related physical exertion. Whooping cough is a predisposing cause in childhood. Hernias are more common in smokers, which may be as a result of an acquired collagen deficiency.

→ Causes of hernia

2. C, E

Femoral hernias are more common in women. Even amongst women it is more common in those who have had children than in nulliparous ones. Pregnancy itself predisposes to hernias due to increased intra-abdominal pressure.

→ Complications of hernia

3. E

Any hernia which is chronically irreducible is probably incarcerated. A hernia with a short history of irreducibility should be viewed with suspicion and treated as an emergency. It is not possible to reliably exclude strangulation and hence these should be explored without delay. Inflammation can occur from inflammation of the contents of the sac, e.g. acute appendicitis and acute salpingitis, or from external causes such as a trophic ulcer developing in the dependent areas of a large hernia.

→ Strangulated hernia

4. D

Strangulation is a genuine surgical emergency and requires prompt surgery. The clinical features may mimic gastroenteritis in a strangulated Richter's hernia, which may delay diagnosis. The initial symptoms in a strangulated omentocele are similar to a strangulated bowel, but vomiting and constipation may be absent.

Anatomy of the inguinal canal

5. A, D

The inferior epigastric vessels lie posterior and medial to the internal ring. Identifying these vessels at operation confirms complete dissection of the sac up to internal ring. In adults, the inguinal ring is about 3.75 cm long. The internal ring is a U-shaped condensation of the transversalis fascia and the external opening is a triangular opening in the external oblique aponeurosis.

Sliding inguinal hernia

6. A, D, E

A sliding hernia (synonym: hernia-en-glissade) is one in which part of the wall is formed by some abdominal viscera which has slipped down along with the posterior parietal peritoneum. It is rare and occurs approximately once in 2000 cases. It occurs almost exclusively in men and the patient is nearly always more than 40 years of age. It is usually the posterior wall that is involved. The most common structure involved is the sigmoid colon but the caecum and the urinary bladder can also be involved. It is to be remembered that these structures are not within the sac but are actually forming part of its wall. Hence, utmost care should be taken, as these structures can be injured while opening the sac or excising it. The sac should not be excised in a sliding hernia but any opening made should be closed carefully and reduced back. A sliding hernia should be suspected in a very large globular hernia descending into the scrotum.

Femoral hernia

7. A, D

The femoral hernia is the third most common type of primary hernia, accounting for about 20 per cent of hernias in women and 5 per cent in men. This occurs through the femoral canal which occupies the medial most compartment of the femoral sheath. It is related to the femoral vein laterally and the lacunar ligament medially. The overriding importance is that this hernia cannot be controlled by a truss and has an increased tendency to get strangulated. Hence an operation is usually advised.

Umbilical hernia

8. A, C

The umbilical hernia in adults is really a paraumbilical hernia, as the defect is in the linea alba just above or below the umbilicus. It is five times more common in women, and obesity and repeated pregnancies are predisposing factors. Ninety-five per cent of infantile hernias resolve spontaneously and hence conservative treatment is indicated under the age of 2 years. Mayo repair is a primary herniorrhaphy with overlapping of the margins. A mesh repair is required if the hernia is large, recurrent or the patient has predisposing factors which might increase the risk of recurrence.

Umbilical discharge

9. A, B, C, D, E

The stump of the umbilical cord is colonised by staphylococci in 50 per cent of the babies by the third or fourth day after delivery. This can get clinically infected, especially in communities not practising aseptic severance of the umbilical cord. This is called omphalitis and usually responds to antibiotics leaving behind a granulating surface. Persistent vitellointestinal duct causes a small-bowel fistula at the umbilicus, while a persistent urachus results in urinary discharge. Occasionally, a part of the duct is patent, leading to recurrent infections and discharge of serous or purulent fluid. Hence it is aptly remarked that the umbilicus is a creek into which many fistulous streams may open.

→ Burst abdomen

10. B, D

Burst abdomen (also known as abdominal dehiscence) occurs in 1–2 per cent of cases around the 6th and 8th days after the operation. The disruption of the sutures usually occurs a few days earlier and is associated with a serosanguinous discharge. The most important causes are poor closure technique, deep wound infection, and patient factors such as persistent cough, vomiting, abdominal distension and poor metabolic state. An emergency operation is required to replace the bowel, relieve any obstruction and resuture the wound. While awaiting operation, the wound is covered with a sterile towel and the anxious patient is given analgesics and reassured.

Answers: Extended matching questions

→ 1. Diagnosis of various abdominal wall hernias

1C

The incidence in black infants is eight times higher. Ninety-five per cent of infantile hernias resolve spontaneously and hence conservative treatment is indicated under the age of 2 years.

2E

An early operation would be required as it is likely to affect his work and because of the higher incidence of irreducibility in indirect inguinal hernias.

3F

Pain and irreducibility are the usual symptoms. The smaller ones contain omentum while the larger ones may involve bowel and hence strangulation can be a problem.

4B

The clinical appearance can be deceptive. It is easy to miss a small lump clinically or it can be confused with a lymph node. Beware of the palpable medial groin 'lymph node' – a femoral hernia has to be ruled out.

5D

An incisional hernia has to be considered when a medial groin hernia overlying a previous Pfannenstiel incision is seen.

6A

A direct hernia is less likely to strangulate and is more often bilateral. The patient is usually elderly.

7I

This is a rare variety of interparietal hernia occurring at the level of the arcuate line. The hernia spreads out like a mushroom between the internal and external oblique muscles. An ultrasound or CT scan is sometimes helpful in diagnosis. Operation is advised due to the risk of strangulation.

8H

The patient presents because of the obvious bulge. This is wide-based and does not have a sac. Hence it cannot strangulate and an operation is not needed. The divarication is sometimes associated with a discrete hernia which may need to be repaired.

9G

Pain is the predominant (and sometimes the only) symptom. The lump is usually small and contains extraperitoneal fat. There is no risk of bowel strangulation but an operation is advised to sort out the pain.

2. Complications of hernia

1C
Long-standing and large inguinoscrotal hernias are difficult to reduce completely. This is as a result of adhesions developing between the sac and its contents as well as the surrounding structures.

2A
This is a surgical emergency and requires urgent exploration.

3B
It is impossible to rule out strangulation and hence it should be operated on urgently without the usual trial of conservative treatment for small-bowel obstruction.

4E
It is not possible to reliably exclude strangulation in an irreducible hernia.

5D
Long-standing (usually incisional hernia) hernias can develop closed-loop obstruction and perforate. The leakage is contained within the sac and discharges as a faecal fistula. The peritoneal cavity is usually not affected and the patient can still remain remarkably well.

3. Treatment of abdominal wall hernias

1C
There are no significant advantages in doing a laparoscopic repair for an unilateral inguinal hernia and hence the present guidelines still recommend an open operation. A laparoscopic repair may, however, still be appropriate in selective patients.

2F
The morbidity and time off work are less compared with a bilateral open repair and hence this should be the technique of choice.

3F
Adhesions due to previous open operation make this a suitable case for laparoscopic repair through a virgin territory.

4A
Ninety-five per cent of these spontaneously resolve. Hence a conservative approach is advised up to 2 years of age.

5B
A TEP repair is difficult as the planes are obliterated.

6E
A repair is unnecessary. An associated discrete hernia, if definitely confirmed, will need to be repaired.

7D
Use of mesh in primary repair is recommended in view of the increased incidence of recurrence.

8H
The defect is usually small and only requires a couple of sutures. Mesh is rarely required.

9G
A mesh repair is considered in big defects, recurrent cases and in the presence of predisposing factors.

58 The peritoneum, omentum, mesentery and retroperitoneal space

Multiple choice questions

➜ Peritoneum

1. **Which of the following statements are true?**
   - A The surface area of the peritoneal membrane is nearly equal to that of the skin.
   - B The parietal peritoneum is poorly innervated.
   - C The peritoneum has the capacity to absorb large volumes of fluid.
   - D The peritoneum has the ability to produce fibrinolytic activity.
   - E When injured, the peritoneum produces an inflammatory exudate.

➜ Peritonitis

2. **Which of the following organisms is not a gastrointestinal source of peritonitis?**
   - A *Escherichia coli*
   - B *Streptococcus*
   - C *Bacteroides*
   - D *Chlamydia*
   - E *Clostridium*
   - F *Klebsiella pneumoniae*
   - G *Staphylococcus*

3. **Which of the following statements are true?**
   - A Peritonitis in perforated duodenal ulcer is initially sterile.
   - B Immunocompromised patients may present with opportunistic peritoneal infection.
   - C *Bacteroides* are sensitive to penicillin.
   - D In perforated duodenal ulcer there may be signs of peritonitis in the right iliac fossa.
   - E Children can localise infection effectively.

4. **Which of the following statements are false?**
   - A Perforation proximal to an obstruction is associated with severe generalised peritonitis.
   - B Stimulation of peristalsis helps in localisation of peritonitis.
   - C The greater the virulence of the organism, the lesser the chance of localisation.
   - D The patient with diffuse peritonitis writhes around in pain unable to assume a comfortable position.
   - E Systemic inflammatory response syndrome (SIRS) is a late manifestation of peritonitis.

➜ Diagnostic aids

5. **Which of the following statements are true?**
   - A Raised serum amylase is always diagnostic of acute pancreatitis.
   - B There is always gas under the right dome of the diaphragm in perforated duodenal ulcer.
   - C Ultrasound (US) and computed tomography (CT) scan are often diagnostic.
   - D On diagnostic peritoneal lavage (DPL), bile aspiration indicates perforated duodenal ulcer or perforated gall bladder.

Extended matching questions

→ 1. Intra-abdominal infection

A Pelvic abscess
B Subphrenic abscess
C Postoperative peritonitis
D Bile peritonitis
E Basal pneumonia

Choose and match the correct diagnosis with each of the scenarios given below:

1 A 72-year-old patient underwent an emergency right hemicolectomy and ileotransverse anastomosis for carcinoma of the caecum presenting as acute intestinal obstruction. He progressed satisfactorily until the fifth postoperative day when he developed pyrexia, generalised abdominal tenderness and rigidity with rebound tenderness.

2 A 50-year-old patient underwent a laparoscopic closure of a perforated duodenal ulcer. On the fourth postoperative day, he developed pyrexia, looked toxic, complained of pain in his right shoulder tip and was tender and rigid over his right upper quadrant.

3 Following emergency appendicectomy for acute perforated appendicitis, a 30-year-old female patient progressed well for about 6 days. After that she felt unwell, was pyrexial and complained of tenesmus and foul-smelling vaginal discharge.

4 A 14-year-old boy has been brought with right upper quadrant pain of 3 days' duration. He is pyrexial, tachypnoeic and tender in the right upper quadrant. There is reduced air entry in the right lower chest which is dull on percussion.

5 After an uneventful laparoscopic cholecystectomy, a 35-year-old female patient was sent home on the first postoperative day. While at home the same evening she developed sudden onset of severe right upper abdominal pain and pain in the right shoulder tip. On examination she had a tinge of jaundice and was extremely tender in the right upper quadrant with guarding and rebound tenderness.

→ 2. Ascites

A Tuberculous peritonitis
B Peritoneal malignancy
C Portal hypertension
D Congestive cardiac failure

Choose and match the correct diagnosis with each of the scenarios given below:

1 A 70-year-old woman, who is known to have had a myocardial infarct in the past, complains of shortness of breath and abdominal distension. She has a raised jugular venous pressure.

2 A 50-year-old patient who is an alcoholic complains of abdominal distension. He has distended veins around his umbilicus (caput medusa), palmar erythema and spider naevi. He is slightly jaundiced.

3 A 60-year-old male patient complains of feeling generally unwell for 3–4 months. During this period he has felt gradual distension of his abdomen, weight loss and generalised malaise. He has recently returned from the subcontinent after living there for 2 years.

4 A 70-year-old female patient has had weight loss, abdominal distension, malaise and anorexia for almost 4 months. Abdominal examination shows massive ascites. US shows solid bilateral ovarian masses.

3. The mesentery

A Mesenteric cyst
B Mesenteric tear
C Torsion of omentum
D Retroperitoneal sarcoma

Choose and match the correct diagnosis with each of the scenarios given below

1 A 55-year-old female patient presents with vague abdominal and back pain for 3 months. She feels her abdomen is enlarging and is constipated. On examination there is a large mass in the left loin, smooth in consistency, tender and bimanually palpable.

2 A 20-year-old male patient presents with recurrent attacks of periumbilical abdominal pain and intermittent vomiting. Abdominal examination reveals a 5–6 cm fluctuant mass in the umbilical region which is mobile in an oblique plane.

3 A 30-year-old male patient has been brought in after a road traffic accident complaining of abdominal pain. He was a front-seat passenger wearing a seatbelt. In the accident there was a sudden deceleration and a head-on collision. In the A&E department, on assessment, he had no injuries except for abdominal wall bruising from the seatbelt. He has marked abdominal tenderness, rigidity and rebound tenderness.

4 A 50-year-old obese man has been brought in as an emergency complaining of sudden onset of severe periumbilical abdominal pain. On examination he is writhing around in pain and very tender in the umbilical region with rigidity.

Answers: Multiple choice questions

Peritoneum

1. A, C, D, E

The peritoneal cavity is the largest cavity in the body, the surface area of the membrane being equal to that of the skin, almost 2 square metres in the adult. This aspect of a large surface area which can absorb large volumes of fluid is used for peritoneal dialysis. The parietal peritoneum is richly innervated so that pain arising from it is severe and localised to the area.

Peritonitis

2. D

3. A, B, D

For several hours immediately after perforation of a duodenal ulcer, there is sterile chemical peritonitis. A few hours after perforation, the leaking duodenal contents may track along the right paracolic gutter giving signs of peritonitis in the right iliac fossa, mimicking acute appendicitis. *Bacteroides* are resistant to penicillin and sensitive to metronidazole, clindamycin, lincomycin and cephalosporins. Children, by virtue of their poor development of the greater omentum, do not localise peritonitis.

4. B, D

Stimulation of peristalsis by food, water or administration of an enema hinders localisation and spreads the infection. The patient with diffuse peritonitis likes to lie still as any movement causes exacerbation of the pain.

➜ Diagnostic aids

5. C, D

The serum amylase may be raised in perforated peptic ulcer and therefore not diagnostic of acute pancreatitis. In perforated duodenal ulcer there may not be gas under the right dome of the diaphragm in early cases, if the perforation is small or if it is plugged by omentum at an early stage. US and CT scan are very reliable diagnostic aids, as is DPL.

Answers: Extended matching questions

➜ 1. Intra-abdominal infection

1C

This patient who underwent an emergency right hemicolectomy has now developed postoperative peritonitis from anastomotic leak. This needs to be assessed by contrast CT or a gastrograffin enema and dealt with accordingly.

2B

The patient has the hallmarks of a classical subphrenic abscess – pain in the shoulder tip and the right upper quadrant and toxic after an intra-abdominal operation. This is confirmed by US or CT and drained under US/CT guidance by the radiologist. This may require more than one aspiration because of the abscess being multilocular.

3A

This young female has the features of a pelvic abscess that is about to drain naturally through the posterior fornix of the vagina. The diagnosis can be confirmed by a pelvi- or intravaginal US and progress can be assessed by serial US. This may require US-guided drainage if the abscess does not resolve naturally.

4E

The young boy has right basal lobar pneumonia. Pain in the right upper quadrant is a classical presentation of such a condition. A chest X-ray will confirm the diagnosis and is treated with intravenous antibiotics.

5D

Following an uneventful laparoscopic cholecystectomy, this patient after going home had slippage of the clip on the cystic duct resulting in bile peritonitis. This requires emergency resuscitation, imaging with US or CT followed by drainage either laparoscopically or by open method.

➜ 2. Ascites

1D

This woman has the hallmarks of ascites from cardiac failure and should be referred to a physician.

2C

The patient's history of alcohol abuse should give the suspicion of portal hypertension. The external features of caput medusa, palmar erythema and spider naevi with ascites are the classical clinical features. The patient should be referred to a physician.

3A

A patient who has recently returned from the subcontinent after a stay of 2 years should be suspected of having tuberculous peritonitis and investigated as such: US of abdomen may show loculated ascites, raised erythrocyte sedimentation rate (ESR), C-reactive protein (CRP), analysis of ascitic fluid and chest X-ray.

4B
This 70-year-old woman has peritoneal malignancy (carcinoma peritonei) from ovarian carcinoma. She should be referred to a gynaecologist.

3. The mesentery

1D
This woman with vague abdominal pain has the features of a retroperitoneal mass. Usually they are retroperitoneal liposarcoma and need to be managed in a tertiary cancer centre. An MRI followed by guided core biopsy gives the answer. It is then staged and managed accordingly.

2A
A mesenteric cyst occurs in the younger age group. The characteristic physical finding is a fluctuant swelling near the umbilicus which is non-tender and moves freely along a line from the right upper quadrant to the left iliac fossa – at right angles to the attachment of the mesentery. US will confirm the diagnosis. Sometimes such a patient may present as an emergency due to torsion, haemorrhage into the cyst or infection.

3B
This patient, who has no other external injury except for bruising over the abdominal wall, should be suspected of having a mesenteric tear, a condition referred to as 'seatbelt syndrome'. A contrast CT scan or a diagnostic peritoneal lavage may help in the diagnosis. In 60 per cent of cases the mesenteric laceration is associated with a tear in the intestine.

4C
Such an obese male patient could easily be mistakenly diagnosed as having acute appendicitis. Most often such a patient is operated on for 'acute appendicitis' and the diagnosis of torsion of the omentum is made at operation.

59 The oesophagus

Multiple choice questions

Anatomy

1. Which of the following statements are true?

A The oesophagus is 30 cm long.
B The oesophagus has three natural constrictions.
C It is lined throughout by columnar epithelium.
D The lower oesophageal sphincter (LOS) is a zone of high pressure.
E The pressure at the LOS is 50 mmHg.

Dysphagia

2. Which of the following statements are false?

A Difficulty on swallowing (dysphagia) is a cardinal symptom of oesophageal carcinoma.
B Retrosternal pain on swallowing (odynophagia) is always of cardiac origin.
C Heartburn is a common symptom of gastro-oesophageal reflux disease (GORD).
D Dysphagia in the oral or pharyngeal (voluntary) phase, when patients say they cannot swallow, is usually from neurological or muscular diseases.
E Regurgitation and reflux are the same and are caused by obstruction to the oesophagus.

3. Which of the following statements regarding investigations in dysphagia are false?

A Barium swallow is the investigation of choice in GORD.
B Flexible oesophagogastroduodenoscopy (OGD) is the initial investigation of choice in suspected carcinoma.
C Endosonography (EUS) should be carried out when a carcinoma is seen in the oesophagus.
D Oesophageal manometry should be done when motility disorder is suspected.
E 24 h pH recording is an accurate method of evaluating GORD.

Oesophageal emergencies

4. Which of the following statements are true?

A In a suspected foreign body (FB) in the oesophagus, water-soluble contrast examination should be carried out.
B When a food bolus is stuck in the oesophagus, always suspect an underlying disease.
C Most iatrogenic perforations of the oesophagus can be treated conservatively.
D Most spontaneous perforations of the oesophagus (Boerhaave's syndrome) require an operation.
E In Mallory–Weiss syndrome the tear is usually in the lower end of the oesophagus

Cancer of the oesophagus

5. Which of the following conditions are precancerous?

A Pharyngeal (Zenker's) diverticulum
B GORD
C Achalasia
D Corrosive stricture
E Barrett's oesophagus
F Schatzki's ring
G Oesophageal candidiasis

6. One of the curative operations for carcinoma of the oesophagus is called

A Whipple's operation
B Anderson–Hynes operation
C Heller's operation
D Ivor–Lewis operation
E Hartmann's operation

Complications of GORD

7. Which of the following are not complications of GORD?

A Stricture
B Barrett's oesophagus
C Oesophageal shortening
D Diffuse oesophageal spasm
E CREST syndrome
F Plummer–Vinson syndrome
G Carcinoma
H Iron deficiency anaemia

Extended matching questions

1. Dysphagia

A Peptic stricture
B Carcinoma
C Achalasia
D Diffuse oesophageal spasm
E Schatzki's ring
F Pharyngeal (Zenker's) diverticulum

Choose and match the correct diagnosis with each of the scenarios given below:

1 A 50-year-old patient complains of chest pain on swallowing. This is usually episodic. He has had these symptoms for many years but recently they have become more frequent and severe.

2 A 45-year-old male patient complains of dysphagia of 2 years' duration. He seems to have greater difficulty swallowing liquids than solids. Recently he has noticed that at night he is woken up by coughing. He has lost about 7–8 kg in weight in 6 months.

3 A 35-year-old female complains of occasional dysphagia with food sticking in the lower retrosternal region. She has had occasional heartburn for many years.

4 A 65-year-old male, a heavy smoker, complains of dysphagia to solid food of 2 months' duration. At present he can only take fluids. He has quite severe cough when he tries to swallow any food or fluids. He feels this is different to his 'smoker's cough' which he has suffered for many years. He has lost about 10 kg in weight since the onset of these symptoms.

5 A 65-year-old male patient complains of dysphagia, with food sticking in the lower retrosternal region. He has suffered from heartburn all his life and occasionally has a sour and bitter taste in his mouth with waterbrash. He also has cough on occasions. He has not lost any weight.

6 A 60-year-old male complains of quite a severe cough which occurs when he lies in bed. At times he is woken up because of incessant cough when food material seems to project out. He is embarrassed by bad breath. He also has some dysphagia. His doctor has been treating him for chest infections.

Answers: Multiple choice questions

Anatomy

1. B, D

The oesophagus is 25 cm long. It has three natural constrictions: cricopharyngeal junction, aortic and bronchial constriction, and diaphragmatic and sphincter constriction. These are 15, 25 and

40 cm, respectively, from the incisor teeth. It is lined throughout by squamous epithelium. The LOS is a zone 3–4 cm long of relatively high pressure of 10–25 mmHg.

→ Dysphagia

2. B, E

Oesophageal dysphagia (during the involuntary phase of swallowing) with a history of 'food sticking' is a sinister symptom and carcinoma must be ruled out initially. Odynophagia is primarily a symptom of inflammation and ulceration although a cardiac origin of the pain should be excluded. Difficulty in swallowing in the voluntary (oral or pharyngeal) phase is of muscular or neurological aetiology. Regurgitation actually occurs when there is obstruction of the oesophagus and the contents (food or saliva) overflow into the tracheobronchial tree. Reflux classically indicates gastric contents entering the oesophagus or mouth and causing heartburn, indicating GORD.

3. A

Barium swallow is not a good investigation to evaluate GORD. The preliminary ideal investigation is OGD. It will indicate the site of the LOS from the incisors, thereby assessing if there is any shortening of the oesophagus, see the degree of oesophagitis, the quality of refluxing fluid, the presence of a hiatus hernia (HH) and enable a biopsy to be taken. Endoluminal ultrasound (EUS) should always be carried out during OGD in carcinoma. This would assess the local spread and the state of the mediastinal lymph nodes. The biopsy should be done after the US so as not to distort the US images.

→ Oesophageal emergencies

4. B, C, D

In suspected FB in the oesophagus a contrast study is not indicated; it may actually hinder the treatment. When a food bolus is stuck, one must suspect a mechanical obstruction such as peptic stricture or carcinoma as an underlying cause.

Most iatrogenic perforations of the oesophagus can be managed conservatively as they are small perforations in a clean oesophagus without obstruction and leakage is likely to be localised. Cervical oesophageal perforations are almost always treated conservatively. On the other hand, Boerhaave's syndrome usually requires an operation after thorough evaluation with a contrast CT scan. In Mallory–Weiss syndrome in 90 per cent the tear, in the form of a vertical split, occurs in the stomach.

→ Cancer of the oesophagus

5. A, B, C, D, E

The mucosa in a long-standing pharyngeal diverticulum may have dysplastic changes resulting in squamous carcinoma in situ. GORD may go on to develop Barrett's oesophagus, which is precancerous. The increased risk of adenocarcinoma is about 25 times that of the general population. In corrosive stricture there is a lifetime risk of less than 5 per cent of developing carcinoma in the damaged segment. In achalasia, the large oesophagus develops oesophagitis due to retention and fermentation of food accounting for the increased incidence of carcinoma.

6. D

→ Complications of GORD

7. D, E, F

Answers: Extended matching questions

→ 1. Dysphagia

1D

Chest pain on swallowing and dysphagia should alert one to the motility disorder of diffuse oesophageal spasm. A barium swallow followed by oesophageal manometry will confirm the diagnosis. An ECG should be done to exclude any cardiac pathology.

2C

A patient with long-standing dysphagia, particularly for liquids with some weight loss, is indicative of achalasia. The patient also has typical symptoms of regurgitation at night when in bed. The diagnosis is confirmed by OGD and biopsy.

3E

A patient who has occasional heartburn on and off for years and complains of occasional dysphagia which is not unduly disabling should arouse the suspicion of a Schatzki's ring. OGD will confirm the diagnosis and treatment by dilatation is carried out at the same time.

4B

This patient, a chronic smoker, has the hallmarks of an oesophageal carcinoma – dysphagia of recent onset, weight loss and typical symptom of a tracheo-oesophageal fistula. He needs an urgent OGD with EUS, CT scan of chest and abdomen and laparoscopic staging (if resection is contemplated, although unlikely in view of the impending tracheo-oesophageal fistula).

5A

This patient's symptoms are typical of GORD causing a peptic stricture – heartburn, waterbrash and nasty taste in the mouth. He has not lost any weight. He requires an urgent OGD and biopsy to exclude carcinoma. At the same time he can be treated by balloon dilatation.

6F

Classical features of food regurgitation when a person lies down are typical of a pharyngeal pouch. This results in repeated attacks of chest infection and is treated as such. Dysphagia with halitosis should alert one to the diagnosis, which is confirmed by a barium swallow.

60 Stomach and duodenum

Multiple choice questions

Anatomy of the stomach and duodenum

1. Which of the following statements are true?

A The right gastric artery is a branch of the coeliac artery.
B Vagal fibres to the stomach are afferent.
C The parietal cells are in the body of the stomach and are the acid-secreting cells.
D The venous drainage of the stomach ends in the inferior vena cava (IVC).
E The chief cells secrete pepsinogen.

Physiology of the stomach and duodenum

2. Which of the following statements are true?

A The 'gastric phase' of gastric acid secretion is mediated by the vagus nerve.
B Hydrogen ions are exported from the parietal cells via the proton pump.
C Cholecystokinin is secreted by the duodenal endocrine cells.
D The gastric motor activity is propagated from the fundus and moves caudally at a rate of three per minute.
E Secretin increases gastric acid secretion.

Gastric mucosal barrier

3. Which of the following can damage the gastric mucosal barrier?

A Non-steroidal anti-inflammatory drugs (NSAIDs)
B Alcohol
C Trauma
D Bile
E Shock.

Helicobacter pylori

4. Which of the following statements regarding *H. pylori* are true?

A The organism is round in shape.
B It has the ability to hydrolyse urea with the production of ammonia.
C Some strains produce the cytokinins cagA and vacA, which are associated with the ability to cause gastritis, ulceration and cancer.
D The incidence of infection in a general population appears to be high.
E Treatment is recommended for infected patients who are asymptomatic.

Gastritis

5. Which of the following statements are true?

A Type B gastritis is an autoimmune condition.
B Type A gastritis affects the antrum.
C Both types A and B gastritis predispose to malignancy.
D Erosive gastritis due to NSAIDs is mediated via inhibition of Cox1 enzyme.
E Reflux gastritis is commonly seen after gastric surgery.

Peptic ulcers

6. Which of the following regarding peptic ulcers are true?

A The term 'peptic ulcer' is a misnomer.
B Patients with gastric ulceration have increased levels of gastric acid production.
C 'Kissing ulcers' refers to adjacent gastric and duodenal ulcers.

D There is a greater association between gastric ulcers and malignancy than duodenal ulcers.
E All peptic ulcers can be healed by using proton pump inhibitors (PPIs).

7. Common sites for peptic ulcers include:
A First part of duodenum
B Fundus of stomach
C Oesophagus
D Jejunum, such as a stomal ulcer after gastric surgery
E Meckel's diverticulum.

8. Which of the following are predisposing factors for gastric ulcer?
A Gastric acid
B *H. pylori* infection
C NSAIDs
D Smoking
E High socioeconomic groups.

9. Which of the following are true with regard to the clinical features of peptic ulcers?
A The pain never radiates to the back and this differentiates this from biliary colic.
B Vomiting is a notable feature.
C Bleeding is rare.
D They may cause gastric outlet obstruction.
E Weight loss is a typical symptom.

10. Which of the following statements regarding treatment of peptic ulceration are true?
A Surgery remains the mainstay treatment.
B Eradication therapy is given routinely to all patients with peptic ulceration.
C Late dumping syndrome occurring after gastric surgery is due to a sudden increased osmotic load in the small bowel.
D Biopsy of the ulcer margins is mandatory when dealing with a duodenal ulcer.
E All peptic ulcers can be healed by PPI therapy.

➜ Sequelae/complications after gastric operations

11. Which of the following are true with regard to sequelae/complications after gastric operations?
A Recurrent ulceration is rare after gastric surgery for peptic ulcer.
B Early satiety can occur even in the absence of gastric resection.
C Early dumping syndrome is due to a sudden high osmotic load to the small bowel.
D Late dumping syndrome is due to reactive hypoglycaemia.
E The lag-phase between the gastric operation and development of malignancy is usually 10 years.

➜ Haematemesis

12. Which of the following are true with regard to haematemesis?
A The in-patient mortality is about 5 per cent.
B Oesophageal varices are the most common cause.
C It is better to avoid surgery in elderly patients.
D Mallory–Weiss tear is a longitudinal tear below the gastro-oesophageal junction.
E Dieulafoy's lesion is a gastric arteriovenous malformation.

➜ Gastric outlet obstruction

13. Which of the following are true in respect of gastric outlet obstruction (GOO)?
A It is most commonly associated with long-standing peptic ulcer disease and gastric cancer.
B The usual metabolic abnormality is hyperchloraemic alkalosis.
C Endoscopy has no role in management.
D Surgery is the mainstay of treatment.
E Hypokalaemia may occur due to paradoxical renal aciduria.

Gastric cancer

14. **Which of the following are important in the causation of gastric cancer?**
   - A *H. pylori* infection
   - B Gastric atrophy
   - C Pernicious anaemia
   - D Previous gastric surgery
   - E Smoking.

15. **Which of the following statements regarding clinical features of gastric cancer are true?**
   - A They may be non-specific in the early stages.
   - B Anaemia can be a presenting symptom.
   - C Troiser's sign refers to a palpable 'Virchow's node' in the right supraclavicular fossa.
   - D This is a rare cause of GOO.
   - E Trousseau's sign is diagnostic.

16. **Which of the following are associated with the molecular pathology of gastric cancer?**
   - A Mutation or loss of heterozygosity in APC gene
   - B Mutation in gene coding for beta-catenin
   - C Mutations in gene coding for E-cadherin
   - D Inactivation of p53
   - E Microsatellite instability.

17. **Which of the following are true with regard to spread of gastric cancer?**
   - A Tumour reaching the serosa usually indicates incurability.
   - B Blood-borne metastases commonly occur in the absence of lymph node spread.
   - C Krukenberg's tumours are always associated with other areas of transcoelomic spread.
   - D Sister Joseph's nodule is diagnostic of gastric cancer.
   - E The lymphatic vessels related to the cardia have no relation to the oesophageal lymphatics.

18. **Which of the following are unequivocal evidence of incurability in gastric cancer?**
   - A Haematogenous metastases
   - B Involvement of distant peritoneum
   - C N3 nodal disease
   - D Involvement of adjacent organs
   - E Gastric outlet obstruction.

19. **Which of the following are true regarding the treatment of gastric cancer?**
   - A D1 resection is superior to a D2 resection.
   - B The 5-year survival in the UK is between 50 and 75 per cent.
   - C There is a definite role for neoadjuvant chemotherapy.
   - D Gastrointestinal continuity is established after total gastrectomy by a Roux loop.
   - E Radiotherapy to the gastric bed is a useful adjunct.

Gastric conditions

20. **Which of the following statements are true?**
   - A Gastrointestinal stromal tumours (GIST) are associated with tyrosine kinase c-kit oncogene mutation.
   - B GIST tumours show a poor response to imatinib.
   - C Gastric lymphoma is more common in young people.
   - D Primary gastric lymphomas are T-cell-derived and arise from mucosa-associated lymphoid tissue (MALT).
   - E Trichobezoars are more common in female patients.

21. **Which of the following statements regarding gastric volvulus are true?**
   - A In organoaxial volvulus the rotation occurs in a horizontal direction.
   - B Mesenteroaxial rotation is more common than organoaxial rotation.
   - C The condition is usually associated with a diaphragmatic defect.
   - D The condition is usually chronic.
   - E Management is essentially medical and symptomatic.

Extended matching questions

1. Differential diagnosis of upper GI presentations

A Carcinoma of the oesophagus
B Gastro-oesophageal reflux disease (GORD)
C Duodenal ulcer
D Gastritis
E Gastric outlet obstruction
F Achalasia cardia

Choose and match the correct diagnosis with each of the scenarios given below:

1 A 63-year-old male presents with repeated non-bilious vomiting containing ingested food. He has upper abdominal fullness and has lost 3 stones in weight. He is found to be pale and cachectic.

2 A 42-year-old executive presents with upper abdominal discomfort and heartburn. Smoking and stress seem to make it worse. Clinical examination reveals him to be overweight but otherwise normal.

3 A 40-year-old male presents with right upper quadrant pain radiating to the back. It is episodic, burning in nature and aggravated by spicy food. He mentions that his stools are sometimes black.

4 A 52-year-old female presents with a history of slowly progressive dysphagia. She tends to regurgitate ingested food after a few hours. She has occasionally woken up with a choking sensation. She is also concerned about her persistent halitosis.

5 A 78-year-old female presents with upper GI bleed and melaena. She has been on long-term NSAIDs for her arthritis.

6 A 63-year-old male presents with rapidly progressive dysphagia and profound weight loss. He is pale and cachectic.

2. Sequelae of gastric surgery

A Recurrent ulceration
B Early dumping syndrome
C Malignancy
D Late dumping syndrome
E Postvagotomy diarrhoea
F Vitamin B12 deficiency

Choose and match the correct diagnosis with each of the scenarios given below:

1 A 48-year-old male who has had previous gastric resection for his peptic ulcer presents with tremor, faintness and prostration 1.5 h after eating. This lasts for 30 min and is relieved by food and aggravated by exercise.

2 A 50-year-old male with a previous operation for a duodenal ulcer was fully relieved of his symptoms for a few years but now presents with similar symptoms as before. He has upper abdominal pain which is burning in nature. This is episodic and aggravated by alcohol.

3 A 54-year-old male who has had a previous total gastrectomy presents with anaemia and tingling in his arms and legs. He is found to have macrocytic anaemia on blood tests.

4 A 58-year-old male who has had previous gastric resection for his peptic ulcer presents with epigastric fullness, sweating, light-headedness and diarrhoea almost immediately after eating. The attack last for half an hour and is relieved by lying down and aggravated by more food.

5 A 46-year-old male who has had a previous operation for peptic ulcer presents with severe and explosive diarrhoea. This is associated with urgency and not responding to usual antidiarrhoeal medications.

6 A 70-year-old male who underwent a partial gastrectomy 30 years ago presents with recent-onset abdominal pain, vomiting and weight loss.

➔ 3. Gastric conditions

A Trichobezoar
B GIST
C Mallory–Weiss tear
D Dieulafoy's lesion
E Gastric lymphoma
F Gastrinoma
G Gastric volvulus
H Gastric cancer
I Gastric polyps

Choose and match the correct diagnosis with each of the descriptions given below:

1 It is a rare cause of upper GI bleed and is essentially a gastric arteriovenous malformation which is covered by normal mucosa.

2 This is a longitudinal tear below the gastro-oesophageal junction induced by repetitive and strenuous vomiting.

3 The most common type of this condition is the metaplastic type, which is associated with *H. pylori* infection. The other types include inflammatory and fundic gland type. The true adenoma type has a malignant potential.

4 These are principally of two types – intestinal and diffuse. *H. pylori* infection, pernicious anaemia and gastric atrophy are some of the predisposing factors.

5 These are associated with a mutation in the tyrosine kinase c-kit oncogene and commonly occur in the stomach and duodenum. Their biological behaviour is difficult to predict.

6 They arise from the MALT and are more prevalent in the sixth decade. Bleeding and perforation are two common complications after chemotherapy.

7 This causes Zollinger–Ellison syndrome. These may be sporadic or a part of multiple endocrine neoplasia (MEN) type 1 syndrome. These are usually found in the duodenal loop or the pancreas.

8 These are unusual and almost exclusively found in young female psychiatric patients. This can lead to ulceration, perforation, bleeding and obstruction.

9 This is one cause of upper abdominal pain, vomiting and difficulty in eating. This is of two types: organoaxial and mesenteroaxial. It is commonly associated with a diaphragmatic defect.

➔ 4. Gastric operations

A Lap band procedure
B Total gastrectomy

C Gastrojejunostomy
D Cystogastrostomy
E Gastric bypass
F Billroth 1 procedure
G Truncal vagotomy
H Highly selective vagotomy
I Billroth 2 procedure

Choose and match the correct operations with each of the descriptions given below:

1 This has the best long-term results for morbid obesity. It can be done laparoscopically and is becoming a standard procedure for the morbidly obese. The operative mortality is around 2 per cent.

2 This involves resection of part of the stomach followed by closure of the duodenal stump. The continuity is restored by doing an anastomosis with the jejunum.

3 This is a non-selective operation used previously for peptic ulcers. Gastric stasis is a common postoperative problem and hence this was combined with a drainage procedure.

4 The was a common gastric drainage procedure used in peptic ulcer surgery and is presently more often used as a palliative procedure in malignancies. It can be anterior or posterior and isoperistaltic or antiperistaltic. Diarrhoea is a common postoperative sequela.

5 The lower half of the stomach is resected and the gastric remnant is directly anastomosed to the first part of the duodenum. This has a higher rate of anastomotic leak.

6 This procedure selectively denervates the parietal cell mass and has a low incidence of side-effects and acceptable rate of recurrence.

7 This is a popular procedure for morbid obesity with a mortality rate of less than 1 per cent. Slippage and dysphagia are two common complications.

8 This is an operation to treat chronic pancreatic pseudocysts and involves creating a wide and direct communication between the posterior wall of the stomach and the cyst.

9 This is a complex major operation usually done for malignancies. Continuation is restored by a Roux-en-Y loop of jejunum. Vitamin B12 injections are necessary after this operation to prevent deficiency. Patients are advised to eat small amounts at a time after this surgery.

Answers: Multiple choice questions

→ Anatomy of the stomach and duodenum

1. C, E

The stomach has a rich blood supply with excellent anastomotic arcades among all arteries. The blood supply of the stomach is derived mainly from five arteries – on the lesser curve, the left gastric artery and the right gastric artery branches of coeliac axis and common hepatic artery, respectively. On the greater curvature are three arteries, the right gastroepiploic artery, branch of the gastroduodenal artery and the left gastroepiploic and short gastric arteries, which are both branches of the splenic artery. The venous drainage of the lesser curve is into the portal vein and that of the greater curve is into the splenic vein. Apart from parietal and chief cells, the stomach also has numerous endocrinal cells such as G cells producing gastrin, enterochromaffin (ECF) cells producing histamine and D cells producing somatostatin.

Physiology of the stomach and duodenum

2. B, C, D

Classically three phases of gastric secretion are described: the cephalic phase, mediated by the vagus nerve; the gastric phase, mediated principally by gastrin; and the intestinal phase, mediated by secretin, somatostatin and the presence of chyme in the duodenum.

Gastric mucosal barrier

3. A, B, C, D, E

The gastric mucous layer is essential to the integrity of the gastric mucosa. It is a viscid layer of mucopolysaccharides produced by the mucus-producing cells of the stomach. Many factors can lead to the breakdown of this barrier. Tonometry studies have shown that in the entire gastrointestinal tract the stomach is the most sensitive to ischaemia and also the slowest to recover. This explains the high incidence of stress ulceration.

Helicobacter pylori

4. B, C, D

Helicobacter pylori is spiral shaped and resides in the mucous layer of the stomach. Its ability to produce ammonia, an alkali, results in increased gastrin release due to a negative feedback. *H. pylori* infection is very common and population infection rates of 80–90 per cent are not unusual. It appears that most infection is acquired in childhood and the probability of infection is inversely related to socioeconomic group. At present, eradication therapy is recommended for patients with duodenal ulcer disease, but not for non-ulcer dyspepsia or in asymptomatic patients who are infected. *H. pylori* is now classified by the WHO as a class 1 carcinogen.

Gastritis

5. C, D, E

Type A gastritis is an autoimmune condition in which there are circulating antibodies to the parietal cell. This results in the atrophy of the parietal cell mass followed by hypochlorhydria and finally achlorhydria. This also affects the intrinsic factor which can lead to vitamin B12 deficiency and pernicious anaemia. In type A gastritis, the antrum is not affected and the hypochlorhydria leads to increased gastrin production and enterochromaffin-like (ECL) hypertrophy. Patients with type A gastritis are prone to gastric cancer.

Type B gastritis is associated with *H. pylori* infection. This commonly affects the antrum and the patient is prone to peptic ulcer disease. Intestinal metaplasia is seen in gastritis with atrophy. Patients with pangastritis and those with dysplastic changes have malignant potential.

Reflux gastritis is caused by enterogastric reflux and is common after gastric surgery. Bile chelating or prokinetic agents may be helpful in management.

Erosive gastritis is caused by all agents that disrupt the gastric mucosal barrier. NSAIDs and alcohol are common causes. Stress gastritis is a common sequel after serious illness or injury and is characterised by reduction in blood supply to the superficial mucosa of the stomach.

Peptic ulcers

6. A, D, E

The common sites for peptic ulcers are the first part of duodenum and the lesser curve of stomach, but they may occur in the oesophagus, the stoma following gastric surgery and Meckel's diverticulum. It is now widely accepted that *H. pylori* is the most important factor in the development of peptic ulceration. The other major factor is the ingestion of NSAIDs. Patients with gastric ulcers have relatively normal levels of gastric acid secretion. Kissing ulcers refer to two adjacent ulcers on the anterior and posterior walls of the duodenum.

7. A, C, D, E

The peptic ulcers tend to occur at a junction between two different types of epithelium, the ulcer occurring in the epithelium least resistant to acid damage.

8. B, C, D

Gastric ulcers are more prevalent in lower socioeconomic groups and are considerably more common in the developing world. The incidence is equal between the sexes and patients with gastric ulcers tend to be older.

9. D

The pain is epigastric and may radiate to the back. It is intermittent and demonstrates periodicity. Vomiting is not a notable feature unless stenosis has occurred. Weight gain may sometimes be seen, although patients with gastric ulcers tend to be underweight. All peptic ulcers may bleed. Some may present with chronic anaemia while others may have acute GI bleed.

10. B, E

The vast majority of uncomplicated peptic ulcers are treated medically. Late dumping syndrome is due to reactive hypoglycaemia and early dumping syndrome is due to sudden increased osmotic load. Biopsy of the ulcer margins of a perforated duodenal ulcer is not required as there is no risk of malignancy, unlike gastric ulcers.

→ Sequelae/complications after gastric operations

11. B, C, D, E

The important sequelae after gastric surgery are recurrent ulceration, small stomach syndrome, bilious vomiting, early and late dumping syndrome, diarrhoea and malignant transformation. Approximately 30 per cent of patients can expect to suffer a degree of dysfunction following peptic ulcer surgery, and in about 5 per cent of these patients, the symptoms are intractable.

→ Haematemesis

12. A, D, E

The most common causes of haematemesis are bleeding peptic ulcer (60 per cent), erosions (26 per cent), Mallory–Weiss tear (4 per cent) and oesophageal varices (4 per cent).

Whatever the cause, the principles of management are identical – initial resuscitation followed by urgent investigations to determine the cause of bleeding and definitive therapy. There are numerous endoscopic measures to control peptic ulcer bleeding, such as injections and argon diathermy. The criteria for surgical intervention – patients continuing to bleed, rebleed, visible vessel at ulcer base, a spurting vessel or an ulcer with a clot on the base – are statistically likely to require surgical treatment. Elderly and unfit patients are more likely to die from the bleed than younger patients and hence should have early surgery. In general, anyone needing more than 6 units of blood needs surgery.

→ Gastric outlet obstruction

13. A, D, E

In recent years, the most common cause of GOO is gastric cancer. The patient commonly loses weight, and appears unwell and dehydrated. The vomiting of hydrochloric acid results in hypochloraemic alkalosis. As dehydration progresses, hypokalaemia ensues along with reduced circulating ionised calcium, which may cause tetany. Treatment involves correcting the metabolic abnormalities and dealing with the mechanical problem. Endoscopic treatment with balloon dilatation has been tried in benign pyloric stenosis but surgery remains the mainstay of management.

Gastric cancer

14. A, B, C, D, E

The aetiology of gastric cancer is multifactorial. The other predisposing factors are gastric polyps, duodenogastric reflux and reflux gastritis. It is also associated with cigarette smoking and ingestion of dust from industrial sources. Diet is also important and excessive salt intake, deficiency of antioxidants and exposure to N-nitroso compounds are also implicated. Genetic factors are also important but imperfectly elucidated.

15. A, B

The key to improving outcome is early diagnosis. The symptoms are non-specific in early cases and it thus requires a high index of suspicion and use of screening programmes in places of high incidence (e.g. Japan). In advanced cancer, early satiety, bloating, distension and vomiting may occur. The tumour frequently bleeds leading to iron deficiency anaemia. Obstruction leads to dysphagia, epigastric fullness or vomiting. Virchow's lymph node may be palpable in the left supraclavicular fossa, signifying metastases. Non-metastatic effects such as thrombophlebitis (Trousseau's sign) and deep vein thrombosis may be seen, but are not diagnostic.

16. A, B, C, D, E

The molecular pathology of gastric cancer is still to be completely worked out but several genetic events have been established. Several growth factors are also over-expressed, including c-Met, k-Sam, c-ErbB2, TGF-alpha, EGF ad VEGF. Well known syndromes, such as hereditary non-polyposis colorectal cancer (HNPCC), have gastric cancer as part of their spectrum.

17. A

Carcinoma of the stomach spreads by all modes, including direct spread, lymphatic spread, blood and transperitoneal routes. It is important to note that distant spread is unusual before the disease spreads locally and blood-borne metastases are uncommon in the absence of lymph node metastases. Krukenberg's tumours in the ovaries may be the sole site of transcoelomic spread. Tumour may spread via the falciform ligament to the umbilicus (Sister Joseph's nodule), which is also seen in many other abdominal malignancies. The lymphatics at the cardia communicate freely with the lymphatics of the oesophagus.

18. A, B

It is important that patients with incurable disease are not subjected to radical therapy that cannot help them. Unequivocal evidence of incurability is haematogenous metastases, involvement of the distant peritoneum, N4 nodal disease and fixation to structures that cannot be removed. Involvement of another organ *per se* does not imply incurability provided that it can be removed. There are debates on the question of operability in N3 involvement.

19. C, D

D2 gastrectomy involves en-bloc resection of the second tier of nodes (clearance of the major arterial trunks) and is superior to D1 resections (removal of the perigastric nodes only). This may, however, be associated with a higher level of morbidity and mortality. The 5-year survival in the West is 25–50 per cent. In Japan, approximately 75 per cent of patients have a curative resection with a 5-year survival between 50 and 75 per cent. There are a number of radiosensitive tissues in the gastric bed, which limits the dose of radiotherapy that can be given.

Gastric conditions

20. A, E

An 80 per cent objective response rate can be observed after Imatinib therapy of GIST tumours. This has dramatically improved the prognosis of advanced metastatic GIST. Primary gastric lymphomas account for 5 per cent of all gastric neoplasms and is most prevalent in the 6th decade of life. Primary gastric lymphomas are B-cell derived, the tumour arising from the MALT. This remains in the stomach for a prolonged period before involving lymph nodes. The treatment is somewhat controversial but surgery alone seems appropriate for localised disease process.

Trichobezoars are almost exclusively found in young females, often with psychiatric problems.

21. A, C, D

Rotation of the stomach usually occurs around an axis between two fixed points – the cardia and the pylorus. Organoaxial volvulus is the most common type. If the problem is causing symptoms, surgical treatment is the only satisfactory approach.

Answers: Extended matching questions

→ 1. Differential diagnosis of upper GI presentations

1E, 2B, 3C, 4F, 5D, 6A

→ 2. Sequelae of gastric surgery

1D, 2A, 3F, 4B, 5E, 6C

→ 3. Gastric conditions

1D, 2C, 3I, 4H, 5B, 6E, 7F, 8A, 9G

→ 4. Gastric operations

1E, 2I, 3G, 4C, 5F, 6H, 7A, 8D, 9B

61 The liver

Multiple choice questions

➜ Liver anatomy

1. **Which of the following statements are false?**

A The liver is fixed in its place by peritoneal reflections called ligaments.
B The major part of the blood supply of the liver is derived from the hepatic artery.
C The portal vein lies posterior to the hepatic vein and common bile duct.
D The bile duct, portal vein and hepatic artery are contained in the lesser omentum.
E The portal vein is formed by the union of the superior mesenteric and left gastric veins.

2. **Which of the following statements are true?**

A The left hepatic duct has a longer extrahepatic course than the right.
B The major venous drainage is by three veins – right, middle and left hepatic veins draining directly into the inferior vena cava (IVC).
C All the three major veins join the IVC within the liver parenchyma.
D The functional lobes of the liver are divided by the falciform ligament.
E The liver is divided into eight functional segments – I to IV in the left hemi-liver and V–VIII in the right hemi-liver.

➜ Liver function

3. **Which of the following liver function tests (LFTs) are abnormal?**

A Bilirubin 5–17 μmol/L
B Alkaline phosphatase (ALP) 35–130 IU/L
C Aspartate transaminase (AST) 55–80 IU/L
D Alanine transaminase (ALT) 135–240 IU/L
E Gamma-glutamyl transpeptidase (GGT) 110–148 IU/L
F Albumin 35–50 g/L
G Prothrombin time (PT) 12–16 s

➜ Clinical features of chronic liver disease

4. **Which of these clinical features are not primarily a feature of chronic liver disease?**

A Jaundice
B Muscle wasting
C Bruising
D Oliguria
E Ascites and splenomegaly
F Thirst
G Confusion.

➜ Liver imaging

5. **Which of the following statements are true for imaging of the liver?**

A Ultrasound (US) is the first-line investigation.
B Radioisotope liver scan gives an idea of the extent of anatomical derangement.
C The 'gold standard' is contrast-enhanced computed tomographic scan (CECT).
D Magnetic resonance imaging (MRI) has advantages over CECT.
E Angiography is best reserved when embolisation is contemplated.

➜ Liver trauma

6. **Which of the following statements are false?**

A Liver injuries are common.

B Blunt trauma is often associated with splenic, mesenteric and renal injuries.
C Penetrating trauma is often associated with pericardial or chest injuries.
D CECT scan must be carried out in every case of liver trauma.
E Laparoscopy as an investigation has a role.

7. Which of these statements are true?
A Penetrating injuries should be explored.
B Blunt injuries are usually treated conservatively.
C Exploration for a liver injury is best done by a long midline incision.
D Severe crush injury is ideally treated by packing.
E Venovenous bypass should be considered in major liver vascular injury.
F A subcapsular or intrahepatic haematoma requires urgent laparotomy.

➜ Portal hypertension

8. Which of the following statements are false?
A Acute haematemesis from portal hypertension occurs most commonly from gastric varices.
B Initial endoscopic treatment of oesophageal varices with banding as opposed to injection sclerotherapy has less chance of oesophageal ulceration.
C Long-term beta-blocker therapy coupled with sclerotherapy regime or endoscopic banding is the mainstay of treatment of portal hypertension.
D In failed drug or endoscopic treatment, the ideal choice is the surgical shunt of portocaval anastomosis.
E Ascites in cirrhosis can be treated by a peritoneovenous shunt.

Extended matching questions

➜ 1. Chronic liver conditions

A Budd–Chiari syndrome
B Primary sclerosing cholangitis
C Primary biliary cirrhosis
D Caroli's disease
E Simple cystic disease

Choose and match the correct diagnosis with each of the scenarios given below:

1 A 30-year-old patient has a history of recurrent attacks of fever with rigors, right upper quadrant pain and jaundice with itching. Biochemistry shows a jaundice of obstructive nature. CT scan shows intrahepatic ductal dilatation with stones.

2 A 40-year-old female presents with recurrent episodes of right upper quadrant pain with jaundice. Biochemistry shows an obstructive pattern of the jaundice. Five years ago she underwent a panproctocolectomy for ulcerative colitis and has been well since, except for these attacks. Endoscopic retrograde cholangiopancreatography (ERCP) shows irregular narrowed intra- and extrahepatic bile ducts.

3 A 50-year-old female complains of general malaise, lethargy, pruritus and jaundice, the latter being present over the last 3 months. The LFTs show a rise in bilirubin, the transaminases and prothrombin time. She has had recurrent small haematemesis and has ascites.

4 A 30-year-old female complains of abdominal discomfort and distension. She has had 3 episodes of small haematemesis in the past 6 months. On examination she has hepatomegaly and ascites. All the LFTs are deranged. CT scan of the liver shows a large congested liver.

5 A fit-looking 50-year-old male complains of recent onset of dull, aching, right upper quadrant pain of 3–4 months' duration. Examination shows no abnormality. Liver function tests are

normal, as is an upper gastrointestinal endoscopy. An ultrasound of the liver shows a 6 cm solitary cystic lesion.

→ 2. Liver infections

A Viral hepatitis
B Ascending cholangitis
C Pyogenic liver abscess
D Amoebic liver abscess
E Hydatid liver disease

Choose and match the correct diagnosis with each of the scenarios given below:

1 A 25-year-old male complains of generally feeling unwell with fever and weight loss. He has had bloodstained motions on and off for the last 6 weeks after he returned from the subcontinent where he was working for 6 months. On examination he has a tender right upper quadrant with hepatomegaly. US shows a hypoechoic cavity in the right lobe with ill-defined borders.

2 A 50-year-old female patient has had recurrent attacks of colicky right upper quadrant and epigastric pain with jaundice, high temperature with rigors and itching. Ten months ago she underwent an uneventful laparoscopic cholecystectomy. On examination she is jaundiced with scratch marks all over her body and hepatomegaly. She has raised serum bilirubin and the ALP is 1100 IU/L. US shows a dilated common bile duct with stones.

3 A 35-year-old male patient presents with general ill-health, weight loss, anorexia and malaise for several weeks. He has developed jaundice for the last 2 weeks; he has no pruritus. Abdominal examination shows a tender hepatomegaly. Liver function tests show raised bilirubin and transaminases.

4 A 75-year-old male diabetic patient complains of anorexia, fever, malaise and right upper quadrant discomfort. On examination there is weight loss and tender hepatomegaly. US shows a multiloculated cystic mass, a finding confirmed on CT scan.

5 A 50-year-old male patient, a native of Cyprus, presents with a painful mass in the right upper quadrant. The pain is a continuous dull ache and has the features of a mass arising from the right lobe of the liver. The blood count shows raised eosinophils. The CT scan shows a smooth space-occupying lesion with multiple septa within it.

→ 3. Liver tumours

A Haemangioma
B Hepatic adenoma
C Focal nodular hyperplasia
D Secondary liver metastasis
E Hepatocellular carcinoma (HCC)

Choose and match the correct diagnosis with each of the scenarios given below:

1 A 35-year-old woman who is on the contraceptive pill presents with right upper quadrant aching pain. She is fit without any physical findings. Her LFTs and other blood tests are normal. US of the liver shows a single well-demarcated hyperechoic mass and CT scan demonstrates a well-circumscribed vascular solid tumour.

2 A 40-year-old male patient presents with dull, persistent upper abdominal pain, weakness, weight loss and occasional fever. He had one episode of haematemesis. Abdominal examination shows an enlarged liver with a mass in the right lobe. Liver function tests show elevation of the transaminases and much raised alpha-fetoprotein (AFP).

3 A 60-year-old male patient presents with dragging pain in the right upper quadrant for 3 months and weight loss. On examination he is slightly jaundiced. He has an enlarged liver. Three years ago he underwent a right hemicolectomy for cancer of the caecum. LFTs show elevation of all the parameters. US shows a solid mass in the right lobe and a CECT confirms the mass with lack of enhancement.

4 In a 30-year-old female patient, during laparoscopic cholecystectomy, the surgeon noticed that the under-surface of the liver has several lesions which are blue in colour.

5 A 45-year-old female patient underwent an US for suspected biliary pain. The US of the biliary tract was normal but showed a solid lesion in the liver. Therefore she had a CECT scan which showed a vascular lesion surrounding a solid mass with central scarring.

Answers: Multiple choice questions

→ Liver anatomy

1. B, E

The liver is fixed inside the peritoneal cavity by its ligaments which are the various peritoneal reflections. These are falciform ligament, right and left triangular ligaments. The major (80 per cent) blood supply of the liver comes from the portal vein and the rest from the hepatic artery. The bile duct, portal vein and the hepatic artery are contained within the lesser omentum (hepatoduodenal ligament). The bile duct lies lateral to the hepatic artery and both lie anterior to the portal vein. The portal vein is formed by the union of the superior mesenteric vein and the splenic vein behind the neck of the pancreas.

2. A, B, E

The left hepatic duct has a longer extrahepatic course whereas the right one is entirely intrahepatic. This anatomical situation is made use of in the repair of high common bile duct strictures where a side-to-side anastomosis is carried out between the left intrahepatic duct and a Roux loop of jejunum. The major venous drainage is by three major hepatic veins – right, middle and left. The right hepatic vein joins the IVC outside the liver while the other two empty into the IVC within the liver substance.

The functional lobes of the liver are divided by a line between the gall bladder fossa and the middle hepatic vein (Cantlie's line) and not the falciform ligament, which divides the liver into anatomical lobes. The liver is divided into eight functional segments: segments I–IV in the left and V–VIII in the right.

→ Liver function

3. C, D, E

The normal transaminase (ALT and AST) levels are 5–40 IU/L. The normal GGT is 10–48 IU/L. Derangement of these enzymes indicate hepatocellular damage.

→ Clinical features of chronic liver disease

4. D, F

→ Liver imaging

5. A, C, D, E

Ultrasound is the first-line investigation as it is safe and universally available. It detects liver tumours and biliary pathology. It is operator-dependent. Radioisotope liver scanning does not show anatomical derangement but shows up functional derangement and is a useful non-invasive screening test in suspected bile leak or biliary obstruction. When a radioactive sulphur colloid is used, an adenoma or a haemangioma can be diagnosed, as these do not take up sulphur colloid.

CECT is the 'gold standard' for liver imaging in most clinical situations – trauma, tumour, infections and inflammations. Triple-phase, multi-slice, spiral CECT provides fine detail of liver lesions. Oral contrast shows up the anatomical relationship of the stomach and duodenum to the liver hilum. Intravenous contrast gives the arterial and venous phases. MRI has the following advantages over CECT: no risk of allergic reaction as iodine-containing contrast is not used; there is no radiation; magnetic resonance cholangiopancreatography (MRCP) provides excellent images of the biliary tract; and magnetic resonance angiography (MRA) gives high-definition images of hepatic artery and portal vein without recourse to arterial cannulation. As vascular information can be obtained from CECT and MRI, hepatic angiography is mostly reserved when therapeutic embolisation is contemplated, as in trauma or tumour.

Liver trauma

6. A, D

Liver injuries are rare because of its anatomical position under the diaphragm where it is protected by the lower thoracic cage. Therefore when the liver is damaged, the overall injury is serious. Blunt trauma is often associated with damage to neighbouring structures, such as the spleen, kidneys and mesentery. Stab and gunshot wounds causing penetrating injuries are associated with chest trauma.

CECT scan is not done in every case of liver trauma. If unstable, the patient needs to be taken to theatre forthwith without wasting time on a scan. On the other hand, stable patients who are suspected of having liver damage should undergo a CECT scan. When haemoperitoneum is suspected, in the stable patient, a laparoscopy is carried out to look for diaphragmatic rupture.

7. A, B, D, E

A penetrating injury, such as a lower right chest and abdominal stab wound, requiring large amounts of blood replacement will need urgent exploration. The patient should be transferred to the operating theatre while active resuscitation is underway. Blunt injuries are mostly treated conservatively. Stable patients need to undergo a CECT scan and be treated conservatively as long as they continue to be stable. Exploration for liver injury is ideally carried out by a rooftop incision which can be extended upwards for a median sternotomy.

Severe crush injury is treated by packing and re-exploration after 48 h. In major liver vascular damage, the patient is put on a venovenous bypass. In this a cannula is passed from the femoral vein to the superior vena cava; this allows the IVC to be safely clamped to facilitate caval or hepatic vein repair. A subcapsular or intrahepatic haematoma does not need any intervention and usually resolves spontaneously.

Portal hypertension

8. A, D

Acute haematemesis from portal hypertension most often occurs from lower oesophageal varices. The initial definitive treatment is endoscopic sclerotherapy or banding, the latter having a lesser incidence of oesophageal ulceration. Long-term beta-blocker therapy with endoscopic sclerotherapy or banding is the main treatment for portal hypertension. When this fails, transjugular intrahepatic portosystemic stent shunt (TIPSS) is the treatment of choice in preference to the operation of portocaval anastomosis. Ascites can be treated by insertion of a peritoneovenous shunt – either a Le Veen or a Denver shunt. The latter helps to evacuate any debris blocking the shunt.

Answers: Extended matching questions

→ 1. Chronic liver conditions

1D

This patient has recurrent attacks of obstructive jaundice with features of sepsis – typical of bile duct stones. The CT scan confirms the diagnosis of this congenital condition.

2B

This patient who has suffered from ulcerative colitis suffers from primary sclerosing cholangitis. Although her ulcerative colitis has been treated successfully by surgery, her primary sclerosing cholangitis has continued unabated. The ERCP is diagnostic. A close surveillance should be carried out because she may develop a cholangiocarcinoma in future.

3C

This female patient suffers from primary biliary cirrhosis, a condition of gradual onset. The liver function tests show hepatocellular dysfunction. Confirmation is by liver biopsy.

4A

This is Budd–Chiari syndrome where there is hepatic vein thrombosis caused by an underlying myeloproliferative disorder or a procoagulant state due to antithrombin 3, protein C or protein S deficiency. The hepatic venous outflow obstruction causes a congested liver, impaired liver function, portal hypertension, ascites and oesophageal varices. CT scan is diagnostic. Confirmation is by hepatic venography via the transjugular route which may allow a biopsy.

5E

This patient has a simple solitary hepatic cyst confirmed on ultrasound with typical findings: a regular, thin-walled unilocular space-occupying lesion without any surrounding tissue response or variation in density within the cavity. Asymptomatic cysts are left alone. But as this patient has symptoms from it, laparoscopic deroofing should be considered.

→ 2. Liver infections

1D

Having returned from a stay in the subcontinent, this patient has amoebic dysentery with an amoebic abscess. The diagnosis is confirmed by stool examination and isolation of the parasite. US of the liver followed by diagnostic aspiration of the contents are both therapeutic and diagnostic – the contents are usually sterile but the aspirate is characteristically chocolate-coloured.

2B

This patient has classical Charcot's intermittent hepatic triad almost certainly from a retained stone as seen on the US. The LFTs will show an obstructive picture. She needs to be treated with antibiotics, vitamin K and an ERCP and endoscopic papillotomy.

3A

Viral hepatitis can be due to hepatitis A, B and C. Hepatitis C is one of the most common causes of liver disease worldwide. Hepatitis B is the most serious and later can cause a hepatoma. Some patients may present acutely with fulminating liver failure or at a late stage with cirrhosis, variceal bleeding and ascites. Diagnosis is confirmed by the antibody titre to the infective agent.

4C

Pyogenic liver abscess usually occurs in the elderly and infirm who are immunocompromised, as is this patient. The US and CT scan findings are diagnostic. The patient is treated with antibiotics and aspiration.

5E
As a native of a Mediterranean country, this patient has a hydatid cyst of the right lobe of the liver. The diagnosis is confirmed by eosinophilia on haematological examination, serological test for antibodies to hydatid antigen in the enzyme-linked immunosorbent assay (ELISA) and typical CT scan findings of a floating membrane within the cyst and multiple septa.

3. Liver tumours

1B
This woman on the contraceptive pill has a hepatic adenoma confirmed on the US and CT findings. Biopsy is contraindicated because of the extreme vascularity of these tumours. Stopping the pill is known to have produced tumour regression. They are thought to have a malignant potential and therefore large symptomatic tumours are best resected.

2E
This male patient clinically has the features of a HCC. He needs to be thoroughly staged with contrast MRI, CECT, bone scan and CT scan of chest. Most patients are not amenable for resection. Therefore, one of the choices for non-surgical treatment is considered.

3D
This patient who had a colonic cancer removed 3 years ago now has the clinical features of secondaries in the liver: jaundice, hepatomegaly and a liver mass on imaging. He now needs a thorough reassessment so that he can be considered for hepatic resection.

4A
This is a liver haemangioma, the commonest benign liver lesion, increasingly being diagnosed with the availability of expertise in US reporting. MRI will show the classical 'light bulb' sign. They are best left alone in the vast majority.

5C
Focal nodular hyperplasia is the second commonest benign liver lesion, an incidental finding, increasingly diagnosed with improvements in US and CT imaging. US and CT images are typical. Focal nodular hyperplasia contains both hepatocytes and Kupffer cells which are very few in tumours. Thus a sulphur colloid scan which is taken up by Kupffer cells would be diagnostic.

62 The spleen

Multiple choice questions

Anatomy

1. Which of the following ligaments are connected to the spleen and keep it in its place?

A Gastrocolic omentum
B Lienorenal ligament
C Phrenicocolic ligament
D Gastrophrenic ligament
E Gastrosplenic ligament.

2. Which of the following statements are false?

A The spleen lies in front of the left 10th, 11th and12th ribs.
B The splenic artery arises from the coeliac axis.
C The inferior mesenteric vein empties into the splenic vein.
D The tail of the pancreas lies in the lienorenal ligament.
E The inner surface of the spleen has two impressions – gastric and colic.

Splenectomy

3. Which of the following statements are true?

A Partial splenectomy can result in splenic regeneration.
B During splenectomy the tail of the pancreas can be damaged.
C A gastric or pancreatic fistula can occur as a post-splenectomy complication.
D In a left hemicolectomy the spleen can be in danger.
E The risk of opportunist post-splenectomy infection (OPSI) is greatest after the first 6 months of splenectomy.

Splenic abnormalities

4. Which one of the following statements is false?

A Splenunculi are present in approximately 10–30 per cent of the population.
B Splenic artery aneurysm can occur as a complication of acute pancreatitis.
C Plain abdominal X-ray is the ideal imaging modality.
D A massively enlarged spleen is prone to infarction.
E The splenic hilum is a common site for the development of a pseudocyst of the pancreas.

Extended matching questions

1. Splenic pathology

A Idiopathic thrombocytopenic purpura (ITP)
B Hereditary spherocytosis
C Splenic infarction
D Splenic artery aneurysm
E Splenic rupture

Choose and match the correct diagnosis with each of the scenarios given below

1 A male patient of 55 years, known to suffer from myelofibrosis, presents with onset of severe left upper quadrant and shoulder tip pain of 8 h duration. On examination he has a

temperature and marked tenderness over an enlarged spleen. A contrast-enhanced computed tomography scan (CECT) shows a perfusion defect in an enlarged spleen.

2 An 18-year-old male presents with intermittent generalised abdominal pain, mild jaundice and anorexia. On examination he has pallor, jaundice and splenomegaly. An ultrasound of his abdomen shows multiple small gallstones and confirms splenomegaly.

3 A 30-year-old female patient presents with petechial haemorrhagic spots in her skin. She suffers from menorrhagia. Abdominal examination shows no organomegaly but many areas of skin ecchymoses. The coagulation and bleeding times are normal. The blood tests show anaemia and low platelet count. Bone marrow reveals large number of platelet-producing megakaryocytes.

4 A 25-year-old male was kicked in his abdomen accidentally while playing football. He got up and continued to play for another few minutes, but then he felt dizzy with intense pain in his left upper abdomen. In hospital he complained of pain in his left shoulder tip and had rigidity and rebound tenderness in his left hypochondrium. Until the age of 18 years he lived in a tropical country when he had suffered from malaria.

5 A 30-year-old woman during her ultrasound for pregnancy was found to have a calcified 1 cm mass in the epigastrium. A bruit was heard in the epigastric region. She does not have any symptoms.

Answers: Multiple choice questions

Anatomy

1. B, C, E

The spleen is connected to the posterior abdominal wall by the lienorenal ligament, which contains the splenic artery and vein; to the anterolateral abdominal wall by the phrenicocolic ligament; and, anteriorly, it is the gastrosplenic ligament that contains the short gastric vessels.

2. A, E

The spleen lies in front of the left 9th, 10th and 11th ribs. Therefore in a fracture of these ribs, splenic injury should be suspected. The inner (visceral) surface of the spleen has gastric, colic, renal and pancreatic impressions.

Splenectomy

3. A, B, C, D

If possible, partial splenectomy in trauma should always be attempted because there is rapid regeneration of lost tissue with no reduction in splenic function. The tail of the pancreas can be damaged while ligating the splenic artery and vein at the hilum. The greater curve of the stomach can be damaged during ligation and division of the short gastric arteries. If damage to the pancreatic tail and the stomach is not recognised, then a gastric or pancreatic fistula can occur as a postoperative complication. The commonest cause of iatrogenic injury to the spleen is a left hemicolectomy. The period during which a person is most at risk for OPSI is during the first 2–3 years after splenectomy.

Splenic abnormalities

4. C

The ideal imaging modality for splenic pathology is CECT. Magnetic resonance imaging (MRI) is similarly useful. Radioisotope scanning is useful to find out if the spleen is an important site for destruction of red blood cells.

Answers: Extended matching questions

1. Splenic pathology

1C

This patient has splenic infarction, a condition that occurs in those with massive splenomegaly, such as in myeloproliferative disorders, portal hypertension or splenic vein thrombosis. CECT confirms the diagnosis. Conservative management is tried but if the patient continues to be septic, denoting a splenic abscess, splenectomy is carried out.

2B

This patient has hereditary spherocytosis, an autosomal dominant disorder. He has unconjugated hyperbilirubinaemia, splenomegaly and gallstones (almost certainly pigment stones). The blood picture will show anaemia, a positive fragility test and a large number of reticulocytes. Radioactive chromium labelling of the patient's own red cells will show the spleen to be site of red cell sequestration. Splenectomy and cholecystectomy should be carried out.

3A

This 30-year-old female has signs of petechial haemorrhages and generalised bleeding tendency. Her low platelet count points to the diagnosis of ITP. The spleen is palpable in a minority of cases. If the platelet count remains low and the patient has two relapses on steroid therapy, splenectomy is considered. Response to steroids indicates a good response to splenectomy. Up to two-thirds of patients will be cured by splenectomy; a further 15 per cent will be improved, whilst in the remainder the operation will make no difference.

4E

This young man has the hallmarks of a ruptured spleen. He spent the early part of his life in a tropical country where he suffered from malaria, which would have caused an enlarged spleen. Trivial trauma during a game of contact sport caused rupture of his spleen. Resuscitation followed by an US or CECT (if time permits), followed by operation, is the definitive management.

5D

This pregnant woman has the incidental finding of a splenic artery aneurysm. These are usually silent unless they rupture. Fifty per cent of cases of rupture occur in patients younger than 45 years and 25 per cent occur in pregnant women usually in the third trimester or during labour. Hence a serious consideration should be given to prophylactically treat this splenic artery aneurysm by interventional radiology.

63 The gall bladder and bile ducts

Multiple choice questions

➜ Anatomy of the gall bladder and bile ducts

1. Which of the following statements are true?

A The normal capacity of the gall bladder is 250 mL.
B The cystic duct always joins the common hepatic duct (CHD) above the duodenum.
C The cystic artery is a branch of the right hepatic artery.
D Moynihan's hump refers to the neck of the gall bladder.
E The lymphatics from the gall bladder drain into the cystic lymph node of Lund.

➜ Physiology of the gall bladder

2. Which of the following statements are true?

A The approximate water content of bile when it leaves the liver is 50 per cent.
B The liver excretes bile at an approximate rate of 40 mL/h.
C The rate of bile secretion is primarily controlled by secretin.
D The sole function of the gall bladder is to act as a reservoir for bile.
E The gall bladder secretes about 20 mL of mucus daily.

➜ Investigations on the biliary tract

3. Which of the following statements are true?

A CT scan is more sensitive than ultrasound for gallstones.
B A plain radiograph can show radio-opaque gallstones in 10 per cent of patients.
C An 'end-viewing' endoscope is used during endoscopic retrograde cholangiopancreatography (ERCP) to cannulate the ampulla.
D Biliary scintigraphy can be helpful in the diagnosis of cholecystitis, bile leaks and iatrogenic obstruction.
E Magnetic resonance cholangiopancreatography (MRCP) has excellent diagnostic and therapeutic applications in bile duct disorders.

➜ Congenital abnormalities of the gall bladder and bile ducts

4. Which of the following statements are true?

A The gall bladder is never absent.
B The 'Phrygian cap' refers to the septum present in the gall bladder in approximately 2–6 per cent.
C An accessory cholecystohepatic duct may be present, passing directly into the gall bladder from the liver.
D Caroli's disease refers to the multiple saccular dilatations of the extrahepatic ducts.
E Choledochal cyst increases the risk of cholangiocarcinoma.

➜ Gallstones

5. Which of the following statements regarding gallstones are true?

A Cholesterol stones are more common than pigment stones in the UK.
B Biliary colic is typically present in 10–25 per cent of patients.
C The risk of having acute cholecystitis in a person with asymptomatic gallstones is 10 per cent/year.

D Courvoisier's law is usually associated with gallstones.
E Murphy's sign suggests the presence of acute inflammation.

6. Which of the following statements regarding the treatment of gallstones are true?
A Patients with asymptomatic gallstones should routinely be advised to have a cholecystectomy.
B Ninety per cent of patients with acute cholecystitis respond to conservative treatment.
C Antibiotics are not required in the management of acute cholecystitis in the absence of jaundice.
D Urgent laparoscopic cholecystectomy in a patient with acute cholecystitis is associated with a five times greater conversion rate compared with elective surgery.
E Acalculous cholecystitis has a mild clinical course.

➜ Gall bladder conditions

7. Which of the following statements are true?
A A 'porcelain gall bladder' has no clinical significance.
B 'Strawberry gall bladder' is due to the submucous aggregations of cholesterol crystals and esthers.
C Typhoid carriers can excrete typhoid bacteria in their bile.
D Surgery is advised if gall bladder polyps >1 cm are identified.
E Diverticulosis of the gall bladder can be demonstrated by cholecystography.

➜ Cholecystectomy

8. Which of the following statements regarding cholecystectomy are true?
A The incidence of bile-duct injury is 0.05 per cent.
B A fundus-first approach is helpful in difficult open operations.
C Routine Per-Operative Cholangiogram is mandatory.
D Post-cholecystectomy syndrome occurs in 15 per cent of the patients.
E The cystic duct is free and easily dissected in Mirizzi's syndrome.

➜ Obstructive jaundice

9. Which of the following statements regarding obstructive jaundice are true?
A The incidence of symptomatic bile duct stones varies from 5 to 8 per cent.
B Charcot's triad consists of pain, stones and jaundice.
C Primary sclerosing cholangitis (PSC) is associated with hypergammaglobulinaemia and elevated smooth muscle antibodies.
D Clonorchiasis can predispose to bile duct carcinoma.
E Bismuth type 3 biliary stricture is a hilar stricture.

➜ Bile duct carcinoma

10. Which of the following predispose to bile duct carcinoma?
A Ulcerative colitis
B Gall bladder stones
C Sclerosing cholangitis
D Choledochal cyst
E Colorectal carcinoma.

➜ Gall bladder carcinoma

11. Which of the following regarding gall bladder carcinoma are true?
A It is a rare disease.
B The majority are adenocarcinomas.
C The CA19–9 is elevated in 80 per cent of the cases.
D A palpable mass is an early sign.
E Prognosis is generally good.

Extended matching questions

➜ 1. Clinical conditions caused by gallstones

A Biliary colic
B Cholangitis
C Pancreatitis
D Gallstone ileus
E Empyema of the gall bladder
F Acute cholecystitis
G Gall bladder mucocele
H Gall bladder perforation/biliary peritonitis

Choose and match the correct diagnosis with each of the scenarios given below:

1 A 30-year-old female presents with a 2-day history of constant pain over the right upper quadrant (RUQ) associated with vomiting. She is febrile with a positive Murphy's sign.

2 A 56-year-old male presents with a week-long history of severe upper abdominal pain. He is very unwell with spiking fever. He has signs of right upper quadrant peritonism with an underlying, vaguely palpable, tender lump. Blood tests reveal an increased white cell count.

3 A 60-year-old male presents with a 6 h history of severe and constant generalised abdominal pain. On examination he is very unwell and in shock. The abdomen is distended with generalised guarding and rebound tenderness.

4 A 38-year-old female presents with a 6 h history of colicky abdominal pain over the RUQ. This radiates to the back and right shoulder. On examination she is afebrile with a soft abdomen.

5 A 40-year-old female being treated for acute cholecystitis is observed to have a non-tender palpable gall bladder. She is afebrile and systemically well.

6 A 78-year-old female with known gallstones for several years presents with central colicky abdominal pain and vomiting. She has also been constipated for the past few days. Clinical examination reveals a distended abdomen with increased bowel sounds.

7 A 42-year-old male presents with a sudden onset of severe epigastric pain radiating to the back. This is associated with repeated vomiting and retching. He is very uncomfortable and in shock. Clinical examination reveals upper abdominal tenderness with some guarding.

8 A 60-year-old male presents with a history of episodic abdominal pain, jaundice and fever with chills.

➜ 2. Types of biliary stones

A Mixed stones
B Cholesterol stones
C Black pigment stones
D Brown pigment stones

Choose and match the correct gallstone type with each of the descriptions given below:

1 They are usually solitary and pale and ovoid in appearance. Obesity, high-calorie diets and certain medications increase the risk of these stones.

2 Bile stasis and infected bile predispose to these stones. This stone formation is related to deconjugation of bilirubin diglucuronide by bacteria. These are also associated with the presence of foreign bodies such as endoprosthesis or parasites.

3 These are the commonest variety and are usually multiple and faceted. They have a crystalline structure on cross-section.

4 These are usually amorphous and contain an insoluble bilirubin polymer. They are associated with haemolytic conditions such as sickle cell anaemia and hereditary spherocytosis.

→ 3. Management of biliary problems

A Laparoscopic cholecystectomy
B ERCP – stenting
C Percutaneous transhepatic cholangiography (PTC) and antegrade stenting
D ERCP – stone extraction followed by cholecystectomy
E Surgery – palliative bypass
F Laparotomy – enterotomy and removal of stone
G Cholecystectomy and choledocholithotomy
H No active treatment
I Whipple's operation
J Subtotal cholecystectomy
K Cholecystostomy

Choose and match the correct management with each of the scenarios given below:

1 A 79-year-old female with a long history of gallstones presents with central colicky abdominal pain and vomiting. She has also been constipated for the past few days. Clinical examination reveals a distended abdomen with increased bowel sounds. Abdominal X-ray confirms features of small-bowel obstruction with pneumobilia.

2 A 92-year-old female with multiple co-morbidities is found to have incidental gallstones on abdominal ultrasound.

3 A 40-year-old female has been having episodes of colicky RUQ pain for the past 3 months. The pain radiates to her back and is associated with dyspeptic symptoms. Ultrasound scan confirms gall bladder stones with normal bile ducts. Blood tests show normal liver functions.

4 A 60-year-old male presents with progressive painless jaundice. Examination reveals a palpable non-tender gall bladder. Ultrasound and CT scans show a dilated bile duct with a pancreatic head tumour which is not resectable.

5 A 59-year-old female presents with progressive painless jaundice. Examination reveals a palpable non-tender gall bladder. Ultrasound and CT scans show a dilated bile duct with a small, malignant-looking tumour at the ampulla. Biopsies confirm malignancy and the tumour is considered to be resectable with no evidence of spread.

6 A 40-year-old female has been having episodes of colicky RUQ pain for the past 3 months. The pain radiates to her back and is associated with dyspeptic symptoms. Ultrasound scan confirms gall bladder stones and dilated bile ducts with stones. Blood tests show abnormal liver functions.

7 A 76-year-old male presents with progressive painless jaundice. Examination reveals a palpable tender liver. Ultrasound and CT scans show dilated intrahepatic bile ducts with a mass at the hilum. A contracted gall bladder and normal bile duct are seen. Attempts at ERCP are unsuccessful in stenting the stricture.

8 A 53-year-old man has presented with an acute abdomen and has been diagnosed to have an empyema of the gall bladder. Percutaneous drainage is unsuccessful and hence it is decided to

operate on him. At operation the gall bladder is tense and distended. Aspiration reveals frank pus. There are dense vascular adhesions around the gall bladder which makes dissection very difficult.

9 A 58-year-old male was admitted for an elective laparoscopic cholecystectomy. At operation, dense adhesions were present in the Calot's triangle and hence had to be converted to an open operation. A fundus-first technique is used but it is still difficult to dissect the Calot's triangle and reliably identify the structures.

10 A 46-year-old male has been having episodes of colicky RUQ pain for the past 8 months. The pain radiates to his back and is associated with dyspeptic symptoms. Ultrasound scan confirms gall bladder stones and dilated bile ducts with stones. Blood tests show abnormal liver functions. Attempts at ERCP to remove the bile duct stones are unsuccessful.

11 A 62-year-old male presents with progressive painless jaundice. He also has vomiting and is unable to tolerate orally. Examination reveals a palpable non-tender gall bladder and features of gastric outlet obstruction. Ultrasound and CT scans show a dilated bile duct with a pancreatic head tumour which is not resectable. ERCP is unsuccessful.

Answers: Multiple choice questions

➔ Anatomy of the gall bladder and bile ducts

1. C, E

The gall bladder is a pear-shaped structure, 7.5–12 cm long, with a normal capacity of about 35–50 mL. The cystic duct length can be variable but is around 3 cm long. The mucosa of the cystic duct is arranged in spiral folds known as the valves of Heister and is surrounded by a sphincteric structure called the sphincter of Lutkens. It joins the supraduodenal segment in 80 per cent of cases but may extend down into the retroduodenal or even retropancreatic part of the bile duct before joining it. The term 'Moynihan's hump' refers to 'caterpillar turn' – a tortuous course of the right hepatic artery which may run in front of the cystic duct. The mucosa of the gall bladder may show multiple indentations called the crypts of Luschka.

➔ Physiology of the gall bladder

2. B, E

The composition of the bile as it leaves the liver is approximately 97 per cent water, 1–2 per cent bile salts and 1 per cent pigments, cholesterol and fatty acids. The rate of bile secretion is controlled by cholecystokinin (CCK), which is released from the duodenal mucosa. The hepatic bile gets concentrated 5 to 10 times, with a corresponding increase in bile salts, bile pigments, cholesterol and calcium. The functions of the gall bladder include acting as a reservoir for the bile, concentrating the bile and the secretion of mucus.

➔ Investigations on the biliary tract

3. B, D

Abdominal ultrasound is the initial imaging modality of choice as it is accurate, readily available, inexpensive, non-invasive, involves no radiation and is quick to perform. It can also give information on the size of the gall bladder, the thickness of the gall bladder wall, presence of inflammation around the gall bladder, size of the common bile duct (CBD) and, occasionally, the presence of stones in the bile duct. A side-viewing endoscope is used during an ERCP to help locate the position of the ampulla and help in cannulation. Magnetic resonance cholangiopancreatography (MRCP) is helpful in evaluation and diagnosis of biliary disorders but has no therapeutic application.

Congenital abnormalities of the gall bladder and bile ducts

4. B, C, E

Extrahepatic biliary atresia is present in approximately 1 in 12 000 births. The extrahepatic bile ducts are progressively destroyed by inflammation and, if untreated, liver failure ensues by 3 years. This can involve the CBD, the CHD or the right and left hepatic ducts. Portoenterostomy (Kasai procedure) is the preferred operation in most cases. Caroli's disease is a rare condition characterised by multiple irregular saccular dilatations of the intrahepatic ducts with a normal extrahepatic biliary system. The aetiology is unknown but is thought to be hereditary. Associated conditions include biliary stasis, stones and cholangiocarcinoma. Treatment usually involves antibiotics for infections, removal of stones and occasionally lobectomy. Choledochal cysts are congenital dilatations of the intra- or extrahepatic biliary system. Sixty per cent of cases are diagnosed before the age of 10 years. Usual presentations are jaundice, fever, abdominal pain and a lump.

Gallstones

5. A, B, E

In the UK, 80 per cent of the stones are cholesterol or mixed, while in some parts of Asia 80 per cent are pigment stones. Pigment stones contain less than 30 per cent cholesterol. There are two types: black and brown. The black stones are largely composed of an insoluble bilirubin pigment polymer mixed with calcium phosphate and calcium bicarbonate. Overall 20–30 per cent of stones are black and this incidence rises with age. Black stones accompany haemolysis, usually hereditary spherocytosis and sickle cell disease. Brown pigment stones contain calcium bilirubinate, calcium palmitate and calcium stearate, as well as cholesterol. Brown pigment stones are rare in the gall bladder but are formed in the bile duct and are related to bile stasis, infected bile and the presence of foreign bodies in the bile duct.

The risks of having biliary colic and acute cholecystitis in a person with asymptomatic gallstones are 1–2 and 0.2 per cent/year, respectively. The risk of developing acute cholecystitis in a patient with biliary colic is 5 per cent/year. Courvoisier's law is usually associated with a pathology other than gallstones.

6. B, D

Most authors would suggest that it is safe to observe patients with asymptomatic gallstones. Prophylactic cholecystectomy, however, should be considered in diabetic patients, those with congenital haemolytic anaemia and those due to undergo surgery for morbid obesity. A broad-spectrum antibiotic is advised during the management of acute cholecystitis. Acute acalculous cholecystitis is seen particularly in patients recovering from major surgery, trauma, burns and multiple organ failure (MOF). The mortality can be high.

Gall bladder conditions

7. B, C, D, E

The porcelain gall bladder is associated with malignancy in up to 25 per cent of patients. It is therefore an indication for cholecystectomy.

Cholecystectomy

8. A, B, D

Routine Per-Operative Cholangiogram (POC) is not performed but may be helpful in selected patients and to clarify anatomy. Calot's triangle dissection may be hazardous in Mirizzi's syndrome (stone ulcerating through into the bile duct) and, if this is suspected, the infundibulum of the gall bladder should be opened, the stone removed and the infundibulum oversewn.

Obstructive jaundice

9. A, C, D, E

Charcot's triad consists of intermittent jaundice, abdominal pain and fever with chills. PSC is an idiopathic fibrosing inflammatory condition of the biliary tree that affects both the intra- and extrahepatic ducts. It is more common in males and usually occurs between the ages of 30 and 60 years.

Bile duct carcinoma

10. A, C, D

The other associations include hepatolithiasis and liver fluke infestations. Overall, only 10–15 per cent are suitable for surgical resection and the median survival is 18 months.

Gall bladder carcinoma

11. A, B, C

A palpable mass is a late sign. Gall bladder carcinoma has a very poor prognosis with a median survival of less than 6 months and a 5-year survival of 5 per cent.

Answers: Extended matching questions

1. Clinical conditions caused by gallstones

1F, 2E, 3H, 4A, 5G, 6D, 7C, 8B

2. Types of biliary stones

1B, 2D, 3A, 4C

3. Management of biliary problems

1F, 2H, 3A, 4B, 5I, 6D, 7C, 8K, 9J, 10G, 11E

64 The pancreas

Multiple choice questions

Anatomy

1. Which of the following statements are true?

A The pancreas weighs 200 g.
B The uncinate process lies behind the superior mesenteric vessels.
C The vast majority of pancreatic tissue is composed of exocrine acinar tissue.
D Of the endocrine cells, 75 per cent are B cells, 20 per cent are A cells and the remainder are D cells
E The accessory pancreatic duct drains the head and uncinate process.

Investigations

2. Which of the following statements are false?

A Ultrasonography (US) is the initial investigation of choice in the jaundiced patient.
B When doing a computed tomography (CT) scan, initially an unenhanced scan must be done followed by a scan after intravenous contrast injection (CECT).
C While doing a magnetic resonance cholangiopancreatography (MRCP), intravenous secretin injection helps to determine any obstruction to the pancreatic duct.
D An increase in serum amylase is diagnostic of acute pancreatitis.
E Endoscopic retrograde cholangiopan-creatography (ERCP) should always be preceded by a plain radiograph.

Pancreatic injury

3. Which of the following statements are true?

A Pancreatic injury is common following blunt abdominal trauma.
B Pancreatic injury is often accompanied by damage to the liver, spleen and duodenum.
C The serum amylase is raised in most cases of pancreatic injury.
D A CECT scan will delineate the damage.
E In doubtful cases, urgent ERCP is helpful.

4. Which of the following statements is false?

A All patients with pancreatic trauma should undergo an exploratory laparotomy.
B Pancreatic duct disruption requires surgical exploration.
C Severe injury to the duodenum and the head of the pancreas requires a pancreatoduodenectomy.
D After conservative management for pancreatic injury, duct stricture and pseudocyst may occur as complications.
E During splenectomy, iatrogenic injury to the pancreatic tail can occur.

Acute pancreatitis

5. Which of the following statements is false?

A Acute pancreatitis accounts for 3 per cent of hospital admissions in the UK for abdominal pain.
B Acute pancreatitis is classified into mild and severe.
C 80 per cent of cases are mild acute pancreatitis, with a mortality rate of 1 per cent.
D 20 per cent are severe acute pancreatitis, with a mortality of 20–50 per cent.
E In all cases of acute pancreatitis, there is a marked rise in serum amylase.

6. **Which one of the following causes of acute pancreatitis is due to a congenital anatomical variation?**
A Gallstones
B Hereditary pancreatitis
C Pancreatic divisum
D Autoimmune pancreatitis
E Hyperparathyroidism.

7. **Which of the following statements are true regarding the aetiology of postoperative acute pancreatitis?**
A Following ERCP the incidence of acute pancreatitis is 10 per cent.
B Therapeutic intervention during ERCP has a higher incidence.
C Patients after cardiothoracic surgery may develop acute pancreatitis.
D The post-gastrectomy patient may develop acute pancreatitis.
E In a post-cholecystectomy patient, acute pancreatitis may be due to a retained stone.

8. **Which of the following are not parameters to assess the severity of acute pancreatitis in either Ranson or Glasgow score?**
A Age
B White cell count
C Serum amylase
D Serum calcium
E Blood urea
F Lactate dehydrogenase (LDH) and aspartate transaminase (AST).

9. **Which of the following signs have been known to occur in acute pancreatitis?**
A Trousseau's sign
B Courvoisier's sign
C Boas' sign
D Grey–Turner's sign
E Cullen's sign.

10. **Which of the following statements are true with regard to pseudocysts?**
A Pseudocysts occur within the first week of onset of acute pancreatitis.
B They can be confused with cystic neoplasms.
C The majority of them require intervention.
D Gastrointestinal bleeding may be a complication of a pseudocyst.
E They can arise after blunt trauma to the upper abdomen.

11. **Which of the following statements are true with regard to complications in acute pancreatitis?**
A Patients with severe acute pancreatitis require a CECT scan to detect pancreatic necrosis.
B In severe acute pancreatitis, a laparotomy must be done in all cases of pancreatic necrosis.
C Aneurysm of the superior mesenteric artery can occur.
D The vast majority of patients with peripancreatic sepsis can be treated conservatively.
E Pleural effusion is seen in 10–20 per cent of patients.

→ Surgical treatment

12. **The radical curative operation of pancreatoduodenectomy for carcinoma of the head of the pancreas, periampullary carcinoma or the lower end of CBD goes by which name?**
A Millin
B Billroth
C Whipple
D Wertheim
E Ombrédanne.

Extended matching questions

→ 1. Pancreatic pathology

A Acute pancreatitis
B Chronic pancreatitis
C Carcinoma of the head of the pancreas

D Pseudocyst of the pancreas
E Periampullary carcinoma

Choose and match the correct diagnosis with each of the scenarios given below:

1 A 65-year-old man complains of intense itching and jaundice of 6 weeks' duration. He has upper abdominal discomfort and has noticed of late that his urine is deep yellow in colour and his stools are pale. He has some weight loss. On examination he is deeply jaundiced with scratch marks all over his body; abdominal examination reveals a globular discrete mass in the right upper quadrant.

2 A 10-year-old boy presents with upper abdominal pain of 2 weeks' duration. This is associated with upper abdominal distension, nausea, intermittent vomiting and some weight loss, which he puts down to his loss of appetite. On abdominal examination he looks unwell, with a smooth mass in his epigastrium which is tense and does not move with respiration. There is bruising over the skin of the epigastrium and, when questioned about it, he says it was the result of his falling off his bike and the handlebar sticking into his tummy.

3 A 45-year-old woman, who is on the waiting list for a laparoscopic cholecystectomy, presents as an emergency with severe epigastric pain radiating to the back and the rest of the abdomen of 3 h duration. She has nausea, has vomited a few times and has retching. On examination she is tachypnoeic, has tachycardia and a blood pressure of 110/60 mmHg. She is slightly icteric. Abdominal examination reveals a Cullen's sign, extreme tenderness all over the abdomen with rebound and rigidity.

4 A 55-year-old man complains of intermittent jaundice associated with itching. This is associated with anorexia, weight loss and upper abdominal discomfort. On examination the patient is anaemic, has scratch marks over his body, is slightly jaundiced and has a gall bladder that is just palpable.

5 A 50-year-old male patient presents with dull aching pain in his epigastrium and umbilical areas radiating to the back for the last 6 months. He has episodes of exacerbation of this pain which lasts for a day or two. This is associated with nausea and occasional vomiting and diarrhoea most days. He has lost some weight over this period. Two months ago he was diagnosed with type 2 diabetes and is on oral medication. He admits to more than average alcohol consumption. Clinical examination shows no abnormality except for generalised tenderness.

Answers: Multiple choice questions

→ Anatomy

1. B, C, D, E

→ Investigations

2. D

A markedly increased serum amylase is highly suggestive of acute pancreatitis, but not diagnostic, as other conditions, such as perforated peptic ulcer, mesenteric vascular occlusion, ruptured ectopic pregnancy and a retroperitoneal haematoma, can produce a raised amylase. An unenhanced CT always precedes a CECT to look for pancreatic or biliary calcification. After contrast injection, arterial and venous phases delineate accurately space-occupying lesions. During an magnetic resonance cholangiopancreatography (MRCP), secretin injection will show emptying of the pancreatic duct, thereby showing the absence or presence of obstruction. A plain X-ray of the abdomen should precede an ERCP to look for calcification.

Pancreatic injury

3. B, C, D, E

Pancreatic injury is rare in blunt upper abdominal trauma because of the retroperitoneal position of the organ. Therefore, for the pancreas to be injured, the force of trauma has to be severe. Thus the liver, duodenum and spleen are frequently damaged. A raised serum amylase indicates damage to the pancreas. A CECT scan will delineate the damage, failing which an urgent ERCP should be done.

4. A

All pancreatic injuries do not need a laparotomy. A stable patient following a blunt injury should be thoroughly assessed. Disruption of the main pancreatic duct is an indication for an operation. Penetrating injury in an unstable patient needs urgent surgical exploration. Severe injuries to the head of the pancreas and duodenum require an emergency pancreatoduodenectomy – a procedure to be carried out by the expert hepatobiliary surgeon.

Stricture of the pancreatic duct may occur later, resulting in recurrent acute pancreatitis. A pseudocyst may develop in the aftermath of the injury. Unrecognised damage to the pancreatic tail during splenectomy may cause a pancreatic fistula.

Acute pancreatitis

5. E

All cases of acute pancreatitis do not cause a rise in serum amylase. A normal amylase in acute pancreatitis may occur when the disease is so severe that the entire pancreas has been destroyed and there is not enough pancreatic tissue left to elaborate the enzyme. A normal amylase level may also be because the blood has been taken too late and the patient has recovered from the acute attack, which has been transient.

6. C

During the development of the pancreas, most of the dorsal duct drains into the proximal part of the ventral duct. The proximal part of the dorsal duct persists as accessory pancreatic duct. Late in the development or in the postnatal period, the ducts fuse. Eighty-five per cent of infants have patent accessory ducts, while in only 40 per cent of adults is it patent. In 10 per cent the duct may not fuse. In such a situation, separate drainage occurs into the duodenum – pancreatic divisum, in which the ventral duct drains the uncinate process.

7. B, C, D, E

The incidence of acute pancreatitis following ERCP is 1–3 per cent. This incidence rises if therapeutic intervention such as sphincterotomy or balloon dilatation is carried out.

8. C

Serum amylase is not one of the blood results for assessing severity. Besides the other tests mentioned in the list, serum albumin and arterial oxygen saturation are the other important factors.

9. D, E

The above signs are not pathognomonic although, if present, are very suggestive of acute haemorrhagic pancreatitis. Grey–Turner's sign (described in leaking abdominal aortic aneurysm) is a bluish discoloration of the flanks as a result of blood tracking along the fascial planes. Cullen's sign (described in ruptured ectopic pregnancy) is haemorrhage around the umbilicus, the blood having tracked there through the falciform ligament.

10. B, D, E

After acute pancreatitis, a pseudocyst usually takes up to 4 weeks or more to develop. Occasionally a chronic pseudocyst can be confused with a cystic neoplasm. Endoscopic ultrasound (EUS)-guided aspiration of the cyst fluid, which is sent for carcinoembryonic antigen (CEA), amylase levels and cytology, helps in arriving at a diagnosis.

Spontaneous resolution of a pseudocyst occurs in most cases because the majority have a communication with the main pancreatic duct. Gastrointestinal bleeding can occur if the pseudocyst ruptures into the stomach or duodenum.

11. A, C, D, E

Patients with severe acute pancreatitis are treated in the ITU and, while they are there, a CECT is carried out at least every other day to look for pancreatic necrosis. If the CECT shows areas of reduced enhancement and peripancreatic fluid collection with pockets of gas within, it means that the necrosis is infected. Confirmation of infection is carried out by fine-needle aspiration cytology. If the fluid is purulent and obviously infected, the patient is treated by antibiotics and insertion of the widest possible tube drains. The fluid can be viscous and the drain may require regular flushing and repeated replacement. If the sepsis worsens despite vigorous measures, a pancreatic necrosectomy should be undertaken – a challenging procedure which is not often encountered.

A superior mesenteric artery aneurysm can occur. The anatomical position of the superior mesenteric vessels behind the neck and between the inferior border and uncinate process of the pancreas makes these vessels vulnerable to compression and inflammation, resulting in an aneurysm (sometimes referred to as a pseudoaneurysm) of the artery and thrombosis of the vein.

➜ Surgical treatment

12. C

Answers: Extended matching questions

➜ 1. Pancreatic pathology

1C

This patient has painless obstructive jaundice with a distended gall bladder and weight loss – classical features of a carcinoma of the head of the pancreas. Besides all the usual blood tests, he needs an US followed by a CT scan to see the solid mass in the head of the pancreas obstructing the lower end of the CBD. If there is evidence of secondaries in the abdomen, as there usually are, he should be treated by insertion of a stent in the CBD to alleviate his intense pruritus.

2D

This young boy has developed a pseudocyst of the pancreas. About 4 weeks ago his bicycle injury produced blunt upper abdominal trauma with transient acute pancreatitis. Although his symptoms at that time were not severe enough for him to seek help, there was a contused pancreas which later resulted in a pseudocyst. He needs an US and CT scan for confirmation. This is to be followed by a decision as to the best method of treating him, whether by percutaneous or endoscopic drainage, or the open operation of cystogastrostomy.

3A

This patient has acute pancreatitis of biliary origin. She needs to be resuscitated forthwith with analgesia and intravenous fluids, and blood investigations need to be carried out, in particular serum amylase. This would be elevated to well over 1000 IU. If the serum amylase is not elevated, the diagnosis of acute pancreatitis should then be confirmed by a CECT scan. The patient is then stratified as mild or severe acute pancreatitis and managed accordingly. An US of the biliary tract is repeated or an magnetic resonance cholangiopancreatography (MRCP) is done to look for a stone in the common bile duct (CBD). If there is a stone in the CBD, an ERCP and endoscopic papillotomy are carried out with laparoscopic cholecystectomy at the same admission a few days later.

4E

This patient has intermittent obstructive jaundice (where the icterus waxes and wanes) with a gall bladder that is minimally palpable. His anaemia and weight loss should point to an underlying malignant lesion in the region of the lower end of the CBD. As the jaundice is intermittent, the diagnosis is obviously a periampullary carcinoma. In this condition, as the tumour grows, the patient's jaundice gets deeper; as the carcinoma outgrows its blood supply, there is necrosis of the cancer, resulting in alleviation of the jaundice. He needs an US, CECT, EUS and biopsy of the lesion. If the staging shows no distant spread, the patient should next undergo the final staging procedure of laparoscopy and laparoscopic US to look for small peritoneal or liver secondaries. If there are no secondaries, the patient should then be considered for radical pancreatoduodenectomy.

5B

This patient has alcoholic chronic pancreatitis with exocrine and endocrine dysfunction (diarrhoea and diabetes). He should have all the usual haematological and biochemical investigations including estimation of 24-hours faecal fat. Confirmation is by US and CECT and ERCP to visualise the anatomy of the pancreatic duct. He should be managed by the physicians for his pancreatic insufficiency and the pain clinic for analgesia.

65 The small and large intestines

Multiple choice questions

➜ Anatomy

1. **Which of the following statements are false?**

A The small bowel is approximately 10 metres long.
B The colon is approximately 3 metres long.
C The most fixed part of the small bowel is the duodenum.
D The jejunum is wider, thicker and more vascular than the ileum.
E Peyer's patches are contained in the ileum.

➜ Diverticula of small intestine

2. **Which of the following statements are true?**

A Duodenal diverticulum may result from a long-standing duodenal ulcer.
B Jejunal diverticula may give rise to malabsorption problems.
C A Meckel's diverticulum can cause severe lower gastrointestinal haemorrhage.
D A suspected Meckel's diverticulum is best imaged by a barium meal and follow through.
E Pain originating in a Meckel's diverticulum is located around the umbilicus

➜ Diverticular disease of colon

3. **Which of the following statements are false?**

A In the Western world, 60 per cent of the population over the age of 60 have diverticular disease.
B A low-fibre diet causes the disease.
C These diverticula consist of mucosa, muscle and serosa.
D Those with perforation have a 10 times higher mortality than those with an inflammatory mass.
E Sepsis is the principal cause of morbidity.

4. **Which of the following is not a complication of diverticular disease of the colon?**

A Paracolic abscess
B Fistulae
C Lower gastrointestinal haemorrhage
D Carcinoma
E Stricture.

5. **Which of the following are not true in complicated diverticular disease?**

A Urinary symptoms may be the predominant presentation at times.
B Profuse colonic haemorrhage may occur in 17 per cent.
C Fistulae occur in 5 per cent of cases.
D The commonest fistula is coloenteric.
E In acute diverticulitis, CT scan is the 'gold standard' for imaging.

6. **Which of the following is not a cause of vesicocolic fistula?**

A Carcinoma of rectosigmoid
B Radiation enteritis
C Crohn's colitis
D Diverticular disease
E Amoebic colitis.

7. **In the surgical treatment of diverticular disease, which of the following statements are true?**

A Colonoscopy must be carried out in all elective cases.
B Barium enema is essential prior to elective operation.
C Primary resection and end-to-end anastomosis mustt be carried out in all cases.

D Hartmann's operation is the procedure of choice in perforated diverticulitis.
E In vesicocolic fistula, a one-stage operation can usually be done.

➜ Ulcerative colitis

8. Which of the following statements are true in ulcerative colitis (UC)?
A In 95 per cent of cases, the disease starts in the rectum and spreads proximally.
B It is a diffuse disease affecting all the layers of the large bowel.
C Granulomas are a typical microscopic feature.
D The transverse colon is affected in toxic megacolon.
E Patients may present as an emergency with fulminating colitis in 5–10 per cent.

9. Which of the following is not a complication of UC?
A Carcinoma
B Primary sclerosing cholangitis
C Internal fistulae
D Ankylosing spondylitis
E Perforation.

10. Which of the following is not a barium enema finding in UC?
A Loss of haustrations
B Narrow contracted colon
C Increase in the presacral space
D Cobblestone appearance
E Backwash ileitis.

11. What is colonoscopy routinely used for in UC?
A To assess the extent of the disease
B To distinguish it from Crohn's disease
C To monitor the response to treatment
D To carry out surveillance for the development of cancer
E To assess severity in acute cases.

12. Which of the following criteria do not indicate severe disease in UC?
A More than four motions a day
B Pyrexia of over 37.5°C
C Tachycardia >90/min
D Tachypnoea >20/min
E Hypoalbuminaemia <30 g/L.

13. Which UC patients have an enhanced risk of developing cancer?
A Those who have had the disease since childhood.
B Those who have had the disease for over 10 years.
C Those who have had a very severe first attack.
D Those who have the entire colon involved.
E Those who have another member of the family with the disease.

14. Which of the following drugs are not used in the medical treatment of UC?
A Prednisolone
B 5-ASA compounds
C Predsol enema
D Azathioprine
E Isoniazid.

15. In the management of a severe attack of UC, which of the following is not true?
A Every patient needs a proctocolectomy after resuscitation.
B Daily plain abdominal X-ray is taken to assess transverse colon dilatation.
C Parenteral high-calorie alimentation is instituted.
D Intravenous hydrocortisone is given.
E Azathioprine or cyclosporin A is given.

16. What are the indications for surgery in UC?
A Severe fulminating disease not responding to vigorous medical treatment.
B Severe dysplastic change or cancer on biopsy.
C Non-compliance of medical treatment.
D Chronic steroid-dependent disease requiring large doses.
E Extraintestinal disease.

17. Which of the following statements regarding surgery in UC is false?
A In the emergency situation, total abdominal colectomy and ileostomy should be the procedure of choice.
B Proctocolectomy and ileostomy are associated with the lowest complication rate.

C Restorative proctocolectomy with an ileoanal pouch should be considered in all patients.
D Colectomy with ileorectal anastomosis is the most favoured procedure.
E Ileostomy with a continent intra-abdominal pouch is not often done.

➜ Crohn's disease

18. Which of the following statements is not true of Crohn's disease (CD)?
A The ileum is affected in 60 per cent of cases.
B It affects the entire thickness of the bowel.
C Non-caseating granulomas are found in only 60 per cent of patients.
D One in 10 patients have a first-degree relative with the disease.
E A patient can be cured of CD once the diseased small or large bowel is removed.

19. Which of the following pathological features is not found in CD?
A Internal fistulae
B Serpiginous and aphthous ulcers
C Chronic inflammation involves all layers of the bowel wall
D Pseudopolypi
E Cobblestone mucosa.

20. Which of the following can cause acute presentation of CD?
A Mimicking acute appendicitis
B Perforation
C Intestinal obstruction
D Toxic megacolon
E All of the above.

21. Which of the following are true of large-bowel CD?
A 50–70 per cent will have an anal lesion.
B Non-caseating giant-cell granulomas are most common in perianal disease.
C In a strictured area, malignancy can occur.
D A perianal abscess or a fissure may be the first presenting feature.
E Surgery is usually indicated.

22. Which of the following is not a clinical presentation of CD?
A Bloodstained diarrhoea
B Intermittent abdominal pain
C Mass in the right iliac fossa
D Typical evening rise of temperature
E Pneumaturia and urinary tract infections.

23. Which of the following statements about imaging in CD are true?
A Small-bowel enema is the imaging of choice in small-bowel disease.
B Barium enema and colonoscopy should be done for large-bowel disease.
C MRI is the 'gold standard' for perianal fistulae.
D CT scan is used for suspected intra-abdominal abscess and internal fistulae.
E All of the above.

24. Which of the following drugs are used in the treatment of CD?
A Steroids
B 5-ASA compounds
C Azathioprine
D Infliximab
E Metronidazole
F All of the above.

25. Which of the following operations is not done in CD?
A Segmental resections
B Strictureplasty
C Proctocolectomy and ileostomy
D Colectomy and ileorectal anastomosis
E Restorative proctocolectomy with ileoanal pouch.

26. Which of the following statements about inflammatory bowel disease (UC and CD) is not true?
A Patients must be managed jointly by the physician and surgeon.
B Surgery, when indicated, must be as radical as possible.
C Patients must be given a good trial of optimum medical treatment prior to surgery.
D There is more chance of a cure after surgery in UC than in CD.
E In emergency presentation, patients must be vigorously resuscitated prior to operation and managed in the ITU postoperatively.

Tumours of the large intestine

27. **In familial adenomatous polyposis (FAP), which of the following statements is false?**
   - A It is inherited as a Mendelian dominant condition.
   - B More than 80 per cent occur in patients with a positive family history.
   - C The majority will become malignant.
   - D The condition usually manifests by the age of 15 years.
   - E Family members should be offered genetic testing in their early teens.
   - F At-risk family members should be offered annual colonoscopic surveillance from the age of 12 years.

28. **In FAP, which of these statements are true?**
   - A 20 per cent of FAP arise as a result of new mutations in the adenomatous polyposis coli (APC) gene.
   - B Large-bowel cancer occurs 15–20 years after the onset of the disease.
   - C On surveillance, if there are no polyps by the age of 30 years, FAP is unlikely.
   - D Polyps do not develop anywhere else other than the colon.
   - E Colectomy with ileorectal anastomosis may result in rectal cancer later.

Carcinoma of the colon

29. **Which of the following are true in hereditary non-polyposis colorectal cancer (HNPCC)?**
   - A The lifetime risk of developing colorectal cancer is 80 per cent.
   - B The mean age of diagnosis is 44 years.
   - C Females with HNPCC have a 30–50 per cent risk of developing endometrial cancer.
   - D It can be diagnosed by genetic testing.
   - E It is a much more malignant type of cancer.
   - F The majority occur in the proximal colon.

30. **Which of the following statements are true with regard to colorectal cancer?**
   - A Almost 60 per cent occur in the rectosigmoid region.
   - B Reduced dietary fibre is associated with an increased risk.
   - C The least malignant form is the cauliflower type.
   - D 20 per cent present as an emergency with intestinal obstruction.
   - E All of the above.

31. **Which of the following statements are false?**
   - A Right colonic cancers present with features of anaemia.
   - B Left colonic cancers present with rectal bleeding and obstructive symptoms.
   - C Even for an experienced colonoscopist, the failure rate to visualise the caecum is 10 per cent.
   - D Intravenous urography (IVU) should be routinely done.
   - E Synchronous cancers occur in 5 per cent.

32. **In large bowel cancer, which of the following statements are true?**
   - A Thorough preoperative assessment and staging should be done with colonoscopy, US and spiral CT.
   - B Resection is not done if the patient has liver metastases.
   - C If, at operation, hepatic metastases are found, biopsy should be done.
   - D Hepatic resection for metastases should be considered as a staged procedure.
   - E Over 95 per cent of colonic carcinomas can be resected.

Enterocutaneous or faecal fistula

33. **Which of the following is false with regard to an enterocutaneous fistula?**
   - A The commonest cause is postoperative.
   - B A high-output fistula is defined as one where there is >1 L/day.
   - C They should be thoroughly assessed with barium studies and CT scans.
   - D They always need an operation to cure the problem.
   - E Hypoproteinaemia and sepsis often accompany the condition.

→ Stoma

34. With regard to a stoma, which of the following statements are true?

A An anterior resection is better de-functioned by a loop ileostomy than by a transverse loop colostomy.
B A stoma is always spouted.
C Fluid and electrolyte problems are more often encountered in ileostomy patients.
D Most colostomy complications are due to poor technique.
E When fashioning a colostomy, it is essential to close the lateral paracolic gutter to prevent internal herniation.

Extended matching questions

→ 1. Clinical presentations of small and large intestine pathology

A Diverticular disease
B Crohn's disease
C Ulcerative colitis
D Carcinoma of the caecum
E Carcinoma of the descending colon

Choose and match the correct diagnoses with each of the scenarios given below:

1 A 60-year-old woman complains of feeling tired while doing her usual household work over the last 3 months. She has been short of breath climbing one flight of stairs at home. Her haemoglobin is 8.5 g/L. Abdominal examination reveals a mobile mass in the right iliac fossa.

2 A 45-year-old male patient complains of diarrhoea with mucus and blood. He has three to four such motions a day, which are associated with dull aching in his lower abdomen. He has had these symptoms for the past 4 months during which time he has lost about 10 pounds in weight. Abdominal examination reveals some vague tenderness. Rectal examination shows blood and mucus, and sigmoidoscopy shows hyperaemic mucosa, which bleeds easily.

3 A 60-year-old male patient complains of frequency of micturition, discomfort while passing urine which is very foul smelling and sometimes contains brown material. On questioning he admits to passing air bubbles in his urine and recently has been constipated. On examination of his abdomen there is nothing to find. Urine examination shows heavy growth of *E. coli*.

4 A 55-year-old male has presented as an emergency with an acute perianal abscess. He has had frequent loose motions occasionally mixed with blood on and off for many months. He also suffers from colicky abdominal pain. He has a feeling of heaviness in his right iliac fossa. On examination he has an acute perianal abscess and a mass in the right iliac fossa.

5 A 70-year-old man complains of constipation for 4 months. He has to take increasing amounts of laxatives to have a bowel action. Following a bowel action, he is left with a feeling of insufficient evacuation. On straining at stools, he passes blood from his anus. On examination there is nothing to find except some evidence of weight loss, as seen by his loose trousers requiring an extra notch in his belt.

→ 2. Imaging of small and large intestine pathology

A Foreign body in rectum
B Diverticular stricture
C Carcinoma of the ascending colon
D Crohn's disease
E Intussusception
F Ulcerative colitis
G Intestinal obstruction

Choose and match the correct diagnoses with each of Figs 65.1–65.7 below:

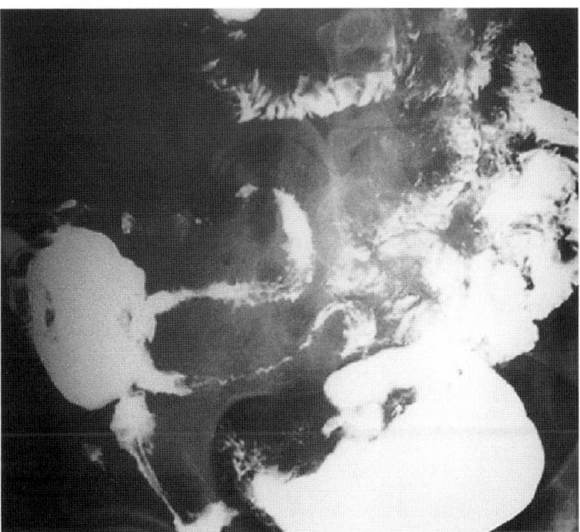

Figure 65.1a

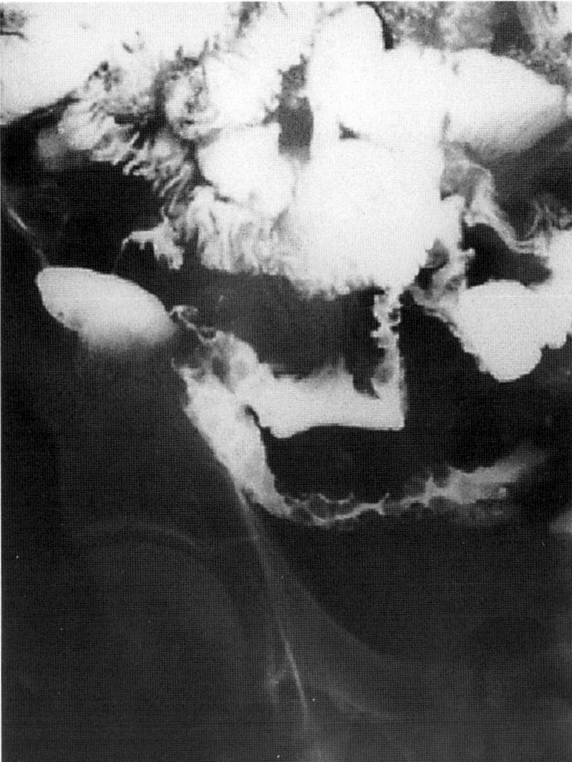

Figure 65.1b

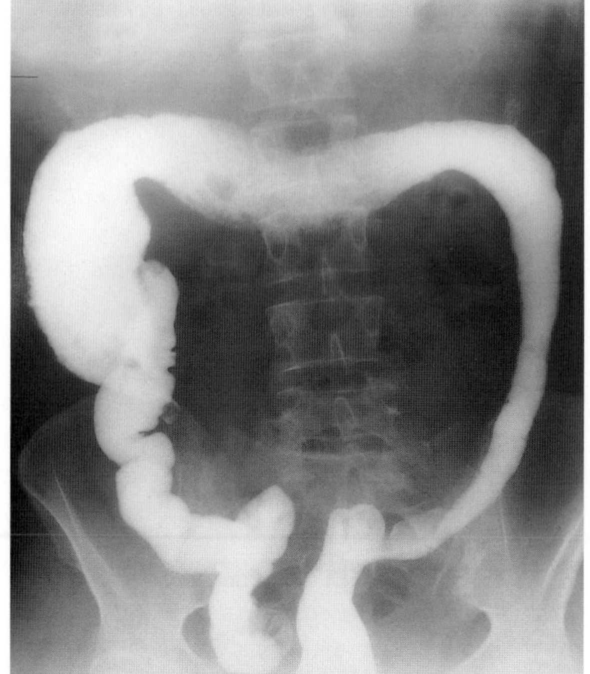

Figure 65.2

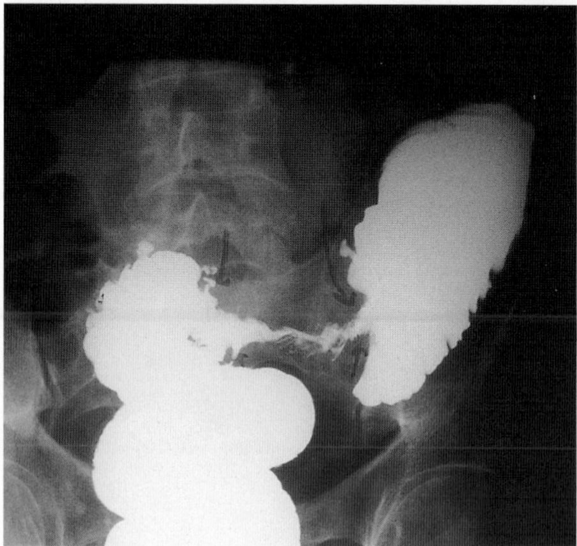

Figure 65.3a

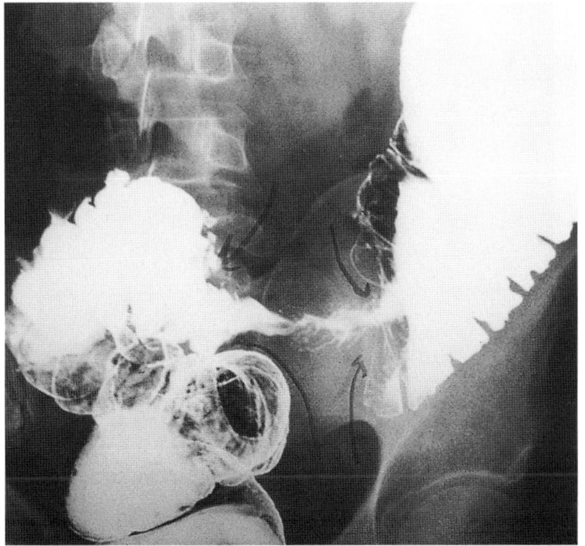

Figure 65.3b

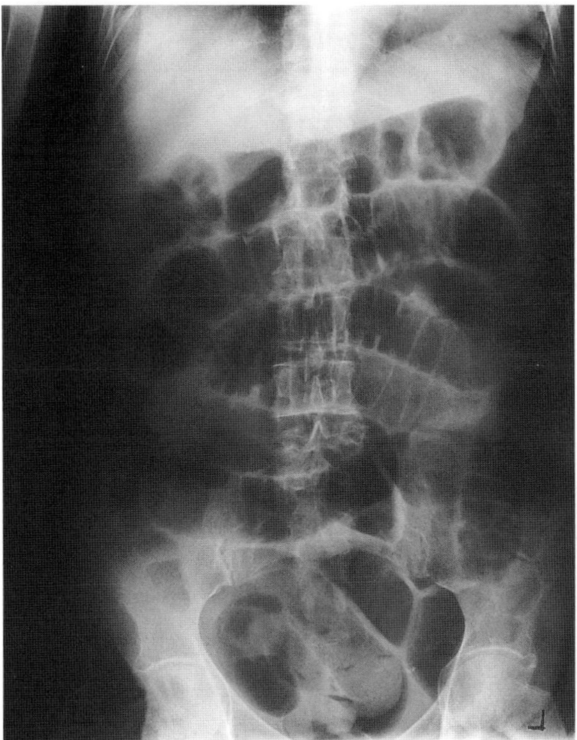

Figure 65.4

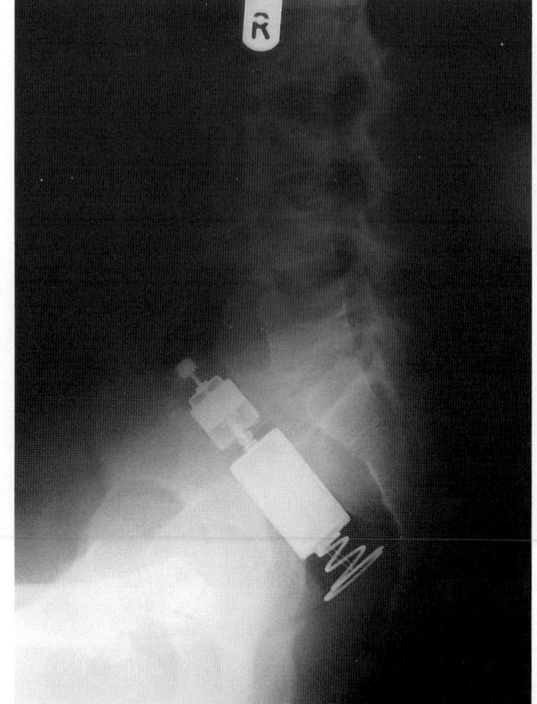

Figure 65.5

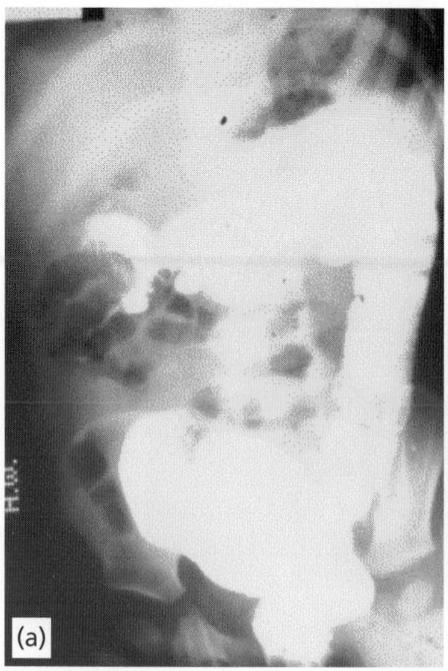

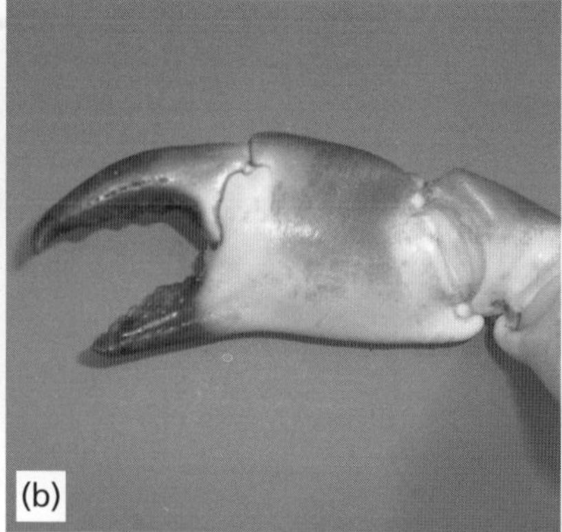

Figure 65.6

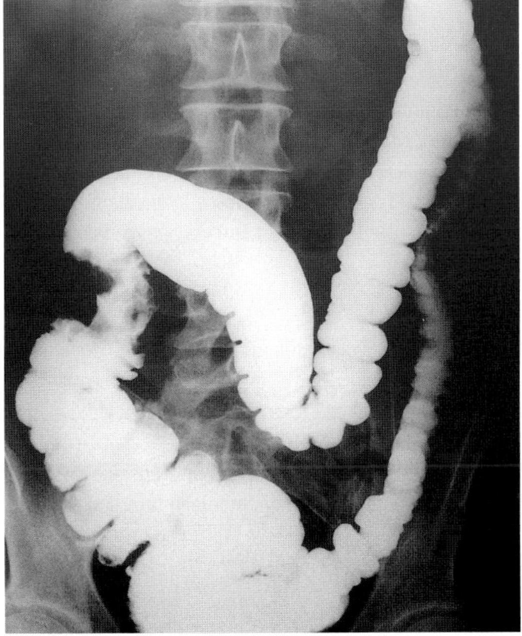

Figure 65.7

Answers: Multiple choice questions

Anatomy

1. A, B

The small bowel is approximately 7 metres long and the colon is 1.5 metres long. The duodenum is devoid of mesentery and therefore the most fixed part of the small bowel. This anatomical fact makes it vulnerable to injury from severe blunt abdominal trauma.

Diverticula of small intestine

2. A, B, C, E

An acquired duodenal diverticulum is always the outcome of a long-standing duodenal ulceration causing duodenal stenosis. Jejunal diverticula, although they may be asymptomatic, can cause malabsorption problems: anaemia, steatorrhoea, hypoproteinaemia and vitamin B12 deficiency.

A Meckel's diverticulum can be the source of a major lower gastrointestinal bleed from a peptic ulcer arising from ectopic gastric mucosa. The ideal imaging method would be a small-bowel enema. Scanning after a patient's own red blood cells are labelled with technetium-99 is an accurate method of identifying such a source of bleeding. As the diverticulum is part of the midgut, pain originating from it would be felt initially around the umbilicus.

Diverticular disease of colon

3. C

Colonic diverticula are acquired. Therefore they consist of mucosa only, covered by serosa. They protrude through the circular muscle where the blood vessels enter the colonic wall, a point of weakness.

4. D

Whilst carcinoma is not a complication of diverticular disease, it coexists in 12 per cent.

5. D

When a patient presents with urinary symptoms in diverticular disease, it indicates a vesicocolic fistula, which is the commonest type of fistula that occurs. Profuse colonic haemorrhage may occur and usually settles with conservative management. In acute diverticulitis a CT scan is the imaging of choice as it demonstrates bowel wall thickening, abscess formation and any other coincidental disease. CT guidance can also be used to drain an abscess percutaneously.

6. E

7. A, B, D, E

In the elective situation, a colonoscopy and barium enema must be done to exclude a coincidental carcinoma. Because of narrowing of the bowel, it may not always be possible to do a full colonoscopy. Primary resection and anastomosis can be done in the elective patient but not in the patient with perforated diverticulitis; only in selected cases can it be attempted in an emergency after intraoperative colonic irrigation. Hartmann's operation is the safest alternative. In a vesicocolic fistula, after thorough investigation, a one-stage resection and anastomosis can be done.

Ulcerative colitis

8. A, D, E

In 95 per cent of cases, the disease affects the rectum and spreads proximally. It is a diffuse inflammatory bowel disease that affects the mucosa and superficial submucosa only; in severe disease the deeper layers are involved. Granulomas do not occur in UC; crypt abscesses are the typical microscopic feature. In acute toxic megacolon, the transverse colon is affected. Up to 10 per cent of patients may present as an emergency with acute fulminant UC.

9. C

10. D

11. A, B, C, D

Colonoscopy has a vital role in the management of UC. It should not be used in the acute case for fear of causing perforation. A plain abdominal X-ray can help to assess the severity of the disease.

12. D

13. A, B, C, D

14. E

15. A

A severe case of UC is a medical emergency but every patient does not require a proctocolectomy. Vigorous medical treatment is instituted according to the above regimen and if improvement does not occur within 3–5 days, surgery should be undertaken. Prolonged high-dose steroid treatment is dangerous because silent perforation can occur.

16. A, B, D, E

17. D

Colectomy with ileorectal anastomosis is a rare procedure because the rectum is diseased in the vast majority. The patient needs regular rectal surveillance for malignancy. Although the operation avoids a stoma and has minimal risk of sexual dysfunction, it has largely been replaced by restorative proctocolectomy.

Crohn's disease

18. E

Crohn's disease is not a curable disease. It can recur in other parts of the gastrointestinal tract even after removal of a diseased section of the bowel. Hence resection for CD must always be conservative, and as little bowel as possible should be sacrificed.

19. D

Pseudopolypi do not occur in CD. It is a feature seen in advanced chronic UC due to regeneration of normal mucosa, also called inflammatory polyps.

20. E

21. A, B, C, D

22. D

Evening pyrexia is not a clinical feature of CD. It is suggestive of abdominal tuberculosis.

23. E

24. F

Crohn's disease is mainly treated medically, with all the above drugs used from time to time. Steroids are the mainstay of treatment and help in remission in 70–80 per cent of cases. 5-ASA compounds are particularly useful in colonic disease. Immunosuppressive agents are used for their steroid-sparing effect. Infliximab is a monoclonal antibody that is useful in fistulae, particularly perianal ones. Metronidazole is known to control disease activity in ileocolic and colonic disease.

25. E

In proven CD, restorative proctocolectomy with ileoanal pouch is not done because of the high incidence of recurrence. Moreover, the ileum to be used for a pouch may be involved with the disease. Perianal disease, which is common in colonic CD, prevents this operation being carried out.

26. B

Surgery must be as conservative as possible in CD. In UC, in emergency situations such as toxic megacolon or perforation, a total abdominal colectomy and ileostomy is performed, avoiding a pelvic dissection. The rectal stump is brought out as a mucous fistula or closed just beneath the skin.

Tumours of the large intestine

27. C

In all (100 per cent) of untreated patients, carcinoma of the large bowel will result.

28. A, B, C, E

In a fifth of patients where there is no family history, FAP occurs as a result of new mutations in the APC gene. Onset of the disease is around the age of 15 years and cancer develops 15–20 years later. If, on annual colonoscopic surveillance, polyps have not developed by the age of 30 years, FAP is unlikely. Polyps do develop in the stomach and duodenum; hence, postoperatively, patients should have gastroscopies carried out. The risk of cancer developing in the rectal stump is 10 per cent over 30 years.

Carcinoma of the colon

29. A, B, C, D, F

30. E

31. D

Intravenous urography is not a routine investigation for colorectal cancer. It is done in left colonic cancers when an US or CT shows left hydronephrosis to see the function of the right kidney and the extent of involvement of the left ureter.

32. A, D, E

Thorough preoperative assessment with confirmation by biopsy and staging is essential. Even with liver secondaries, the appropriate hemicolectomy is carried out as there is no better palliation than to remove the original tumour. Biopsy of a liver secondary should never be done as this may cause tumour dissemination.

→ Enterocutaneous or faecal fistula

33. D

All enterocutaneous fistulae do not always need an operation. Low-output fistulae heal spontaneously if there is no distal obstruction. A fistula will fail to heal spontaneously if there is epithelial continuity between the gut and the skin, if there is active disease or an associated complex abscess.

→ Stoma

34. A, C, D

An ileostomy is always spouted but a colostomy is flush with the skin. While making a left iliac fossa end colostomy, most surgeons still close the lateral paracolic gutter, but there is no evidence that it is effective.

Answers: Extended matching questions

→ 1. Clinical presentations of small and large intestine pathology

1D

This woman has the classical presentation of a carcinoma of the caecum – symptoms from anaemia and a mass in the right iliac fossa. She needs confirmation by colonoscopy and biopsy, a barium enema if full colonoscopy is unsuccessful, and CT scan of the abdomen. The treatment is right hemicolectomy.

2C

This patient's symptoms are suggestive of ulcerative colitis, which is clinically confirmed on sigmoidoscopic findings. A biopsy will give the final diagnosis. He needs assessment by barium enema and colonoscopy with medical management thereafter.

3A

This patient has severe symptoms of urinary tract infections from a vesicocolic fistula – gross *E. coli* infection, pneumaturia and faecaluria. He has suffered from constipation due to diverticular disease, causing stricture. He needs a barium enema, flexible sigmoidoscopy and biopsy to find the cause, CT scan of the pelvis and a cystoscopy. In diverticular disease, after thorough bowel preparation, the affected bowel is dissected off the urinary bladder, the hole in the bladder closed and a one-stage resection and end-to-end anastomosis done.

4B

This patient who has had symptoms of inflammatory bowel disease has a mass in the right iliac fossa which is suggestive of Crohn's disease. He presents as an emergency with an acute perianal abscess. He needs an emergency drainage of the abscess followed by an examination under anaesthesia (EUA) and investigations for thorough assessment – colonoscopy and biopsy, barium enema, small-bowel enema and a CT scan to exclude any areas of sepsis inside the abdomen. The aftermath of the drainage of the perianal abscess would almost certainly lead to a fistula-in-ano which will require MRI. He is managed medically.

5E
This patient, who has increasing constipation and a feeling of incomplete emptying after a bowel action, should be suspected of having a left colonic carcinoma. He needs a colonoscopy and biopsy. A full colonoscopy may not be possible, as his symptoms suggest an annular or tubular lesion. A barium enema is then necessary to exclude a synchronous cancer, followed by a CT scan. A radical left hemicolectomy is the treatment.

➜ 2. Imaging of small and large intestine pathology

Fig. 65.1a and b, D
These two pictures are a series of a barium meal and follow-through. It shows all the features of typical Crohn's disease – narrowing of the terminal ileum (string sign of Kantor), skip lesions with normal bowel interspersed with diseased bowel, radiating spicules, cobblestone appearance and an enteroenteric fistula.

Fig. 65.2, F
This is a barium enema showing complete loss of haustrations of the entire colon with a hosepipe appearance, shortening of the colon and backwash ileitis, features typical of total long-standing ulcerative colitis.

Fig. 65.3a and b, B
These two barium enema pictures show an irregular stricture in the sigmoid colon. This is suggestive of a carcinoma. A flexible sigmoidoscopy and biopsy were done at which no malignancy was seen. The diagnosis was diverticular stricture. This is a classical example of a stricture from diverticular disease mimicking a carcinoma. The patient presented with constipation and features of intermittent large-bowel obstruction.

Fig. 65.4, G
This is a plain X-ray of the abdomen showing gross distension of the entire small bowel in the centre of the abdomen. In the upper part, there are valvulae conniventes from jejunal distension. In the lower part there is characterless distended bowel, which is the hallmark of ileal obstruction. The patient turned out to have a carcinoma of the caecum presenting as an emergency with acute distal small-bowel obstruction.

Fig. 65.5, A
This a plain X-ray showing a foreign body (vibrator) in the rectum. The patient needed a laparotomy, at which the foreign body was milked through the rectum out of the anus.

Fig. 65.6, E
This is a barium enema in a child, as is obvious by the skeletal features. It shows complete arrest of barium just distal to the hepatic flexure with a crab-claw deformity. This is an ileocaecocolic intussusception.

Fig. 65.7, C
This is a barium enema showing an irregular filling defect in the terminal ascending colon just proximal to the hepatic flexure – typical of a polypoid carcinoma. The patient presented with clinical features of anaemia and a mass in the right upper quadrant of the abdomen.

66 Intestinal obstruction

Multiple choice questions

➜ Adynamic intestinal obstruction

1. Which of the following are causes of adynamic intestinal obstruction?

A Paralytic ileus
B Hernia
C Mesenteric vascular obstruction
D Pseudo-obstruction
E Adhesions.

➜ Fluid and electrolyte changes in intestinal obstruction

2. Which of the following cause dehydration and electrolyte loss in intestinal obstruction?

A Reduced oral intake
B Defective intestinal absorption
C Vomiting
D Diarrhoea
E Sequestration in the bowel lumen.

➜ Strangulation in intestinal obstruction

3. Which of the following statements regarding strangulation in intestinal obstruction are true?

A The common causes are hernial orifices, adhesions, volvulus and closed-loop obstruction.
B The arterial supply is compromised before the venous return.
C Marked translocation and systemic exposure to anaerobic organisms occur.
D The morbidity of strangulation due to an external hernia is greater than intraperitoneal strangulation.
E The morbidity and mortality in strangulation are independent of patient age.

➜ Internal herniation

4. Which of the following are potential sites for internal herniation?

A A hole in the transverse mesocolon
B Defects in the broad ligament
C A hole in small bowel mesentery
D Foramen of Winslow
E Paracaecal fossae.

➜ Bolus obstruction

5. Which of the following are examples of bolus obstruction?

A Gallstones
B Phytobezoar
C Trichobezoar
D Stercoliths
E Worms.

➜ Postoperative adhesions

6. Which of the following are associated with increased postoperative adhesions?

A Ischaemic areas
B Good surgical technique
C Foreign material
D Covering anastomosis and raw areas
E Crohn's disease.

➜ Intussusception

7. Which of the following statements regarding intussusception are true?

A It is most common in children with a peak incidence between 5 and 10 months of age.
B About 10 per cent of infantile intussusceptions are idiopathic.
C It causes obstruction but not strangulation.
D Meckel's diverticulum can be a cause in older children.

E The ileocolic region is the most common site in adults.

Sigmoid volvulus

8. Which of the following statements are true about sigmoid volvulus?

A This is the most common site of volvulus in adults.

B The predisposing factors include constipation, long pelvic mesocolon and narrow attachment of the mesocolon.

C The rotation is usually in a clockwise direction.

D Flatus tube decompression is associated with a low rate of recurrence.

E There is no role for emergency surgery.

Clinical features of intestinal obstruction

9. Which of the following statements regarding clinical features of intestinal obstruction are true?

A Vomiting occurs early in high small-bowel obstruction.

B The development of severe pain is indicative of strangulation.

C Distension is a late feature in large-bowel obstruction.

D Some patients may pass flatus or faeces even after the onset of obstruction.

E Constipation is a predominant feature of Richter's hernia.

Imaging in intestinal obstruction

10. Which of the following statements regarding imaging in intestinal obstruction are true?

A Erect abdominal films should routinely be obtained.

B The ileal loops are characterised by valvulae conniventes.

C Small-bowel loops can be dilated in colonic obstruction.

D Barium follow-through is helpful in the diagnosis of small-bowel obstruction.

E A water-soluble enema is helpful in differentiating mechanical obstruction from pseudo-obstruction.

Treatment of intestinal obstruction

11. Which of the following statements regarding treatment of intestinal obstruction are true?

A Gastrointestinal drainage and fluid/electrolyte replacement are always necessary before attempting surgical treatment.

B Indications for early surgery include obstructed external hernia and suspected internal strangulation.

C Division of all the adhesions is mandatory during surgery for adhesive obstruction.

D The treatment of pseudo-obstruction is initially non-surgical.

E Infantile intussusception can be reduced non-operatively in more than 70 per cent of cases.

Extended matching questions

1. Causes of intestinal obstruction

A Adhesions

B Recurrence of malignancy

C Strangulated external hernia

D Primary colonic tumour

E Faecal impaction

F Sigmoid volvulus

G Pseudo obstruction

H Congenital malrotation

Choose and match the correct diagnosis with each of the scenarios given below:

1 A 70-year-old male is brought to the A&E with a history of abdominal pain, distension and absolute constipation. He had noticed increasing constipation over the last 3 months and had lost a stone in weight. Clinical examination reveals a tense and tympanic abdomen. Abdominal X-ray shows a dilated caecum and proximal colon up to the splenic flexure.

2 A 42-year-old female presents with a 4-day history of abdominal pain, distension and vomiting. She had an operation for an ovarian malignancy 2 years ago and has recently received chemotherapy.

3 A 30-year-old male presents with on-and-off abdominal pain and vomiting over the previous week. He has been managing to pass small amount of stools occasionally. He has been admitted to the hospital four times with similar symptoms after his laparotomy for a perforated appendix 5 years ago.

4 An 86-year-old female presents with increasing abdominal distension and vomiting for the past 3 days. Abdominal examination reveals signs of small-bowel obstruction. A 2 cm tender and irreducible lump is palpable over the medial aspect of her right groin.

5 A 90-year-old demented female has been brought from her nursing home. Her carer says that she seems to have abdominal discomfort. She has been having diarrhoea and incontinence for several days. Clinical examination reveals a distended abdomen with multiple palpable masses in her colon. Per rectal examination reveals that her rectum is full of soft stools.

6 A 10-year-old boy is brought to the hospital with recurrent episodes of abdominal pain ever since he was young. This episode has been more severe and associated with vomiting and abdominal distension. Chest X-ray reveals dextrocardia.

7 You are called to see a 70-year-old man who underwent coronary artery bypass graft (CABG) 2 weeks previously. He has not opened his bowels for more than a week and has developed massive abdominal distension. Clinically the abdomen is very distended and tympanic. Bowel sounds are absent. Abdominal X-ray reveals massively dilated large bowel up to the rectum with no cut-off.

8 A 68-year-old female with chronic constipation is brought with a history of rapid distension of the abdomen and constipation. She has had previous similar episodes which have been treated conservatively. Abdominal X-ray reveals 'coffee bean' sign.

→ 2. Radiological signs in intestinal obstruction

A Claw sign
B Coffee bean sign
C Step-ladder pattern
D Pneumobilia
E Rigler's sign

Choose and match the correct radiological sign with each of the diagnoses below:

1 Small-bowel obstruction

2 Bowel perforation

3 Intussusception

4 Sigmoid volvulus

5 Gallstone ileus

3. Management of various types of obstruction

A Emergency laparotomy
B Trial with conservative management
C Flatus tube insertion
D Manual disimpaction
E Colonic stenting
F Urgent exploration

Choose and match the correct intervention with each of the diagnoses below:

1 Sigmoid volvulus

2 Irreducible inguinal hernia

3 Obstructing left colonic carcinoma

4 Adhesive small-bowel obstruction

5 Faecal impaction

6 Signs of peritonitis

Answers: Multiple choice questions

Adynamic intestinal obstruction

1. A, C, D

This type of intestinal obstruction is characterised by the absence of the typical features of mechanical obstruction such as colicky abdominal pain and hyperactive bowel sounds. The obstruction is due to the absence of propulsive movements in the bowel as a result of paralysis of the enteric nervous system. This can be a primary bowel problem or a systemic condition. The abdomen is typically distended, soft or tense and very quiet.

Paralytic ileus is characterised by a failure of transmission of peristaltic waves as a result of neuromuscular failure. This has a variety of causes, including abdominal operations, electrolyte (commonly potassium) abnormalities, infections, reflex (after spinal operations, retroperitoneal haemorrhage) and metabolic conditions such as uraemia.

Pseudo-obstruction usually affects the colon. It is associated with various conditions, such as myocardial infarction, shock, burns, drugs and various metabolic conditions that have an element of myopathy or neuropathy. This occurs in both acute (Ogilvie's syndrome) and chronic forms.

Mesenteric ischaemia can be occlusive or non-occlusive and can have venous or arterial causes. The most important thing in management is correction of the predisposing cause. Surgery may be needed for complications.

Hernia and adhesions are examples of dynamic intestinal obstruction.

Fluid and electrolyte changes in intestinal obstruction

2. A, B, C, E

All patients with intestinal obstruction will have some degree of dehydration and electrolyte abnormalities. It is therefore important to resuscitate them promptly with IV fluids and appropriate electrolyte supplementation. A close monitoring of the fluid balance is vital.

Strangulation in intestinal obstruction

3. A, C

When strangulation occurs, the viability of the bowel is threatened secondary to compromised blood supply. The venous return is compromised before the arterial supply. As the viability of the bowel is compromised, there is marked translocation and systemic exposure to anaerobic organisms with their associated toxins.

The morbidity and mortality associated with strangulation are dependent on age and extent. In strangulated external hernia, the segment involved is short and the resultant blood and fluid loss is small. In some internal strangulation, the bowel involvement can be extensive and the loss of blood and fluid will cause peripheral circulatory failure.

→ Internal herniation

4. A, B C, D, E

Internal herniation occurs when a portion of the small bowel becomes entrapped in one of the retroperitoneal fossae or congenital mesenteric defect, or defects created after previous operations. Internal herniation can also be caused by congenital or acquired diaphragmatic hernias, duodenal retroperitoneal fossae and intersigmoid fossae.

→ Bolus obstruction

5. A, B, C, D, E

Bolus obstruction may occur after partial or total gastrectomy when unchewed articles can pass directly into the small bowel. Fruit and vegetables are particularly liable to cause obstruction. Gallstone obstruction tends to occur in the elderly secondary to erosion of a large gallstone through the gall bladder into the duodenum. Trichobezoars and phytobezoars are firm masses of undigested hair and fruit/vegetable fibre, respectively. Stercoliths are usually found in the small bowel in association with a jejunal diverticulum or ileal stricture. *Ascaris lumbricoides* can cause low small-bowel obstruction, particularly in children.

→ Postoperative adhesions

6. A, C, E

Adhesions and bands are the most common cause of small-bowel obstruction in the Western world. Any source of peritoneal irritation results in local fibrin production, which produces adhesions between apposed surfaces. The common cause of intra-abdominal adhesions are ischaemic areas, foreign material, infection, inflammatory conditions, radiation enteritis, sites of anastomoses, raw areas, Crohn's disease, talc, starch, gauze, silk and any other cause of trauma.

Several factors have been shown to reduce adhesions, including good surgical technique, washing of the peritoneal cavity with saline to remove clots and the like, minimising contact with gauze and covering anastomosis and raw areas. Numerous substances have been instilled in the peritoneal cavity to prevent adhesion formation, including hyaluronidase, hydrocortisone, silicone, dextran and polyvinylpropylene (PVP). Currently no single agent has been shown to be particularly effective. Postoperative adhesion giving rise to intestinal obstruction usually involves the lower small bowel. Operations for appendicitis and gynaecological procedures are common precursors for adhesions.

→ Intussusception

7. A, D

Intussusception occurs when one portion of the bowel becomes invaginated within an immediately adjacent segment. It is most commonly seen in children between 5 and 10 months of age when 90 per cent of cases are idiopathic. It is believed that hyperplasia of Peyer's patches in the terminal ileum may be the initiating event. Weaning, loss of passively acquired immunity and common viral pathogens have all been implicated in the pathogenesis. After the age of 2 years, a pathological point is found in at least one-third of cases and the likely causes are Meckel's diverticulum, polyp, duplication and Henoch–Schönlein purpura. In adults, an intussusception is invariably associated with a lead point and a tumour has to be ruled out.

In most children, the intussusception is ileocolic, whereas colocolic intussusception is more common in adults. The intussusception can cause obstruction, which can lead to strangulation if not reduced.

→ Sigmoid volvulus

8. A, B

A volvulus is a twisting or axial rotation of a portion of bowel about its mesentery. When complete it forms a closed loop of obstruction with resultant ischaemia secondary to vascular occlusion. Sigmoid volvulus is the most common variety and the twist occurs in an anticlockwise direction. Flatus tube or colonoscopic decompression may provide temporary relief but has a high incidence of recurrence. Surgery may become necessary in the emergency setting to deal with complications such as perforation or strangulation. Failure of non-surgical measures may also need surgical intervention.

→ Clinical features of intestinal obstruction

9. A, B, C, D

The more distal the obstruction, the longer the interval between the onset of symptoms and the appearance of nausea and vomiting. Intestinal obstruction typically causes colicky abdominal pain. The development of constant and severe pain should alert one to the possibility of strangulation. The degree of distension is dependent on the site of the obstruction and is greater the more distal the lesion. Distension is delayed in colonic obstruction and may be minimal or absent in the presence of mesenteric vascular occlusion. It is not uncommon for patients with small-bowel obstruction to continue opening their bowels even after the onset of symptoms. The rule that constipation is present in intestinal obstruction does not apply in Richter's hernia, gallstone obstruction, mesenteric vascular obstruction, obstruction associated with pelvic abscess and partial obstruction due to faecal impaction (there may be overflow diarrhoea).

→ Imaging in intestinal obstruction

10. C, E

Erect abdominal films are no longer routinely obtained and the radiological diagnosis is based on a supine abdominal film. The jejunum is characterised by its valvulae conniventes, which completely pass across the width of the bowel and are regularly placed, giving a 'concertina' effect. The distal ileum does not have these lines and is described as featureless. A distended caecum is shown by a rounded gas shadow in the right iliac fossa. Small-bowel loops can be dilated in large-bowel obstruction when associated with an incompetent ileocaecal valve. A barium follow-through is contraindicated if obstruction is suspected, as this can precipitate complete obstruction and worsen matters. A water-soluble enema is useful in confirming large-bowel obstruction. CT scan is another alternative in this situation.

→ Treatment of intestinal obstruction

11. A, B, D, E

Although multiple adhesions are usually found, only one may be causative. This should be divided and the remaining adhesions left in situ unless severe angulation is present.

During operative intervention for bowel obstruction, three things need to be assessed – the site of obstruction, the cause of obstruction and the viability of the gut.

Answers: Extended matching questions

1. Causes of intestinal obstruction

1D, 2B, 3A, 4C, 5E, 6H, 7G, 8F

2. Radiological signs in intestinal obstruction

1C

This appearance occurs as a result of stacking of small-bowel loops one upon another in the central abdomen.

2E

Bowel perforation with resultant leakage of air into the peritoneal cavity outlines both the inner and outer margins of the bowel wall.

3A

This characteristic appearance occurs as some of the contrast enters the outer tube, giving rise to the claw shape.

4B

This was also known as 'bent inner tube sign'.

5D

The pneumobilia is due to the cholecystoduodenal fistula which helped the gallstones to pass on into the bowel.

3. Management of various types of obstruction

1C, 2F, 3E, 4B, 5D, 6A

67 The vermiform appendix

Multiple choice questions

➜ Anatomy

1. **Which of the following statements is false?**
   A The appendicular artery arises from the right colic artery.
   B The commonest position of the appendix is retrocaecal.
   C The position of the base of the appendix is constant.
   D The submucosa is rich in lymphoid aggregates.
   E Argentaffin cells are found in the base of the crypts.

➜ Clinical aspects

2. **Which of the following statements are true?**
   A The peak incidence of acute appendicitis is in the teens and early 20s.
   B The incidence of acute appendicitis is lowest in those who have a high intake of dietary fibre.
   C Obstruction of the appendix lumen by a caecal carcinoma may give rise to acute appendicitis.
   D Aerobic and anaerobic organisms are responsible for acute appendicitis.
   E A mucocele of the appendix is a clinical variation of acute appendicitis.

3. **Which of the following types of patients do not have an increased risk of perforation?**
   A Extremes of age
   B Immunosuppressed
   C Diabetes mellitus
   D Pelvic position of appendix
   E Obese patient.

4. **Which of the following is not a sign of acute appendicitis?**
   A Rovsing's sign
   B Pointing sign
   C Obturator sign
   D Psoas sign
   E Murphy's sign.

5. **Which of the following statements are true in acute appendicitis?**
   A Perforation is more common in acute obstructive appendicitis than in acute catarrhal appendicitis.
   B Acute appendicitis in pregnancy will result in fetal loss in 3–5 per cent.
   C An Alvarado score of 7 or more is suggestive of the diagnosis.
   D Routine use of contrast-enhanced CT scan will reduce the incidence of removal of a normal appendix.
   E Cancer of the caecum may masquerade as acute appendicitis.

6. **In children, which of the following is not part of the differential diagnosis of acute appendicitis?**
   A Gastroenteritis
   B Mesenteric adenitis
   C Meckel's diverticulitis
   D Intussusception
   E Urinary tract infection
   F Lobar pneumonia.

7. **In the adult male, which of the following is not part of the differential diagnosis of acute appendicitis?**
   A Regional ileitis
   B Ureteric colic
   C Perforated peptic ulcer
   D Acute pancreatitis
   E Torsion of testis
   F Mesenteric cyst.

8. **In the adult female, which of the following is not part of the differential diagnosis of acute appendicitis?**

A Mittelschmerz
B Pelvic inflammatory disease
C Pyelonephritis
D Biliary colic/acute cholecystitis
E Ruptured ectopic pregnancy
F Torsion or ruptured ovarian cyst.

9. In the elderly, which of the following is not part of the differential diagnosis of acute appendicitis?

A Diverticulitis
B Intestinal obstruction
C Mesenteric infarction
D Leaking abdominal aortic aneurysm
E Carcinoma of the caecum
F Bladder calculus.

Extended matching questions

→ 1. Differential diagnosis of acute appendicitis

A Acute appendicitis
B Right ureteric colic
C Carcinoma of caecum
D Ruptured ectopic pregnancy
E Crohn's disease
F Perforated peptic ulcer
G Mittelschmerz

Choose and match the correct diagnoses with each of the scenarios given below:

1 A 25-year-old female complains of severe pain in her central lower abdomen of 4 h duration. It started with some initial discomfort around her suprapubic area. She feels faint and is very thirsty. She is not sure about her last menstrual period and is on the oral contraceptive pill (OCP). On examination she is in agony, looks pale and is cold, clammy and sweaty. She is apyrexial and has marked tenderness, rigidity and rebound tenderness over her entire lower abdomen. She has some discoloration around her umbilicus.

2 A 35-year-old female complains of colicky pain in the right iliac fossa for the last 6 h. In between the attacks she is left with a dull ache. She has vomited a few times and feels feverish. In the past she has had diarrhoea on and off for almost a year. On examination she has a temperature of 38°C, is in discomfort from her pain and has tenderness, rigidity and minimal rebound tenderness in the right iliac fossa.

3 A 40-year-old male complains of pain in his right iliac fossa over the last 2 days. His pain in the right iliac fossa was preceded by a bout of sudden-onset severe epigastric and right upper quadrant pain 3 days ago that lasted for a few hours. This initial pain subsided with some antacids which he has been taking on and off for 'indigestion' for almost 18 months. On examination he is pyrexial (39°C) and very tender and rigid over the right iliac fossa.

4 An 18-year-old female complains of generalised colicky abdominal pain for about 6 h. She feels unwell, has vomited a couple of times and is anorexic. The pain has shifted to the right iliac fossa. On examination she has pyrexia of 38°C, is tender over the right iliac fossa with rigidity and has rebound tenderness.

5 A 28-year-old female complains of sudden onset of severe right-sided abdominal pain which he is unable to localise. He is in agony, writhing around and cannot find a comfortable position in which to get any relief from his pain. He has some strangury. On examination he is tender all over the right side of his abdomen with some rigidity but no rebound. On percussion there is a tympanitic note.

6 A 22-year-old female patient complains of pain in the right iliac fossa. The pain started suddenly and has spread all over the lower abdomen. Her last menstrual period was 2 weeks ago. On examination she looks slightly pale, apyrexial and is tender with rigidity and rebound tenderness in the right iliac fossa.

7 A 60-year-old male patient complains of pain in his right iliac fossa of 24 h duration. The pain has been constantly in the right iliac fossa. He has felt unwell for a few months, being unduly short of breath during his normal activities. On examination he looks pale and is tender with rigidity and rebound tenderness in the right iliac fossa.

Answers: Multiple choice questions

Anatomy

1. A

The appendicular artery arises from the lower branch of the ileocolic artery.

Clinical aspects

2. A, B, C, D

A mucocele is not a variation of acute appendicitis. It occurs when acute inflammation of the appendix resolves. This causes the appendix to distend with mucus, resulting in a mucocele.

3. E

The obese patient will have ample greater omentum. This will help localise the acutely inflamed appendix and reduce the risk of perforation.

4. E

Murphy's sign is found in acute cholecystitis

5. A, B, C, E

Contrast-enhanced CT scan is not used routinely. Selective use, particularly in an equivocal Alvarado score of 5–6, helps to exclude acute appendicitis and thus prevents an unnecessary appendicectomy.

6. E

7. F

8. D

9. F

Answers: Extended matching questions

1. Differential diagnosis of acute appendicitis

1D

This is a young female who is unsure about her menstrual periods. She has had a sudden onset of very severe lower abdominal pain and has presented with features of hypovolaemic shock. Although she is on the OCP, the clinical picture is typical, particularly with Cullen's sign (bloodstained discoloration around the umbilicus), of a ruptured ectopic pregnancy.

2E

This female patient complains of colicky right-sided abdominal pain from the start, denoting an obstructive feature. Her past history of diarrhoea should alert one to the possibility of primary bowel pathology. She is generally feeling unwell with acute signs in the right iliac fossa. These features should point to a diagnosis of acute terminal ileitis from Crohn's disease.

3F

This patient who has suffered from indigestion in the past, for which he has taken antacids, has had a sudden attack of epigastric and right hypochondrial pain from a leaking peptic ulcer. This pain was thought by the patient to be an acute episode of his indigestion for which he tried to get relief by taking some more antacids. However, he did not get better and has come in with signs of peritonitis in the right iliac fossa. This scenario is typical of a leaking peptic ulcer that has been closed off by omentum and the leaked contents have gravitated to the right iliac fossa along the right paracolic gutter, mimicking acute appendicitis.

4A

This 18-year-old female has the classical features of acute appendicitis. The clinical examination is in keeping with her history of visceral-somatic sequence of pain. When asked to point to the site of her pain, she would almost certainly point to where the pain started (periumbilical) and where it subsequently moved (right iliac fossa).

5B

This young man has sudden onset of severe right-sided abdominal pain which he is unable to localise. He is in agony and writhing around in pain, unable to find a position of comfort. Abdominal examination shows a tympanitic abdomen which is due to ileus, a common accompaniment of ureteric colic.

6G

This young woman has developed pain in the right iliac fossa halfway through her menstrual period. She has signs in her lower abdomen of bleeding from a ruptured lutein cyst. The diagnosis is Mittelschmerz.

7C

This 60-year-old patient has pain and signs of an acute abdominal episode in the right iliac fossa. He has felt short of breath in his daily routine and looks pale – features of anaemic hypoxia. He has signs in the right iliac fossa. The scenario is very typical of a carcinoma of the caecum masquerading as acute appendicitis. It is important to remember that true acute appendicitis will not cause anaemia.

68 The rectum

Multiple choice questions

Anatomy

1. Which of the following statements are false?

A The adult rectum is approximately 15 cm long.
B The anorectal angle is 120°.
C The fascia in front of the rectum is Waldeyer's fascia.
D The fascia at the back of the rectum is Denonvilliers' fascia.
E Waldeyer's and Denonvilliers' fascias prevent the spread of cancer.

2. Which of the following statements are true?

A The part of the rectum below the middle valve of Houston is called the ampulla.
B The superior rectal artery arises from the internal iliac artery.
C The middle rectal artery is contained in the lateral ligaments.
D The superior rectal veins ultimately drain into the portal system.
E The usual drainage flow of the lymphatics is upwards.

Clinical aspects

3. What are the main symptoms of rectal disease?

A Rectal bleeding
B Tenesmus
C Altered bowel habit
D Mucous discharge
E Anorexia
F Urinary frequency
G Prolapse.

4. In clinical examination, which of the following statements are true?

A Visual examination of the perianal region is essential to exclude fissures, fistulae or other painful conditions.
B A cancer in the upper third of the rectum can be felt by the index finger.
C A proctoscope visualises the lower 10 cm of the rectum.
D A rigid sigmoidoscope is 25–30 cm in length.
E A flexible sigmoidoscope visualises 45–50 cm of the terminal large bowel.

Rectal injury

5. Which of the following is not a mechanism of rectal injury?

A Falling over a pointed object, causing impalement
B Sexual assault
C Crush injury during prolonged childbirth from the fetal head
D Penetrating injuries, including gunshot trauma
E Road traffic accidents.

6. Which of the following statements regarding the treatment of rectal injuries are false?

A A computed tomography (CT) scan with rectal contrast is useful for assessment.
B Intraperitoneal tear is treated by closure and defunctioning left iliac proximal colostomy.
C In extraperitoneal injury, debridement of the external wound with left iliac defunctioning colostomy is carried out.
D In a large defect, resection of the damaged bowel with end-to-end anastomosis is done.
E Broad-spectrum antibiotic cover is mandatory.

Rectal prolapse

7. **In rectal prolapse which of the following statements are true?**
   A In children the prolapse is partial or mucosal.
   B Full-thickness prolapse commences as an intussusception.
   C Full-thickness prolapse is much more common in women.
   D Children are treated conservatively.
   E All of the above.

8. **Which of the following procedures are not done for complete rectal prolapse?**
   A Thiersch operation
   B Hartmann's operation
   C Delorme's operation
   D Ripstein's operation
   E Milligan–Morgan operation.

Proctitis

9. **In proctitis, which of the following statements are true?**
   A The condition is always limited to the rectum
   B It causes bleeding, diarrhoea and tenesmus.
   C It can be due to specific infections.
   D Proctoscopy and biopsy are the mainstay in the diagnosis.
   E Treatment is usually conservative.

Rectal cancer

10. **In the pathology of rectal cancer, which of the following statements are false?**
   A Low-grade well-differentiated cancers account for almost 50 per cent.
   B Mucoid adenocarcinomas have a poor prognosis.
   C Circumferential local spread is the most important.
   D Synchronous cancers are seen in 5 per cent.
   E Lymphatic spread occurs along the blood vessels to the para-aortic, iliac and inguinal nodes.

11. **Assessment in rectal cancer should include:**
   A Sigmoidoscopy and biopsy
   B Colonoscopy or CT colonography or barium enema to exclude synchronous cancer
   C CT scan of liver and chest
   D Magnetic resonance imaging (MRI) of pelvis and endoluminal ultrasound
   E All of the above.

12. **In all patients with rectal cancer, which of the following is not part of routine preoperative preparation?**
   A Mechanical bowel preparation
   B Counselling and siting of stoma
   C Radiotherapy
   D Prophylactic antibiotics
   E Prophylaxis for deep vein thrombosis

13. **In surgery for rectal cancer, which of the following statements are false?**
   A The vast majority are treated by abdominoperineal resection.
   B Locally advanced tumours are treated preoperatively by chemoradiotherapy.
   C Anterior resection with total mesorectal excision is possible in a selected few.
   D In node-positive disease, adjuvant chemotherapy should be given.
   E Liver resection for secondaries at a subsequent operation offers a chance for cure in a selected group.

14. **In the staging for rectal cancer, which of the following are true?**
   A The incidence of Dukes' stage A is 15 per cent.
   B The incidence in Dukes' stage C is 50 per cent.
   C Dukes' stage D indicates distant metastasis, usually to the liver.
   D In the TNM (tumour, node, metastasis) staging, T3 indicates invasion through the serosa or mesorectal fascia.
   E In the TNM staging, N1 indicates the involvement of one to three lymph nodes.

Extended matching questions

1. Clinical conditions affecting the rectum

A Proctitis
B Solitary rectal ulcer
C Rectal prolapse
D Carcinoma of rectum
E Villous adenoma
F Amoebic granuloma

Choose and match the following diagnosis with each of the scenarios given below

1 A 45-year-old male complains of mucous discharge from the rectum for several months. Recently this has become profuse and has made him feel very weak. On examination he has lost some weight and on rectal examination there is a fronded large growth that is palpable. He has a serum potassium of 2.2 mmol/L.

2 A 35-year-old male complains of bleeding per rectum and tenesmus. On examination there is nothing to find in the abdomen. On rectal examination, a fleshy mass is felt in the mid-rectum. On sigmoidoscopy there is a mass with an ulcerated surface. A biopsy has been taken. A year ago he returned to Britain after living in the Far East for a few years.

3 A 50-year-old female complains of bleeding from the rectum associated with defaecation. During a motion she passes flatus, mucus and blood and very little faecal matter. On rectal examination there is blood on the finger; sigmoidoscopy shows inflamed rectal mucosa up to about 15 cm without any ulceration.

4 A 40-year-old female complains of rectal bleeding and passage of mucus for several months with occasional incontinence. During this time she has been constipated and feels a lump protruding from her anus which she can reduce herself. On examination she has a partial rectal prolapse. On sigmoidoscopy at about 10 cm, there is an ulcer on the anterior wall. A biopsy has been taken.

5 A 55-year-old female complains of a lump protruding from her anus for almost 10 months. She has to push the lump back but it reappears when she passes a motion. On examination she has a 5 cm length of rectum outside the anus, and when it is pushed back it reduces with a gurgle.

6 A 65-year-old male complains of early morning diarrhoea for the last 4 months. He has urgency of defaecation and a feeling of insufficient evacuation of his rectum with tenesmus. He passes blood and mucus in his stools. On abdominal examination he has indentable masses in his left iliac fossa. On rectal examination there is a hard indurated mass which can be seen at 8 cm on sigmoidoscopy. A biopsy has been taken.

Answers: Multiple choice questions

Anatomy

1. C, D

The fascia at the back is called Waldeyer's fascia and separates the rectum from the coccyx and the lower two sacral vertebrae. The fascia in the front is called Denonvilliers' fascia and separates the rectum from the prostate and seminal vesicles or the vagina.

2. A, C, D, E
The superior rectal artery is a continuation of the inferior mesenteric artery. The middle rectal artery arises from the internal iliac artery.

Clinical aspects

3. A, B, C, D, G

4. A, B, C, D
When doing a digital rectal examination, if a patient is asked to strain, a cancer in the upper third of the rectum can be felt. Proctoscopy is an integral part of clinical examination. This should be followed by a rigid sigmoidoscopy or, better still, a flexible sigmoidoscopy (after giving the patient an enema). A flexible sigmoidoscope is 60 cm long and can visualise up to the splenic flexure in ideal circumstances.

Rectal injury

5. E

6. D
Primary anastomosis should never be done in extensive injuries. The injured bowel is excised and the proximal end is brought out as an end colostomy and the distal end closed as a Hartmann's procedure. After all the wounds have healed (and this may take several months), bowel continuity is restored.

Rectal prolapse

7. E

8. B, E
In Hartmann's operation the sigmoid colon is excised and the rectum is closed, not an operation done for prolapse. Milligan and Morgan described one of the original operations for haemorrhoids.

Proctitis

9. B, C, E
Although the disease is limited to 5–15 cm from the anus in the majority, in 10 per cent the condition extends to involve the entire colon – total ulcerative colitis. To obtain a diagnosis, proctoscopy is not sufficient. Sigmoidoscopy and biopsy are done, supplemented by bacteriological examination and stool culture. This should be followed by a full colonoscopy and multiple biopsies to determine the extent of the disease.

Rectal cancer

10. A, E
Low-grade (well-differentiated) cancers account for only 11 per cent; average grade cancers (moderately differentiated) occur in 64 per cent; and high-grade anaplastic cancers occur in 25 per cent. Although the lymphatics drain along the blood vessels, spread of cancer occurs principally upwards via the superior rectal vessels to the para-aortic nodes.

11. E

12. B, C
While all patients require thorough counselling, they do not require routine counselling for stoma because in an anterior resection a stoma is not required. However, if a low anterior resection is contemplated then the patient should be counselled about the possibility of a loop ileostomy. Pre-operative radiotherapy is not routinely used in all patients. It is used in cases of local extra-rectal spread.

13. A, C

Abdominoperineal resection is performed in only a minority of patients with rectal cancer. The vast majority are suitable for restorative anterior resection with total mesorectal excision. In a low anterior resection, a temporary defunctioning ileostomy is sometimes carried out. This is closed after about 6 weeks, having confirmed the integrity of the anastomosis by a barium enema.

14. A, B, C, E

In TNM staging, which is the internationally recognised staging system, T3 indicates tumour invasion through the muscularis propria but not through the serosa or mesorectal fascia. If the growth has invaded the serosa or mesorectal fascia, it is T4.

Answers: Extended matching questions

1. Clinical conditions affecting the rectum

1E

This is a villous adenoma which causes profuse mucous discharge that is rich in potassium – hence the hypokalaemia. These have a tendency to become malignant. A colonoscopy is carried out to exclude another lesion higher up. If malignancy has been excluded, these tumours can be resected endoscopically by submucosal resection.

2F

Amoebic granuloma (sometimes called amoeboma) can be easily mistaken for a carcinoma. A biopsy confirms the diagnosis. Microscopic examination of the scrapings with a spoon helps establish the diagnosis. The condition can rarely be seen in a patient who has not visited a country where it is endemic. The treatment is medical.

3A

This patient is suffering from proctitis. A biopsy is done on sigmoidoscopy to determine the cause. A full colonoscopy with multiple biopsies is then carried out. Diagnosis of specific infection (*Clostridium difficile*, bacillary or amoebic dysentery, tuberculosis, *Gonococcus*, lymphogranuloma venereum, Aids, bilharziasis) is excluded by bacteriological examination and culture of the stools, examination of scrapings or swabs from ulcers, and serological tests.

4B

This is a solitary rectal ulcer (syndrome) which peaks in the third to fourth decades. The condition is associated with rectal prolapse and an ulcer on the anterior wall at 7–10 cm from the anal verge. There is an internal rectal intussusception caused by chronic straining from constipation. Confirmation is by histology.

5C

This is full-thickness rectal prolapse, which is six times more common in women and may be associated with uterine prolapse. There is a peritoneal pouch, like a hernia, accompanying the anterior wall of the prolapse. This contains loops of small bowel, which cause the gurgling sound during manual reduction of the prolapse.

6D

This patient's symptoms of early morning diarrhoea along with a feeling of insufficient evacuation are typical of a carcinoma of the rectum. It is referred to as spurious diarrhoea as there is no proper motion but only wind and water. The abdominal lumps are inspissated faeces proximal to an obstructing rectal cancer. Confirmation is by biopsy at sigmoidoscopy. This is followed by full colonoscopy, CT colonography or barium enema to exclude a synchronous cancer (5 per cent) and staging by CT of abdomen and MRI of pelvis. Most patients are suitable for restorative anterior resection.

69 The anus and anal canal

Multiple choice questions

➜ Anal canal anatomy

1. Which of the following are true regarding anal canal anatomy?

A The anorectal ring marks the junction between the rectum and the anal canal.
B The puborectalis muscle is not concerned with the continence mechanism.
C The intersphincteric plane is not of much significance.
D The internal sphincter is the thickened distal continuation of the circular muscle layer of the rectum.
E The dentate line is an important landmark representing the site of fusion of the proctodaeum and postallantoic gut.

➜ Anal glands

2. Which of the following are true regarding anal glands?

A These are found in the anal mucosa.
B They normally number between 20 and 25 in an individual.
C They drain via ducts into anal sinuses at the level of the dentate line.
D They are widely considered as the potential source of anal sepsis.
E They secrete mucus, which helps to ease defaecation.

➜ Congenital anomalies of anal canal

3. Which of the following statements regarding the congenital anomalies of the anal canal are true?

A The dorsal part of the cloacal membrane is called the anal membrane.
B Imperforate anus is divided into two types – high and low – depending on the level of rectal termination in relation to the urinary bladder.
C Low defects are easier to correct but more prone to constipation.
D Postanal dermoid usually remains asymptomatic until adult life.
E A postanal dimple is of no clinical significance.

➜ Pilonidal sinus

4. Which of the following statements regarding pilonidal sinus are true?

A It is usually congenital.
B The primary sinuses are always in the midline between the sacrococcygeal joint and the tip of coccyx.
C Bascom's procedure involves a midline incision directly over the sinus cavity.
D The Karydakis operation avoids a midline scar.
E It is more common in women.

➜ Anal incontinence

5. Which of the following statements about anal incontinence are true?

A The most common cause of anal sphincter disruption is obstetric damage.
B Anal incontinence cannot occur in the absence of sphincter disruption.
C Double overlap repair is the standard technique to repair discrete muscle disruption.
D Gracilis muscle transposition can be effective in approximately 20 per cent of patients in the long term.
E Sacral nerve stimulation works by neurophysiological modulation of the hindgut by stimulation of the sacral nerve roots.

Anal fissure

6. Which of the following statements regarding anal fissure are true?

A It is a longitudinal split in the lower rectal mucosa.
B It is most common in the posterior wall.
C The common finding is a hypotonic anal sphincter.
D Operation can be avoided in about 50 per cent of patients by the use of local agents like glyceryl trinitrate (GTN) or Diltiazem.
E The most important complication after lateral internal sphincterotomy is incontinence, which may affect up to 30 per cent of patients.

Haemorrhoids

7. Which of the following statements about haemorrhoids are true?

A Most haemorrhoids are congenital.
B Pain is rare in uncomplicated grade 1 haemorrhoids.
C Piles which remain permanently prolapsed are called grade 3 haemorrhoids.
D Portal pyaemia is a rare but known complication of haemorrhoids.
E Profuse haemorrhage is never seen.

8. Which of the following statements regarding management of piles are true?

A Submucosal injection of 50 per cent phenol is an effective treatment for grade 1 piles.
B Banding of piles involves application of tight elastic bands onto the base of the pedicle which cause ischaemic necrosis of the piles.
C Cryotherapy and infrared coagulation are also methods of treating piles.
D Milligan–Morgan haemorrhoidectomy is a closed technique where the piles are excised and the mucosa completely closed.
E Stapled haemorrhoidectomy is a method where a special stapling gun is used to excise a strip of mucosa and submucosa.

Pruritus ani

9. Which of the following statements regarding pruritus ani are true?

A It is a common problem.
B The perianal skin is usually normal.
C Threadworms need to be excluded, especially in young patients.
D Skin biopsies may sometimes be needed to confirm diagnosis.
E Washing the area with soap can be helpful.

Perianal abscess

10. Which of the following statements regarding perianal abscesses are true?

A They present as a painful, throbbing swelling in the perianal area.
B They are always associated with an underlying anal fistula.
C Fistulotomy is advised if a fistula is found at the time of draining the abscess.
D Treatment of abscess involves a cruciate incision over the most fluctuant point, deroofing the cavity and finger curettage.
E Finding Gram-positive organisms on pus culture is associated with an underlying anal fistula.

Anal fistula

11. Which of the following statements about anal fistula are true?

A It may be found in association with ulcerative colitis.
B Trans-sphincteric fistulae usually have an external opening close to the anal verge.
C Posterior fistulae are more likely to have a curved track and a horseshoe communication.
D Fistulotomy is the treatment of choice in trans-sphincteric fistula involving more than 30 per cent of the external sphincter.
E Setons can either be 'loose' or 'tight'.

Anal warts

12. Which of the following statements regarding anal warts are true?

A They are associated with HPV infection.

B HPV subtypes 4 and 8 are associated with greater risk of progression to malignancy.
C The incidence has decreased over the last three decades.
D Acetic acid is helpful in diagnosis.
E Treatment options include 25 per cent podophyllin and surgical excision.

Anal cancer

13. The risk factors for anal squamous cell carcinoma (SCC) include:

A Human papillomavirus (HPV) infection
B HIV infection
C Renal transplant
D Other genital cancers
E Rectal cancer.

14. Which of the following statements regarding anal cancers are true?

A They constitute less than 2 per cent of all bowel cancers.
B They are usually SCCs.
C The primary group of lymph nodes are the iliac nodes in the pelvis.
D Treatment is usually surgical.
E Pain and bleeding are the most common symptoms.

Extended matching questions

1. Diagnosis of rectal bleeding

A Haemorrhoids
B Anal fissure
C Proctitis
D Rectal cancer
E Ulcerative colitis
F Infective colitis
G Ischaemic colitis
H Diverticulitis

Choose and match the correct diagnosis with each of the scenarios given below:

1 A 68-year-old male presents with bright red painless bleeding. He has an associated history of recent change in bowels and a sensation of incomplete defaecation.

2 A 32-year-old female complains of fresh blood per rectum and some discomfort following a recent pregnancy. She mentions a tendency towards constipation.

3 A 28-year-old male is referred with a history of severe anal pain associated with defaecation. He also has streaks of fresh blood per rectum. He has a long history of hard stools and straining.

4 An 82-year-old male who has had three previous myocardial infarctions and a recent abdominal aortic aneurysm (AAA) repair complains of abdominal pain and darkish rectal bleeding.

5 A 90-year-old female with a long history of constipation is referred to the hospital with lower abdominal pain on and off and painless dark blood per rectum.

6 An 18-year-old student who has just returned from travelling in his gap year presents with bloody diarrhoea and colicky abdominal pain.

7 A 24-year-old female presents with a 6-month history of diarrhoea along with blood and mucus. She has lost a stone in weight. She says that her mother has also had chronic bowel problems and presently has a stoma.

8 A 30-year-old male presents with a 2-week history of severe tenesmus and fresh blood per rectum. He is known to be HIV-positive.

→ 2. Investigations in anorectal symptoms

A Rigid sigmoidoscopy
B Colonoscopy
C Flexible sigmoidoscopy
D Magnetic resonance imaging (MRI) scan
E Examination under anaesthesia (EUA)
F Biopsy
G Anorectal physiology

Choose and match the correct investigations with each of the scenarios given below:

1 A 70-year-old male is referred with a history of recent change in bowels and weight loss.

2 A 36-year-old male is referred with a history of recurrent anal fistulae needing several operations.

3 A 26-year-old female is referred with fresh blood per rectum following a recent pregnancy. Her bowels are normal and she has no abdominal symptoms.

4 A 28-year-old male presents with severe anal pain persisting despite local medications. Clinical examination reveals anal sphincter spasm and hence further examination is not possible.

5 A 58-year-old female presents with urge incontinence progressively getting worse over the last 2 years. She has had a perineal tear during a previous delivery several years ago.

6 A 65-year-old male is referred with history of a lump in the anus. Examination reveals a 1.5 cm hard lump at the anal verge.

7 A 30-year-old male presents with history of dark-coloured rectal bleeding associated with diarrhoea and left-sided abdominal pain.

→ 3. Treatment of anorectal disorders

A Stapled anopexy
B Excision biopsy
C Lateral internal sphincterotomy
D Glyceryl trinitrate
E Altemeier's procedure
F Lay open/seton insertion

Choose and match the correct operation with each of the conditions given below:

1 Rectal prolapse

2 Primary treatment of anal fissure

3 Anal polyp

4 Anal fissure resistant to medical therapy

5 High anal fistula

6 Grade 3 piles

→ 4. Aetiology of anorectal disorders

A Anal fissure
B Haemorrhoids
C Anal fistula
D Urge incontinence

E Anal SCC
F Rectal prolapse
G Anismus
H Solitary rectal ulcer syndrome (SRUS)

Choose and match the correct diagnosis with each of the descriptions given below:

1 This is essentially due to failure of supports of the rectum usually compounded by straining.

2 The most common cause is an occult obstetric sphincter injury.

3 AIN and HPV infection virus can predispose to this.

4 This is usually caused by the failure of relaxation of the puborectalis muscle during defaecation.

5 This is evidence of straining during defaecation with an internal intussusception in most cases.

6 This is caused by a hypertonic anal sphincter with resultant mucosal ischaemia.

7 This is associated with dilatation and prolapse of the anal vascular cushions usually due to straining.

8 The cause is usually cryptogenic and associated with sepsis in the terminal part of the anal glands.

Answers: Multiple choice questions

→ Anal canal anatomy

1. A, D, E

The anal canal commences at the level where the rectum passes through the pelvic floor and ends at the anal verge. This is marked by the anorectal bundle (or ring), which can be felt with the finger as a thickened ridge. It is formed by the joining of the puborectalis, deep part of the external sphincter, conjoined longitudinal muscle and the highest part of the internal sphincter. The puborectalis is an important component of the continence mechanism. It maintains the anorectal angle. Relaxation of this facilitates defaecation, and failure to relax causes anismus. The intersphincteric plane is an important potential space and contains intersphincteric anal glands. This is the route for the spread of pus. This plane can be opened up surgically to provide access for operations on the sphincter muscles.

→ Anal glands

2. C, D, E

The anal glands are found in the submucosa and the intersphincteric space. They normally number between 0 and 10 in an individual.

→ Congenital anomalies of anal canal

3. A, C, D, E

Imperforate anus has historically been divided into high and low types depending on the level of termination of the rectum in relation to the pelvic floor. Treatment and prognosis are influenced by the type and the associated abnormalities of the sacrum and the genitourinary systems. Careful examination is helpful. Presence of meconium on the perineum indicates a low defect. The finding of a single perineal orifice indicates a persistent cloaca – a common opening for the rectum, vagina and urinary tract – and is usually associated with complex abnormalities. A lateral prone X-ray at 24 h after birth indicates the distance between the rectum and the perineum. Low anomalies can be treated by anoplasty, while complex abnormalities require a defunctioning colostomy followed by definitive surgery (posterior sagittal anorectoplasty – PSARP) later on.

➜ Pilonidal sinus

4. B, D

The term pilonidal sinus describes a condition found in the natal cleft overlying the coccyx, consisting of one or more midline openings. These openings communicate with a fibrous track lined by granulation tissue and containing hair lying loosely within the lumen. It is more common in men and the predisposing factors include a hairy area, deep natal cleft and occupational factors which involve prolonged sitting, e.g. long-distance drivers, cab drivers and work involving prolonged hours in front of a computer. Cultural factors may also be important. Bascom's procedure involves an incision lateral to the midline to gain access to the sinus cavity along with excision and closure of the midline pits. Karydakis's procedure involves a lateral advancement flap and aims to remove the affected tissues, flatten the deep natal cleft and bring new tissues to close the gap with a wound off the midline.

➜ Anal incontinence

5. A, C, E

Obstetric damage is the most common cause of anal incontinence due to sphincter disruption followed by anal surgery and trauma. Faecal incontinence can occur without sphincter disruption due to neuropathy and urge incontinence due to various reasons. Double overlap sphincter repair is successful in about 80 per cent of patients which may reduce to 50 per cent in the long term. If direct repair is not possible gracilis muscle transposition has been found to be effective in about 60 per cent of patients in the long term.

➜ Anal fissure

6. B, D, E

An anal fissure is a longitudinal split in the anoderm of the distal anal canal. The location in the posterior midline perhaps relates to the exaggerated shearing forces acting at that site at defaecation, less elastic anoderm and relatively small blood supply. The most common associated finding is a hypertonic anal sphincter. Lateral internal sphincterotomy is the 'gold standard' but has potential risks of anal incontinence. Alternative methods such as anal advancement flaps have hence been tried with equally good results.

➜ Haemorrhoids

7. B, D

Internal haemorrhoids are symptomatic anal vascular cushions which typically lie in the 3, 7 and 11 o'clock positions. External haemorrhoids relate to venous channels of the inferior haemorrhoidal plexus deep in the skin surrounding the anal verge. The four degrees of haemorrhoids are as follows:

- first degree – bleed only, no prolapse
- second degree – prolapse but reduce spontaneously
- third degree – prolapse and have to be manually reduced
- fourth degree – permanently prolapsed.

Haemorrhoids are acquired, and numerous predisposing factors, such as anal hypertonia, repeated infection of the anal lining and a higher proportion of collagen than muscle due to ageing, may be contributory. It is currently believed that shearing forces acting on the anus lead to caudal displacement of the anal cushions and mucosal trauma. Bleeding is the most common symptom and can be profuse or sustained, leading to anaemia. Portal pyaemia is a rare complication after strangulation. The grade 1 and 2 piles can be managed by injection sclerotherapy or banding, but grade 3 and 4 varieties are more likely to need open/stapled haemorrhoidectomy.

8. B, C, E
Injection sclerotherapy involves injecting 5–10 mL of 5 per cent phenol in almond/arachis oil submucosally at the apex of each pile. Milligan–Morgan haemorrhoidectomy (open technique) involves dissection and ligation of the piles and leaving the wound open. The closed technique is more popular in the USA.

➜ Pruritus ani

9. A, C, D
This is a common and embarrassing condition which can be difficult to treat. The perianal skin is usually reddened and hyperkeratotic. It can also become cracked and moist. A useful mnemonic for the causes is 'pus, polyps, parasites, piles and psyche'. Cotton wool should be substituted for toilet paper. Soap is avoided and replaced by water alone. Anal intraepithelial neoplasia (AIN) may need to be ruled out by biopsy. Symptomatic treatment remains the mainstay, although every effort is made to find and treat the cause.

➜ Perianal abscess

10. A, D
Acute sepsis in the anal region is common and men are more affected. Not all cases are associated with an underlying anal fistula. This can arise from a simple boil or skin appendage infection. In about half of the cases, however, it is as a result of sepsis in the intersphincteric space (cryptoglandular) and may be followed by a persistent anal fistula. Finding Gram-negative organisms on pus swab further suggests an underlying anal fistula, and Gram-positive organisms point to a superficial skin source. Treatment involves draining the abscess under general anaesthetic. It is not recommended to do immediate fistulotomy except in the most experienced hands.

➜ Anal fistula

11. C, E
An anal fistula is an abnormal chronic communication between the anal canal and the surrounding perianal skin. This may be found in association with specific conditions such as Crohn's disease. They are divided into various types depending on the relation of the primary track into trans-sphincteric, intersphincteric, suprasphincteric and extrasphincteric varieties. They are classified as 'high' or 'low' depending on the level of the internal opening in relation to the dentate line. Intersphincteric fistulae usually have an external opening close to the anal verge. Goodsall's rule predicts the type of track and location of internal opening – an anterior external opening is more likely to have a straight track while a posteriorly placed external opening is more likely to have a curved track with an internal opening in the midline posteriorly. A fistulotomy (laying open of the fistula) is done in intersphincteric and some trans-sphincteric fistulae involving less than 30 per cent of the external sphincter. The safer option when the track involves the sphincter muscles is to do a partial lay-open with a seton insertion. The seton can be 'loose' – for drainage/marker – or 'tight', for cutting. Anal flaps and plugs can also be useful in selected patients.

➜ Anal warts

12. A, D, E
Condyloma accuminata is the most common sexually transmitted disease encountered by colorectal surgeons. There has been an increase in this condition over the last three decades. They

are caused by HPV. There are more than 80 subtypes of this virus but the subtypes associated with a greater risk of malignancy are 16, 18, 31 and 33. Many are asymptomatic but pruritus, discharge, bleeding and pain are the usual symptoms. The warts are initially discrete but later on coalesce to carpet the skin. Relentless growth may lead to giant condylomata (Buschke–Lowenstein tumour). Staged excision is done in extensive warts.

➔ Anal cancer

13. A, B, C, D

Rectal adenocarcinoma is not a risk factor for anal SCC. AIN is a virally induced dysplasia of the perianal or intra-anal dermis. This can be asymptomatic and confirmed on biopsy. It is classified according to the degree of dysplasia into three types – AIN 1, AIN 2 and AIN 3 according to the lack of keratocyte maturation and the extension of the proliferative zone from the lower third (AIN 1) to the full thickness (AIN 3). The natural history is uncertain but progression to invasive carcinoma has been observed. The term Bowen's disease, though often used, is best avoided to prevent confusion.

14. A, B, E

Anal cancer is an uncommon cancer associated with HPV and more common in HIV-positive patients. This may affect the verge or the anal canal. The primary group of lymph nodes are the inguinal group, although sometimes retrograde and alternative spreads may occur. Treatment is by chemoradiotherapy in the first instance (Nigro regimen), and major ablative surgery if that fails.

Answers: Extended matching questions

➔ 1. Diagnosis of rectal bleeding

1D

Rectal cancer should be ruled out in any patient in this age group presenting with new-onset bowel symptoms. Piles and diverticuloses frequently coexist with malignancy.

2A

Most piles in females start during pregnancy.

3B

The typical symptom of anal fissure is severe anal pain aggravated by defaecation. Only limited examination is possible, which usually reveals anal sphincter spasm and a sentinel skin tag.

4G

Consider ischaemic colitis in a known arteriopath presenting with lower gastrointestinal bleed. The most common differential diagnosis is diverticular bleed. The presence of peritonitis or raised lactate should alert the surgeon.

5H

Most diverticular bleeds are self-limiting and very rarely require emergency surgery. This may be painless as they are not often associated with acute inflammation.

6F

Recent international travel might suggest an infective cause – amoebiasis and *Shigella* are common causes of bloody dysentery.

7E

Inflammatory bowel disease will need to be ruled out in the young patient presenting with bleeding and change in bowel habits.

8C
Tenesmus is usually associated with proctitis. An EUA may be required for detailed evaluation.

→ 2. Investigations in anorectal symptoms
1B, 2D, 3A, 4E, 5G, 6F, 7C

→ 3. Treatment of anorectal disorders
1E, 2D, 3B, 4C, 5F, 6A

→ 4. Aetiology of anorectal disorders
1F, 2D, 3E, 4G, 5H, 6A, 7B, 8C

PART 12 Genitourinary

70 Urinary symptoms and investigations 515

71 The kidneys and ureters 521

72 The urinary bladder 533

73 The prostate and seminal vesicles 541

74 The urethra and penis 546

75 The testis and scrotum 549

76 Gynaecology 554

70 Urinary symptoms and investigations

Multiple choice questions

→ Haematuria

1. Which of the following statements are false?

A Microscopic haematuria is not always abnormal.
B Haematuria at the start of urinary stream indicates a cause in the lower urinary tract.
C Haematuria where the urine is uniformly mixed with the urine points to a cause in the upper urinary tract.
D Terminal haematuria is caused by bladder irritation or infection.
E Painful haematuria indicates malignant pathology.

→ Pain of urological origin

2. Which of the following statements are true?

A Pain of renal origin is a deep-seated, sickening ache.
B Pain from a ureteric stone is colicky and the patient rolls around in agony.
C Pain from the urinary bladder is a suprapubic discomfort.
D Perineal pain is a penetrating ache and can occur in both sexes
E All of the above.

→ Preliminary investigations and renal failure

3. Which of the following statements are false?

A If 30 per cent of kidney function is lost, renal failure becomes evident by blood results.
B In hypertension and renal artery stenosis, the plasma flow is impaired, causing renal failure.
C In glomerulonephritis or acute cortical necrosis, loss of glomeruli causes renal failure.
D In pyelonephritis, tubular function is impaired, causing renal failure.
E Cytological examination of urine is more likely to be abnormal in poorly differentiated rather than well-differentiated transitional cell cancer of bladder.

→ Imaging in urological conditions

4. Which of the following statements are true?

A Most urinary calculi are radiodense.
B Uric acid calculi can be seen on a plain X-ray.
C Ultrasound scanning (US) provides broadly similar anatomical information as an intravenous urogram (IVU).
D IVU has no advantage over US.
E IVU can be dangerous.

→ Renal failure

5. Which of the following statements are false?

A Anuria is defined as complete absence of urine production.
B Oliguria is defined as an urinary output of less than 300 mL in 24 h.
C Certain drugs can cause renal failure.
D All patients with renal failure will require renal replacement therapy.
E Indwelling stents can be used to relieve ureteric obstruction.

Extended matching questions

→ 1. Imaging

A CT scan of urinary bladder
B Renal angiogram
C Antegrade pyelogram
D Intravenous urogram
E Retrograde ureterogram

Match the investigations with Figs 70.1–70.5 below:

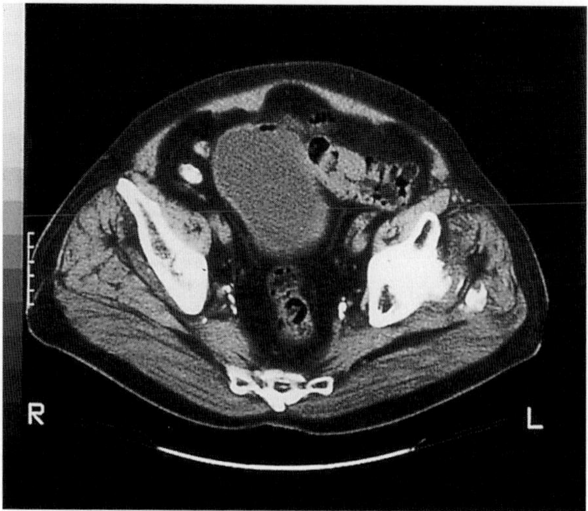

Figure 70.1a

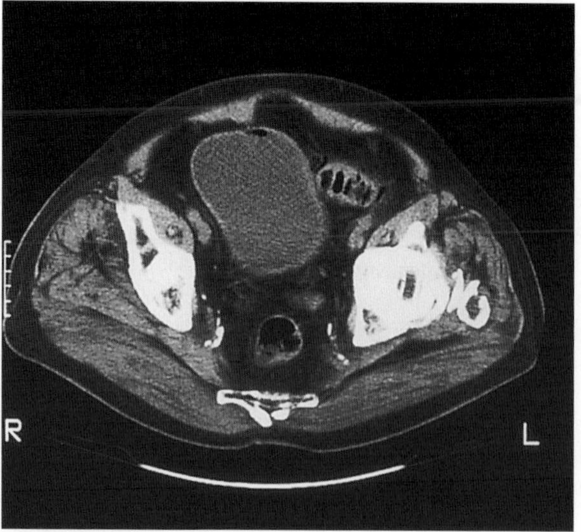

Figure 70.1b

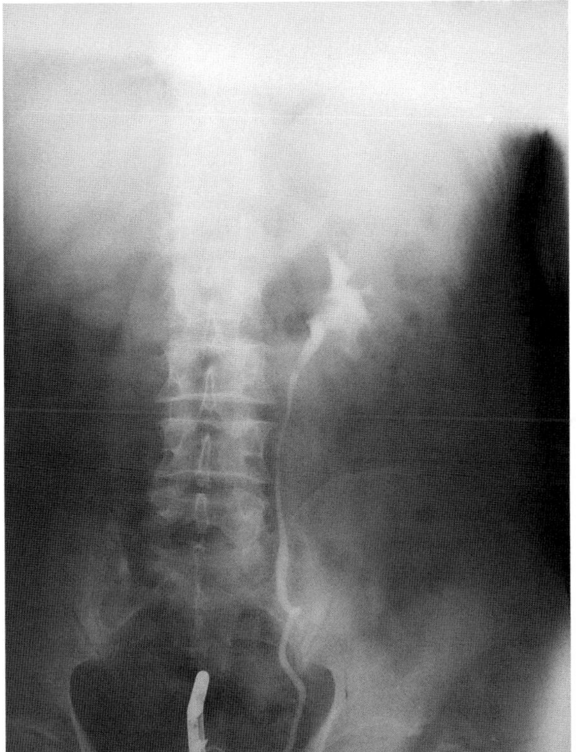

Figure 70.2

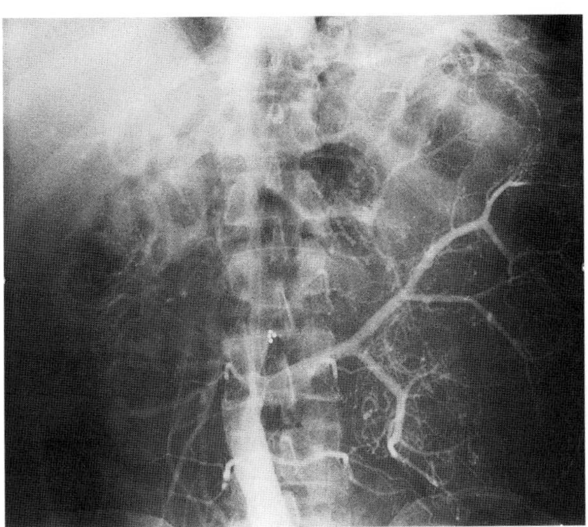

Figure 70.3

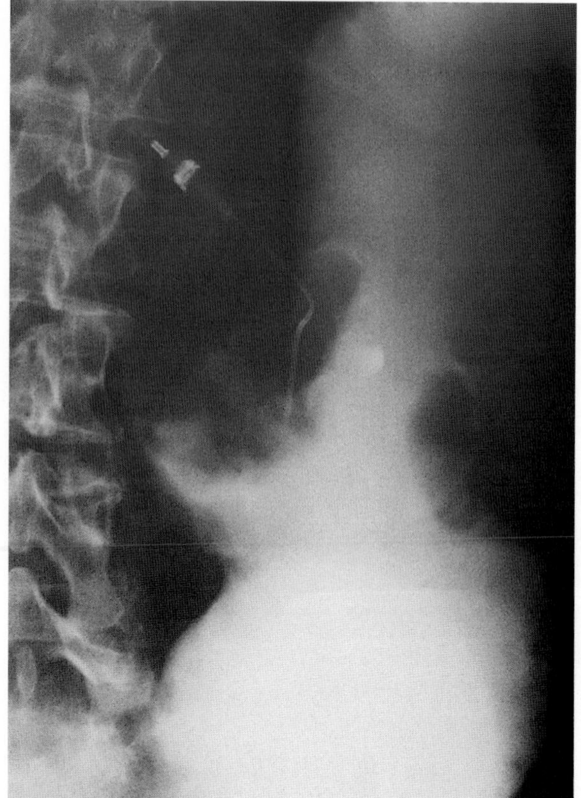

Figure 70.4

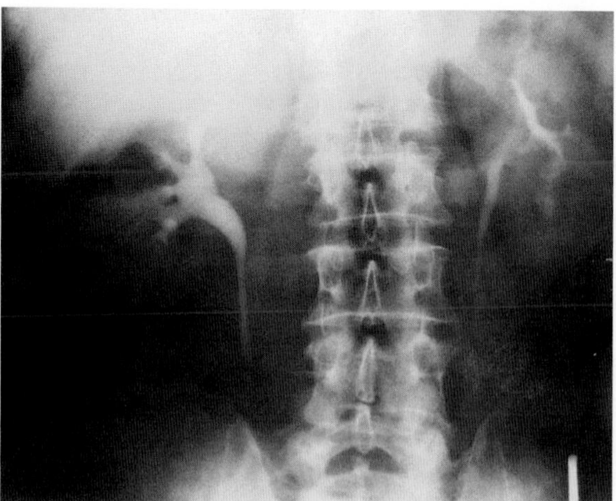

Figure 70.5

Answers: Multiple choice questions

Haematuria

1. A, E

Haematuria, whether macroscopic or microscopic, is always abnormal Haematuria from a malignant cause is usually painless although renal cell carcinoma presents with loin pain.

Pain of urological origin

2. E

Renal pain is a deep ache in the loin and is caused by stretching of the renal capsule. When the cause is inflammatory, there may be deep local tenderness with psoas spasm causing flexion of the hip. Ureteric calculus causes one of the most severe pains ever, with the patient writhing around unable to find a comfortable position, and the pain radiates to groin and genitalia. Bladder pain may take the form of wrenching discomfort at the end of micturition referred to as strangury. Pain in the perineum is a penetrating ache radiating to the rectum. Although it is usually of prostatic origin it is known to occur in women.

Preliminary investigations and renal failure

3. A

More than 70 per cent of kidney function must be lost before renal failure becomes evident because the kidneys have a large functional reserve.

Imaging in urological conditions

4. A, C, E

Uric acid calculi are radiolucent and hence not visible on a plain X-ray. IVU has the advantage over US in that an IVU shows renal function, which US does not. However, IVU can be dangerous as, in a minority of patients, the intravenous contrast can cause severe hypersensitivity reactions.

Renal failure

5. D

All patients with renal failure will not require renal replacement therapy. The cause of renal failure should be established – prerenal, renal or postrenal. The patient is treated depending on the cause. When all conservative measures helped by a nephrologist have failed and the patient has severe life-threatening hyperkalaemia, some form of dialysis is indicated.

Answers: Extended matching questions

1. Imaging

Fig. 70.1a and b, A

Computed tomography (CT) scan showing air in the urinary bladder from vesicocolic fistula.

Fig. 70.2, E

Left retrograde ureterogram showing irregular filling defect in left renal pelvis from transitional cell carcinoma.

Fig. 70.3, B

Left renal angiogram showing a very large and voscular left renal cell carcinoma pushing the aorta to the right.

Fig. 70.4, C
Left antegrade pyelogram showing multiple filling defects from transitional cell carcinoma of renal pelvis.

Fig. 70.5, D
Intravenous urogram showing irregular filling defect in left renal pelvis from transitional cell carcinoma.

71 The kidneys and ureters

Multiple choice questions

Congenital abnormalities of the kidney, renal pelvis and ureters

1. Which of the following statements are true?

A The incidence of absence of one kidney is 1 in 5000.
B The incidence of ectopic kidney is 1 in 1000.
C Horseshoe kidney occurs in 1 in 1000.
D Polycystic kidneys can be transmitted by either parent as an autosomal dominant trait.
E Polycystic kidneys present in childhood as renal failure.

2. Which of the following statements are false?

A Duplication of the renal pelvis is found in 4 per cent of patients.
B Duplication of the ureter is found in 3 per cent of patients.
C Ureterocele is a cystic enlargement of the intramural ureter.
D All ureteroceles must be treated by endoscopic diathermy incision.
E Retrocaval ureter can cause obstructive symptoms.

Renal and ureteric injury

3. Which of the following statements are true?

A Haematuria following trivial injury of the kidney indicates a previously pathological kidney.
B Closed renal injury is always extraperitoneal.
C In closed renal injury, surgical exploration is necessary in the majority.
D Intravenous urography or contrast-enhanced computed tomography (CECT) scan should be performed urgently in suspected renal injury.
E Hypertension may be a long-term complication of renal injury.

4. Which of the following statements are false?

A Most ureteric injuries are due to surgical trauma during pelvic surgery.
B Preoperative ureteric catheterisation helps to protect them from injury during operation.
C When recognised during operation, an injured ureter should be repaired immediately.
D When ureteric injury is diagnosed postoperatively, delayed repair is undertaken.
E Urinary fistula through an abdominal or vaginal wound indicates a damaged ureter.

Clinical conditions

5. In hydronephrosis from pelviureteric junction (PUJ) obstruction (idiopathic or congenital hydronephrosis), which of the following statements are false?

A The condition may be asymptomatic.
B It can be diagnosed in utero.
C Ultrasound scanning is the least invasive method of imaging.
D An intravenous urogram (IVU) is the ideal imaging.
E If there is more than 5 per cent of function in the obstructed kidney, a procedure to preserve the kidney is carried out.

6. With regard to renal stones, which of the following statements are true?

A The common bacteria found as a nidus for urinary stones are staphylococci and *E. coli.*

B Hyperparathyroidism is found in 5 per cent or less of those presenting with radio-opaque calculi.

C If a parathyroid adenoma is found to be the cause of renal calculi, it should be removed before treatment of the calculus.

D Pure uric acid stones are radio-opaque.

E A staghorn calculus is composed of calcium-ammonium-magnesium phosphate.

7. Which of the following statements are false?

A Renal stones are usually visible on a plain X-ray.

B The severity of pain of ureteric colic is related to the size of stone.

C Hydronephrosis and/or pyonephrosis with a palpable loin swelling is common.

D Haematuria is common.

E There are very few physical signs.

8. Which of the following imaging techniques are used for urinary calculus disease?

A Plain kidney, ureter and bladder (KUB) X-ray

B CECT

C IVU

D Ultrasound (US)

E Retrograde pyelography.

9. Which of the following statements regarding the management of urinary calculi are false?

A Ureteric calculi smaller than 1 cm will pass spontaneously.

B Infection in the presence of upper urinary tract obstruction due to a stone requires surgical intervention.

C Most urinary calculi can be treated by minimal-access techniques.

D In bilateral renal stones, the kidney with poorer function is treated first.

E Open operations for renal stones are performed through an extraperitoneal loin approach.

10. Which of the following statements are true in ureteric stones?

A The majority pass spontaneously.

B If obstruction persists after 6 weeks, the stone should be removed.

C Stones are commonly arrested at the two sites of ureteric narrowing.

D Most stones are treated by ureteroscopic electrohydraulic fragmentation.

E Severe renal pain subsiding after a day or two suggests that the stone has passed.

→ Infections

11. Which of the following statements are false?

A Ascending infection in the urinary tract is the most common route.

B *E. coli* and other Gram-negative organisms are most commonly responsible.

C *Proteus* and staphylococci thrive in acidic urine.

D Up to 50 per cent of children with urinary infection have an underlying abnormality.

E All patients present electively with dysuria and frequency of micturition.

12. Which of the following statements are true?

A Sterile pyuria should alert one to the possibility of renal tuberculosis.

B Chronic pyelonephritis is often associated with vesicoureteric reflux.

C Pyonephrosis is an infected hydronephrosis and is most commonly due to a stone causing obstruction.

D Renal carbuncle is most commonly seen in the immunocompromised.

E Perinephric abscess may occur from extension of a retrocaecal appendix abscess.

F All of the above.

G None of the above.

Renal neoplasms

13. Which of the following statements about Wilms' tumour is false?

A It is a tumour of embryonic nephrogenic tissue occurring below the age of 5 years.
B Haematuria and fever are the commonest presentations.
C Lymphatic spread is rare.
D Imaging modalities are US, CT and MRI.
E Treatment is by chemotherapy, surgery and radiotherapy.

14. Which of the following statements are true about hypernephroma?

A It occurs more commonly in women.
B In 25 per cent of patients there are no local symptoms.
C A left-sided varicocele may be a presenting feature in a male.
D Haematuria and clot colic are the commonest presentations.
E IVU, US and CECT are the imaging methods of choice.
F Following nephrectomy, chemotherapy and radiotherapy should be given.

Extended matching questions

1. Renal pathology

A Renal stone
B Hypernephroma
C Congenital (idiopathic) hydronephrosis
D Pyonephrosis
E Ureteric calculus

Choose and match the following diagnoses with each of the scenarios given below:

1 A 40-year-old man has come to the A&E department complaining of a sudden onset of very severe pain in his left loin of 4 h duration, radiating to the front of the lumbar area and groin and the left testis. He has vomited a couple of times and has urinary frequency. On examination he is writhing around in pain and cannot find a comfortable position.

2 A 60-year-old man complains of haematuria associated with pain in his left loin radiating to the lower abdomen. He passes clots which are 'worm-like'. On examination he has an enlarged left kidney, and scrotal examination reveals a varicocele which he finds uncomfortable.

3 A 45-year-old female patient complains of nagging pain in her right loin and urinary frequency for several months. On examination she has tenderness in her loin over the kidney. Urine examination shows red blood cells and a growth of *Proteus* and staphylococci.

4 A 20-year-old fit young man had a game of rugby, following which he passed frank blood in his urine in the changing room. He felt some discomfort in his left loin. On going home, his haematuria became worse and he noticed some fullness in his left loin. He then came to the A&E department. His blood pressure was 110/60 mmHg, pulse 110/min and he had fullness in his left loin.

5 A 60-year-old female patient was seen as an emergency with high temperature, rigors and pain in her right loin. She had a blood pressure of 160/70 mmHg, bounding pulse of 90/min and extreme tenderness in her right loin.

2. Renal pathology imaging

A Renal trauma
B Staghorn calculus
C Hypernephroma
D Horseshoe kidney
E Hydronephrosis

Choose and match the diagnoses with the images (Figs 71.1–71.5) shown below:

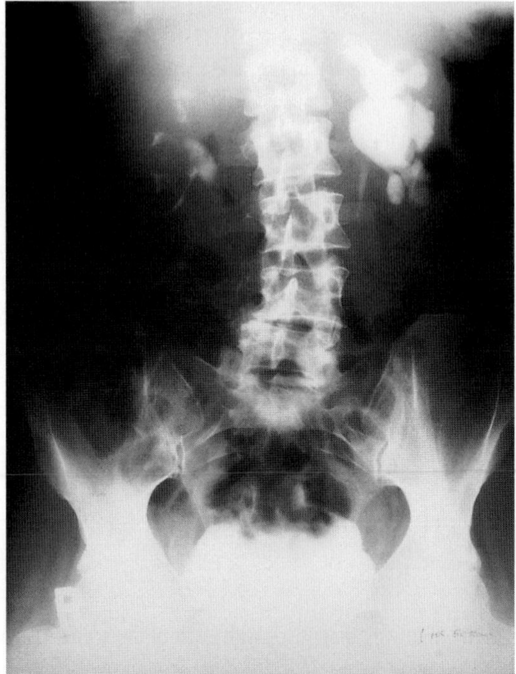

Figure 71.1

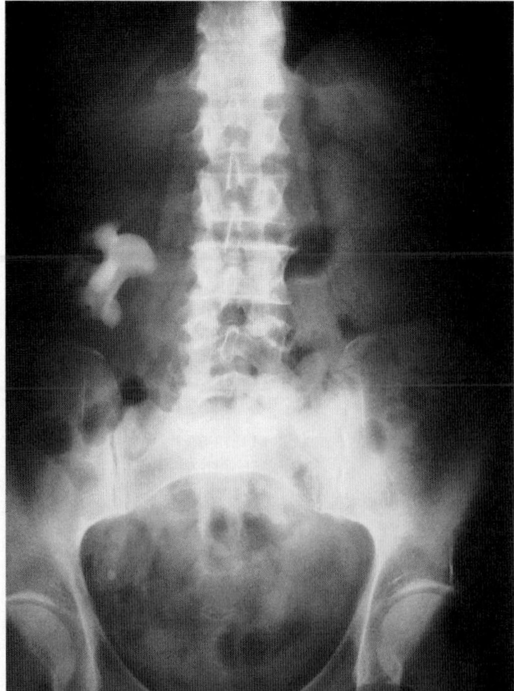

Figure 71.2

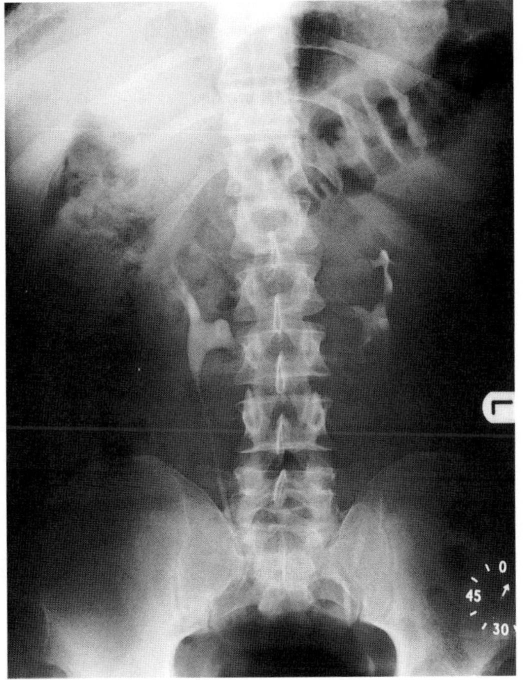

Figure 71.3

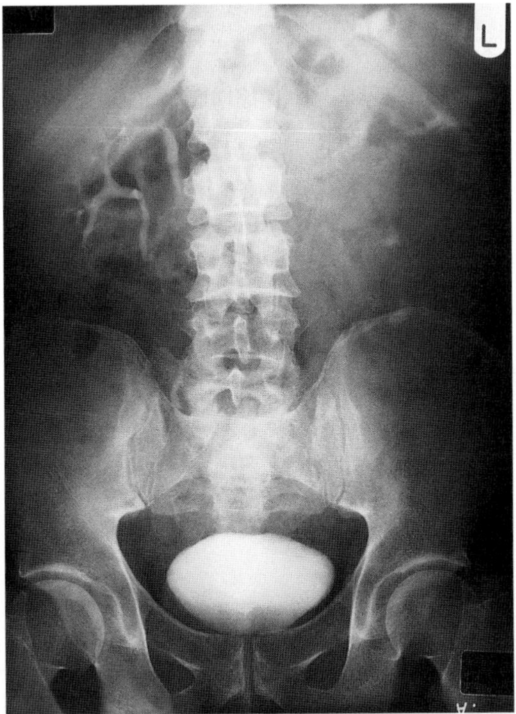

Figure 71.4

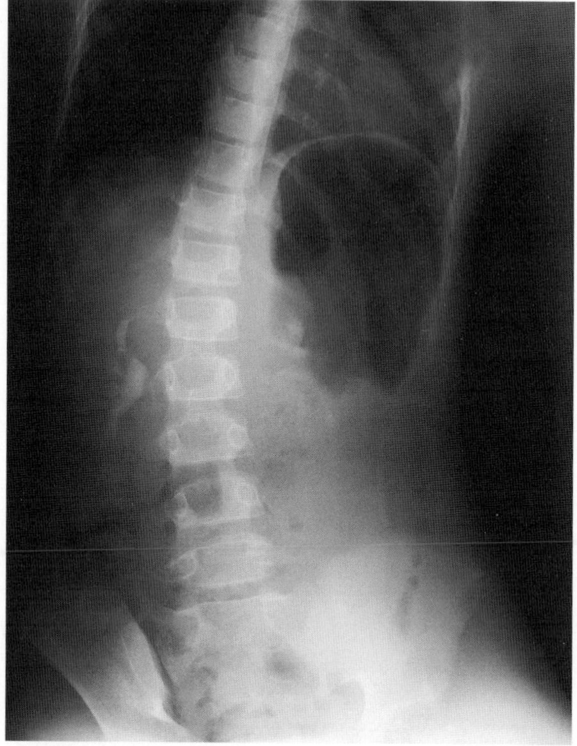

Figure 71.5

3. Ureteric pathology imaging

A Carcinoma of the ureter
B Retrograde pyelogram showing transitional cell carcinoma of the renal pelvis
C Left ureteric calculus
D IVU showing transitional cell carcinoma of the left renal pelvis
E Antegrade pyelogram showing transitional cell carcinoma of the renal pelvis

Choose and match the diagnoses with the images (Figs 71.6–71.10) shown below:

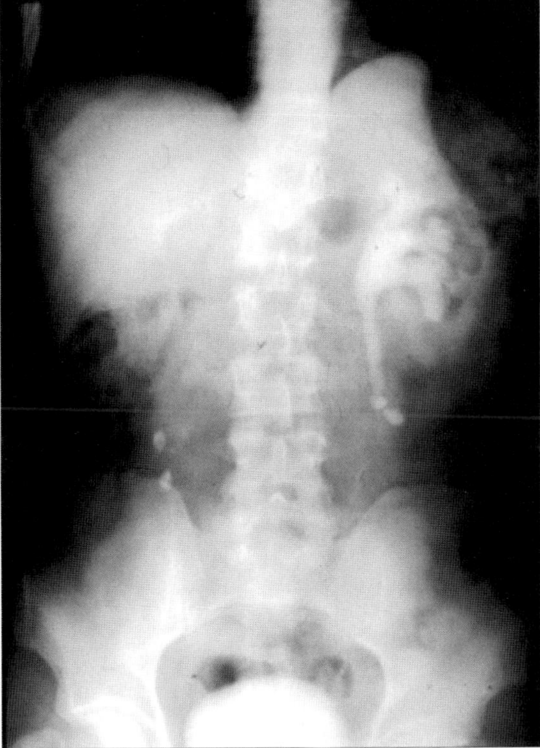

Figure 71.6

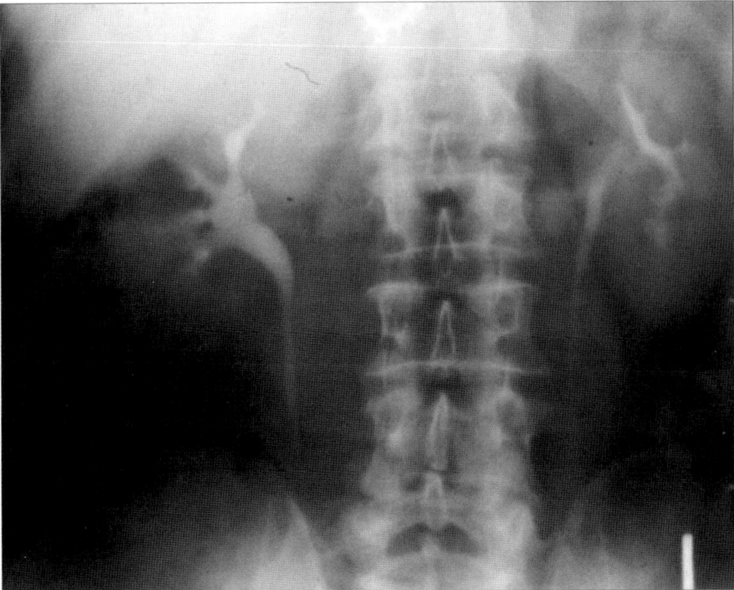

Figure 71.7

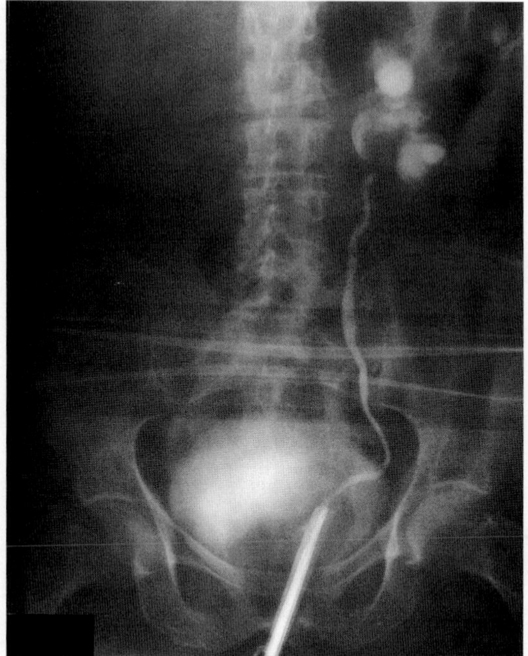

Figure 71.8

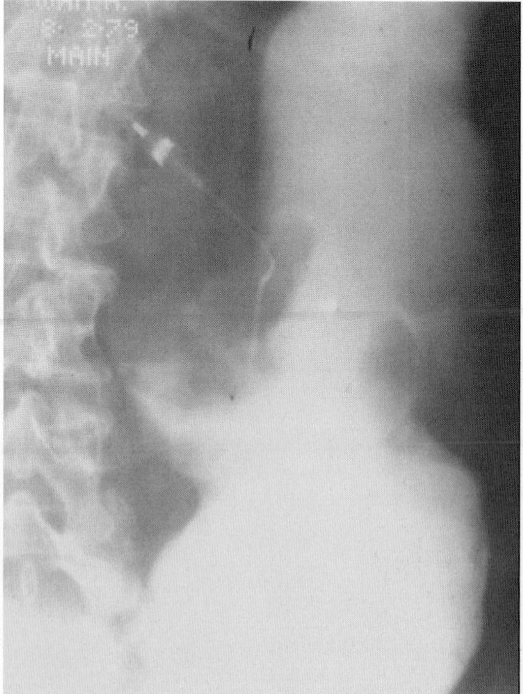

Figure 71.9

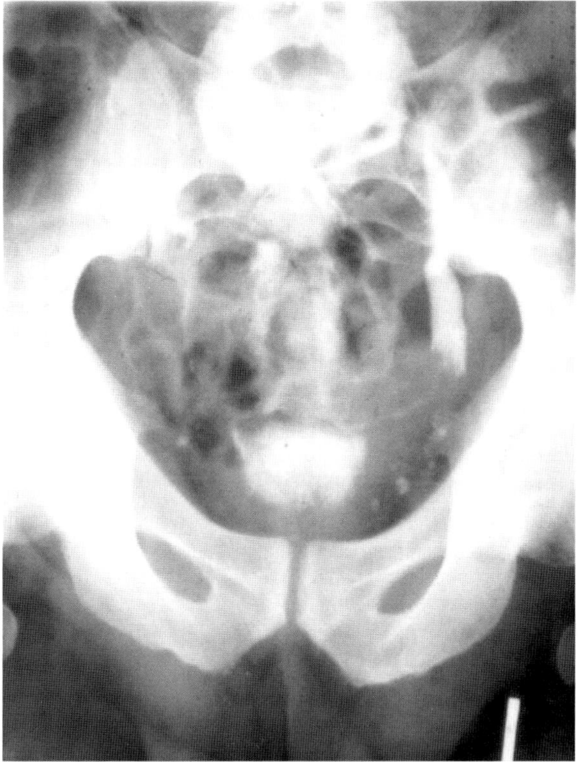

Figure 71.10

Answers: Multiple choice questions

Congenital abnormalities of the kidney, renal pelvis and ureters

1. B, C, D

The incidence of renal agenesis is 1 in 1400 and is most often diagnosed incidentally. Horseshoe kidneys are usually fused by its isthmus at the lower pole. Polycystic kidneys are usually detected on standard imaging in the second and third decades. The condition does not manifest itself clinically before the age of 30 years.

2. D

Ureteroceles do not always produce symptoms, in which case they should be left alone. If there is recurrent infection and stone formation, it is treated by endoscopic diathermy incision. This can result in postoperative vesicoureteric reflux.

Renal and ureteric injury

3. A, D, E

Closed renal injury is usually extraperitoneal in adults. However, in children, because they have very little extraperitoneal fat, the peritoneum, which is closely adherent of the kidney, can tear with the renal capsule causing urine and blood to leak into the peritoneum. The mainstay of management of renal injury is conservative. Surgical exploration is necessary in less than 10 per cent of closed renal injury cases.

4. D

When ureteric injury is diagnosed postoperatively, early repair is safe provided the patient's general condition is good. The patient should undergo an IVU or a CECT to evaluate the nature of injury and repair undertaken.

Clinical conditions

5. D, E

Isotope renography is the best test to establish that dilatation is caused by obstruction. It would also determine the percentage function of the kidney. IVU is not the ideal imaging method. It is useful only when there is significant renal function of the obstructed kidney. A procedure to preserve the kidney is carried out when a renogram shows that there is more than 20 per cent of renal function. The operation of choice is Anderson–Hynes pyeloplasty, a procedure which is now being carried out laparoscopically. Minimal-access surgical techniques such as endoscopic pyelotomy and balloon dilatation are also being done.

6. A, B, C, E

Pure uric acid stones are radiolucent and show up as a filling defect on an IVU, mimicking a transitional cell carcinoma of the renal pelvis. Most uric acid stones contain some calcium and therefore cast a faint shadow on plain X-ray. Confirmation is done by a CT scan.

7. B, C

The severity of ureteric colic is not related to the size of the stone. The pain is agonising, typically passing from the loin to the groin with the patient writhing round unable to find a comfortable position. Hydronephrosis or pyonephrosis is rare. Most stones pass spontaneously.

8. A, B, C, D

Plain radiography has a limited place as opacities from calcified mesenteric lymph nodes, gallstones, foreign bodies, phleboliths and calcified adrenal gland may cause confusion. Spiral CECT is the gold standard of investigation in acute ureteric colic. IVU has a role if CECT is not available and also shows up the anatomical site of the stone. Ultrasound is essential for treatment with extracorporeal shock wave lithotripsy (ESWL).

9. A, D

Ureteric calculi smaller than 0.5 cm will pass spontaneously, larger stones requiring surgical intervention. In bilateral renal stones, the kidney with better function is treated first. The exception is that the kidney with pain or pyonephrosis is treated first by decompression by nephrostomy.

10. A, D

If obstruction from a ureteric stone persists after 1 or 2 weeks, the stone should be removed; otherwise it may cause renal atrophy and loss of function. In the ureter, stones are commonly arrested at one of the 5 anatomical sites of narrowing: pelviureteric junction, crossing of the iliac vessels, proximity of vas deferens or broad ligament, entrance to the bladder wall and ureteric orifice. Severe renal pain subsiding after a day or so is a sinister symptom: it denotes complete ureteric obstruction.

Infections

11. C, E

Proteus and staphylococci are urea-splitting organisms and form ammonia, which makes the urine alkaline, predisposing to stone formation. While patients may present electively, often they are seen as an emergency with septicaemia presenting with high temperature, rigors, tachycardia and features of shock.

12. F

Renal neoplasms

13. B

The commonest presentation is an abdominal mass noticed by the mother when bathing the child. Haematuria is a late symptom and denotes extension of the tumour into the renal pelvis and thus a poor prognosis.

14. B, C, D, E

Hypernephroma is twice as common in men as in women. Chemotherapy and radiotherapy have no role in adjuvant treatment. The cytokine interleukin-2 has had some encouraging outcomes.

Answers: Extended matching questions

1. Renal pathology

1E

This patient has typical ureteric colic. He needs immediate analgesia with diclofenac and indomethacin. Confirmation of the diagnosis is made by CECT and IVU, and appropriate definitive treatment should be instituted.

2B

This male patient has the classical presentation of a left hypernephroma (adenocarcinoma): haematuria, loin pain and clot colic and an enlarged kidney. He also has a left varicocele caused by growth extending into the left renal vein, obstructing the entry of left testicular vein. He needs an IVU, CECT and a chest X-ray and radical nephrectomy.

3A

This patient with nagging pain in her right loin and urinary frequency has symptoms suggestive of a kidney stone. The growth of urea-splitting organisms of *Proteus* and staphylococci indicate alkaline urine which is conducive to the formation of phosphate calculi. An IVU, US and CT scan should be done to confirm the diagnosis, and appropriate treatment of percutaneous nephrolithotomy (PCNL), extracorporeal shockwave lithotripsy (ESWL) or a combination of both instituted.

4C

This 20-year-old man developed haematuria following minor trauma while playing rugby. He was completely unaware of the trauma and surprised to have haematuria. He did notice some left loin discomfort. Haematuria following minor trauma occurs typically in a pathological kidney. In a fit young man this would be a hydronephrosis from a PUJ obstruction which has ruptured with urinary extravasation. He needs an US, IVU and CECT followed by urgent exploration and possible Anderson–Hynes operation.

5D

This woman has all the features of septicaemia: shock and hyperdynamic circulation (large pulse pressure) and bounding pulse. Loin tenderness points to a diagnosis of pyonephrosis. She needs urgent resuscitation, blood cultures, appropriate antibiotics, IVU, US and CECT. This should be followed by nephrostomy. In due course, she should have isotope renogram to assess function of the kidney and appropriate definitive treatment.

2. Renal pathology imaging

Fig. 71.1, E

This IVU shows normal excretion from the right kidney. On the left side there is gross pelvicalyceal dilatation with clubbing of the calyces. The upper end of the ureter is normal, indicating a PUJ obstruction – idiopathic or congenital hydronephrosis.

Fig. 71.2, B
This is a plain X-ray showing a typical staghorn calculus in the right kidney.

Fig. 71.3, D
This IVU shows the renal pelvis and calyces facing medially, a 'flower vase' appearance of a typical horseshoe kidney, an abnormality found in 1 in 1000. This is most often discovered incidentally.

Fig. 71.4, C
This IVU shows normal excretion from the right kidney with a bifid renal pelvis. On the left side there is a huge soft-tissue shadow with irregular excretion of contrast. The urinary bladder is filled normally. The diagnosis is left hypernephroma.

Fig. 71.5, A
This IVU in a child shows marked scoliosis with concavity to the left, elevated left dome of diaphragm, the stomach and colonic gas bubbles pushed up, left psoas shadow obliterated, good excretion from right kidney and extravasated contrast in the left renal area. These features are suggestive of a left perirenal haematoma from left renal injury.

→ 3. Ureteric pathology imaging

Fig. 71.6, C
This IVU shows left hydronephrosis and hydroureter proximal to a stone in the middle third of the ureter. The right kidney has completely excreted and the bladder is filled. There are calcified lymph nodes on both sides.

Fig. 71.7, D
This IVU shows an irregular filling defect in the left renal pelvis classical of a transitional cell carcinoma of the left renal pelvis.

Fig. 71.8, B
This is a left retrograde pyelogram showing the cystoscope in the urinary bladder and dye injected into the left ureter and renal pelvis. There is an irregular filling defect in the renal pelvis denoting a transitional cell carcinoma.

Fig. 71.9, E
This is an antegrade pyelogram showing a hugely dilated renal pelvis containing a large number of irregular filling defects – typical of a transitional cell carcinoma of the renal pelvis.

Fig. 71.10, A
This IVU shows the cystographic phase. There is dilatation of the lower end of the left ureter showing an irregular filling defect distal to the dilatation with minimal contrast going through the area of filling defect. This is typical of a transitional cell carcinoma of the lower end of the left ureter. Some phleboliths are also seen.

72 The urinary bladder

Multiple choice questions

Anatomy

1. Which of the following anatomical statements are true?

A The bladder is lined by transitional epithelium.
B Hypertrophy of the detrusor muscle results in bladder trabeculation.
C The epithelium of the trigone extends into the lower ends of ureters and proximal urethra.
D The internal sphincter prevents urinary incontinence.
E The distal urethral sphincter is supplied by S2–S4 fibres via the pudendal nerves.

Bladder injury

2. In bladder trauma, which of the following statements are false?

A Extraperitoneal rupture is more common than intraperitoneal rupture.
B Extraperitoneal rupture mimics rupture of membranous urethra.
C CT scan is the investigation of choice.
D Retrograde cystography is useful in making a diagnosis.
E Laparotomy is required in all cases of bladder rupture.

Detrusor instability

3. Which of the following statements about detrusor instability is false?

A 50 per cent of men with bladder outflow obstruction have detrusor instability.
B In 50 per cent the detrusor instability resolves after prostatectomy.
C Patients with neurogenic bladder may have detrusor instability.
D Genuine stress incontinence (GSI) is indistinguishable from detrusor instability.
E Urodynamic studies are essential for evaluation of detrusor instability.

Bladder stones

4. With regard to bladder stones which of the following statements are false?

A Men are more often affected than women.
B An oxalate calculus develops in sterile urine.
C A cystine calculus is not radio-opaque.
D Treatment is crushing with an optical lithotrite in all cases.
E In men with stones and outflow obstruction from enlarged prostate, both can be dealt with at the same time.

Bladder diverticula

5. Which of the following are true about bladder diverticula?

A They are diagnosed when they produce double micturition and repeated urinary tract infections.
B All bladder diverticula must be excised.
C Trabeculation and sacculation precede diverticula formation.
D The normal intravesical pressure during voiding is 35–50 cmH_2O.
E The majority occur in males.
F Haematuria is a symptom in 30 per cent.

Urinary fistulae

6. Which of the following statements about urinary fistulae is false?

A Most urinary fistulae are vesicovaginal.
B A combined ureterovaginal fistula may be present in 10 per cent of patients.
C Examination under anaesthesia, intravenous urogram (IVU) and cystoscopy are necessary to evaluate them.
D When there are multiple tracts, the causes may be radiation, malignancy or sepsis.

E Conservative management by catheter drainage of the bladder is usually successful.

Urinary tract infection

7. In urinary tract infection (UTI) which of the following statements are false?

A The condition is more common in women.
B In recurrent infections, haematuria and rigors, cystoscopy and imaging are essential.
C Sterile pyuria is a sinister finding.
D In tuberculous cystitis, the route of infection is usually haematogenous or lymphogenous.
E Carcinoma in situ may present as recurrent abacterial cystitis.

Bladder cancer

8. Which of the following are true of bladder cancer?

A 95 per cent of primary bladder cancers are transitional cell carcinomas.
B Painful haematuria is the most significant symptom.
C Depth of invasion (T) in TNM classification and grade (WHO classification I, II, III) are important factors in planning treatment.
D In a quarter of new patients, the muscle is invaded.
E In newly diagnosed patients, 70 per cent do not invade muscle.

9. What are the essential investigations in bladder cancer?

A IVU and US
B Contrast-enhanced computed tomography (CECT) – this is necessary for suspected muscle-invasive tumours
C A bone scan – necessary to exclude bone secondaries
D Cystourethroscopy and bimanual examination – mandatory for staging
E Urine cytology.

10. In the treatment of bladder cancers, which of the following statements are true?

A Superficial tumours are treated by endoscopic resection and a single dose of mitomycin instillation.
B Grade 3 superficial disease is best managed by BCG immunotherapy.
C External beam radiotherapy should be the first-line treatment in muscle-invasive disease.
D In muscle-invasive disease, radical cystectomy and lymphadenectomy should be the primary treatment of choice.
E Neoadjuvant cisplatin-based chemotherapy improves survival in muscle-invasive tumours.

Extended matching questions

1. Bladder pathology

A Bladder stone
B Bladder diverticulum
C Bladder carcinoma
D Tuberculosis of the bladder
E Schistosomiasis of bladder

Choose and match the following diagnoses with each of the scenarios given below:

1 A 35-year-old male, a recent visitor from Egypt, attended the A&E department with painless haematuria at the end of micturition. He had a few similar episodes while at home in Egypt. Clinical examination revealed no abnormality. He was referred to the one-stop haematuria clinic. On flexible cystoscopy he was found to have scattered tubercles and islands of pale patches resembling sand.

2 A 70-year-old male, a heavy smoker for over 50 years, complains of painless, profuse and periodic haematuria for 6 weeks or so. The blood is uniformly mixed with the urine. He has frequency of micturition and some retropubic discomfort. Clinical examination reveals no abnormality.

3 A 70-year-old male complains of poor micturition stream, post-micturition dribbling and a feeling of insufficient emptying of his bladder. He has some dysuria. On occasions he has found that shortly after micturition he again passes a large amount of urine. Clinical examination reveals no abnormality.

4 A 60-year-old man complains of haematuria, painful micturition and occasionally finds that his micturition stream suddenly stops. He has learnt to re-start his stream by changing position. Clinical examination reveals no abnormality.

5 A 35-year-old female patient, a recent visitor from India, complains of frequency of micturition and bilateral loin discomfort. She has evening pyrexia, general malaise and weight loss. Clinical examination reveals no abnormality. Urine examination carried out by her doctor shows sterile pyuria.

2. Bladder imaging

A Benign prostatic hypertrophy (BPH)
B Rupture of the bladder
C Carcinoma of the bladder
D Bladder stone
E Bladder diverticulum

Choose and match the diagnoses with the images (Figs 72.1–72.5) shown below:

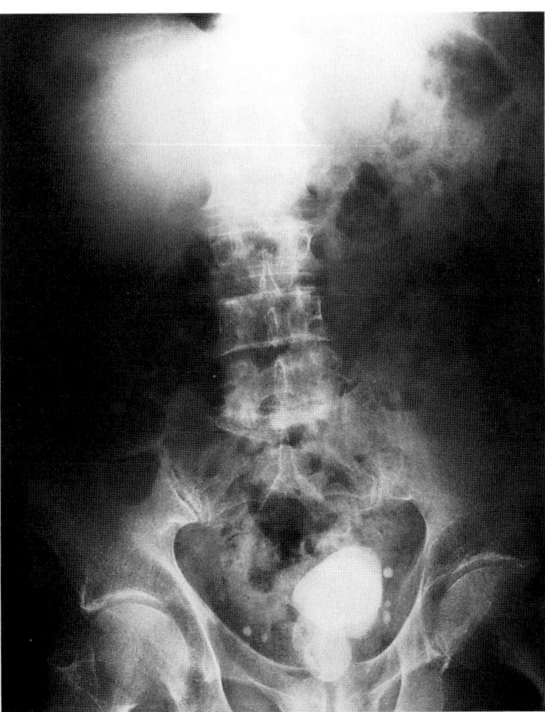

Figure 72.1

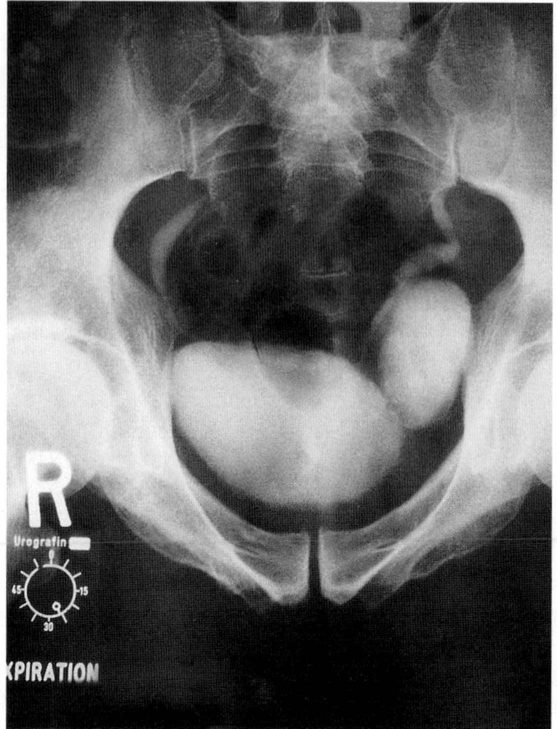

Figure 72.2

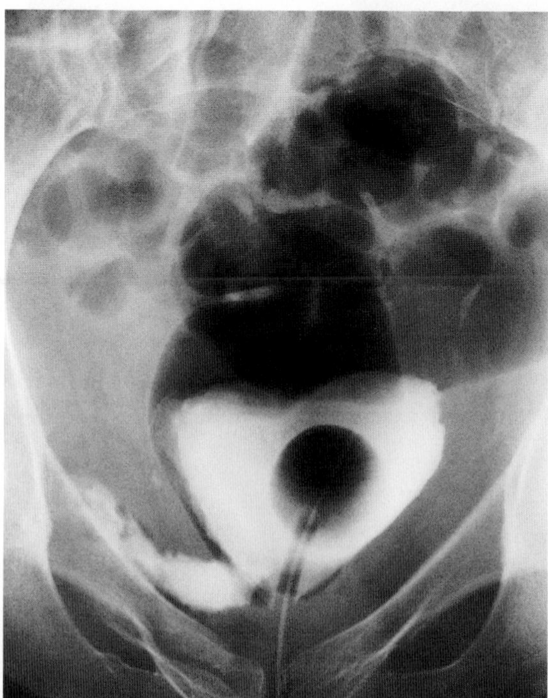

Figure 72.3

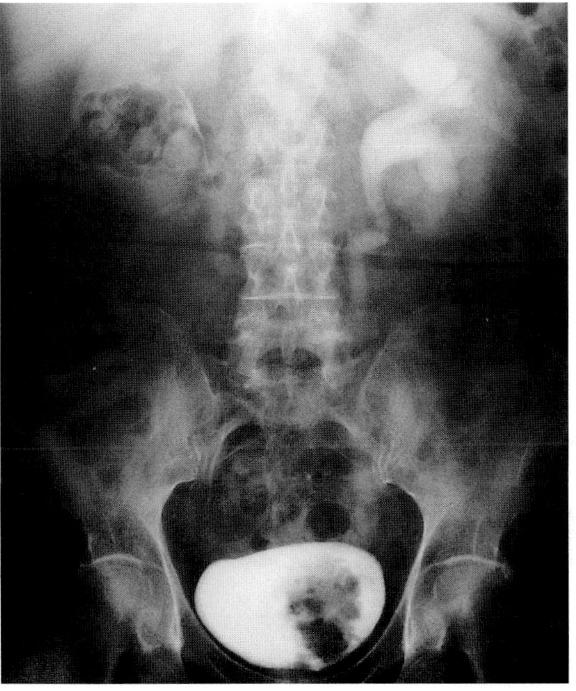

Figure 72.4a

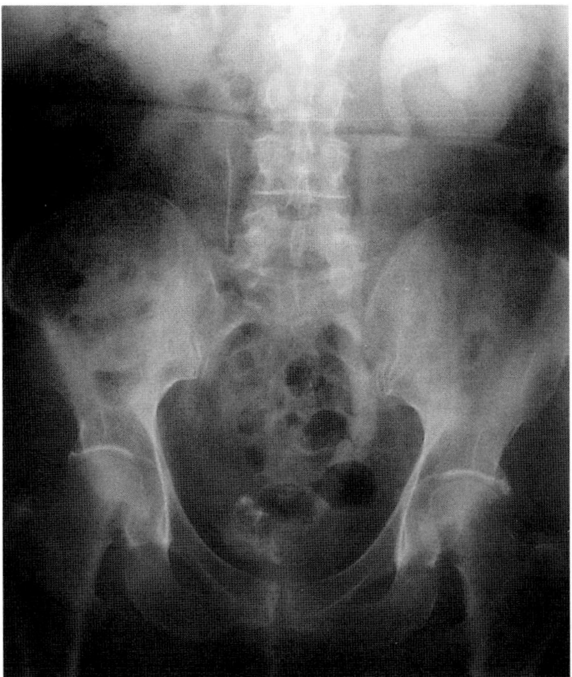

Figure 72.4b

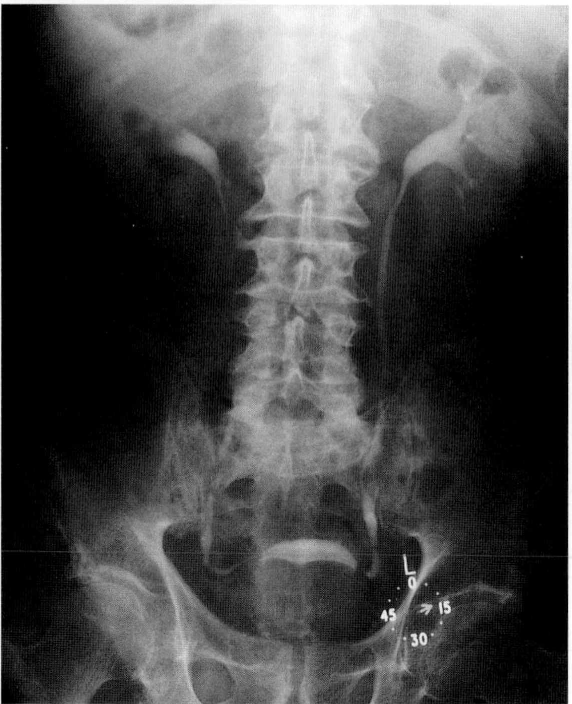

Figure 72.5

Answers: Multiple choice questions

→ Anatomy

1. A, B, C, E

The internal sphincter is the smooth muscle around the male bladder neck which prevents retrograde ejaculation and has no role in urinary continence.

→ Bladder injury

2. E

In intraperitoneal injury, treatment is laparotomy and closure of the perforation. In extraperitoneal rupture, catheter drainage of the bladder for 10 days is the management.

→ Detrusor instability

3. D

Idiopathic detrusor instability can mimic GSI and may coexist. But they are different conditions that can be properly diagnosed by urodynamic studies. Surgical treatment will only be successful in the correctly diagnosed patient with GSI.

→ Bladder stones

4. D

While most bladder stones can be treated by minimal-access surgery by litholapaxy using an optical lithotrite, the procedure is contraindicated in patients below 10 years.

Bladder diverticula

5. C, D, E, F

Bladder diverticula are most often detected incidentally on imaging (US or IVU) or on cystoscopy. Most of them do not need to be excised unless there is a complication such as recurrent infections, stone or tumour. As they are caused by bladder outflow obstruction, TURP is all that is required in the vast majority.

Urinary fistulae

6. E

Conservative management is rarely successful. The principles of repair are good exposure, excision of diseased tissue and tension-free vascularised repair in anatomical layers.

Urinary tract infection

7. D

Tuberculous cystitis is secondary to renal tuberculosis and not due to haematogenous or lymphogenous spread. Therefore, changes commence around the ureteric orifices and trigone in the form of pallor of the mucosa and submucosal oedema. Tubercles appear later.

Bladder cancer

8. A, C, D, E

Painless, periodic, progressive gross haematuria is typical of bladder cancer. If pain occurs in bladder cancer, it denotes extravesical spread.

9. A, B, D

A bone scan is not essential. It is only done when skeletal spread is strongly suspected clinically. Urine cytology is helpful only if positive but a negative result has no value.

10. A, B, D, E

In muscle-invasive disease, the primary treatment of choice should be radical surgery in the form of radical cystectomy with lymphadenectomy. This should be combined with cisplatin-based systemic chemotherapy. This improves survival by about 5–7 per cent. External beam radiotherapy as an option should be considered in those unfit for major surgery or those who decline surgery.

Answers: Extended matching questions

1. Bladder pathology

1E

This patient has schistosomiasis of the urinary bladder. Investigations to determine involvement of the liver should be done. Antibody detection by enzyme-linked immunosorbent assay (ELISA) using *Schistosoma mansoni* adult microsomal antibody (MAMA) is carried out. Medical treatment by praziquantel is effective.

2C

This patient has the typical symptoms of a bladder carcinoma – painless, profuse and periodic haematuria. He needs urgent assessment by IVU, US, CECT followed by cystourethroscopy and bimanual palpation for accurate staging followed by the appropriate treatment.

3B

This man has all the clinical features of bladder outflow obstruction (BOO). The history of double micturition is typical of a bladder diverticulum which is the direct result of BOO. An US is done to confirm the diagnosis, followed by urodynamic studies to assess his BOO. The treatment should be, firstly, cystoscopy to see the inside of the diverticulum. If this shows no abnormality, transurethral resection of his prostate is carried out. Follow-up by US assessment of the diverticulum is done, as most do not require removal.

4A

This man's painful micturition and haematuria are from a bladder stone. The history of sudden cessation of micturition stream is a typical feature. Imaging should be done by US followed by cystoscopy and treatment by optical litholapaxy.

5D

This woman has a history typical of tuberculosis – evening pyrexia, malaise and weight loss. Bilateral loin pain and sterile pyuria would suggest tuberculosis of the kidneys and the bladder. The patient requires urine culture, full haematological and biochemical examination, IVU and chest X-ray. This is followed by cystoscopy, which may show a contracted bladder with 'golf hole' ureters and tubercles studded in the mucosa. She should be managed by a multidisciplinary team.

→ 2. Bladder imaging

Fig. 72.1, D

This is a plain X-ray showing a large, dumbbell-shaped bladder stone lying at the bladder base.

Fig. 72.2, E

This is a cystographic phase of an IVU showing a bladder diverticulum on the left, close to the ureteric orifice.

Fig. 72.3, B

This cystogram shows extravasation of contrast at the bladder neck – typical of extraperitoneal rupture of the bladder. Patient has an indwelling Foley catheter as treatment.

Fig. 72.4a and b, C

These two IVU pictures show an irregular filling defect on the left side of the bladder obstructing the left ureter, causing left hydronephrosis and hydroureter.

Fig. 72.5, A

This IVU shows a regular, smooth filling defect in the base of the bladder. The lower ends of the ureters show a classical 'fish hook' deformity. The picture is typical of benign prostatic hypertrophy.

73 The prostate and seminal vesicles

Multiple choice questions

Anatomy and physiology

1. **Which of the following statements is false?**
   - A The prostate is anatomically divided into a peripheral zone, a central zone and a transitional zone.
   - B The glands of the peripheral zone are lined by transitional epithelium.
   - C Benign prostatic hypertrophy occurs in the transitional zone.
   - D Most carcinomas arise in the peripheral zone.
   - E Denonvilliers' fascia separates the prostate from the rectum.

2. **Which of the following statements regarding androgenic hormones are true?**
   - A Luteinising hormone (LH) from the anterior pituitary controls the secretion of testosterone.
   - B 90 per cent of testosterone is secreted by Leydig cells from the testes.
   - C The enzyme 5α-reductase is found in high concentration in the prostate.
   - D Adrenal androgens have a major effect in the normal male.
   - E 5α-reductase converts testosterone into1,5-dihydrotestosterone (DHT).

Benign prostatic hypertrophy

3. **In benign prostatic hypertrophy (BPH) which of the following statements are false?**
   - A It is the commonest cause of bladder outflow obstruction (BOO) in men >70 years of age.
   - B Decrease in serum testosterone levels and therefore relative increase in serum oestrogens cause BPH.
   - C The condition affects the transitional zone and the central zone.
   - D All lower urinary tract symptoms (LUTS) in men >70 years are due to BPH.
   - E The prostatic urethra is elongated.

Investigations

4. **In urodynamic studies, which of the following statements are true?**
   - A A voided volume >200 mL with a peak flow rate >15 mL/s is normal.
   - B A voiding pressure of <60 cmH_2O is normal.
   - C Increase in voiding pressures with a low flow rate is diagnostic of BOO.
   - D In patients with a residual volume of 250 mL or more, bilateral hydronephrosis will result.
   - E Urodynamically proven BOO only occurs from benign prostatic hypertrophy.

5. **In assessing LUTS in men, which of the following statements are false?**
   - A Charting patient's symptoms according to the International Prostate Symptom Score (IPSS) is routinely used.
   - B Flow rate measurement studies and pressure-flow urodynamic studies are done.
   - C Thorough nervous system examination is mandatory.
   - D The upper urinary tract should always be imaged.
   - E Transrectal ultrasound (US) is carried out.
   - F Cystourethroscopy is a good guide as an indication for surgery.

Management of BPH causing BOO

6. Which of the following statements regarding the management of BPH causing BOO are true?

A All patients with acute retention ultimately require a prostatectomy.
B Chronic retention accounts for 15 per cent of prostatectomies.
C Severe symptoms account for 60 per cent of prostatectomies.
D Drug therapy is with alpha-blockers and/or 5α-reductase inhibitor.
E A low maximum flow rate of <10 mL/s and a residual volume of 100–250 mL are indications for surgery.

7. In the principles of treatment of benign prostatic hypertrophy causing BOO, which of the following statements are true?

A Alpha-adrenergic blocking agents inhibit the contraction of prostatic smooth muscle.
B 5α-reductase inhibitors inhibit the conversion of testosterone to DHT.
C Drug therapy results in 20 per cent improvement in symptom scores.
D Transurethral resection of the prostate (TURP) results in 75 per cent improvement in the symptom scores.
E Retrograde ejaculation occurs in all patients after TURP.

Prostate cancer

8. Which of the following statements are true in carcinoma of the prostate?

A It is the most common cancer in men over the age of 65 years.
B In the younger age group who develop prostate cancer, 10–15 per cent have a positive family history.
C A patient who has had a prostatectomy for benign prostatic hypertrophy can develop prostate cancer.
D Carcinoma mostly originates in the peripheral zone of the prostate
E Prostate-specific antigen (PSA) is an extremely reliable method of screening.

9. In carcinoma of the prostate, which of the following statements is false?

A The histological type is an adenocarcinoma.
B Gleason scoring system is based on the degree of glandular differentiation.
C The Gleason score correlates well with spread and prognosis.
D Prostate cancer is the commonest site for skeletal metastasis.
E Skeletal metastases from prostate cancer are always osteolytic.

10. On rectal examination, which of the following features do not suggest carcinoma?

A Nodules within the prostate
B Obliteration of the median sulcus
C Irregular stony hard induration
D Mobile rectal mucosa over the prostate
E Extension beyond the capsule into the bladder base.

11. Assessment in suspected prostate cancer should include:

A Transrectal ultrasound-guided biopsy (TRUS)
B Cross-sectional MRI imaging
C Bone scan
D General blood tests, PSA and liver function tests
E IVU.

12. Which of the following statements regarding treatment of prostate cancer is false?

A Radical prostatectomy is only suitable for T1 and T2 disease (early cancer).
B Radical external beam radiotherapy is an alternative to radical prostatectomy.
C T3 patients are treated by radical radiotherapy and/or androgen ablation.
D Incidentally diagnosed disease is treated by radical prostatectomy.
E The incidence of severe stress incontinence after radical prostatectomy is about 2 per cent.

Extended matching questions

1. Clinical conditions of the prostate

A Benign prostatic hypertrophy causing BOO
B Chronic urinary retention with overflow
C Carcinoma of prostate
D Acute retention of urine
E Acute prostatitis

Choose and match the diagnoses with the scenarios below:

1 A 40-year-old male complains of feeling unwell with pyrexia of 39°C. He has rigors with aches all over and has flu-like symptoms in general. He has rectal irritation, pain on defaecation and perineal discomfort. He has pain on micturition and passes threads in his urine. Rectal examination reveals a tender, swollen prostate.

2 A 70-year-old male complains of poor stream, frequency of micturition both in the day and at night, hesitancy, intermittent stream, a feeling of incomplete emptying and terminal haematuria. These symptoms of BOO have been there for about 4 months. More recently he has had backache localised to the small of his back. On clinical examination, no abnormality is found. On rectal examination he has a generalised hard, nodular prostate with overlying fixed rectal mucosa.

3 A 72-year-old man has come to the A&E department with severe acute pain in his lower abdomen not having passed urine for almost 10 h. He has been on some medicines which he bought across the counter for cold and flu. This has also made him constipated. On examination he is in severe pain from a large mass in his subumbilical region arising from his pelvis. The mass is dull to percussion.

4 A 70-year-old man complains of urgency, frequency and hesitancy of micturition with a feeling of incomplete emptying. He also has poor flow, intermittent stream and post-micturition dribbling. These symptoms have been going on for 2 years and are gradually getting worse. Clinical examination reveals no abnormality. On rectal examination he has an enlarged smooth prostate with overlying mobile rectal mucosa and the median vertical groove is easily felt.

5 A 75-year-old male complains of general malaise, lethargy, abdominal distension and urinary incontinence. On examination he has a large painless mass in his subumbilical region arising from the pelvis and has continuous urinary dribbling. The mass is dull on percussion. He is a type 2 diabetic and is on medication.

Answers: Multiple choice questions

Anatomy and physiology

1. B

The glands of the peripheral zone are lined by columnar epithelium and hence a cancer arising from there is an adenocarcinoma.

2. A, B, C, E

Testosterone is converted into DHT by the prostatic enzyme 5α-reductase. DHT is five times more potent than testosterone. Luteinising hormone-releasing hormone (LHRH) secreted by the hypothalamus controls the secretion of LH from the anterior pituitary, which in turn controls the output of testosterone. LHRH has a short half-life and is released in a pulsatile manner, a phenomenon utilised for androgen deprivation therapy in prostate cancer. Adrenal androgens play a minor role, accounting for 5–10 per cent of testosterone.

➜ Benign prostatic hypertrophy

3. D

Lower urinary tract symptoms increase in both sexes with age. Therefore, in older men, such symptoms are not always from benign prostatic hypertrophy. It can be due to idiopathic detrusor overactivity or neuropathic bladder dysfunction.

➜ Investigations

4. A, B, C, D

Benign prostatic hypertrophy is not the only cause of BOO proven by urodynamic studies. Besides benign prostatic hypertrophy, bladder neck stenosis, bladder neck hypertrophy, prostate cancer, urethral stricture and functional obstruction from neuropathic conditions are other causes.

5. D, E, F

In the assessment of LUTS as a result of BOO, upper tract imaging by US or IVU is not routinely carried out. It is only done if there is a history of haematuria or if infection is present. Transrectal US scanning is not routine unless, on rectal examination, a carcinoma is suspected. Cystourethroscopy does not give any guide as to the degree of BOO and the need for surgery.

➜ Management of BPH causing BOO

6. B, C, D, E

Only 25 per cent of fit, male patients with acute retention, where no cause for the retention has been found, e.g. constipation, drugs, recent operation, need a prostatectomy. In some patients after initial catheterisation, drug therapy is used for a while followed by trial without catheter. Such management is sometimes successful. The same is true of patients with chronic retention of urine, provided renal function has been stabilised by catheterisation.

➜ Management of BOO

7. A, B, C, D

In counselling men for TURP, the key is the assessment of symptoms. Moreover, good flow rates with low residual volume do not require an operation. Drug therapy over a year produces a 25 per cent shrinkage of the prostate gland. Alpha-blockers act more quickly. 5α-reductase inhibitors work better in patients with adenomas larger than 50 g, need to be taken for at least 6 months and have fewer side-effects. After TURP, retrograde ejaculation occurs in 65 per cent of patients.

➜ Prostate cancer

8. A, B, C, D

There is no consensus about use of PSA as a screening procedure. Detection of cancer using PSA is 2–4 per cent. Thirty per cent of men with a raised PSA will have proven prostate cancer. Twenty per cent of patients with proven prostate cancer will have normal PSA. Population-based screening for prostate cancer is carried out within clinical trials and it remains unclear whether national screening programmes should be established.

9. E

Skeletal metastases from prostate cancer are mostly osteosclerotic, the most frequently involved being the pelvis and lower lumbar vertebrae.

10. D

Mobile rectal mucosa over the prostate is a normal finding. In prostate carcinoma the rectal mucosa will be adherent to the prostate.

11. A, B, C, D

Transrectal ultrasound-guided biopsy is used to confirm the diagnosis by taking 10 systematic biopsy cores. Cross-sectional MRI is the most accurate method of local staging. Bone scan is particularly useful when the PSA is >10 nmol/mL or the biopsy shows high-grade cancer. IVU is not necessary.

12. D

Incidentally discovered disease at TURP for clinically diagnosed benign prostatic hypertrophy is managed by active surveillance with regular digital rectal examination (DRE) and PSA estimation. For metastatic disease, androgen ablation is effective in the majority of patients.

Answers: Extended matching questions

→ 1. Clinical conditions of the prostate

1E

This young male patient has the typical features of acute prostatitis. He needs analgesia; urine is cultured and treatment is started with trimethoprim or ciprofloxacin. If not promptly treated, these patients may develop a prostatic abscess as shown by high temperature with rigors, severe perineal and rectal pain with tenesmus and, on rectal examination, an enlarged, hot, tender fluctuant prostate. The treatment of a prostatic abscess is periurethral resection and deroofing of the abscess cavity.

2C

This patient has LUTS of relatively short duration from BOO. Rectal examination shows a typical prostate carcinoma. He needs PSA, general blood tests, confirmation of the diagnosis by TRUS, local staging by CT or MRI followed by bone scan. Appropriate treatment is instituted after thorough assessment.

3D

This patient has acute retention of urine almost certainly brought on by the drugs and the resultant constipation. He needs analgesia with immediate catheterisation. His constipation should be treated. Assessment of his LUTS is done by the IPSS. If his IPSS is low, he will benefit from a trial without a catheter. A period of drug treatment may precede removal of the catheter. This regime will be successful, particularly if he is shown to have a low residual volume on US.

4A

This patient has features of LUTS from BOO. He has both irritative and obstructive symptoms. Examination shows benign prostatic hypertrophy. His symptoms need to be assessed according to the IPSS. He needs PSA, haematological and biochemical tests, followed by flow rate measurement and pressure-flow urodynamic studies. He should then be considered for drug therapy initially.

5B

This diabetic elderly male has features of chronic renal failure with chronic retention of urine with overflow. He is unaware of his hugely distended bladder. His haematology would show anaemia, his biochemistry would reveal metabolic acidosis with hyperkalaemia and his urine would be infected. He needs immediate catheterisation to relieve back pressure and treat his renal failure. He would have post-obstructive diuresis which would require intravenous hydration. After adequate resuscitation, pressure-flow urodynamic studies should be carried out and his diabetes assessed. He probably has diabetic neuropathy causing the chronic retention.

74 The urethra and penis

Multiple choice questions

➜ Congenital abnormalities

1. Which of the following statements is false?

A The verumontanum marks the proximal end of the external urethral sphincter.
B Posterior urethral valves causing obstruction can be diagnosed antenatally.
C The incidence of hypospadias is 1 in 200–300.
D Hypospadias is the commonest congenital urethral anomaly.
E Glandular hypospadias should be surgically treated early in life.

➜ Urethral rupture

2. In bulbous urethral rupture, which of the following statements are true?

A It is caused by direct blow to perineum.
B Acute retention occurs.
C There is perineal haematoma with blood at the urethral meatus.
D In a full bladder, suprapubic catheterisation is carried out.
E Urethral catheterisation may be attempted as an alternative.

3. In rupture of the membranous urethra, which of the following statements is false?

A It is almost always associated with a pelvic fracture.
B 10–15 per cent of fractured pelvis cases will have associated urethral injury.
C It is usually a part of multiple trauma.
D The prostate may be high-riding and out of reach on rectal examination.
E A urethral catheter is inserted as a part of initial resuscitation.

4. In superficial extravasation of urine, which of the following statements are true?

A It occurs in ruptured bulbous urethra.
B Extravasated urine is confined by the Denonvilliers' fascia.
C Extravasated urine collects around the scrotum and penis.
D A urethrogram is carried out to confirm the diagnosis.
E Suprapubic cystostomy is the immediate treatment.

➜ Urethral stricture

5. Causes of urethral stricture include:

A Inflammation and infection
B Trauma
C Neoplasm
D Postoperative
E Congenital.

6. Which of the following statements about urethral stricture is false?

A The symptoms are those of bladder outflow obstruction (BOO).
B Ascending urethrography is necessary.
C Urethroscopy is mandatory to evaluate.
D Periurethral abscess is a complication.
E Urethral dilatation is the ideal treatment.

Extended matching questions

➜ 1. Conditions of the penis

A Balanoposthitis
B Peyronie's disease

C Persistent priapism
D Carcinoma of penis
E Chordee

Choose and match the correct diagnoses with the scenarios below:

1 A 35-year-old male complains of deformity of his penis during erection. He has increasing difficulty in sexual intercourse. In the past he had urethritis, which was treated successfully with antibiotics.

2 A 38-year-old male complains of bloody, foul-smelling discharge from his penis. He has a hard ulcerated lesion under his prepuce. He also complains of lumps in his groin.

3 A 45-year-old male complains of progressive deformity of his penis which is very pronounced during erection; this has been going on for the past 2 years. On examination, indurated plaques can be palpated around the penile shaft. On questioning he has thickening of his palmar fascia on both hands.

4 A 60-year-old male who is under treatment for leukaemia recently started developing penile erection without any reason. This is prolonged and painful and is now distressing him.

5 A 22-year-old male complains of itching around his glans penis and prepuce. Recently he has developed purulent discharge from the subprepucial area. His glans and foreskin look red and inflamed. He is a type I diabetic on insulin.

Answers: Multiple choice questions

Congenital abnormalities

1. E

Glandular hypospadias does not need surgical treatment unless the meatus is stenosed, in which case a meatotomy is performed.

Urethral rupture

2. A, B, C, D

A fall astride a projecting object, such as may occur in scaffolders, gymnasium accidents caused by a fall across a beam or cycling accidents, are the usual causes of direct blow to the perineum. The clinical triad is acute urinary retention, blood at the external meatus and perineal haematoma. Urethral catheterisation, rarely advocated by some, is best avoided for fear of converting a partial tear into a complete tear. Suprapubic cystostomy is carried out with full assessment later.

3. E

The plain X-ray of the pelvis in a case of multiple trauma will often give an idea of the presence or otherwise of a urethral injury. Urethral catheter should not be inserted. A suprapubic cystostomy is the initial treatment of choice. In case of doubt, an ascending urethrogram with water-soluble contrast may be carried out.

4. A, C, E

The extravasated urine is confined in front of the midperineal point by the attachment of the Colles' fascia to the triangular ligament and by the attachment of the Scarpa's fascia just below the inguinal ligament. Thus urine collects in the scrotum and penis and beneath the deep layer of the superficial fascia of the abdominal wall. The diagnosis is so obvious that urethrogram is not necessary. The patient is treated by urgent suprapubic cystostomy and incisions over the scrotum and thighs to drain the urine.

→ Urethral stricture

5. A, B, D, E

Gonococcal urethritis and non-specific causes such as chlamydial infection can result in inflammatory stricture. External trauma, such as fracture of the pelvis producing rupture of membranous urethra or blow to the perineum causing bulbous urethral rupture, inevitably result in stricture in due course. Postoperative causes are after prostatectomy, urethroscopy, amputation of the penis and prolonged catheterisation. Congenital stricture is very rare and occurs from urethral duplication; symptoms occur in adolescence.

6. E

Urethral dilatation as a form of treatment is not often used, except in elderly men. The ideal treatment is internal visual urethrotomy, which cures 50 per cent of simple strictures. In complicated post-traumatic strictures after pelvic trauma, urethroplasty is the treatment of choice.

Answers: Extended matching questions

→ 1. Conditions of the penis

1E

This patient suffers from chordee, which is a fixed bowing of his penis. While it can be the result of hypospadias, in this patient it is the aftermath of chronic urethritis.

2D

This patient has a carcinoma of the penis with probable secondaries in his inguinal lymph nodes. The usual principles of cancer management should be followed: confirmation of diagnosis, staging of the disease and definitive treatment. In 50 per cent of patients the inguinal lymph node enlargement is from sepsis. He needs a biopsy of the lesion, fine-needle aspiration of his groin nodes, liver ultrasound and chest X-ray. Thereafter, discussion in a multidisciplinary meeting is followed by the appropriate definitive treatment.

3B

This patient has Peyronie's disease, which is often accompanied by Dupuytren's contracture, as in this case. A plain X-ray of the penis may show up calcification. The condition is self-limiting but surgery may be indicated when the condition interferes with sexual function.

4C

This patient, who suffers from leukaemia, has persistent priapism. It can also occur due to sickle cell disease. He can be treated by aspiration of the sludged blood in the corpora cavernosa or injection of adrenaline solution.

5A

This young man has balanoposthitis and needs to be treated with the appropriate antibiotics. One should make sure that his diabetes is under good control. He should be given advice with regard to local hygiene.

75 The testis and scrotum

Multiple choice questions

➜ Incompletely descended testis

1. In incompletely descended testis, which of the following statements is false?

A The incidence is 4 per cent.
B A testis absent from the scrotum after 3 months is unlikely to descend.
C An incompletely descended testis tends to atrophy as puberty approaches.
D Early orchidopexy can preserve function.
E Orchidopexy reduces the chances of developing a testicular tumour.

2. The hazards of incomplete descent of testis include:

A Sterility in bilateral cases
B Trauma
C Torsion
D Increased liability to malignant change in later life
E Epididymo-orchitis.

➜ Testicular torsion

3. Which of the following statements are true with regard to testicular torsion?

A The typical symptom is sudden agonising pain in the scrotum.
B It is most common between 10 and 25 years of age.
C Inversion of the testis and a transverse lie are the commonest cause.
D Doppler ultrasound (US) scan should be done to confirm the diagnosis.
E The emergency operation of fixation of the testis to the tunica albuginea with non-absorbable sutures should be done on both sides.

➜ Hydrocele

4. The following statements are true about a hydrocele except

A A hydrocele is a collection of fluid within the tunica vaginalis.
B A congenital hydrocele causes an intermittent swelling.
C An acute hydrocele in a young man may be a sinister finding.
D Testicular pathology may cause a hydrocele.
E Drainage is an effective treatment.

➜ Epididymo-orchitis

5. In epididymo-orchitis, which of the following are true?

A The causes are chlamydia and gonococci as sexually transmitted infections.
B The initial symptoms are those of urinary tract infection (UTI).
C In mumps 18 per cent of men may develop the condition.
D It is a common postoperative complication after prostatectomy.
E Treatment is doxycycline for chlamydia or a broad-spectrum antibiotic.

➜ Testicular tumour

6. In testicular tumours, which of the following statements are false?

A A scrotal lump that is inseparable from the testis is likely to be a tumour.
B Lymphatic spread is usually to the inguinal lymph nodes.
C Teratomas occur in the third decade and seminomas in the fourth decade.
D Seminomas usually spread via the lymphatics.

E Diagnosis is confirmed by US-guided fine-needle aspiration cytology (FNAC).

7. Which of the following statements are true with regard to the management of testicular tumours?

A Tumour markers are measured and a chest X-ray carried out.
B Initial surgical treatment is orchidectomy through the groin.
C Staging is done by CT scan and MRI.
D Seminomas are radiosensitive.
E Secondaries from teratoma are always treated by surgery.

Extended matching questions

→ 1. Scrotal and testicular conditions

A Vaginal hydrocele
B Epididymal cyst
C Spermatocele
D Testicular tumour
E Acute epididymo-orchitis
F Torsion of the testis
G Torsion of the hydatid of Morgagni
H Varicocele
I Idiopathic oedema of the scrotum
J Encysted hydrocele of the cord

Choose and match the correct diagnoses with the clinical scenarios below:

1 A 22-year-old male complains of acute pain in the top of his left testis for 16 h. On examination the scrotum looks normal and the testis can be felt with care without undue tenderness. There is a small blue pea-sized tender mass on top of the testis.

2 A 30-year-old male complains of a swollen scrotum for almost a year. This is not painful but recently has caused discomfort. On examination he has a tense fluctuant lump in his right scrotum where the testis cannot be felt separately. The swelling transilluminates.

3 A 45-year-old man complains of a painful left testis of 4 days' duration. This is associated with fever and rigors. He has painful micturition and considerable frequency. On examination he looks unwell, has pyrexia of 39°C and has a swollen, red, oedematous and shiny left hemiscrotum; the testis and epididymis feel indurated and tender.

4 An 18-year-old male complains of sudden onset of agonising pain in his right groin and suprapubic area of 6 h duration. He has no urinary symptoms. On examination he is in agony, the right testis is drawn up and the scrotum is red. The testis is impossible to feel because of pain.

5 A 25-year-old male complains of feeling heavy in his left scrotum where he noticed a lump while in the shower. A few days before he felt a lump in the periumbilical region of his abdomen. At the same time he noticed another lump on the left side of his neck. The abdominal and neck lumps do not give him any symptoms. On questioning he admits to coughing up some blood in his sputum a month ago. On examination he has a 2 cm irregular lump over his left supraclavicular area and a 5 cm irregular firm lump in his umbilical region. Examination of the left testis reveals a large lump which is hard and heavy.

6 A 50-year-old man complains of a lump in his right scrotum of a year's duration. This is gradually growing larger in size and gives him some discomfort. Examination of his scrotum

reveals a cystic lump, about 7 cm in diameter, above and behind the left testis, which is minimally tender. Transillumination is positive and shows septa within the lump looking like a Chinese lantern.

7 A 4-year-old boy has been brought by his parents to the A&E department with a red, swollen scrotum. On examination the child is not in any pain and there is redness and oedema around the penis and perineum.

8 A 40-year-old male presents with a swelling in his right scrotum which he says feels like 'a third testis'. He has just noticed it in the shower and is worried that he has got cancer. He has no symptoms. On examination he has a lax, cystic swelling on top of his right testis. It is not tender and does not transilluminate well.

9 A 30-year-old man presents with a swelling in his left hemiscrotum which he discovered by chance in the bath. On examination the testis feel separate from the swelling which is about 2 cm in diameter and above the testis. It transilluminates and comes down on traction to the testis.

10 A 45-year-old male complains of a dragging discomfort in the left side of his scrotum. He noticed an irregular lump in his scrotum separate from the testis. He thinks he has had this for many years but only recently noticed discomfort in the lump. On examination he has a bunch of veins in the scrotum and the testis feels normal. On lying down the veins disappear. Abdominal examination in the left renal area does not show any abnormality.

Answers: multiple choice questions

➜ Incompletely descended testis

1. E

An incompletely descended testis has a much greater chance of developing a tumour in later life. Correcting the abnormality by orchidopexy does not reduce the incidence of a tumour but greatly enhances the chances of early detection. This is because young men will notice changes in the size, weight and feel of a testis much more easily when it is in the scrotum.

2. A, B, C, D

There is no increased risk of epididymo-orchitis. However, should it occur in an incompletely descended testis on the right side, it can be confused with acute appendicitis.

➜ Testicular torsion

3. B, C, E

The typical symptom is sudden agonising pain in the groin and suprapubic area and not the testis. Anatomical abnormalities such as inversion and transverse lie, high investment of the tunica vaginalis and separation of the epididymis from the body of the testis are the usual causes. Doppler US may show lack of blood supply but it should not be done routinely as precious time may be lost. In case of doubt, the scrotum should be explored.

➜ Hydrocele

4. E

A congenital hydrocele is due to a patent processus vaginalis and is therefore continuous with the peritoneal cavity. Hence it can sometimes be emptied and when the child lies down the fluid disappears into the abdomen causing the swelling to disappear. An acute hydrocele in a young man may herald the onset of a testicular tumour. Drainage is not an effective treatment as the condition inevitably recurs and may cause infection.

Epididymo-orchitis

5. A, B, C, E

Initial symptoms are dysuria and frequency followed by tender, red, swollen epididymis and testis. Infection spreads to the epididymis via the vas from primary urethritis or UTI. Post-prostatectomy epididymitis is very rare because of closed catheter drainage and prophylactic antibiotics.

Testicular tumour

6. B, E

The lymphatic drainage of the testis is to the para-aortic group of lymph nodes alongside the blood vessels. Metastasis to inguinal lymph nodes do not occur unless the scrotal skin is involved, which is rare. Diagnosis is confirmed by US where the homogenous tumour tissue produces multiple tumour reflections. FNAC should never be done as it would disseminate tumour cells along the needle track. In case of any doubt about the diagnosis, frozen section during inguinal orchidectomy should be arranged.

7. A, B, C, D

Once testicular tumour is diagnosed on clinical grounds, it is mandatory to measure tumour markers – beta-human chorionic gonadotrophin (β-HCG), alpha-fetoprotein (α-FP) and lactate dehydrogenase (LDH). Treatment is according to the stage, of which there are four. Early stages of seminoma (stages 1 and 2) have excellent results following radiotherapy; later stages are treated by chemotherapy. Secondaries from teratoma are not always treated by surgery. Stage 1 is monitored whilst stages 2–4 are treated by chemotherapy. Surgery in the form of retroperitoneal lymph node dissection is only carried out if secondary lymph nodal masses are still present following chemotherapy.

Answers: Extended matching questions

1. Scrotal and testicular conditions

1G

This 22-year-old man complains of acute pain in his scrotum. On examination the testis is not tender but he is tender over a small swelling at the top of the testis. The blue small lump is the torted hydatid of Morgagni. Removal of the lump cures the condition.

2A

This patient has a vaginal hydrocele – a tense cystic swelling in his scrotum where the testis is not separately palpable and the swelling transilluminates. Confirmation, if necessary, is by US and treatment is by operation.

3E

This patient has urinary tract infection with an enlarged, tender left testis suggestive of acute epididymo-orchitis. Blood and urine cultures and testicular US are carried out. The patient is treated with the appropriate antibiotics. It may take 6–8 weeks to resolve.

4F

This 18-year-old male has testicular torsion. Pain is sudden and excruciating, it starts typically in the groin and lower abdomen and the testis is pulled up. The patient should be explored through a scrotal incision and the testis should be fixed on both sides to the tunica albuginea with non-absorbable sutures.

5D

This 25-year-old man has the hallmarks of a metastatic testicular teratoma – hard enlarged testis, abdominal and supraclavicular lumps from metastatic lymph nodes and haemoptysis from pulmonary secondaries. He needs bloods to be sent for tumour markers, testicular and abdominal US, chest X-ray, high inguinal orchidectomy, staging by abdominal CT and MRI, CT of chest followed by discussion in a multidisciplinary meeting and appropriate treatment.

6B

This patient has an epididymal cyst – a cystic swelling separate from the testis which lies above and behind the testis. Transillumination shows a Chinese lantern appearance. Treatment is by excision.

7I

This 4-year-old boy has idiopathic oedema of the scrotum. This is a self-limiting disease and does not require any active treatment.

8C

This patient who complains of a 'third testicle' has a spermatocele – a lax cystic swelling above and behind the testis which does not transilluminate well because the fluid is opalescent due to the presence of spermatozoa.

9J

This man has an encysted hydrocele of the cord – a cystic swelling separate from and situated above the testis. Traction on the testis brings the swelling down.

10H

This patient has a left varicocele. As it is on the left side, it is important to exclude a left renal carcinoma. Rarely a tumour thrombus may spread along the left renal vein, blocking the left testicular vein causing the varicocele.

76 Gynaecology

Multiple choice questions

→ Anatomy and physiology

1. **Which of the following are true anatomical facts?**

A The cervix divides the vault of the vagina into anterior, posterior and lateral fornices.
B The pouch of Douglas is the area between the uterus anteriorly and the rectum posteriorly.
C The uterus is normally anteverted.
D The fallopian tube is 10 cm long and has four parts.
E The uterine arteries arise from the abdominal aorta.

2. **Which of the following statements regarding reproductive physiology is false?**

A The hypothalamus produces gonadotrophin-releasing hormone (GRH).
B GRH stimulates the pituitary to release follicle-stimulating hormone (FSH) and luteinising hormone (LH).
C FSH and LH control the production of oestrogen and progesterone.
D The proliferative or follicular phase (first half) of the menstrual cycle is controlled by oestrogen and the second half is controlled by progesterone.
E Gestational age is best calculated by the date of the last menstrual period (LMP).

→ Abnormal/excessive vaginal bleeding

3. **In vaginal bleeding, which of the following statements are true?**

A Painless vaginal bleeding in pregnancy denotes a threatened miscarriage.
B In the non-pregnant state it can occur from an intrauterine contraceptive device (IUCD).
C All non-pregnant women >40 years of age should have an ultrasound (US) and endometrial biopsy.
D Women on tamoxifen have a higher incidence of vaginal bleeding as they have a greater risk of developing endometrial cancer.
E Women with hereditary non-polyposis colorectal cancer (HNPCC) have a higher incidence of endometrial cancer and vaginal bleeding.
F All women should undergo endometrial biopsy.

→ Ectopic pregnancy

4. **Which of the following statements about ectopic pregnancy is false?**

A Lower abdominal pain with vaginal bleeding in early pregnancy should alert one to ectopic pregnancy unless otherwise proven.
B Transvaginal US showing absence of intrauterine gestational sac and a positive urinary pregnancy test points to ectopic pregnancy.
C Levels of beta-human chorionic gonadotrophin (β-HCG) are a useful guide.
D Laparoscopy is the best diagnostic test.
E Salpingectomy is the treatment of choice.

5. **Which of the following are risk factors for ectopic pregnancy?**

A Past pelvic inflammatory disease (PID)
B Past history of spontaneous miscarriage

C Previous medical termination
D History of infertility
E Past abdominal operation.

Pelvic inflammatory disease

6. Which of the following statements about pelvic inflammatory disease (PID) is false?

A The majority are caused by sexually transmitted ascending infection.
B *Streptococcus* is the most common organism.
C A low threshold for empirical treatment should be adopted.
D Outpatient antibiotic treatment should be started soon after the diagnosis is suspected.
E Some patients may need to be admitted for treatment.

7. Which of the following patients with suspected PID need to be admitted?

A A surgical emergency, e.g. acute appendicitis, cannot be excluded
B Severe disease with constitutional symptoms
C Tubo-ovarian abscess
D PID in pregnancy
E Fitz-Hugh–Curtis syndrome.

Extended matching questions

1. Gynaecological pathology

A Ectopic pregnancy
B Uterine fibroids
C Endometriosis
D Ovarian cyst
E Carcinoma of ovary
F Pelvic inflammatory disease (PID)

Choose and match the correct diagnoses with each of the scenarios below:

1 A 25-year-old woman has been admitted with severe right-sided lower abdominal pain of 4 h duration. The pain gradually spread to the left side. It was colicky to start with but has now settled to a continuous agonising pain. She is apyrexial, sweaty, with a blood pressure of 110/60 mmHg and a pulse of 120/min. Abdominal examination reveals tenderness, rigidity and rebound tenderness over the entire lower abdomen.

2 A 35-year-old woman has been admitted with sudden onset of severe right-sided lower abdominal pain of 6 h duration. She is unsure about her last menstrual period and has been trying to conceive for the first time. On examination she is apyrexial, looks pale, her blood pressure is 80/50 mmHg, and pulse is 120/min; she is extremely tender over the entire lower abdomen. On vaginal examination there is cervical excitation and the os is closed.

3 In the outpatient clinic, a 38-year-old woman complains of severe dysmenorrhoea for several months. Recently she has developed chronic pain deep in the lower abdomen. She also suffers from mid-menstrual pain. She has not conceived as yet, although she would like to. She has chronic fatigue. On examination she is tender in her lower abdomen, and vaginal and rectal examinations show tenderness in the fornices and irregular nodules are felt in the pouch of Douglas.

4 A 27-year-old woman complains of foul-smelling vaginal discharge of several months' duration. She has frequency of micturition and intermittent lower abdominal pain and fever. She has an IUCD inserted at present. On examination she looks in discomfort and is tender over her lower abdomen. Vaginal examination shows foul-smelling cervical discharge.

5 A 60-year-old woman complains of unexplained gain in weight and increase in her girth over the last 6 months. Recently she found that her clothes are getting tight and she has to wear skirts two sizes larger. She has some generalised abdominal discomfort and shortness of breath. Recently she has been constipated with frequency of micturition. On examination she has generalised abdominal distension and ascites with shifting dullness and fluid thrill.

6 A 40-year-old woman complains of lower abdominal discomfort of several months' duration. She has heavy periods, frequency of micturition, constipation and backache. On examination she looks pale; abdominal examination reveals a firm mass in the suprapubic area about 8 cm long and 5 cm wide. The lower limit of the mass cannot be felt.

Answers: Multiple choice questions

Anatomy and physiology

1. A, B, C, D

The uterine arteries arise from the anterior branch of the internal iliac arteries.

2. E

The woman's date of recollection of LMP may be wrong. Therefore, the alternative practice is to use ultrasound measurements of fetal size.

Vaginal bleeding

3. A, B, C, D, E

Vaginal bleeding can be a sinister symptom and therefore needs to be thoroughly investigated. History of being on tamoxifen or having had HNPCC or a family history of the condition should make the clinician wary of vaginal bleeding as it may herald the onset of endometrial cancer. The patient should undergo US and endometrial biopsy. In women below the age of 40 years without any risk factors, pathology is rarely found and therefore may be treated symptomatically. Women who have been treated for HNPCC should be screened annually from the age of 35 years by transvaginal US to measure endometrial thickness and biopsy when appropriate.

Ectopic pregnancy

4. E

Salpingectomy is not always performed. Salpingostomy may be performed as it is thought that subsequent intrauterine pregnancy rates are higher and recurrent ectopic rates are lower following conservative surgery. This can be carried out by the laparoscopic route.

5. A, B, C, D

A previous abdominal operation does not increase the chance of ectopic pregnancy.

Pelvic inflammatory disease

6. B

Chlamydia trachomatis is the commonest organism responsible for PID. Probably the next common organism is *Neisseria gonorrhoeae*.

7. A, B, C, D, E

Whilst all the above need admission, Fitz-Hugh–Curtis syndrome is interesting as it can be confused with acute cholecystitis. These patients, besides having the usual clinical features of PID, also complain of pain in the right upper quadrant where there is tenderness. The condition is an extrapelvic manifestation of PID as a result of inflammation of the liver capsule and diaphragm. US of the gall bladder will help in making the diagnosis.

Answers: Extended matching questions

→ 1. Gynaecological pathology

1D

This young woman is a surgical emergency with sudden onset of severe lower abdominal pain with clinical features of peritonism – tenderness, rigidity and rebound tenderness. She is apyrexial and has no constitutional symptoms. She has developed a twisted ovarian cyst. Confirmation is by US and/or laparoscopy. This should be followed by an emergency laparotomy.

2A

This woman has the hallmarks of a ruptured ectopic pregnancy – features of hypovolaemic shock, sudden onset of lower abdominal pain and signs of peritonism in the pelvis. She is unsure about her LMP and at 35 years of age, it is her first pregnancy. She should be vigorously resuscitated and operated upon as an emergency. A laparoscopy may be performed prior to laparotomy or the definitive procedure can be carried out by the laparoscopic route if expertise permits.

3C

This woman with dysmenorrhoea has lower abdominal symptoms of deep abdominal pain and internal examination showing tenderness in the vaginal fornices. There are nodules felt in the pouch of Douglas. She has the features of endometriosis, although sometimes a differential diagnosis of irritable bowel syndrome could be entertained. Diagnosis is confirmed by laparoscopy.

4F

This woman has features of pelvic infection – foul-smelling vaginal discharge, lower abdominal pain, pyrexia and abdominal tenderness. Presence of an IUCD in itself can cause PID. Treatment should be started on empirical grounds, a vaginal swab sent, general blood tests done and the condition confirmed by laparoscopy.

5E

This woman, who is 60 years old, has developed gradual abdominal distension due to ascites. She is short of breath, probably from her ascites. She has the features of an ovarian carcinoma unless otherwise proven. Blood should be sent for CA-125 followed by US and CT scan. A chest X-ray is done to look for pleural effusion. After staging, she is treated appropriately.

6B

This woman has heavy periods and symptoms from pressure to neighbouring structures – urinary bladder and rectum causing frequency of micturition and constipation. She has a midline mass arising from the pelvis which is the fibroid. An US would confirm the diagnosis and appropriate treatment is then instituted.

PART 13 Transplantation

77 Transplantation 561

77 Transplantation

Multiple choice questions

→ Transplantation terms

1. **Which of the following definitions are correct?**
   - A Allograft means an organ or tissue transplanted from one individual to another.
   - B Xenograft refers to a cadaveric donor.
   - C Autograft refers to transplants within the same species.
   - D Orthotopic graft refers to a bone graft.
   - E A heterotopic graft is placed in a site different from where the organ is normally located.

→ Human leucocyte antigen

2. **Which of the following statements regarding human leucocyte antigen (HLA) are true?**
   - A They are highly monomorphic.
   - B HLA class 2 antigens are present in all nucleated cells.
   - C HLA antigens present on graft cells activate T-cells.
   - D HLA-A and B (class 1) and HLA-DR (class 2) are the most important in transplantation.
   - E Anti-HLA antibodies may cause hyperacute rejection.

→ Graft rejection

3. **Which of the following statements regarding graft rejection are true?**
   - A Hyperacute rejection is characterised by intravascular thrombosis.
   - B Acute rejection is T-cell-dependent.
   - C Chronic rejection usually happens after a period of 6 months post-transplant.
   - D Acute rejection is irreversible.
   - E Acute rejection is the most common cause of graft failure.

4. **Which of the following statements regarding hyperacute rejection are true?**
   - A It is due to preformed anti-HLA antibodies.
   - B It occurs 2–4 weeks after transplant.
   - C It can also occur due to ABO blood group graft incompatibility.
   - D The liver is resistant to hyperacute rejection.
   - E The antibodies are mainly towards HLA class 2 antigens.

5. **Which of the following statements regarding acute rejection are true?**
   - A It occurs within a month after transplant.
   - B It is usually reversible.
   - C It is predominantly mediated by T cells.
   - D A characteristic finding is mononuclear infiltration of the graft.
   - E Antibodies have no role.

6. **Which of the following statements regarding chronic rejection are true?**
   - A It usually occurs several years after the transplant.
   - B It is a rare cause of rejection.
   - C It is characterised by myointimal proliferation in graft arteries.
   - D Immunosuppressive therapy is not helpful.
   - E The liver is more resistant to this type of rejection.

→ Graft-versus-host disease

7. **Which of the following statements regarding graft-versus-host disease (GVHD) are true?**
   - A It is due to the donor lymphocytes reacting against the host antigens.

B It frequently involves the skin with a rash over the palms and soles.
C GVHD is a minor condition.
D It can also involve the liver and gastrointestinal tract (GIT).
E It commonly occurs after renal transplant.

Immunosuppressive therapy

8. Which of the following statements regarding mode of action of immunosuppressive therapy are true?

A Cyclosporin blocks IL-2 gene transcription.
B Corticosteroids cause widespread anti-inflammatory effects.
C Azathioprine blocks IL-2 receptor signal transduction.
D Tacrolimus blocks IL-2 gene transcription.
E OKT3 monoclonal antibody causes depletion and blockade of T-cells.

9. Which of the following statements regarding complications of immunosuppression are true?

A Risk of viral infection is highest in the first month after transplantation.
B Cytomegalovirus (CMV) is a major problem.
C Chemoprophylaxis has no role.
D There is increased incidence of squamous cancer of the skin.
E Post-transplant lymphoproliferative disorder (PTLD) is a recognised entity.

Brainstem death

10. Which of the following statements regarding brainstem death are true?

A Traumatic head injury should not be present.
B Hypothermia should be ruled out.
C The diagnosis has to be confirmed by two consultant grade doctors.
D Electrophysiological tests are mandatory in the UK.
E The presence of spinal reflexes does not preclude brainstem death.

Organ donation

11. Which of the following statements regarding organ donation are true?

A Primary tumours of the central nervous system (CNS) are an absolute contraindication for donation.
B The usual acceptable upper age limit for heart donation is 65 years.
C The retrieved organs are preserved between 0 and 4°C.
D The safe maximum cold storage time for the kidneys is 8 h.
E The optimal cold storage time for the heart is less than 3 h.

Renal transplantation

12. Which of the following statements regarding renal transplantation are true?

A Living donor transplants account for about 25–30 per cent of all renal transplants in UK.
B The upper age limit to be considered for transplantation is 65 years.
C Peritransplant lymphoceles are usually asymptomatic.
D Delayed graft function is more common after living donor transplant than after cadaveric transplants.
E Graft survival after a cadaveric transplant is about 75 per cent at 5 years.

Transplantation in general

13. Which of the following statements are true?

A The graft survival after heart transplant is 70 per cent at 5 years.
B GVHD is a particular problem after small-bowel transplant.
C Primary hepatic malignancy is not an indication for liver transplant.
D Bladder drainage of the exocrine pancreas is the preferred technique.
E Simultaneous pancreas and kidney transplant (SPKT) has better results than pancreas transplantation alone.

Extended matching questions

1. Types of allograft reactions

A Chronic rejection
B Hyperacute rejection
C Graft-versus-host response
D Acute rejection

Choose and match the correct diagnosis with each of the descriptions given below:

1 This is due to ABO or preformed anti-HLA antibodies. It is characterised by intravascular thrombosis.

2 This is T-cell-dependent and is characterised by mononuclear cell infiltration. It is reversible.

3 This is the most common cause of graft failure and is characterised by myointimal infiltration, leading to ischaemia and fibrosis.

4 This is seen after liver and small-bowel transplants. It frequently involves the skin, causing a characteristic rash on palms and soles. This is serious and it can be fatal.

2. Mechanism of immunosuppressive agents

A Corticosteroids
B Cyclosporin/tacrolimus
C Sirolimus/everolimus
D OKT3
E Antilymphocytic globulin (ALG)/antilymphocytic serum (ALS)
F Azathioprine

Choose and match the correct drug with their mechanism of action below:

1 Depletion and blockade of T-cells

2 Prevents lymphocyte proliferation

3 Widespread anti-inflammatory effects

4 Depletion and blockade of lymphocytes

5 Blocks IL-2 gene transcription

6 Blocks IL-2 receptor signal transduction

3. Post-transplantation complications

A CMV infection
B *Pneumocystis carinii* infection
C Fungal infection
D PTLD
E Squamous cell carcinoma

Choose and match the correct diagnosis with each of the scenarios given below:

1 A 50-year-old male who had a liver transplant 3 months ago presents with severe fever not responding to antibacterial medications. He has also been having cough and finding swallowing painful. Blood culture and sputum culture show organisms with characteristic colonies.

2 A 40-year-old female who had a renal transplant 4 months ago presents with fever, chest pain and persistent cough. The diagnosis is confirmed on bronchoalveolar lavage and lung biopsies. She is started on trimethoprim with good response.

3 A 60-year-old farmer who had a renal transplant 15 years ago presents with a rapidly growing lump on the dorsum of his hand for the past 6 months. It is painless but has recently become ulcerated with some bleeding and discharge. It has not responded to the usual wound care and dressings.

4 A 38-year-old male who had a renal transplant 4 months ago presents with high swinging fever and lethargy. He has cough, right upper quadrant pain and some ocular symptoms. He is found to have leucopenia.

5 A 10-year-old girl with a previous history of renal transplant, a few years ago, presents with an 'infectious mononucleosis' type illness. She is found to have multiple lymphadenopathy, enlarged tonsils and a tender spleen.

Answers: Multiple choice questions

→ Transplantation terms

1. A, E

Xenograft refers to a graft performed between different species. In autografts, the donor and recipient are the same individual. Orthotopic graft is a graft placed in its normal anatomical site.

→ Human leucocyte antigen

2. C, D, E

Human leucocyte antigens are strong transplant antigens by virtue of their special physiological role as antigen recognition units. They are highly polymorphic cell surface molecules. There are two types of HLA molecules: class 1 and class 2. The class 1 antigens are present on all nucleated cells, whereas the class 2 antigens are expressed more strongly on antigen-presenting cells, such as dendritic cells, macrophages and B-lymphocytes.

→ Graft rejection

3. A, B, C

Allografts provoke a powerful immune response that results in rapid graft rejection unless immunosuppressive therapy is given. T lymphocytes play an essential role in mediating rejection.

4. A, C, D

Hyperacute occurs immediately and is mediated by ABO or preformed antibodies against HLA class 1 antigens. This is characterised by intravascular thrombosis and graft destruction within minutes and hours. It can be avoided by ensuring ABO group compatibility and by performing a cross-match test on recipient serum to ensure that there are antibodies against the donor HLA antigens. Liver transplants rarely undergo hyperacute rejection.

5. B, C, D

This usually occurs within the first 6 months of transplantation but may occur later. It is predominantly mediated by T-lymphocytes but alloantibodies may also play an important role. Most episodes of acute rejection can be reversed by additional immunosuppressive therapy.

6. C, D, E

This is the most common cause of graft failure and usually occurs after the first 6 months. The liver appears to be more resistant than other solid organs to the destructive effects of chronic rejection. The pathophysiology of chronic rejection is not completely understood. The underlying mechanisms are immunological, and both alloantibodies and cellular effector mechanisms are involved. The risk factors for chronic rejection after renal transplantation are previous episodes of acute rejection, poor HLA match, long cold ischaemia time, cytomegalovirus (CMV) infection, raised blood lipids and inadequate immunosuppression.

Graft-versus-host disease

7. A, B, D

This is the reciprocal problem of an immunological reaction mounted by the graft against the host. The donor liver and small bowel both contain large numbers of immunocompetent lymphocytes which react against host HLA antigens. This frequently involves the skin, liver and GIT. GVHD is a serious and sometimes fatal complication.

Immunosuppressive therapy

8. A, B, D, E

The agents used to prevent rejection act predominantly on T-cells, and different classes of agents act at different sites during T-cell activation. Most immunosuppressive protocols use a combination of agents. Azathioprine prevents lymphocyte proliferation. Monoclonal antibodies directed against IL-2 receptors on T-lymphocytes (CD25) are used to augment the effects of calcineurin blockade during the early post-transplant period. Polyclonal antibody preparations ALG/ALS cause depletion and blockade of lymphocytes. Sirolimus/everolmus blocks IL-2 receptor signal transduction.

9. B, D, E

Transplant recipients are at high risk of opportunistic infections, especially by viruses. Chemoprophylaxis is important in high-risk patients. The risk of viral infection is highest during the first 6 months of transplantation and the risk of bacterial infection is highest in the first month. Pre-transplant vaccination against community-acquired infection should be considered. The important viral infections include CMV, herpes simplex and herpes zoster. Protozoal infections due to *Pneumocystis carinii* and fungal infections due to *Candida* and *Aspergillus* are other important infections.

Post-transplant lymphoproliferative disorder is an abnormal proliferation of B-lymphocytes, usually in response to Epstein–Barr virus infection. This can present as an infectious mononucleosis type of illness. PTLD is a serious condition with a mortality rate of up to 50 per cent.

Brainstem death

10. B, E

Brainstem death occurs when severe brain injury causes irreversible loss of the capacity for consciousness combined with the irreversible capacity for breathing. In most countries it is accepted that the condition of brain death equates in medical, legal and religious terms with death of the patient. The concept of brain death is important in management of patients with irreversible brain damage on life support with no prospect of recovery and in issues of organ transplantation. Traumatic head injury and sudden intracranial haemorrhage are the most common causes of brainstem death. It is important to exclude hypothermia, profound hypotension, metabolic and hormonal conditions, and drugs should be excluded before the diagnosis of brainstem death is made. The UK guidelines state that the tests to confirm the diagnosis should be performed on two separate occasions by two clinicians experienced in this area. At least one of them should be a consultant and neither should be connected to the transplant team. The tests to determine brainstem death aim to confirm the absence of cranial nerve reflexes, absence of motor response and absence of spontaneous respiration. In the UK there is no need to perform electrophysiological or brain perfusion studies.

→ Organ donation

11. B, C, E

Most of the organs used for transplantation are obtained from brainstem-dead, heart-beating donors, and in the majority of cases multiple organs are procured. The presence of malignancy in the past 5 years is an absolute contraindication, with the exception of primary tumours of the CNS, non-melanotic skin tumours and carcinoma in situ of the uterine cervix. There is no upper age limit for kidney and liver donors. The upper age limit for heart and lung donors is 65 years and it is 60 years for pancreas. Various organ preservation solutions, such as University of Wisconsin (UW) solution, are available. The safe maximum storage times for kidney, liver, heart and lung are 48, 24, 6 and 8 h respectively. The optimal cold storage time, however, is usually half of this.

→ Renal transplantation

12. A, C, E

In the UK, around 80–100 people per million of the population develop end-stage renal disease. The living donor renal transplant activity is much higher in some countries, such as Scandinavia and India. The justification for living donor renal transplant is based on the shortage of deceased donor transplants, superior results and the legislation. There is no upper age limit for a renal donor.

Vascular complications after transplant are uncommon and include renal artery thrombosis (1 per cent), renal vein thrombosis (up to 5 per cent) and renal artery stenosis (up to 10 per cent) which usually occurs years after the transplant. Urological complications occur in about 5 per cent of cases. Peritransplant lymphoceles are usually asymptomatic but may occasionally cause ureteric obstruction and oedema of the ipsilateral leg.

Delayed graft function is defined as the need for dialysis post-transplantation. This is as a result of acute tubular necrosis and occurs in up to 30 per cent of heart-beating deceased donors but is uncommon (<5 per cent) following living donor transplantation.

→ Transplantation in general

13. A, B, E

The 1- and 5-year graft survival rates after heart transplantation are around 85 and 70 per cent, respectively. The indications for liver transplantation are cirrhosis, acute fulminant liver disease, metabolic liver disease and primary hepatic malignancy. Enteric drainage of the pancreas is preferred because bladder drainage is associated with several complications such as anastomotic leaks, cystitis, urethritis/urethral stricture, UTI and reflux pancreatitis.

Answers: Extended matching questions

→ 1. Types of allograft reactions

1B

This occurs immediately and is mediated by ABO or preformed antibodies against HLA class 1 antigens. This is characterised by intravascular thrombosis and graft destruction within minutes and hours.

2D

Most episodes of acute rejection can be reversed by additional immunosuppressive therapy.

3A

The risk factors for chronic rejection after renal transplantation are previous episodes of acute rejection, poor HLA match, long cold ischaemia time, CMV infection, raised blood lipids and inadequate immunosuppression.

4C

This is the reciprocal problem of an immunological reaction mounted by the graft against the host.

2. Mechanism of immunosuppressive agents

1D, 2F, 3A, 4E, 5B, 6C

3. Post-transplantation complications

1C

Fungal infection usually occurs in the first 3 months after transplantation. Early diagnosis and aggressive treatment are essential to avoid fatal infection.

2B

This is the most important protozoal infection after transplantation. It occurs in the first few months after the transplant. Prophylaxis with co-trimoxazole is effective and continued for up to 6 months after transplant.

3E

This is the most common skin cancer after transplantation. The other skin cancers seen less frequently are basal cell carcinoma and melanoma. The risk of skin cancer after transplantation increases with age and exposure to sunlight. It has been predicted that 50 per cent of the transplant patients will develop a skin malignancy within 20 years after transplant.

4A

Cytomegalovirus typically presents with a high swinging fever, lethargy and leucopenia. The clinical picture depends on the organ system affected and may present as pneumonia, gastrointestinal disease, hepatitis, retinitis and encephalitis.

5D

This happens in around 1–3 per cent of kidney and liver transplants and is considerably higher in children.

Index

Note: Reference to individual questions and their answers and given in the form of chapter number followed by question number (e.g. 6.1) with a following letter M or E denoting multiple choice and extended matching questions respectively. Occasionally a significant topic in an answer has been indexed even though there is no mention in the question. Topics covering a whole chapter range are given a normal page range reference without any mention of the chapter number (e.g. head injury 160–5).

abdominal aorta
  aneurysm 53.7–9M
  thrombosis 53.1E
  see also aorto-iliac disease
abdominal compartment syndrome 26.3E
abdominal conditions 421–52
  diagnostic aids 58.5M
  history and examination 423–4
  trauma 176–84, 58.3E
  tropical patients
    distension 5.4E
    lump 5.2E
    pain 5.1E, 5.5E
abdominal pain 56.1M
  causes 56.1M
  child, acute pain 6.2E
  imaging in acute pain 10.6M
  sources 56.2E
  tropical patients 5.1E, 5.5E
abdominal wall hernia *see* hernia
aberrations of normal development and involution (ANDI) 50.1E
ABO blood groups and transplantation 77.4M
abscesses 4.7M
  breast 50.1E
  cerebral 40.10M
  collar-stud 45.28M
  diverticula 4.3E
  liver
    amoebic 5.2E, 5.5E, 5.24M, 5.27M, 5.28M, 61.2E
    pyogenic 61.2E
    ruptured 5.5E
  pelvic 4.3E
  perianal 69.10M
  peritonsillar 45.2E, 45.9M
  psoas 5.9E
  retropharyngeal 45.10M
  subphrenic 20.1
achalasia of cardia 59.1E, 59.5M, 60.1E
Achilles tendon
  rupture 32.2E
  tightness 36.1E
acid–base balance 17.16M
acid burns 28.26M
acidosis 17.14M
acoustic neuroma 44.30M
acromioclavicular joint injury 32.12M
acyanotic heart disease 51.7M, 51.8M
Addison's disease 49.1E
adenocarcinoma
  nasal 43.29M
  spinal metastases 33.5M
adenoidectomy 45.6M
adenoma
  hepatic 61.3E
  parathyroid 48.17M, 48.23M, 48.24M
  parotid, pleomorphic 47.1E
  pituitary 17.3E, 40.16M
  rectal 68.1E
adenomatous polyposis, familial 65.27–8M
ADH (antidiuretic hormone), syndrome of inappropriate secretion 17.2
adhesive capsulitis (frozen shoulder) 34.1E
adhesive intestinal obstruction 66.1E
  management 66.3E
  postoperative 66.6M
  tropical patient 5.4E
adolescent (teenager)
  chondromalacia patellae 32.1E, 38.8E
  rib hump 33.9M
adrenal glands 49.1–2E, 49.1–11M
  anatomy 49.1M
  hormones 49.2–3M
  masses 49.5M
adrenal vein catheterization 49.6M
AIDS *see* HIV disease and AIDS
airway
  acute, investigation and management 45.2E
  burns 28.3M

airway – *continued*
smoke inhalation 28.4M
see also respiratory tract
alcohol
overconsumption, chronic pancreatitis 64.1E
withdrawal, postoperative confusion due to 20.1E
alimentary tract *see* gastrointestinal tract
alkali burns 28.26M, 41.15M
eye 41.4E, 41.15M
allied therapies, burns 28.19M
allografts 77.1M
donation 77.11M
immunosuppressive drug therapy 77.2E, 77.8–9M
reactions 77.1E
graft-vs-host disease 77.1E, 77.7M
rejection 77.1E, 77.3–6M
alveolar bone grafts 42.14M
alveolar nerve injury, inferior 25.2M
amoebiasis (*Entamoeba histolytica*) 5.1E, 5.2E, 5.5E, 5.24–8M
liver 5.2E, 5.5E, 5.24M, 5.26M, 5.27M, 5.28M, 61.2E
rectum 68.1E
ampulla of Vater, carcinoma *see* periampullary carcinoma
amputation 53.12–13M
amylase, serum 64.2M
anaesthesia 14.1–7M
anal canal *see* anus and anal canal
analgesia
chronic 14.10–11M
postoperative, assessing adequacy 14.8M
anaphylactic shock 2.1E
anaplastic thyroid carcinoma 48.5E
anastomoses (surgical)
large bowel *see* large bowel
vascular 18.4E
ANDI (aberrations of normal development and involution) 50.1E
androgenic hormones 73.2M
aneurysm
aortic
abdominal 53.7–9M
thoracic 51.1E, 51.9M
splenic artery 62.1E
subarachnoid haemorrhage due to 40.21–3M
superior mesenteric artery 64.11M
angiofibroma, juvenile nasal 43.14–15M, 45.7M
angiography 53.5M
renal 70.1E
angulated fracture 27.2E
anismus 69.4E
ankle
arthrodesis *see* arthrodesis
examination 31.10M
osteophyte removal 36.2M
replacement 36.2M
sports injuries 32.2E, 32.8–9M
ankle–brachial pressure index (ABPI) 53.4M
ankylosing spondylitis 37.2E
antenatal scan, cleft/lip palate 42.7M
antibiotics/antimicrobials 4.18–19M
prophylactic 4.1E, 4.13–14M
GI endoscopy 11.2M
anticoagulants, deep vein thrombosis 54.4M
antidiuretic hormone, syndrome of inappropriate secretion 17.2
antral lavage, trochar insertion 43.24M
anus and anal canal 504–12
abscess in or near to 69.10M
anatomy 69.1M
cancer 69.1E, 69.4E, 69.13–14M
congenital anomalies 69.3M
fissure 69.1E, 69.4E, 69.4E, 69.6M
fistula 69.4E, 69.11M
glands 69.2M
incontinence 69.5M
investigations of symptoms relating to 69.2E
pruritus 69.9M
treatment of disorders 69.3E
warts 69.12M
aortic disease
abdominal *see* abdominal aorta
thoracic 51.1E, 51.9M
aortic valve disease 51.1E, 51.5M
aorto-iliac disease 53.3M
Apert's syndrome 42.15M
Apley system of examination 31.2–4M
appendix 495–8
acute inflammation (appendicitis) 67.2–8M
child 6.2E
differential diagnosis 67.1E, 67.6–8M
incorrect diagnosis of 58.3E
anatomy 67.1–2M
arm (upper limb), Bier's block 14.6M
arrhenoblastoma 49.3E
arterial disorders 405–10
aneurysm *see* aneurysm
investigations 53.4–5M
ulcers 54.1E
arterial pedicle flaps, oropharyngeal cancer 46.22M
arteriovenous malformations 40.24M
arthritis
degenerative *see* osteoarthritis
diagnosis 37.2E
elbow 34.2E
glenohumeral joint 34.1E

radiohumeral joint 34.2E
rheumatoid *see* rheumatoid arthritis
tuberculous *see* tuberculosis
arthrodesis
ankle 36.2M
rheumatoid arthritis 37.1E
hip 37.2E
knee 37.4E
arthrography, MR 10.4M
arthropathies 37.1–2E, 37.1–3M
arthroplasty (joint replacement)
ankle 36.2M
elbow, in rheumatoid arthritis 37.1E
hip 34.3E, 35.1E, 35.5M
shoulder 34.2M
in trauma 27.4M, 27.6M
arthroscopy, knee 35.7M
ascariasis 5.1–9M, 5.3E, 5.4E
ascites 58.2E
Asiatic cholangiohepatitis 5.29–30M
astrocytoma 40.17M
pilocytic 40.19M
atelectasis, postoperative 20.1E
atrial septal defects 51.7M
audit 8.1M
nasal surgery 42.16M
auricular haematoma 44.9M
auricular nerve, greater, in superficial parotidectomy 47.22M
autoimmune gastritis 60.5M
autoregulation, cerebral, head-injured patient 22.2M
avascular necrosis
2nd metatarsal head (Freiberg's disease) 32.3E, 36.1E
hip 34.1E, 34.2E
spontaneous (Perthes' disease) 35.1E, 38.3M
in systemic lupus erythematosus 37.2E
avulsed teeth 25.7M
axillary node management in breast cancer 50.6M

back
imaging in disorders of 33.3M
pain (predominantly low) 33.1M, 33.7M, 37.2E, 37.3E, 37.5M
nocturnal 5
sudden-onset urinary incontinence and 33.2M
bacterial infections
conjunctiva 41.3E
salivary glands 47.15–16M
surgical wound 4.2E, 4.17M
tropical 5.36–7M
see also specific bacterial infections and diseases
balanoposthitis 74.1E
Bancroftian filariasis (*Wuchereria bancrofti*) 5.6E, 5.7E, 5.9E, 5.31M
barium enema, ulcerative colitis 65.10M
Barrett's oesophagus 11.1E, 59.5M
basal cell carcinoma (rodent ulcer) 39.4E
eyelid 41.2E, 41.5M
basal cell papilloma 39.3E
bed (pressure) sores 3.1E, 3.2E, 3.6M, 3.7M
Bell's palsy 44.29M
benign paroxysmal positional vertigo 44.27M
Bier's block 14.6–7M
bile ducts
anatomy 63.1M
ascariasis 5.9M
carcinoma 63.10M
congenital anomalies 63.4M
obstruction 63.9M
stones *see* gallstones
biliary atresia 6.3E
biliary cirrhosis, primary 61.1E
biliary system 461–7
biopsy
lymph node 55.2E
salivary gland tumours 47.12M
specimens from 12.1M
bladder 533–40
anatomy 72.1M
cancer 70.3M, 72.1E, 72.2E, 72.2M, 72.8–9M
diverticula 72.1E, 72.2E, 72.5M
fistula between colon and 65.6M
imaging 70.1E, 70.4M
injury 72.2E, 72.2M
outflow obstruction (BOO) in males 73.M, 73.4M
due to benign prostatic hypertrophy 73.6–7M
stones 72.1E, 72.2E, 72.4M
blast injuries 30.10M
bleeding *see* haemorrhage
blindness (visual loss), investigations 41.18M
blisters (from burns), treatment 28.19M
blood
in urine (haematuria) 70.1M
in vomit (haematemesis) 60.12M
blood flow, cerebral, head-injured patient 22.1–2M
blood pressure in shock 2.5M
see also hypotension
blood supply/drainage
femoral head 35.1M
flaps 29.8M, 29.9M, 29.11M, 29.12M, 29.14M
nasal septum 43.2M
skin grafts 29.3M
blood transfusion *see* transfusion
blood vessels 405–15
anastomoses 18.4E

blood vessels – *continued*
diseases (peripheral) 405–15
nasal, injury causing epistaxis 43.5M
see also specific (types of) vessel
Blount's disease 38.1E
blunt injury 21.4M
child 6.3M
eye, hyphaema with 41.12M
larynx 45.2E, 45.26M
liver 61.6E
body surface area, total, burns in relation to 28.5M
body water, total (TBW) 17.5M
Boerhaave's syndrome 59.4M
bolus obstruction (bowel) 66.5M
bone
fracture *see* fracture
grafts, alveolar 42.14M
tumours 37.3E, 37.5M
bowel *see* intestine
Bowen's disease 39.4M
brachial plexus injury 38.3E
brain 283–91
abscesses 40.10M
metabolism 40.3M
oedema 40.2M
traumatic injury
incidence 22.8M
primary, timing 22.6M
secondary, causes 22.7M
tumours 40.13M, 40.16–20M
brainstem death 77.10M
branchial cyst 45.23M
breast 385–8
benign disease 50.1E, 50.2M
cancer (carcinoma) 50.3–6M
conditions with risk of 50.3M
investigations 50.1M
treatment 7.3E, 50.6M
breathlessness, postoperative 20.1M
bronchi
anatomy and physiology 52.1M
cancer 49.2E, 52.3–4M
neuroendocrine tumours (carcinoids) 49.16M, 52.5M
bronchoscopy, haemoptysis 52.1E
Brugia 5.6E, 5.7E, 5.9E, 5.31M
bucket-handle tear 32.1E
Budd–Chiari syndrome 61.1E
bulbous urethra, rupture 74.2M
bullae (blisters) from burns, treatment 28.19M
bullet wounds 21.3M
bupivacaine vs lidocaine 14.5M
burns 195–204
chemical *see* chemical burns
consequences 28.7–8M
ischaemic necrosis 41.15M
depth 28.6M, 28.10M, 28.20M
extent (surface area) 28.5M
management 28.9–26M
bursae 32.5M
olecranon bursitis 34.2E
burst abdomen 57.10M
butterfly fragment (wedge) fracture 27.2

C-reactive protein, visual loss 41.18M
cable graft repair of facial nerve 47.25M
caecal carcinoma 65.1E
calcifying tendinitis 34.1E
calcium abnormalities see hypercalcaemia; hypocalcaemia
calculi see stones
calf muscle tear 55.1E
cancer (malignancy) 84–95
biliary 63.10–11M
periampullary see periampullary carcinoma
bone 37.3E, 37.5M
breast see breast
causation 7.3M
cerebral metastases 40.20M
colorectal 7.6M
end-of-life issues 7.12M
gastrointestinal tract (predominantly carcinomas)
anus 69.1E, 69.4E, 69.13–14M
intestine see intestine
oesophagus 11.1E, 59.1E, 59.5–6M, 60.1E
stomach 60.1E, 60.14–19M
growth 7.2M
head and neck 45.1E, 341–50
external ear 44.12M
hypopharyngeal 45.13M
laryngeal 44.2E, 45.21–2M
lymph node dissection 45.5M, 45.30M
middle ear 44.22M
nasopharyngeal 45.8M
ocular/periocular 41.2E, 41.5M, 41.8M, 41.9M
oropharyngeal see oropharyngeal cancer
sinonasal 43.29M, 43.30M
submandibular gland 47.10M, 47.11M
thyroid 48.4E, 48.5E, 48.12M, 48.14–16M
treatment 46.12–17M
imaging 10.7M
liver see liver
lungs 49.2E, 52.3–4M
obesity and 7.4M
ovarian 7.3E, 76.1E
pain relief 14.10M

pancreatic head 64.1E, 64.12M
penile 74.1E
peritoneal 58.2E
prostate see prostate
retroperitoneal 58.3E
screening 7.5M
Sjögren's syndrome-associated 47.28M
skin 39.4E, 39.4M
eyelid 41.2E, 41.5M
spinal metastases 33.5M
transformation to *see* premalignant lesions; transformation
treatment 7.1–3E, 7.7–11M
urinary tract
lower (bladder) 70.3M, 72.1E, 72.2E, 72.2M, 72.8–9M
upper 71.1E, 71.2E, 71.3E, 71.13–14M
see also specific histological types
car accident *see* road traffic accident victims
carcinoids *see* neuroendocrine tumours
carcinoma
anus 69.4E, 69.13–14M
basal cell *see* basal cell carcinoma
biliary 63.10–11M, 64.1E
periampullary *see* periampullary carcinoma
bladder 70.3M, 72.1E, 72.2E, 72.2M, 72.8–9M
breast *see* breast
bronchial 49.2, 52.3–4ME
GI tract *see* cancer
large bowel 65.1E, 65.29–32M
imaging 65.2E
nasal 43.29M
ovarian 7.3E, 76.1E
pancreatic head 64.1E, 64.12M
penile 74.1E
pharyngeal
hypopharyngeal 45.13M
nasopharyngeal 45.8M
oropharyngeal 45.12M
prostate *see* prostate
renal cell (hypernephroma) 71.1E, 71.2E, 71.13M
renal pelvis 71.3E
spinal metastases 33.5M
squamous cell *see* squamous cell carcinoma
thyroid 48.4E, 48.5E, 48.12M, 48.14–16M
cardia, achalasia 59.1E, 59.5M, 60.1E
cardiology *see* heart
cardiopulmonary bypass 51.1M
Caroli's disease 61.1E, 63.4M
carotid body tumours 45.1E, 45.29E
carotid surgery 53.4M
carpal tunnel syndrome 40.28M
rheumatoid arthritis 37.3M
test 31.6M
weight-lifter 32.14M
cassava and chronic tropical pancreatitis 5.1E, 5.35M
catabolism in recovery phase of metabolic response to injury 1.4M
cataracts 41.20M
catheterization, adrenal vein 49.6M
cauda equina lesions 5.10E
cavernous sinus, venous blood from nose and sinuses passing to 43.3M
cell metabolism in shock 2.1M
cellulitis 4.8M, 39.2E, 55.1E
leg 5.6E
preseptal 41.2E
cerebral blood flow, head-injured patient 22.1–2M
cerebral non-vascular lesions *see* brain
cerebral palsy 38.3E
foot problems 36.1E
cerebral perfusion pressure 22.3M
cerebrospinal fluid
lumbar puncture for analysis of 40.8M
nasal discharge 43.6M
physiology 40.6M
cerebrovascular accident, paralysis 5.10E
cervical lymph nodes (lymph nodes of the neck) 45.5M
metastases 46.23–6M
dissection for 45.5M, 45.30M, 46.25M
management 46.23–6M
prognosis 46.15M
suspected metastases 45.2E
tuberculosis 45.28M
cervical spine (incl. cord) lesions
anatomy 24.1M
clearing 24.2M
imaging 24.3M
paralysis 5.10E
types 24.1E
cestodes (tapeworms) 5.10–19M
chalazion (Meibomian cyst) 41.3–4, 41.22MM
Charcot joints 36.2M
chemical burns 28.26M, 41.15M
eye 41.4E, 41.15M
chemodectoma, carotid body 45.1E, 45.29E
chemoradiotherapy 7.1E
neoadjuvant 7.1E
oropharyngeal cancer nodal metastases 46.23M, 46.24M
chemotherapy 7.1E, 7.10M
adjuvant 7.1E
bladder cancer, neoadjuvant 72.10M
breast cancer 7.3E, 50.6M
mechanisms of actions of drugs used 7.2E

chemotherapy – *continued*
 oropharyngeal cancer 46.2E, 46.17M
 selection of drugs 7.3E
chest *see* thorax
children 75–83
 consent 9.2M
 ear
  hearing loss 44.24M
  otitis media with effusion 44.15–16M
 elective orthopaedics 264–70
 epiglottitis 45.2E, 45.14M
 injury 6.3M
  fall from height 22.4M
  non-accidental 21.1M, 21.6M, 38.8M
  Salter-Harris fracture classification 27.4M
  thermal 28.1M
 metabolic presentations 17.3E
 parotitis *see* parotitis
 retinoblastoma 41.8M
 shoulder subluxation/dislocation 34.4M
 see also adolescent; infant
cholangiohepatitis, Asiatic 5.29–30M
cholangiopancreatography, endoscopic retrograde *see* endoscopic retrograde cholangiopancreatography
cholangitis 63.1E
 ascending 61.2E
 primary sclerosing 5.16M, 5.17M, 61.1E, 63.9M
cholecystectomy 63.8M
cholecystitis, acute 63.1E, 63.5M
 tropical patient 5.2E
choledochal cyst 63.4M
cholesteatoma 44.1E, 44.19M
cholesterol embolism 53.1E
cholesterol stones 63.2E, 63.5M
chondromalacia patellae 32.1E, 38.8E
chordee 74.1E
choroidal melanoma 41.9M
cirrhosis, primary biliary 61.1E
claudication
 spinal 33.7M
 vascular 33.7M, 53.2M
  drug therapy 53.6M
claw hands 5.8E
claw-sign in intestinal obstruction 65.2E, 66.2E
claw toes 36.1E
cleft lip and palate 302–8
Clonorchis sinensis 5.29–30M
Clostridium
 C. difficile, and pseudomembranous colitis 4.3E
 C. perfringens, and gas gangrene 4.3E, 30.9M
 C. tetani, and tetanus 4.3E, 30.7M
 wound infections 4.11M
clubfoot (talipes equinovarus) 36.1E, 38.2E
cochlea 319
coeliac disease 56.1M
coffee-bean sign 66.2E
cognitive dysfunction, postoperative 20.2E
colectomy, ulcerative colitis 65.17M
colic
 biliary 63.1E
 ureteric, acute 67.1E
colitis
 infective 69.1E
 ischaemic 69.1E
 pseudomembranous (and *C. difficile*) 4.3E
 ulcerative *see* ulcerative colitis
collar-and-cuff traction 27.4E
collar-stud abscess 45.28M
collateral ligament injuries
 medial (knee), torn 32.1E
 ulnar 32.4M
colon and colorectum *see* large bowel; rectum
colonoscopy, ulcerative colitis 65.11M
colostomy 65.34M
compartment syndrome
 abdominal 26.3E
 limb 3.1E, 3.2E, 27.2M, 55.1E
compensated shock 2.6M
composite skin grafts 29.3M, 29.5M
compound naevus 39.3E
computed tomography (CT) 10.3M
 acute abdomen 10.7M
 back (spinal) disorders 33.3M
 bladder 70.1E
 ear 44.7M
 hydatid cyst 5.15M, 5.16M
 mediastinal mass 52.1E
 oncology 10.7M
  in lymphatic dysfunction 55.2E
  oral/oropharyngeal cancer 46.10M
 sinonasal 43.1E
 trauma 10.5M
  limbs 27.1E
  neck/spinal 24.3M
  thoracoabdominal 26.2E, 26.6M
condyle (mandibular)
 fractures 25.1E, 25.4M
 hyperplasia 42.19M, 42.20M
condyloma acuminata 69.12M
confusion, postoperative 20.2E
congenital adrenal hyperplasia 49.1E, 49.9M
congenital malformations 6.3E
 biliary tract 63.4M
 ear (inner) 44.23M
 GI tract

anal canal 69.3M
bowel 6.3E, 66.1E
hypertrophic pyloric stenosis 6.1E, 6.7M
hand 38.5M
heart 51.7–8M
pancreatitis due to 64.6M
spine 38.3E
urethra 74.1M
urinary tract 71.1E, 71.1–2M, 71.2E
congestion, venous, pelvic tumour 5.6E
congestive heart failure *see* heart
conjunctival sac, tears entering 41.1M
conjunctivitis, bacterial 41.3E
Conn's syndrome (primary hyperaldosteronism) 49.2E, 49.5M
consent 13.8M
in difficult situations 9.2M
informed 9.1M
contaminated wounds *see* wounds
contrast-enhanced CT
sinonasal 43.1E
thoracoabdominal trauma 26.2E, 26.6M
contrast media 10.1M
conus (medullaris) syndromes 5.10E
cornea, HSV infection 41.3E, 41.10M, 41.16M
coronary artery disease (predominantly ischaemic) 51.2M
bypass surgery 51.1E, 51.3M
cortisol levels
excess 49.2E, 49.4E, 49.5E
low 49.3E
measurement 49.8M
covert injury 21.5M
crab-claw (claw) sign in intestinal obstruction 65.2E, 66.2E
cranial base *see* skull base
cranial nerves, ear 44.2E
see also paralysis *and specific nerves*
cretinism 48.E369
Creutzfeldt–Jakob disease 40.12M
cricothyroidectomy 45.18M
Crohn's disease 65.1E, 65.18–26M, 67.1E
imaging 65.2E, 65.23M
Crouzon's syndrome 42.15M
cruciate ligament tear, posterior and anterior 32.1E
crush injury
liver 61.7E
syndrome of 30.11M
cryptorchidism (undescended testis) 6.4M, 75.1–2M
crystal arthropathies 37.4M
Cushing's disease 49.2E, 49.9M
Cushing's syndrome 49.2E, 49.7–8M
cyanotic heart disease 51.7M, 51.8M
cyst
amoebic 5.25M
branchial 45.23M
breast 50.1E
choledochal 63.4M
epididymal 75.1E
hepatic (simple) 61.1E
hydatid 5.4M, 5.10M, 5.12M, 5.14M, 5.15M, 5.16M, 5.17M, 61.2E
Meibomian 41.3–4, 41.22MM
mesenteric 58.3E
mucous retention *see* mucocele
ovarian 76.1E
thyroglossal duct 45.25M
cystic hygroma 45.24M
cytology 12.2M
inflammation 12.4M

dacryocystitis, acute 41.6M
deafness *see* hearing loss
death (mortality)
brainstem 77.10M
ethical issues in matters of life and 9.3M
in high-risk patients, preventable factors of 16.3M
trauma causing 21.1M, 22.1M
see also end-of-life issues; life-threatening situations
debridement of contaminated wounds 30.6M
decompression surgery, dysthyroid exophthalmos 41.7M
decubitus ulcers (pressure sores) 3.1E, 3.2E, 3.6M, 3.7M
deep vein thrombosis 5.6E, 54.2–4M, 55.1E
risk factors 13.7M
laparoscopic 19.1E
postoperative 13.1E, 20.4M
treatment 54.4M
varicose veins and 54.2E
degenerative conditions, salivary glands 47.27–39M
dehiscence, abdominal (burst abdomen) 57.10M
delayed fracture union 27.3E
dentition
avulsed tooth 25.7M
cleft lip/palate
care 42.12M
structure 42.17M
eruption 42.18M
detrusor instability 72.3M
developmental dysplasia of hip 38.1M
developmental malformations *see* congenital malformations
diabetic patients
foot, osteomyelitis 36.2M
surgery 13.6M

diaphragmatic hernia, congenital 6.3E, 52.5M
diaphragmatic injury 26.3E
diarrhoea 17.13M
diathermy 15.1M
Dieulafoy's lesion 60.3E, 60.12M
digestive tract *see* gastrointestinal tract
disaster surgery 212–16
discoid meniscus 38.1E
dislocations
  patellar 32.1E
  shoulder 34.3–4M
    sports-related 32.10M, 34.1E, 34.5M
  spinal/cervical 24.1E
disseminated intravascular coagulation, transfusion-related 2.3E
diverticula/diverticulum
  bladder 72.1E, 72.2E, 72.5M
  bowel 65.1E, 65.2M
  Zenker's 45.1E, 45.11M, 59.1E
diverticular disease 65.1E, 65.3–7M
diverticulitis 69.1E
  abscess 4.3E
Doppler ultrasound, arterial disease 53.4M
dressings 3.4E
  burns 28.15–16M
drooling 47.30M
drugs
  nephrotoxic 20.3E
  ototoxic 44.26M
  therapy
    allograft rejection prophylaxis 77.2E, 77.8–9M
    benign prostatic hypertrophy causing bladder outlet obstruction 73.7M
    cancer *see* chemotherapy
    claudication 53.6M
    Crohn's disease 65.24M
    deep vein thrombosis 54.4M
    hypercalcaemia 48.26M
    hyperthyroidism 48.5M
    perioperative 13.2E
    shock 2.2E, 2.8M
    ulcerative colitis 65.14M
dry mouth (xerostomia) 47.30M
ductal carcinoma 50.5M
ductal ectasia 50.1E
Dukes' staging, rectal cancer 68.14M
dumping syndromes, early and late 60.2E, 60.11M
duodenum
  atresia 6.3E
  carcinoma of ampulla of *see* periampullary carcinoma
  diverticulum 65.2M
  physiology 60.2M
  ulcer 60.1E, 60.6M, 60.7M, 60.8M
    acute abdomen 5.5E
    vomiting 5.3E
  see also pancreaticoduodenal tumours; pancreaticoduodenectomy
duplex ultrasound
  arterial disease 53.4M
  venous disease 55.2E
Dupuytren's contracture 5.8E, 31.6M
dynamic hip screw 27.4E
dysphagia 59.1E, 59.2M
dyspnoea (shortness of breath), postoperative 20.1M
dysthyroid exophthalmos 41.7M

ear 319–29
  anatomy 44.1–6M, 44.2E
  external
    conditions 44.9–12M
    development 44.8M
    sensory supply 44.6M
  inner, conditions 44.23–9M
  middle, conditions 44.13–32M
  radiological investigations 44.7M
Echinococcus granulosus (hydatid disease) 5.4E, 5.10–19M, 61.2E
ectopic pregnancy *see* pregnancy
elbow
  arthroplasty in rheumatoid arthritis 37.1E
  examination 31.6M
  injuries 34.2E
    sports 32.13–14M, 34.2E
elderly (older) patients
  femoral neck fractures 22.5M
  hearing less (presbycusis) 44.24M
  metabolic presentations 17.3E
electrical burns 28.25M
electrolyte imbalances 17.2E, 17.13M
  head injury 22.12M
  intestinal obstruction 66.2M
  postoperative confusion due to 20.2E
electronic information sites for research 8.5M
electrosurgery, laparoscopic 19.15–16M
embolus 53.1E
  acute limb ischaemia due to, causing paralysis 5.10E
  pulmonary *see* pulmonary embolism
emergency care
  field hospital 30.5M
  oesophageal disorders 59.4M
emesis *see* vomiting
empyema 52.2M
end-of-life issues in cancer 7.12M

endocavitary (incl. endoscopic) ultrasonography 10.2M
oncology 10.7M
endocrine system/glands 361–84
shock relating to 2.1E
endometriosis 76.1E
endoscopic retrograde cholangiopancreatography (ERCP) 63.3M
pancreatitis following 11.4M, 64.7M
endoscopic surgery
laparoscopic *see* laparoscopic surgery
natural orifice transluminal 19.17M
endoscopy visualisation
gastrointestinal 103–5
rectal disease 67.5E
ultrasonic *see* endocavitary ultrasonography
see also arthroscopy; colonoscopy
endotracheal tube
correct placement 14.3M
laryngeal mask airway vs 14.2M
energy sources, laparoscopic surgery 19.8M
Entamoeba histolytica see amoebiasis
enterocolitis, necrotising 6.3E
enterocutaneous fistulas 65.33M
epididymal cyst 75.1E
epididymo-orchitis 75.1E, 75.5M
epiglottitis, pediatric 45.2E, 45.14M
epilepsy and epileptic seizures 40.25M
head injury 22.13M
epiphora 25.1E
epiphysis
femoral capital *see* femur
growth plate injuries 27.4M
epistaxis 25.6M, 43.12–14M
life-threatening 43.16M
recurrent obstruction and 45.7M
vessel injury causing 43.5M
Epstein–Barr virus and nasopharyngeal carcinoma 45.8M
erosive gastritis 11.5M
erysipelas 39.2E
erythrocyte sedimentation rate, visual loss 41.18M
escharotomy 28.14M, 28.22M
ethics 74–5
ethmoid artery injury, anterior 43.5M
ethmoid sinusitis 43.26M
evisceration, eyeball 41.21M
examination
abdominal 423–4
orthopaedics 31.2–10M
exophthalmos, dysthyroid 41.7M
explosive (blast) injuries 30.10M
external fixation 27.4E, 27.6M
extradural haematoma, traumatic 22.1E, 22.10M
extremities *see* limbs
eye 292–301
eyeball evisceration 41.21M
eyelid
burns 28.20M, 28.23M
infection, intracranial spread 41.2M
lumps 41.2E
basal cell carcinoma 41.2E, 41.5M
Meibomian cyst 41.3–4, 41.22MM

facial nerve 47.23–5M
anatomy relating to ear 44.2E
temporal bone exit 44.3M
anatomy relating to parotid surgery 47.23–5M
branches 47.24–5M
palsy 44.29M
traumatic 25.1E
varicella zoster virus infection 44.2E
facial tissues and skeleton *see* oromaxillofacial tissues incl. skeleton
faeces
fistulas with discharge of 65.33M
impaction 66.1E, 66.3E
incontinence 69.5M
falls
child 22.4M
elderly 22.5M
spinal injury 24.2M
familial adenomatous polyposis 65.27–8M
familial hypocalciuric hypocalcaemia 48.1E
fasciitis
necrotising 4.3E, 30.8M, 39.2E, 39.3M
plantar 32.2E
fasciocutaneous flaps 29.12M
fat embolism 53.1E
fat necrosis, breast 50.1E
feel stage, Apley system of examination 31.3M
feet *see* foot
females, gynaecology 554–7
femoral hernia 57.1E, 57.7M
femur
blood supply to head of 35.1M
neck fractures, elderly 22.5M
upper/capital
avascular necrosis (=Perthes' disease) 35.1E, 38.3M
slipped 35.1E, 38.4M
fertility problems, varicocele 5.7E
fever (pyrexia), postoperative 20.1E
fibroids, uterine 76.1E
fibromatosis, palmar (Dupuytren's contracture) 5.8E, 31.6M
field hospital, emergency care 30.5M

filariasis 5.31–2M
limbs
deformities 5.9E
swollen leg 5.6E, 55.6M
scrotal swelling 5.7E
fine needle aspiration cytology
oropharyngeal cancer 46.11M
salivary gland tumours 47.12M
firearm injury 21.3M
fissure, anal 69.1E, 69.4E, 69.4E, 69.6M
fistulas
anal 69.4E, 69.11M
to skin 39.1E
from bowel 65.33M
tracheo-oesophageal 6.3E
urinary 72.6M
vesicolic 65.6M
fixation of fractures 27.4E, 27.6
flaps 29.8–15M
complications 29.14M
oropharyngeal cancer 46.21–2M
types 29.17M
flatfoot 36.1E, 36.2M
fluid abnormalities 17.2E
intestinal obstruction 66.2M
transfusion causing 2.3E
fluid compartments 17.5M
fluid management (incl. intravenously) 17.8M
burns 28.11–13M
shock 2.7M
spinal injury 24.2M
flukes 5.29–31M
fluoroscopy, limb trauma 27.1E
focal nodular hyperplasia (liver) 61.3E
focussed assessment with ultrasonography (FAST), trauma 10.5M, 26.2E, 26.5M
follicular thyroid carcinoma 48.4E, 48.14M
foot 252–6
examination 31.10M
paediatric problems 38.3E
sports injuries 32.2E
forearm free flap, oropharyngeal reconstruction 46.21M
foreign body
intraocular 41.4E, 41.14M
oesophageal 59.4M
rectal 65.2E
fractures
classification 27.3M
Salter-Harris classification 27.4M
femoral neck, elderly 22.5M
healing 32.6M
complications (in union) 27.3E
humeral head 34.1E
march (metatarsal) 32.3E
maxillofacial 25.1E, 25.1–5M
nasal bone 43.7M
orbital blow-out 25.1E, 41.11M
patellar 32.1E
skull
base 22.1E, 22.9M
temporal bone *see* temporal bone
stress 32.7M
treatment 27.5–6M
types 24.1E, 27.2E
Frankel Grade 24.2M
free flaps 29.13M, 29.18M
oropharyngeal cancer 46.21–2M
Freiberg's disease 32.3E, 36.1E
Frey's syndrome 47.9M, 47.26M
frontoethmoidal sinusitis 43.26M
frozen shoulder 34.1E
full-thickness grafts 29.3M, 29.5M, 29.7M

gall bladder
anatomy 63.1M
disorders 63.1E, 63.7M
cancer 63.11M
congenital 63.4M
inflammatory *see* cholecystitis
physiology 63.2M
removal 63.8M
gallstones 63.1–2E, 63.5–6M
clinical conditions caused by 63.1E
ileus 63.1E, 66.2E
management 63.3E
types 63.2E
gangrene 53.11M
gas 4.3E, 30.9M
gas(s), pneumoperitoneum 19.3–4M
gas gangrene 4.3E, 30.9M
gastric disorders *see* stomach *and entries below*
gastrinomas 49.13M, 49.14M, 60.1E
gastritis 11.1E, 60.1E, 60.5M
gastrointestinal stromal tumour (GIST) 7.3E, 11.1E, 60.3E, 60.20M
gastrointestinal tract 437–50, 474–512
congenital malformations *see* congenital malformations
differential diagnosis 60.1E
endoscopy (diagnostic) 103–5
lower 474–512
secretions 17.9M
upper 437–50
gastro-oesophageal reflux disease 60.1E
complications 59.1E, 59.7M

general anaesthesia
  suxamethonium 14.4M
  of triad 14.1M
Glasgow Coma Scale and head injury 22.5M
Glasgow score 64.8M
glenohumeral joint arthritis 34.1E
gliomas 40.17–18M
globe (eyeball), evisceration 41.21M
glomerulonephritis 70.3M
glomus tumour, middle ear 44.22M
glue ear (otitis media with effusion) 44.15–17M
gluten-sensitive enteropathy (coeliac disease) 56.1M
goal-directed therapy in high-risk patients 16.5M
goitre 48.4E
  toxic nodular 48.2M, 48.4E
Gompertzian growth 7.2M
gout 37.4M
graft(s)/transplants 561–7
  allogeneic *see* allografts
  alveolar bone 42.14M
  cardiac valve 51.6M
  complications (other than rejection) 77.3E
  nerve *see* nerve
  organ 561–7
    donation 77.11M
  skin *see* skin
  tendon 29.17M
  terminology 77.1M
graft-vs-host disease 77.1E, 77.7M
granulomatosis, Wegener's 43.1E, 43.12M
grasp (grip) 34.3E
Graves' disease 48.2M, 48.4E
great vessels, transposition 51.8M
grip (hand) 34.3E
growth, tumour 7.2M
growth plate injuries 27.4M
gunfire injury 21.3M
gustatory sweating (Frey's syndrome) 47.9M, 47.26M
gynaecology 554–7

haemangioma, hepatic 61.3E
haematemesis 60.12M
haematoma
  adrenal 49.1E
  auricular 44.9M
  extradural, traumatic 22.10E, 22.10M
  nasal septal 43.8M
  soft-tissue 32.2M
  subdural, traumatic 22.1E, 22.11M
haematuria 70.1M
haemolytic transfusion reaction 2.3E
haemoptysis 52.1E
haemorrhage (bleeding)
  nasal *see* epistaxis
  reactionary 2.10M
  rectal 69.1M
  retrobulbar 25.2M
  shock due to 2.1E
  subarachnoid, aneurysmal 40.21–3M
  subconjunctival 41.3E
  trochar site 19.14M
  vaginal 76.3M
haemorrhagic telangiectasia, hereditary 43.17M
haemorrhoids 69.4E, 69.4E, 69.7–8M
haemothorax, massive 26.1E
hair balls (trichobezoars) 60.3E, 60.20M
hallux rigidus 36.1E
hallux valgus 36.1E
hands
  conditions 34.5E
    claw hand 5.8E
    paediatric 38.5M
    rheumatoid arthritis 37.3M
    traumatic 34.4E
  examination 31.6M
  grip 34.3E
Hansen's disease *see* leprosy
head and neck disorders 281–360
  cancer *see* cancer
  see also neck
head injury 160–5
healing (of wounds) 3.1–3M
  bone *see* bone
  phases 3.2M, 3.3E
  poor 13.1E
hearing loss
  age-related (presbycusis) 44.24M
  congenital 44.23M
heart 391–6
  congenital disease 51.7–8M
  failure, congestive
    ascites 58.2E
    lower limb swelling 55.1E
    scrotal swelling 5.7E
  ischaemic disease *see* coronary artery disease
  shock 2.1E
  tamponade 26.1E
  transplantation 77.13M
  valves *see* valves
heel bumps 32.3E
Helicobacter pylori 60.4M, 60.5M, 60.6M
helminths 5.1–17M, 5.29–32M
hemiarthroplasty, hip 27.4E, 35.1E
heparin, deep vein thrombosis 54.4M
hepatic problems *see* liver *and entries below*

hepatitis, viral 61.2E
hepatocellular carcinoma 61.3E
hepatopancreatic ampulla, carcinoma *see* periampullary carcinoma
hepatorenal syndrome, postoperative 20.3E
hereditary haemorrhagic telangiectasia 43.17M
hereditary non-polyposis colorectal cancer 65.29M, 76.3M
hereditary spherocytosis 62.1E
hernia
  abdominal wall 5.7E, 57.1E, 57.1–8M
    causes 57.2M
    complications 57.2E, 57.3M
    pediatric 6.1E, 6.4M
    predisposing factors 57.1M
    strangulated 57.2E, 57.4M, 66.1E
    treatment 57.3E, 66.3E
  diaphragmatic
    congenital 6.3E, 52.5M
    hiatus hernia 11.1M
  internal (bowel) 66.4M
herpes simplex infection of cornea 41.3E, 41.10M, 41.16M
hiatus hernia 11.1M
high-risk surgical patient 124–6
hindfoot problems 36.2M
hip (joint)
  aetiology of disorders 35.1E
  anatomy and physiology 35.1M
  developmental dysplasia 38.1M
  dynamic screw 27.4E
  examination 31.6M
  fractures, elderly 22.5M
  replacement *see* arthroplasty; hemiarthroplasty
  spontaneous avascular necrosis (Perthes' disease) 35.1E, 38.3M
  stability 35.2M
Hirschsprung's disease 6.3E
histology specimens 12.1M
history-taking
  abdominal problems 423–4
  musculoskeletal 31.1M
HIV disease and AIDS 4.20M
  chronic childhood parotitis and 47.18M
HLA and transplantation 77.2M, 77.4M
Hoffa's syndrome 32.1E
homeostasis 1.1M
hormones
  adrenal 49.2–3M
  androgenic 73.2M
  in female reproductive physiology 76.M
  sex 49.3E
horseshoe kidney 71.2E
HPV *see* human papilloma virus
HSV keratitis 41.3E, 41.10M, 41.16M
human immunodeficiency virus *see* HIV disease and AIDS
human leucocyte antigens and transplantation 77.2M, 77.4M
human papilloma virus (HPV)
  laryngeal papillomatosis 45.2E
  wart *see* wart
humerus, fractured head 34.1E
Hurthle cell carcinoma 48.14M
hydatid disease 5.4E, 5.10–19M, 61.2E
hydrocele (vaginal) 5.7E, 75.1E, 75.4M
hydrocephalus 40.5M
  obstructive 40.7M
hydronephrosis 71.2E
  idiopathic/congenital 71.1E, 71.5M
21-hydroxylase deficiency 49.3E
hygroma, cystic 45.24M
hyperacute rejection 77.1E, 77.3M, 77.4M
hyperaldosteronism, primary 49.2E, 49.5M
hypercalcaemia 48.18M, 48.19M
  associated disorders 48.19M
  causes 48.1E
  medical management 48.26M
hypercortisolism 49.2E, 49.4E, 49.5E
hyperextension of knee 32.1E
hypernephroma 71.1E, 71.2E, 71.13M
hyperparathyroidism, primary 48.1E, 48.17M
  biochemical diagnosis 48.18M
  surgery 48.21M
hypertension
  portal 58.2E, 61.8M
  systemic arterial 49.5E
hyperthyroidism (thyrotoxicosis) 48.2–7M
  clinical features/presentation 48.2–4M
  diagnosing cause 48.2E
  treatment 48.5–7M
hypertrophic pyloric stenosis, congenital 6.1E, 6.7M
hyphaema 41.12M
hypoadrenalism 49.1E
hypocalcaemia
  causes 48.1E
  familial hypocalciuric 48.1E
  transfusion-related 2.3E
hypocortisolism 49.3E
hypogonadotrophic hypogonadism 49.3E
hypokalaemia 49.5E
hyponatraemia in head injury 22.12M
hypoparathyroidism 48.1E, 48.25M
hypopharyngeal carcinoma 45.13M
hypoproteinaemia, causes 17.3M
hypospadias 74.1M

hypotension
  postoperative 20.3M
  in shock 2.5M
hypothalamic–pituitary–adrenal axis 49.8M
hypothalamic–pituitary–gonadal axis in women 76.2M
hypothermia, crush syndrome and 30.11M
hypothyroidism 48.8–11M
  biochemical features 48.10M
  conditions presenting with 48.11M
  diagnosing cause 48.3E
  myxoedema 48.9M
  neonatal 48.8M
hypovolaemia 17.12M
  shock due to 2.1E, 2.2M
  in trauma 1.15M

ileoanal pouch, ulcerative colitis 65.17M
ileorectal anastomosis, ulcerative colitis 65.17M
ileostomy 65.34M
  ulcerative colitis 65.17M
ileum, tuberculosis 5.2E, 5.3E, 5.19–23M
ileus
  gallstone 63.1E, 66.2E
  paralytic 5.4E
iliac artery disease 53.3M
imaging, diagnostic 96–9
  arterial disease 53.4M, 53.5M
  back disorders 33.3M
  biliary tract 63.3M
  bladder 72.2E
    cancer 72.2E, 72.9M
  ear 44.7M
  hazards 10.1M
  injury
    limbs 27.1E
    neck/spine 24.3M
    thoracoabdominal 26.2E, 26.6M
  intestine 65.2E
    Crohn's disease 65.2E, 65.23M
    obstruction 65.2E, 66.2E, 66.10M
  liver 61.5M
  lymphatic disorders 55.2E
  nose 43.1E
  oral/oropharyngeal cancer 46.10M
  osteoarthritis 35.3M
  pancreas 64.2M
  paranasal sinuses 43.1E, 43.4M
  parathyroid 48.23M
  urological 70.1E, 70.4M, 71.2E, 71.3E
  see also specific modalities
immunodeficiency, causes 4.3M
immunohistochemistry 12.5M
immunosuppressive drugs, rejection prophylaxis 77.2E, 77.8–9M
impetigo 39.2E
implants *see* prostheses
incontinence
  anal 69.5M
  urinary
    sudden-onset 33.2M
    urge 69.4E
infant
  metabolic presentations 17.3E
  newborn, hypothyroidism 48.8M
infarction
  myocardial *see* myocardial infarction
  splenic 62.1E
infections
  colonic 69.1E
  control, with burns 28.18M
  cutaneous 39.2E
  epididymal/testicular 75.1E, 75.5M
  fracture non-union complicated by 27.3E
  host resistance to, disorders reducing 4.3M
  intra-abdominal 58.1E, 58.2–4M
  joint implant 35.3E, 37.2E
  liver *see* liver
  natural barriers to 4.2M
  ocular and orbital
    cornea 41.3E, 41.10M, 41.16M
    eyelid, intracranial spread 41.2M
    tear sac 41.6M
  parapharyngeal space 45.2M
  parotid 47.14–16M
  pelvic 4.3E, 76.1E, 76.6M
  post-transplant 77.3E
  soft-tissue, necrotising 3.8M
  surgical wound 22–30, 4.3E
    prevention 4.13–15M
    pyrexia with 20.1E
    risk factors 4.4M, 13.1E
    secondary 4.5M
    treatment 4.12M
    types of operation and rates of 4.4E
  transfusion-associated 2.3E
  tropical 5.1–34M
  urinary tract *see* urinary tract
  see also specific (types of) pathogens
infertility, varicocele 5.7E
inflammation, cytology 12.4M
inflammatory disease
  bowel *see* Crohn's disease; ulcerative colitis
  pelvic 76.1E, 76.6M
inflammatory response, systemic (syndrome of) 4.9M
informed consent 9.1M

inguinal canal anatomy 57.5M
inguinal hernia 5.7E, 57.1E, 57.2M
 complications 57.3M
 pediatric 6.1E, 6.4M
 sliding 57.6M
 treatment 57.3E, 66.3E
inguinal region
 children, swellings 6.4M
 hernia *see* hernia
inguinal swellings, children 6.4M
inhalation, smoke 28.4M
injury (trauma) 3–7, 151–216, 224–32
 assessment 21.2M, 22.2–5M
 bladder 72.2E, 72.2M
 blunt *see* blunt injury
 brachial plexus 38.3E
 breast, causing fat necrosis 50.1E
 covert 21.5M
 ear 44.13M
 elbow *see* elbow
 electrosurgical, in laparoscopic surgery 19.16M
 epidemiology 156–9
 extremity 185–94E
 firearm 21.3M
 hand 34.4E
 head 160–5
 imaging 10.5M
 liver 26.3E, 61.6–7M
 mass disasters 212–16
 maxillofacial 171–5
 metabolic response 3–7
 multiple *see* polytrauma
 neck *see* cervical spine
 ocular/orbital 25.1E, 41.4E, 41.11M
 pancreas 26.3E, 64.3–4M
 pediatric *see* children
 rectum 68.5–6M
 renal 26.3E, 71.2E, 71.3–4M
 shoulder *see* shoulder
 sinonasal 43.5–8M
 spinal *see* spine
 spleen 62.1E
 sports 224–32
 thermal *see* burns
 thoracoabdominal 176–84, 58.3E
 ureter 71.3–4M
 urethra 74.2–3M
 see also fractures; wounds
inotropic drugs, shock 2.2E, 2.8M
insulinomas 48.22M, 49.2E, 49.13M, 49.14M
internal fixation 27.4E, 27.6M
intestine (bowel) 474–94
 anastomosis 18.4E
 anatomy 65.1M
 ascariasis, obstruction 5.8M
 atresia 6.3E
 cancer 7.1E, 7.3E, 7.6M, 65.1E, 65.27–32M, 68.1E, 68.10–14M, 69.1E
  hereditary non-polyposis colorectal cancer 65.29M, 76.3M
  imaging 65.2E
  obstruction 66.1E
  recurrence 66.1E
  in ulcerative colitis 65.13M
 imaging *see* imaging
 intussusception 6.1E, 65.2E, 66.2E, 66.7M
 malrotation 6.3E
 obstruction 488–94, 66.11M
  abdominal distension in tropical patients due to 5.4E
  adhesive *see* adhesive intestinal obstruction
  adynamic 66.1M
  causes 66.1E, 66.1M, 66.4–8M
  clinical features 66.9M
  fluid and electrolyte changes 66.2M
  management 66.3E, 66.11M
  radiological investigations 65.2E, 66.2E, 66.10M
  strangulation in 66.3M
 perforation *see* perforation
 resections 17.10M
  diverticular disease 65.7M
  ulcerative colitis 65.17M
 transplantation 77.13M
 tuberculosis 5.2E, 5.19–23M
  obstruction 5.3E
  peritonitis 5.5E
 see also large bowel; small bowel
intracranial drainage of venous blood from nose and sinuses 43.3M
intracranial pressure 40.1M
 intracranial traumatic mass lesion and 22.4M
intracranial spread of eyelid infections 41.2M
intramedullary nails 27.4E, 27.6M
intravenous fluids *see* fluid management
intravenous urogram 70.1E, 70.4M
intubation, tracheal *see* endotracheal tube
intussusception 6.1E, 65.2E, 66.2E, 66.7M
investigations (incl. diagnostic aids) 103–6
 abdominal disorders 58.5M
 airway obstruction (acute airway) 45.2E
 anorectal symptoms 69.2E
 arterial disease 53.4–5M
 biliary tract 63.3M
 breast cancer 50.1M
 bronchial carcinoma 52.4M
 dysphagia 59.3M

limb ischaemia (acute) 5.10M
lymphatic disorders 55.2E
ophthalmological problems 41.1E
visual loss 41.18M
pancreas 64.2M
pharynx/larynx/neck 45.1E
oropharyngeal cancer (and oral cavity) 46.10–11M
preoperative 13.2M
radiological *see* imaging
salivary gland
parotid 47.1E
submandibular 47.2E
shoulder pain 38.6M
thoracoabdominal injury 26.2E, 26.5–6M
urinary tract 515–20
males 73.4–5M
iodine, radioactive, in hyperthyroidism 48.5M
ischaemia, limb (lower limb predominantly)
acute embolic, paralysis due to 5.10E
critical 53.2M, 55.1E
ischaemia–reperfusion syndrome 2.3M
limbs 30.11M
ischaemic colitis 69.1E
ischaemic heart disease *see* coronary artery disease
ischaemic necrosis, burns with 41.15M
islanded flaps 29.9M
isotope scan, parathyroid 48.23M
itch (pruritus), anal 69.9M

jaundice
obstructive 63.9M
surgery in patients with 13.5M
jaw deformities 42.19–20M
see also mandible; maxilla
joints
Charcot 36.2M
replacement *see* arthroplasty
junctional naevus 39.3E
juvenile nasal angiofibroma 43.14–15M, 45.7M
juvenile rheumatoid arthritis 37.2E

keloids 3.2E, 3.10M
keratitis, HSV 41.3E, 41.10M, 41.16M
keratoacanthoma 39.3E
ketoacidosis 17.4M
kidney 521–32
congenital anomalies 71.1–2M
failure 70.2M, 70.5M
postoperative 20.3E
injury 26.3E, 71.2E, 71.3–4M
neoplasms 71.1E, 71.13–14M
stones 71.1E, 71.6–9M
transplantation 77.12M
with pancreas 77.13M
Kirschner wire fixation 27.4E
knee
amputation above/through/below 53.13M
arthroscopy 35.7M
deformities, foot problems and 36.2M
examination 31.9M
management of various conditions 34.4E
paediatric problems 38.1E
sports injuries 32.1E
stability 35.6M
Koch's abdomen (subacute intestinal obstruction) 5.3E
Koch's postulates 4.1M
Krukenberg's tumours 60.17M

laboratory tests, pre-analytical errors 17.11M
lacrimal gland secretions 41.1M
lacrimal (tear) sac
infection 41.6M
mucocele 41.2E
LAHSHAL system 42.6M
laparoscopic diagnosis in trauma 26.2E, 26.6M
laparoscopic surgery 19.8–9M
benefits of robotic surgery over 19.12M
complications 19.1E
electrosurgery in 19.15–16M
energy sources 19.8M
nomenclatures 19.2E
pneumoperitoneum for 19.3–6M
simulators 19.9M
large bowel 474–87
anastomosis 18.4E, 65.17M
anatomy 65.1M
cancer 7.1E, 7.3E, 7.6M, 65.1E, 65.27–32M, 68.1E, 68.10–14M, 69.1E
hereditary non-polyposis colorectal cancer 65.29M, 76.3M
laryngeal mask airway 14.2M
laryngeal nerves
recurrent 45.3M
damage/lesions 45.1E, 45.20M
superior 45.3M
laryngectomy 45.22M
larynx
anatomy and physiology 45.3–4M
blunt injury 45.2E, 45.26M
disease 45.14–22M
malignant 44.2E, 45.21–2M
papillomatosis 45.2E
investigation 45.1E
LASIK 41.19M
Le Fort II maxillary fractures 25.1M

leg *see* lower limb
leiomyoma, uterine (=fibroids) 76.1E
lens cataracts 41.20M
leprosy 5.33–4M
  limb deformities 5.9E
    claw hands 5.8E
lidocaine vs bupivacaine 14.5M
life and death, ethical issues in matters of 9.3M
life-threatening situations
  epistaxis 43.16M
  thoracoabdominal injury 26.3–4M
ligament injuries 32.4M
limbs (extremities) 238–56
  amputation 53.12–13M
  claudication *see* claudication
  compartment syndrome 3.1E, 3.2E, 27.2M, 55.1E
  deformities 5.9E
  ischaemia *see* ischaemia
  lower *see* lower limb
  paralysis
    due to acute embolic ischaemia 5.10E
    due to spinal injury 24.2M
  reperfusion injury 30.11M
  trauma 185–94
  upper *see* upper limb
lingual artery ligation 43.16M
lingual nerve, submandibular gland attachments 47.8M
linitis plastica 11.1M
lip
  cancer
    clinical features 46.7M
    treatment 46.14M
  cleft, and palate 302–8
liver 451–7
  anatomy 61.1–2M
  cancer 61.3E
    secondary *see* metastases
  chronic disease/conditions 61.1E
    clinical features 61.4M
  function tests 61.3M
  imaging 61.5M
  infections 61.2E
    amoebiasis 5.2E, 5.5E, 5.24M, 5.26M, 5.27M, 5.28M, 61.2E
    hydatid disease/cyst 5.10M, 5.12M, 5.15M, 5.16M, 61.2E
  injury 26.3E, 61.6–7M
  transplantation 77.13M
  tumours 61.3E
lobar pneumonia 5.1E
lobular carcinoma 50.5M
local anaesthesia
  lidocaine vs bupivacaine 14.5M
  lower limb 14.7M
  upper limb 14.6M
Loeffler's syndrome 5.1M, 5.4M, 5.5M, 5.7M, 5.13M
look stage, Apley system of examination 31.2M
lower limb (leg) 246–56
  amputation 53.12–13M
  Bier's block 14.7M
  claudication *see* claudication
  compartment syndrome 27.2M
  ischaemia *see* ischaemia
  length inequality 38.3E
  paralysis
    due to acute embolic ischaemia 5.10E
    due to spinal injury 24.2M
  swollen 5.6E, 55.1E
    filariasis 5.6M, 55.6M
  ulcers 54.1E
    venous 54.1M
lower motor neuron VII nerve palsy 25.1E
Ludwig's angina 45.27M
lumbar cord lesions, paralysis 5.10E
lumbar puncture 40.8M
lungs
  anatomy and physiology 52.1M
  atelectasis, postoperative 20.1E
  cancer 49.2E, 52.3–4M
  neuroendocrine tumours (carcinoids) 49.16M, 52.5M
  resection, fitness for/extent of 52.1E
lymph nodes
  biopsy 55.2E
  breast cancer (metastases), management 50.6M
  cervical *see* cervical lymph nodes
  see also TNM staging
lymphangitis 39.2E, 55.2M
lymphatic system 416–19
  anatomy and physiology 55.1M
  disorders 55.1–2E, 55.2–7M
    investigations 55.2E
lymphoedema 55.1E, 55.3–7M
  filariasis 5.6M, 55.6M
  primary 5.5E, 55.3M
lymphoma 7.3E
  gastric 60.3E, 60.20M
  Sjögren's syndrome and 47.28M

magnetic resonance angiography 53.5M
magnetic resonance arthrography 10.4M
magnetic resonance imaging (MRI) 10.3M
  back (spinal) disorders 33.3M
  ear 44.7M
  lymphatic disorders 55.2E
  oral/oropharyngeal cancer 46.10M

orthopaedics 10.4M
trauma 10.5M
limbs 27.1E
neck/spinal 24.4M
major incidents/disasters 212–16
malabsorption 17.6M
male genitourinary conditions 541–5, 546–53
malignant tumour *see* cancer
Mallory–Weiss syndrome/tear 11.1E, 59.4M, 60.3E, 60.12M
malrotation and volvulus
gastric 60.3E, 60.21M
intestinal 6.3E, 66.1E, 66.2E, 66.3E, 66.3M, 66.8M
congenital 66.1E
malunion 27.3E
mandible
developmental abnormalities 42.19M
fractures 25.1E, 25.3M
march fractures 32.3E
Marfan's syndrome, cardiac disease 51.1E
Marjolin's ulcer 54.1E
mass disasters 212–16
maxilla
developmental abnormalities 42.19M
Le Fort II fractures 25.1M
see also oromaxillofacial tissues
maxillary sinusitis 43.23M
Meckel's diverticulum 65.2M
median nerve lesions/palsy 31.6M
claw hands 5.8E
compression at wrist *see* carpal tunnel syndrome
weight-lifter 32.14M
mediastinal mass 52.1E
mediastinitis 45.2M
mediators in metabolic response to injury 1.3M
medullary thyroid carcinoma 48.5E, 48.12M, 48.16M
megacolon, congenital (Hirschsprung's disease) 6.3E
Meibomian cyst 41.3–4, 41.22MM
melanoma, malignant 39.3M, 39.4E
choroidal 41.9M
membranous urethra, rupture 74.3M
men, genitourinary conditions 541–5, 546–53
Ménière's disease 44.29M
meningiomas 40.19M
meningitis, tuberculous 40.11M
meningococcal sepsis 49.1E
meniscus
discoid 38.1E
torn 32.1E
mental paraesthesia 25.2E
mesenteric artery aneurysm, superior 64.11M
mesentery 58.3E
mesh grafts 29.7M
metabolism
brain 40.3M
changes (incl. disturbances)
cells, in shock 2.1M
in injury 3–7
in vomiting 17.15M
young and old patients 17.3E
metastases
bone 37.3E, 37.5M
cerebral 40.20M
hepatic 61.3E
from carcinoids 49.4E
lymph node *see* lymph node
oral 46.6M
spinal 33.5M
from stomach 60.17M
see also TNM staging
metatarsal
fatigue (march) fracture 32.3E
second, avascular necrosis of head (Freiberg's disease) 32.3E, 36.1E
metatarsalgia 32.3E
microscopic diagnosis 12.3M
midfoot problems 36.2M
minimal access surgery
advantages 19.1M
limitations 19.2M
missile (firearm) injury 21.3M
mitral valve disease 51.1E, 51.4M
Mittelschmerz 67.1E
mixed venous saturation 2.9M
mobility assessment, Apley system of examination 31.4M
molluscum contagiosum, eyelid 41.2E
Mondor's disease 50.1E
mortality *see* death
Morton's neuroma 32.3E, 36.1E
mouth *see* oral cavity; oromaxillofacial tissues; oropharyngeal cancer
move stage, Apley system of examination 31.4M
mucocele (mucous retention cyst)
gallbladder 63.1E
lacrimal sac 41.2E
salivary *see* sialocele
mucosa, gastric, damage 60.3M
mucous retention cyst *see* mucocele
multiple endocrine neoplasia (MEN) 48.22M, 49.12M, 49.14M
MEN-1 48.17M, 48.24M, 49.12M, 49.13M, 49.14M
MEN-2 49.12M, 49.16M
multiple injury *see* polytrauma
multiple myeloma 17.2E, 37.3E
mumps 47.14M

muscle in clefts 42.5E
Pierre Robin syndrome and 42.7M
muscular dystrophy 38.3E
musculocutaneous (myocutaneous) flaps 29.12M, 29.17M
musculoskeletal system *see* orthopaedics
Mycobacterium
M. leprae see leprosy
M. tuberculosis see tuberculosis
mycotic embolism 53.1E
myeloma, multiple 17.2, 37.3E
myocardial infarction
perioperative risk 13.1E
tropical patients 5.1E
myocutaneous (musculocutaneous) flaps 29.12M, 29.17M
myxoedema 48.9M

naevus
compound 39.3E
junctional 39.3E
nails, intramedullary 27.4E, 27.6M
nasal tissue *see* nose
nasopharyngeal carcinoma 45.8M
natural orifice transluminal surgery 19.17M
neck 45.23–30M
anatomy and physiology relating to 45.1–5M
injury, blunt 45.26M
see also cervical spine
investigation *see* investigations
lymph nodes *see* cervical lymph nodes
see also head and neck disorders
necrosis
avascular *see* avascular necrosis
fat, breast 50.1E
ischaemic, burns with 41.15M
necrotising infections 3.2E
enterocolitis 6.3E
fasciitis 4.3E, 30.8M, 39.2E, 39.3M
otitis externa 44.1E, 44.11M
soft-tissue infections 3.8M
needles 18.3E
Nelson's syndrome 49.1E, 49.9M
nematodes 5.1–9M, 5.31–3M
neonatal hypothyroidism 48.8M
neoplasm *see* tumour
nephroblastoma (Wilms' tumour) 71.13M
nephrotoxin, postoperative renal failure due to 20.3E
nerves
grafts 29.17M
facial nerve repair 47.25M
palsies *see* paralysis
neuroendocrine response to injury 1.2M
neuroendocrine tumours (incl. carcinoids) 49.4EM, 49.15–16
bronchi 49.16M, 52.5M
neurogenic (spinal) claudication 33.7M
neurogenic shock 2.1E
neurological conditions in children, musculoskeletal complications 38.3E
neuroma
acoustic 44.30M
Morton's 32.3E, 36.1E
neuropathy, ulceration 54.1E
neurosurgery, elective 283–91
night-time waking with back pain 33.5M
nipple
discharge 50.4M
Paget's disease 50.5M
nocturnal back pain 33.5
non-accidental injury, children 21.1M, 21.6M, 38.8M
non-steroidal anti-inflammatory drugs, shin injury 32.1M
non-thyroidal illness (sick euthyroid) syndrome 48.1M
non-union of fracture 27.3E
nose 309–18
anatomy 43.1M, 43.2E
bleeding from *see* epistaxis
imaging 43.1E
polyps 43.18–22M
recurrent obstruction and epistaxis 45.7M
septum 43.9–11M
blood supply and drainage 43.2M
deviation 43.9M
haematoma 43.8M
perforation 43.10–11M
surgery 42.16M
trauma 43.5–8M
tumours 43.14–15M, 43.27–30M, 45.7M
NOTES (natural orifice transluminal surgery) 19.17M
nutritional problems in cleft lip/palate, prenatal scan 42.7M
nutritional support 127–34
perioperative 1.4M

oat cell carcinoma, bronchial 49.2E, 52.3M
obesity
cancer and 7.4M
surgery in obese patients 13.4M
oblique fracture 27.2E
observation (look) stage, Apley system of examination 31.2M
obstructive hydrocephalus 40.7M
obstructive jaundice 63.9M
occlusive arterial disease 53.10M
ocular conditions 292–301

oculomotor (IIIrd cranial) nerve palsy in head injury 22.14M
oedema
cerebral 40.2M
lymphatic *see* lymphoedema
optic disc (papilloedema) 40.4M
scrotal, idiopathic 75.1E
oesophagotracheal fistula 6.3E
oesophagus 437–40
anatomy 59.1M
Barrett's 11.1E, 59.5M
cancer 11.1E, 59.1E, 59.5–6M, 60.1E
endoscopy 11.1E
Mallory–Weiss syndrome/tear 11.1E, 59.4M, 60.3E, 60.12M
varices 11.1E, 60.12M
older people *see* elderly
olecranon bursitis 34.2E
oliguria, postoperative 20.5M
omental torsion 58.3E
operating room, care in 122–3
operating table, set-up on 15.3M
ophthalmic conditions 292–301
optic disc oedema (papilloedema) 40.4M
oral cavity (mouth)
cancer *see* oropharyngeal cancer
dryness (xerostomia) 47.30M
floor defects, reconstruction 46.19M
posterior border 46.1M
orbit 292–301
blow-out fracture 25.1E, 41.11M
orbital fissure syndrome, superior 25.2M
oromaxillofacial tissues incl. skeleton
developmental abnormalities 302–8
injury 171–5
oropharyngeal cancer (and oral cavity) 45.12M, 341–50
anatomy and physiology 46.1E, 46.1–6M
clinical features/investigations/staging 46.7–11M
field change 46.2E, 46.5M, 46.17M
treatment 46.2E, 46.12–17M
complications and outcomes 46.2E, 46.27–8M
orthodontic care, clefts 42.12M
orthognathic surgery 42.15M
orthopaedics (musculoskeletal system) 217–70
elective surgery 217–70
paediatric 264–70
imaging 10.4M
Osgood–Schlatter disease 38.1E
Osler–Weber–Rendu syndrome (hereditary haemorrhagic telangiectasia) 43.17M
osteoarthritis 34.1E, 35.1E
radiological features 35.3M
upper limb 34.1E
osteochondritis dissecans 38.1E
osteochondroma 37.3E
osteomyelitis 37.2E
child 38.7M
diabetic foot 36.2M
osteophyte removal, ankle 36.2M
otalgia, laryngeal cancer 44.2E
otitis externa 44.1E, 44.10M
necrotising 44.1E, 44.11M
otitis media 44.1E, 44.14–18M
acute 44.1E
chronic 44.1E, 44.18M, 44.20M
with effusion 44.15–17M
suppurative 44.14M
otosclerosis 44.2E, 44.21M
ovaries
cancer 7.3E, 76.1E
cyst 76.1E
polycystic disease 49.3E

paediatrics *see* children
Paget's disease
of breast/nipple 50.5M
extramammary 39.4M
pain
abdominal *see* abdominal pain
back *see* back
Pain
knee, anterior (chondromalacia patellae) 32.1E, 38.1E
red eye with 41.3E, 41.17M
relief *see* analgesia
scrotal (pain), child 6.6M
shoulder, child 38.6M
urological origin 70.2M
see also colic; metatarsalgia; otalgia; trigeminal neuralgia
palate
cleft lip and 302–8
mobility (traumatic) 25.2E
palatine artery 43.2M
palliative therapy, cancer 7.1E, 7.11M
palmar fibromatosis (Dupuytren's contracture) 5.8E, 31.6M
palpation (feel) stage, Apley system of examination 31.3M
pancreas 468–73
anatomy 64.1M
injury 26.3E, 64.3–4M
investigations 64.2M
transplantation ± kidney 77.13M
pancreaticoduodenal tumours 48.22M, 49.13M

pancreaticoduodenectomy (Whipple operation) 20.3E, 63.3E, 64.12E
pancreatitis 64.5–11M
 acute 64.1E, 64.5–11M
  complications 64.11M
  congenital causes 64.6M
  gallstones causing 63.1E
  postoperative/post-procedure 11.4M, 64.7M
  severity scoring 64.8M
  signs 64.9M
 chronic
  alcoholic 64.1E
  tropical 5.1E, 5.35M
 fluid and electrolyte abnormalities 17.2E
papillary thyroid carcinoma 48.5E, 48.12M, 48.14M
papilloedema 40.4M
papilloma
 basal cell 39.3E
 transitional cell, nasal 43.28M
papillomatosis, recurrent respiratory 45.2E
paraesthesia
 mental 25.2E
 supraorbital 25.1E
paralysis (palsy) 5.10E
 cranial nerve
  IIIrd 22.14M
  VIIth *see* facial nerve
 limbs *see* limbs
 median nerve *see* median nerve lesions
 ulnar nerve *see* ulnar nerve lesions
 vocal cord 45.1E, 45.20M
paralytic ileus 5.4E
paranasal sinuses 309–18
 anatomy 43.1M, 43.2E
 imaging 43.1E, 43.4M
 inflammation (sinusitis) 43.23–6M
 trauma 43.5–8M
parapharyngeal space infection 45.2M
parasites 5.1–17M, 5.24–31M
parathyroid 48.17–26M
 imaging 48.23M
 surgery 48.20–1M, 48.24M
parenteral nutrition, total 17.2M
parietal lobe lesions, dominant 40.14M
parietal peritoneum 56.2M
Parkinson's disease 40.26M
Parkland formula for burns 28.12M
parotid gland 47.13–26M
 disorders 47.13–21M
  sialocele 25.2E
 investigation of mass 47.1E
 surgery (incl. parotidectomy) 47.22–6M
  complications 47.9M, 47.26M
parotitis
 bacterial 47.15–16M
 children
  chronic 47.18M
  recurrent 47.17M
 epidemic (mumps) 47.14M
paroxysmal positional vertigo, benign 44.27M
patella
 chondromalacia 32.1E, 38.1E
 dislocations 32.1E
 fracture 32.1E
patients
 high-risk 124–6
 in preoperative care
  management 13.3M
  preparation 13.1M
 set-up on operating table 15.3M
 transport from disaster scene 30.4M
pelvic inflammatory disease 76.1E, 76.6M
pelvic region
 abscess 4.3E
 tumour, venous congestion 5.6E
pelvis, supporting structures with standing on one leg 35.3M
pelviureteric junction obstruction, hydronephrosis from (=idiopathic/congenital hydronephrosis) 71.1E, 71.5M
penile conditions 74.1E
peptic stricture 11.1E, 59.1E, 59.7M
peptic ulcer 60.1E, 60.6–10M
 acute abdomen 5.5E
 perforated 5.5E, 67.1E
 vomiting 5.3E
perforation
 appendix 67.3M
 bowel
  laparoscopy risk of 19.1E
  radiological signs 66.2M
  tuberculosis 5.5E, 5.23
  typhoid 5.5E, 5.38M
 gallbladder 63.1E
 nasal septum 43.10–11M
 peptic ulcer 5.5E, 67.1E
perfusion pressure, cerebral 22.3M
periampullary carcinoma 64.1E
 operation 20.3E, 63.3E, 64.12E
perianal abscesses 69.10M
pericardial effusion 51.9M
pericardial tamponade (cardiac tamponade) 26.1E
perioperative care 111–50
 optimal 1.5M
peripheral neuropathy, ulceration 54.1E
peripheral vascular disease 405–15

peritoneal cavity
  diagnostic lavage (DPL) 58.5M
    trauma 26.2E, 26.6M
  excess fluid (ascites) 58.2E
peritoneum 58.1M
  parietal 56.2M
peritonitis 58.1E, 58.2–4M, 66.3E
  biliary 63.1E
  tuberculous 5.5E, 58.2E
peritonsillar abscess 45.2E, 45.9M
peroneal tendon subluxations 32.2E
Perthes' disease 35.1, 38.3M
pes deformities *see* talipes
petrous temporal bone fractures 22.1E
Peyronie's disease 74.1E
pharynx
  anatomy and physiology 45.1–2M
  diseases 45.6–13M
    malignant *see* cancer
  investigation *see* investigations
  pouch 45.1E, 45.11M, 59.1E
physeal (growth plate) injuries 27.4M
physical abuse (non-accidental injury), children 21.1M, 21. 6M, 38.8M
physical examination *see* examination
physiotherapy, burns 28.19M, 28.22M
Pierre Robin syndrome 42.4M, 42.8M
piles (haemorrhoids) 69.4E, 69.4E, 69.7–8M
pilocytic astrocytoma 40.19M
pilonidal sinus 69.4M
pinna (auricle), haematoma 44.9M
pituitary tumour (adenoma) 17.3E, 40.16M
  see also hypothalamic–pituitary–adrenal axis; hypothalamic–pituitary–gonadal axis
plain films *see* X-ray
plantar fasciitis 32.2E
plantarflexor mechanism of ankle, injuries 32.9M
plasma proteins, causes of low levels 17.3M
plasmacytoma 37.3E
plaster of Paris 27.4E, 27.6M
plastic surgery *see* reconstructive and plastic surgery
plate and screw fixation 27.4E, 27.6M
pleomorphic adenoma, parotid 47.1E
pleural space disease 52.2M
pneumobilia 66.2E
pneumonia
  lobar 5.1E
  postoperative confusion due to 20.2E
pneumoperitoneum for laparoscopic surgery 19.3–6M
pneumothorax
  open 26.1E
  tension 26.1E, 52.2E
poliomyelitis 5.18M, 38.3E
  limb deformities 5.E9
    claw hands 5.8E
  paralysis 5.10E
polycystic ovarian disease 49.3E
polyp(s)
  gastric 60.3E
  nasal 43.18–22M
polyposis, familial adenomatous 65.27–8M
polytrauma 21.7M
  assessment 22.2–5M
popliteal artery embolism 53.1E
portal hypertension 58.2E, 61.8M
positional vertigo, benign paroxysmal 44.27M
postoperative care 144–50
  pain relief, assessing adequacy 14.8M
  risk factors in 13.1E
potassium, low blood levels 49.5E
Pott's disease 5.10E
pre-analytical errors in laboratory tests 17.11M
precancer *see* premalignant lesions
pregnancy
  ectopic 76.1E, 76.4–5M
    ruptured 67.1E
  hyperthyroidism 48.1E
premalignant lesions and disorders (predisposed to transformation)
  breast 50.3M
  oesophagus 59.5M
  oropharynx 46.4M, 46.13M, 46.17M
  skin 39.4M
prenatal scan, cleft/lip palate 42.7M
preoperative care/management 113–17
  high-risk patients 16.4M
presbycusis 44.24M
preseptal cellulitis 41.2E
pressure sores 3.1E, 3.2E, 3.6M, 3.7M
priapism, persistent 74.1E
prion disease 40.12M
proctitis 68.1E, 68.9M, 69.1E
proctocolectomy, ulcerative colitis 65.17M
proctoscopy 68.4E
prolapse, rectal 68.1E, 68.7M, 69.4E
prostate 541–5
  anatomy and physiology 73.1–2M
  benign hypertrophy 72.1E, 72.2E, 73.3M, 73.6–7M
  cancer (carcinoma) 7.3E, 72.1E, 73.8–12M
    bone metastases 37.3E
prostatitis, acute 72.1E
prostheses and implants
  cardiac valves 51.6M
  joint, infected 35.3E, 37.2E

proteins, serum, causes of low levels 17.3M
pruritus ani 69.9M
pseudocysts, pancreatic 64.1E, 64.10M
pseudogout 37.4M
pseudomembranous colitis (and *C. difficile*) 4.3E
pseudo-obstruction, intestinal 66.1E
psoas abscess 5.9E
psoriatic arthropathies 37.2E
psychological care, burns 28.19M
pulmonary embolism
  laparoscopic risk 19.1E
  postoperative 13.1E
pulmonary non-vascular problems *see* lung
pulmonary venous drainage, totally anomalous 51.8M
pupillary irregularities 41.13M
purpura, idiopathic thrombocytopenic 62.1E
purpura fulminans 39.3E
pus-forming (suppurative/pyogenic) conditions
  acute sinusitis 43.25M
  liver abscess 61.2E
  otitis media 44.14M
  urinary tract 71.1E, 71.12M
pyelogram
  antegrade 70.1E, 71.3E
  retrograde 71.3E
pyelonephritis 70.3M, 71.12M
pyloric stenosis, congenital hypertrophic 6.1E, 6.7M
pyogenic lesions *see* pus-forming conditions
pyonephrosis 71.1E, 71.12M
pyrexia, postoperative 20.1E
pyrophosphate arthropathy (pseudogout) 37.4M

radiation hazards
  burns 28.26M
  in imaging 10.1M
radiography, plain film *see* X-ray
radiohumeral joint arthritis 34.2E
radioiodine in hyperthyroidism 48.5M
radioisotope scan, parathyroid 48.23M
radiology, diagnostic *see* imaging
radiotherapy 7.8M
  bladder cancer 72.10M
  breast cancer 50.6M
  gastric cancer 60.20M
  head and neck cancer
    complications 46.28M
    oropharyngeal cancer 46.2E, 46.17M
  prostatic cancer 73.12M
  see also chemoradiotherapy
Ramsay Hunt syndrome 44.2E
Ranson score 64.8M
Raynaud's phenomenon 53.14M
rearfoot problems 36.2M
reconstructive and plastic surgery 205–11
  cleft lip/palate 42.9M
    revisional surgery 42.13M
  nose 42.16M
  oropharyngeal cancer 46.18M
recovery process, metabolic response to injury 1.4M
rectum 499–503
  anatomy 68.1–2E
  cancer of colon and 7.1E, 7.3E, 7.6M, 65.1E, 65.27–32M, 68.1E, 68.10–14M
  foreign body 65.2E
  injury 68.5–6M
  prolapse 68.1E, 68.7M, 69.4E
  prostatic examination via 73.10M
  symptoms of disease 68.3E
    investigations 69.2E
  treatment of disorders 69.3E
  ulcers, solitary 68.1E, 69.4E
  see also ileorectal anastomosis; large bowel
rectus abdominus free flap, oropharyngeal reconstruction 46.21M
red eye, painful 41.3E, 41.17M
reduction
  ankle injury 32.8M
  fracture 27.5M
refeeding syndrome 17.1E
reflux gastritis 11.1E, 11.5M
rejection, allografts 77.1E, 77.3–6M
renal artery stenosis 70.3M
renal cell carcinoma (hypernephroma) 71.1E, 71.2E, 71.13M
renal pelvis
  congenital anomalies 71.1–2M
  transitional cell carcinoma 71.3E
  see also entries under pyelo-
renal problems *see* kidney
Rendu–Osler–Weber syndrome (hereditary haemorrhagic telangiectasia) 43.17M
reperfusion syndrome *see* ischaemia–reperfusion syndrome
reproductive tract
  female 554–7
  male 541–5, 546–53
research 8.2–5M
  electronic information sites 8.5M
  statistical analysis 8.2E, 8.3M
  types of studies 8.1M
respiratory tract
  anatomy and physiology 52.1M
  papillomatosis, recurrent 45.2E
  problems/symptoms

burns 28.3–4M
cleft lip/palate, prenatal scans 42.7M
see also airway; bronchi; lungs
resuscitation
fluid *see* fluid management
in shock 2.7M
retinoblastoma 41.8M
retrobulbar haemorrhage 25.2M
retroperitoneal mass 58.3E
retropharyngeal abscess 45.10M
rewarming 30.11M
rheumatic heart disease 51.5M
rheumatoid arthritis 37.1–2E
extrarticular manifestations 37.2M
hands 37.3M
juvenile 37.2E
treatment 37.1E
upper limb 34.6M
rhinoplasty 42.16M
rhinorrhoea 43.6M
rib hump, teenager 33.9M
Rigler's sign 66.2E
road traffic accident victims 22.1M
assessment 22.3M
chest trauma 26.1E
femoral fracture fixation 27.4E
head injury 23.1E
knee injury 32.1E
ocular and orbital trauma 41.13M
orofacial trauma 25.1E
pelvic fracture 27.1E
seatbelt syndrome 58.3E
shock 2.1E
robotic surgery 19.10–13M
nomenclatures 19.2E
rodent ulcer *see* basal cell carcinoma
rotated fracture 27.2E
rotator cuff 34.1M
impingement 34.1E
tears 32.11M, 34.1E
roundworms 5.1–9M, 5.31–3M

sacral cord lesions, clinical picture 5.10E
safety issues, radiation *see* radiation
salivary glands 351–60
anatomy and physiology 47.1M, 47.3M
degenerative conditions 47.27–39M
minor 47.1M
sialocele *see* sialocele
Salmonella typhi and typhoid 5.1E, 5.2E, 5.3E, 5.5E, 5.10E, 5.36E, 5.36–8M
Salter-Harris fracture classification 27.4M
sarcoma, retroperitoneal 58.3E
scars 3.9M
with burns 28.24M
keloid 3.2E, 3.10M
Schatzki's ring 59.1E
Scheuermann's disease 38.3E
schistosomiasis, bladder 72.1E
schwannoma, vestibular (acoustic neuroma) 44.30M
scleritis 41.3E
sclerosing cholangitis, primary 5.16M, 5.17M, 61.1E, 63.9M
scoliosis, idiopathic 33.9M, 38.3E
screening, cancer 7.5M
screw and plate fixation 27.4E, 27.6M
scrotum 549–53
pain (acute), child 6.6M
swelling 5.7E
child 6.4M
scrubbing 15.4M
seatbelt syndrome 58.3E
sedation, GI endoscopy 11.1M
segmental fracture 27.2E
seizures *see* epilepsy and epileptic seizures
semicircular canals, vestibular 44.5M
seminal vesicles 541–5
seminoma 75.6M
sensorineural deafness 44.23M
sepsis
meningococcal 49.1E
otological 44.1E
see also otitis
severe 4.10M
septic arthritis 37.2E
septic shock 2.1E
postoperative 20.2E, 20.3E
sex hormones 49.3E
shin injury 32.1M
shock 8–15
compensated 2.6M
drug therapy 2.2E, 2.8M
responses in 2.4–5M
resuscitation in 2.7M
types 2.1E
sepsis *see* septic shock
short synacthen test 49.11M
shortened fracture 27.2E
shoulder
examination 31.6M
frozen 34.1E
injuries 34.1E, 34.5M
sports 32.10–12M, 34.1E, 34.5M
pain, child 38.6M
replacement 34.2M

sialadenitis
- bacterial 47.15–16M
- viral (mumps) 47.14M

sialocele (ranula; mucous retention cyst) 47.4M
- parotid 25.2E
- plunging 47.4M

sialolisthesis (salivary stones) 47.2E, 47.19M
sialorrhoea (drooling) 47.30M
sick euthyroid syndrome 48.1M
sigmoid volvulus 66.1E, 66.2E, 66.8M
single photon emission computed tomography scan, parathyroid 48.23M
sinus (tract) 39.1E
- pilonidal 69.4M

sinuses, paranasal *see* paranasal sinuses
Sjögren's syndrome 47.27–8M
skills (surgical), basic 135–6
skin 29.2M, 273-8
- anatomy 39.1M
- characteristics 29.2M
- eyelid *see* eyelid
- fistulas to *see* fistulas
- grafts 29.3–7M
  - burns 28.21M, 28.22M, 28.23M
- preparation (for surgery) 15.4M
- ulcers *see* ulcers

skin and fascia (fasciocutaneous) flaps 29.12M
skin and muscle (myocutaneous) flaps 29.12M, 29.17M
skip metastasis, oral 46.6M
skull base
- fractures 22.1E, 22.9M
- pharynx extending from level of 45.1M

small bowel 474–87
- anatomy 65.1M
- diverticula 65.2M
- transplantation 77.13M
- tuberculosis 5.2E, 5.19–23M
  - obstruction 5.3E

small cell (oat cell) lung carcinoma 49.2E, 52.3M
smoke inhalation 28.4M
sodium, low blood levels in head injury 22.12M
soft tissue
- haematoma 32.2M
- necrotising infections 3.8M

sonography *see* ultrasonography
spasm, diffuse oesophageal 59.1E
specimens, histology 12.1M
SPECT scan, parathyroid 48.23M
speech problems, cleft lip/palate 42.11M
spermatocele 75.1E
spherocytosis, hereditary 62.1E
spina bifida 38.3E
spinal claudication 33.7M
spine (spinal column) 166–70, 233–7
- examination 31.6M
- injury (incl. spinal cord) 166–70
  - anatomy 24.1M
  - paralysis 5.10E
- paediatric problems 38.3E
- tuberculosis 5.10E

spiral fracture 27.2E
spleen 458–60
- abnormalities/pathology 62.1E, 62.4M
- anatomy 62.1–2M
- excision 62.3M

splenic artery aneurysm 62.1E
splenic injury 26.3E
split-skin grafts 29.4M, 29.5M, 29.6M, 29.7M
spondylitis, ankylosing 37.2E
spondylolisthesis 38.3E
spongiform encephalopathy 40.12M
sports injuries 224–32
- elbow 32.13–14M, 34.2E
- shoulder 32.10–12M, 34.1E, 34.5M

squamous cell carcinoma
- anus 69.4E, 69.13–14M
- head and neck 45.1E
  - hypopharyngeal 45.13M
  - management and degree of differentiation 46.16M
  - middle ear 44.22M
  - oropharyngeal 45.12M, 46.3M
- leg (Marjolin's ulcer) 54.1E

stabilisation of fracture 27.5M
stability
- hip joint 35.2M
- knee 35.6M

staging
- bladder cancer 72.8M
- oropharyngeal cancer 46.7–11M
- rectal cancer 68.14M

starvation 1.5M, 17.1M, 17.7M
statistical analysis in research 8.2E, 8.3M
step-ladder pattern (intestinal obstruction) 66.2E
stitches (sutures) 18.2E
stoma 65.34M
- ulcerative colitis 65.17M

stomach 441–50
- anatomy 60.1M
- conditions 60.3E, 60.5–10M, 60.13–21M
- mucosal barrier, damage 60.3M
- outlet obstruction 60.1E, 60.13M
  - with duodenal ulcer 5.3E
- physiology 60.2M
  - secretions 17.9M, 60.2M

surgery 60.4E
sequelae/complications 60.2E, 60.11M
stones
biliary *see* gallstones
salivary 47.2E, 47.19M
urinary 70.4M, 71.1E, 71.2E, 71.3E, 71.6–10M, 72.1E, 72.2E, 72.4M
stress fractures 32.7M
stress response to injury 1.2M
stroke, paralysis 5.10E
stromal tumour, gastrointestinal (GIST) 7.3E, 11.1E, 60.3E, 60.20M
subarachnoid haemorrhage, aneurysmal 40.21–3M
subconjunctival haemorrhage 41.3E
subcutaneous tissue 273–8
subdural haematoma, traumatic 22.1E, 22.11M
sublingual glands 47.5–10M
anatomy 47.3M
subluxations
peroneal tendon 32.2E
shoulder, child 34.4M
spinal/cervical 24.1E
submandibular duct 47.6M
submandibular glands 47.5–10M
anatomy 47.5M, 47.8M
investigations and management of disease 47.2E
surgical approaches and incisions 47.6–7M
surgical complications 47.9M
subphrenic abscesses 20.1
succinylcholine 14.4M
superior orbital fissure syndrome 25.2M
supernumerary teeth 42.17M, 42.18M
suppurative conditions *see* pus-forming conditions
supraorbital paraesthesia 25.1E
sutures 18.2E
suxamethonium 14.4M
swallowing problems (dysphagia) 59.1E, 59.2M
sweating, gustatory (Frey's syndrome) 47.9M, 47.26M
synacthen test, short 49.11M
systemic inflammatory response syndrome 4.9M
systemic lupus erythematosus
avascular necrosis 37.2E
ulcers 54.1E

tachycardia in shock 2.4M
talipes (pes) cavus 31.10M, 36.1E, 36.2M
talipes (pes) equinovarus 36.1E, 38.2E
talipes (pes) planus (flatfoot) 36.1E, 36.2M
tapeworm 5.10–19M
tapioca and chronic tropical pancreatitis 5.1E, 5.35M
tarsal coalition 36.1E, 38.2E
tear(s) (lacrimal secretions) 41.1M
tear sac *see* lacrimal sac
teeth *see* dentition
temporal bone
facial nerve exiting 44.2M
fractures 44.25M
petrous 22.1E
temporal lobe lesions, dominant 40.14M
tendinitis
calcifying 34.1E
tibialis anterior 32.2E
tendon
grafts 29.17M
injuries 32.3M
ankle 32.2E
tennis elbow 32.13M, 34.2E
tension pneumothorax 26.1E, 52.2E
teratoma 49.3E
testicular 75.6M
terminal care in cancer 7.12M
testis 549–53
atrophy with varicocele 5.7E
torsion 6.6M, 75.1E, 75.3M
tumours 75.1E, 75.6–7M
undescended 6.4M, 75.1–2M
testosterone 73.2M
tetanus 4.3E, 30.7M
thermal injury *see* burns
thoracic aortic disease 51.1E, 51.9M
thoracic spine (incl. cord)
anatomy 24.1M
lesions, paralysis 5.10E
thoracotomy 52.1E
thorax (chest) 397–401
drains 52.1E, 52.3M
trauma 176–84
throat *see* larynx; pharynx
thrombocytopenic purpura, idiopathic 62.1E
thrombophelebitis of superficial veins of chest wall (Mondor's disease) 50.1E
thrombosis
aortic, acute 53.1E
venous *see* venous thrombosis
thyroglobulin 48.13M
thyroglossal duct cyst 45.25M
thyroid disease 48.1–16M, 48.2–5E
exophthalmos 41.7M
tibialis anterior tendinitis 32.2E
tibialis posterior tendon rupture 32.2E, 36.2M
tissue apposition 18.1M
tissue defects *see* wounds
tissue diagnosis 107–9
TNM staging
bladder cancer 72.8M
rectal cancer 68.14M

toes
  claw 36.1E
  great *see* hallux
  injuries 32.3E
tonsilitis 45.2E
tooth *see* dentition
torsion
  omental 58.3E
  testicular 6.6M, 75.1E, 75.2M
torticollis 38.3E
total body surface area, burns in relation to 28.5M
total body water (TBW) 17.5M
total parenteral nutrition 17.2M
tourniquet 15.2M
toxic nodular goitre 48.2M, 48.4E
tracheal tube *see* endotracheal tube
tracheo-oesophageal fistula 6.3E
tracheostomy 45.15–17M
  advantages 45.16M
  indications 45.15M
  tubes, features 45.17M
traction 27.4E, 27.6M
transformation, malignant 7.1M
  lesions predisposed to *see* premalignant lesions
transfusion (blood and blood product) 2.11–12M
  complications 2.3E
    of massive transfusion 2.12M
  products 2.11M
transitional cell carcinoma
  bladder 70.3M, 72.8M
  renal pelvis 71.3E
transitional cell papilloma, nasal 43.28M
translated fracture 27.2E
transplants *see* grafts
transport of patients from disaster scene 30.4M
transposition flap 29.10M
transposition of great vessels 51.8M
transverse fracture 27.2E
trauma *see* injury
Treacher Collins syndrome 42.20M
trematodes (flukes) 5.29–31M
triage 30.3M
trichobezoars 60.3E, 60.20M
trigeminal nerve supply to external ear 44.6M
trigeminal neuralgia 40.27M
trochar
  antral lavage 43.24M
  bleeding from site of 19.14M
trophozoites, amoebic 5.25M, 5.27M
tropical surgery 31–74
tuberculosis (*M. tuberculosis* infection)
  arthritis 37.2E
    elbow 34.2E
  bladder 72.1E
  breast 50.1E
  cervical node 45.28M
  intestinal 5.2E, 5.3E, 5.5E, 5.19–23M
  meningeal 40.11M
  peritoneal 5.5E, 58.2E
  spinal 5.10E
tumour
  benign/unspecified/in general
    bone 37.3E, 37.5M
    brain 40.13M, 40.16–20M
    endocrine 49.12–15M
    inner ear 44.30M
    liver 61.3E
    middle ear 44.22M
    neck 45.29–30M
    ocular 41.8–9M
    pancreaticoduodenal 48.22M, 49.13M
    parotid gland 47.20–1M
    pelvic, venous congestion 5.6E
    rectal 68.1E
    renal 71.1E, 71.13–14M
    sinonasal 43.14–15M, 43.27–30M, 45.7M
    skin 39.3E
    submandibular gland 47.10–12M
    testicular 75.1E, 75.6–7M
  malignant *see* cancer
  see also specific histological types
turf toe 32.3E
tympanic membrane 44.2M
typhoid 5.1E, 5.2E, 5.3E, 5.5E, 5.10E, 5.36–8M

ulcer(s)
  cutaneous 39.1E, 39.2M, 54.1E
    decubitus (pressure sores) 3.1E, 3.2E, 3.6M, 3.7M
    lower limb *see* lower limb
    rodent ulcer *see* basal cell carcinoma
  peptic *see* peptic ulcer
  rectal, solitary 68.1E, 69.4E
ulcerative colitis 65.1E, 65.8–18M, 65.26M
  imaging 65.2E
  rectal bleeding 69.1E
ulnar collateral ligament injuries 32.4M
ulnar nerve lesions and palsy 34.2E
  claw hands 5.8E, 31.6M
ultrasonography (sonography) 10.2M, 10.3M
  acute abdomen 10.6M
  hepatic hydatid cyst 5.14M, 5.16M
  intracavitary *see* endocavitary ultrasonography

oncology 10.7M
orthopaedics 10.4M
parathyroid 48.23M
prenatal, cleft/lip palate 42.7M
trauma 10.5M
focussed assessment with 10.5M, 26.2E, 26.5M
limbs 27.1E
urinary tract 70.4M
vascular disease
arterial 53.4M
lymphatic 55.2E
venous 55.2E
umbilical discharge 57.9M
umbilical hernia 57.8M
upper limb 238–45
Bier's block 14.6M
urate crystal arthropathy (gout) 37.4M
ureter
acute colic 67.1E
imaging 71.3E
stones 71.1E, 71.3E, 71.7M, 71.9M, 71.10M
trauma 71.3–4M
ureterogram, retrograde 70.1E
urethra
congenital abnormalities 74.1M
rupture 74.2–3M
stricture 74.5M
urge incontinence 69.4E
urinary incontinence, sudden-onset 33.2M
urinary tract 513–48
infection 71.11–12M, 72.1E, 72.7M
child 6.2E
postoperative 20.1E
investigations *see* investigations
symptoms
investigations 515–20
lower (LUTS), in men 73.5M
urine
blood in (haematuria) 70.1M
retention, acute and chronic 72.1E
superficial extravasation 74.4M
uterine fibroids 76.1E
uveitis 41.3E

vaginal bleeding, abnormal excessive 76.3M
vaginal (tunica vaginalis) hydrocele 5.7E, 75.1E, 75.4M
vagus (Xth cranial) nerve, branches 45.3M
valves (cardiac)
disease 51.1E, 51.4–5M
prosthetic 51.6M
varicella zoster virus, facial nerve 44.2E
varices, oesophageal 11.1E, 60.12M
varicocele 5.7E, 75.1E
varicose veins 54.5–7M
management 54.2E, 54.6M
complications 54.7E
vasculature *see* blood supply; blood vessels; lymphatic system
vasoactive intestinal peptide (VIP)-secreting tumours 49.13M
vasopressin (ADH), syndrome of inappropriate secretion 17.2
vasopressor agents, shock 2.8M
Vater's ampulla, carcinoma *see* periampullary carcinoma
venous blood, intracranial drainage from nose and sinuses 43.3M
venous catheterization, adrenal 49.6M
venous congestion, pelvic tumour 5.6E
venous disease 411–15
ultrasound 55.2E
venous saturation, mixed 2.9M
venous thrombosis
deep *see* deep vein thrombosis
hepatic 61.1E
ventricular septal defects 51.7M
ventriculoperitoneal shunt complications 40.9M
vertebrae
collapsed 33.4M
congenital abnormality 38.3E
pharynx extent in relation to 45.1M
see also spine
vertigo 44.27–8M
vesicolic fistula 65.6M
vestibular schwannoma (acoustic neuroma) 44.30M
vestibular semicircular canals 44.5M
video-assisted thoracoscopic surgery 52.2M
villous adenoma, rectal 68.1E
VIPomas 49.13M
viral hepatitis 61.2E
visual loss, investigations 41.18M
vitamin D deficiency 48.1E
vocal cord palsy 45.1E, 45.20M
vocal fold nodules 45.19M
volvulus *see* malrotation and volvulus
vomiting (emesis)
of blood 60.12M
child 6.1E
metabolic consequences 17.15M
postoperative 20.5M
tropical patients 5.3E
warfarin, deep vein thrombosis 54.4M
wart (viral papillary) 39.3E
anal 69.12M
water, total body (TBW) 17.5M

wedge fracture 27.2E
Wegener's granulomatosis 43.1E, 43.12M
weight-lifter, median nerve injury 32.14M
Whipple operation 20.3E, 63.3E, 64.12E
Wilms' tumour 71.13M
wire fixation 27.4E
women, gynaecology 554–7
wounds (and tissue defects) 16–21
  abdominal, dehiscence (burst abdomen) 57.10M
  chronic 3.6M
  contaminated 4.16M
    debridement 30.6M
  dressings *see* dressings
  healing *see* healing
  infections *see* infections
  management/repair 3.2E, 3.4E, 3.4–5M
    major defects 29.18M
  types 3.1E, 4.16M
  see also injury
wrist
  examination 31.6M
  median nerve compression at *see* carpal tunnel syndrome
Wuchereria bancrofti 5.6E, 5.7E, 5.9E, 5.31M

X-ray (plain films) 10.2M
  intestinal tuberculosis 5.21M
  limb trauma 27.1E
  orthopaedics 10.4M
  osteoarthritis 35.3M
  sinonasal 43.1E
  spine 33.3M
    injury 24.3M
    vertebral collapse 33.4M
xerostomia 47.28M

yersinial arthritis 37.2E

Z-plasties 29.10M
Zenker's diverticulum (pharyngeal pouch) 45.1E, 45.11M, 59.1E
zygomatic fractures 25.2M